AF704015

Oncology: Targeted Therapies for Tumors

Oncology: Targeted Therapies for Tumors

Editor: Adelina Brando

AMERICAN
MEDICAL PUBLISHERS
www.americanmedicalpublishers.com

AMERICAN
MEDICAL PUBLISHERS
www.americanmedicalpublishers.com

Cataloging-in-Publication Data

Oncology : targeted therapies for tumors / edited by Adelina Brando.
p. cm.
Includes bibliographical references and index.
ISBN 979-8-88740-351-9
1. Cancer--Treatment. 2. Tumors--Treatment. 3. Drug targeting.
4. Drug resistance in cancer cells. 5. Oncology. I. Brando, Adelina.
RC270.8 .O53 2023
616.994 06--dc23

© American Medical Publishers, 2023

American Medical Publishers,
41 Flatbush Avenue,
1st Floor, New York,
NY 11217, USA

ISBN 979-8-88740-351-9 (Hardback)

This book contains information obtained from authentic and highly regarded sources. Copyright for all individual chapters remain with the respective authors as indicated. All chapters are published with permission under the Creative Commons Attribution License or equivalent. A wide variety of references are listed. Permission and sources are indicated; for detailed attributions, please refer to the permissions page and list of contributors. Reasonable efforts have been made to publish reliable data and information, but the authors, editors and publisher cannot assume any responsibility for the validity of all materials or the consequences of their use.

Trademark Notice: Registered trademark of products or corporate names are used only for explanation and identification without intent to infringe.

Contents

Preface

This book was inspired by the evolution of our times; to answer the curiosity of inquisitive minds. Many developments have occurred across the globe in the recent past which has transformed the progress in the field.

Tumor, also known as neoplasm, is a mass or group of tissues that is formed as a result of abnormal growth. It can appear anywhere on the body. Bone, tissues, skin, glands, and organs, all can be affected by tumors. They may be cancerous (malignant), non-cancerous (benign), or precancerous. Malignant tumors can spread to adjacent tissues, glands, or other body parts. Benign tumors pose a low risk of death. They are isolated and do not spread to other body parts or impact neighboring tissues. Precancerous tumors are non-cancerous tumors which may become cancerous if left untreated. Most common types of cancer treatments include targeted therapy (molecularly targeted therapy), hormonal therapy and cytotoxic therapy. There exist two types of targeted therapies, namely, small molecule medicines and monoclonal antibodies. The small molecule medicines are biopharmaceuticals that are so small that they can enter the cancer cells and destroy them. Targeted therapy makes use of monoclonal antibodies which cannot enter into the cells. However, these monoclonal antibodies attack targets outside of cells. In various cases, monoclonal antibodies are used to launch chemo and radiation straight into tumors. This book aims to provide the readers a comprehensive overview of the applications of targeted therapies for the treatment and management of tumors. For all readers who are interested in understanding this therapeutic procedure, it will serve as an excellent guide.

This book was developed from a mere concept to drafts to chapters and finally compiled together as a complete text to benefit the readers across all nations. To ensure the quality of the content we instilled two significant steps in our procedure. The first was to appoint an editorial team that would verify the data and statistics provided in the book and also select the most appropriate and valuable contributions from the plentiful contributions we received from authors worldwide. The next step was to appoint an expert of the topic as the Editor-in-Chief, who would head the project and finally make the necessary amendments and modifications to make the text reader-friendly. I was then commissioned to examine all the material to present the topics in the most comprehensible and productive format.

I would like to take this opportunity to thank all the contributing authors who were supportive enough to contribute their time and knowledge to this project. I also wish to convey my regards to my family who have been extremely supportive during the entire project.

Editor

1

A Natural Isoquinoline Alkaloid with Antitumor Activity: Studies of the Biological Activities of Berberine

Da Liu[1,2], Xue Meng[1,2], Donglu Wu[1,2], Zhidong Qiu[1,2] and Haoming Luo[1,2*]*

[1] *Department of Pharmacy, Changchun University of Chinese Medicine, Changchun, China,* [2] *Key Laboratory of Effective Components of Traditional Chinese Medicine, Changchun University of Chinese Medicine, Changchun, China*

Correspondence:
Zhidong Qiu
Qiuzd@ccucm.edu.cn
Haoming Luo
luo.haoming@163.com

Coptis, a traditional medicinal plant, has been used widely in the field of traditional Chinese medicine for many years. More recently, the chemical composition and bioactivity of Coptis have been studied worldwide. Berberine is a main component of Rhizoma Coptidis. Modern medicine has confirmed that berberine has pharmacological activities, such as anti-inflammatory, analgesic, antimicrobial, hypolipidemic, and blood pressure-lowering effects. Importantly, the active ingredient of berberine has clear inhibitory effects on various cancers, including colorectal cancer, lung cancer, ovarian cancer, prostate cancer, liver cancer, and cervical cancer. Cancer, ranked as one of the world's five major incurable diseases by WHO, is a serious threat to the quality of human life. Here, we try to outline how berberine exerts antitumor effects through the regulation of different molecular pathways. In addition, the berberine-mediated regulation of epigenetic mechanisms that may be associated with the prevention of malignant tumors is described. Thus, this review provides a theoretical basis for the biological functions of berberine and its further use in the clinical treatment of cancer.

Keywords: berberine, biological activities, antitumor, autophagy, epigenetic effects

INTRODUCTION

Natural medicine plays a very important role in novel drug discovery (Zhang et al., 2013; Zhang L. et al., 2017). In recent years, many natural products have been confirmed to play an important role in cancer prevention and therapy (Tao et al., 2015; Zhang et al., 2015, 2016; Meng et al., 2018). Coptis chinensis is a valuable Chinese medicine used commonly in China. The medicinal parts are the dried rhizome of *Coptis chinensis* Franch., *Coptis deltoidea* C.Y.Cheng, and P.K.Hsiao, or *Coptis teeta* Wall (Wang et al., 2015b). It has been reported that Coptis exerts antibacterial, immune-enhancing, anti-ulcer, hypoglycemic, detoxifying, antitumor, and other pharmacological

Abbreviations: AP-1, activating protein 1; AMPK, AMP-activated protein kinase; BTG2, B-cell translocation gene 2; Bax, BCL2 associated X; BBC3, BCL2-binding component 3; CCNB, cyclin B; CCND, cyclin D; CCNE, cyclin E; CDK, cyclin-dependent kinases; CDKN1A/p21, cyclin-dependent kinase inhibitor; COX2, cyclooxygenase-2; DNMT, DNA methyltransferase; EGFR, epidermal growth factor receptor; GMCSF, granulocyte-macrophage colony-stimulating factor; GADD45, growth arrest and DNA damage-inducible 45; HCC, hepatocellular carcinoma cells; HAT, histone acetyltransferase; HDAC, histone deacetylase; HIF1α, hypoxia-induced factor α; INOS, inducible NO synthase; IL-8, interleukin-8; MMPs, matrix metalloproteinases; NSCLC, non-small cell lung cancer cells; NF-κB, nuclear factor kappa B; PARP, poly-ADP ribose polymerase; PGE2, prostaglandin E2; STAT3, signal transducer and activator of transcription 3; SIRT, sirtuins; Bcl-2, the B cell lymphoma-2; TNF, tumor necrosis factor; uPA, urokinase-type plasminogen activator; VEGF, vascular endothelial growth factor.

effects (Imenshahidi and Hosseinzadeh, 2016). Coptis is mainly used for the adjuvant treatment of depression, coronary heart disease, diabetes, liver cancer, and other malignant tumors. There are several active ingredients of Coptis chinensis, such as berberine (BBR), palmatine, coptisine, jatrorrhizine, worenine, columbamine, cedarone, obakunone, obakulactone, magnoflorine, and ferulic acid; berberine is the main bioactive component of Coptis chinensis and is present at a content of 5.20–7.69%. Consequently, it has become one of the natural small-molecule drugs used commonly in the clinical setting treatment for chronic disease such like diabetes (Cicero and Baggioni, 2016; Tabeshpour et al., 2017).

Berberine hydrochloride, the more commonly available salt form of berberine, is a quaternary ammonium isoquinoline alkaloid with the chemical formula $C_{20}H_{18}ClNO_4$ (**Figure 1**) that forms yellow needle-like crystals (Neag et al., 2018). Berberine was originally used as a broad-spectrum antibacterial drug. Extensive research revealed a wide range of pharmacological activities, including antibacterial, anti-inflammatory, antihypertensive, hypolipidemic, and antidiarrheal effects. In addition, berberine exhibits inhibitory effects on a variety of tumors (Xu et al., 2017), such as esophageal cancer. Many studies (Kumar et al., 2015; Foroutan F. et al., 2018; Foroutan T. et al., 2018; Mirhadi et al., 2018) have confirmed that berberine affects the development of tumor cells through the inhibition of tumor cell growth and the induction of apoptosis and cell cycle arrest (Iizuka et al., 2000; Kong et al., 2004; Tang and Feng, 2009; Xue et al., 2013; Signorelli et al., 2017).

It is reported that 8.2 million people die of cancer every year globally and that this number is continuously rising; according to the American Cancer Society, cancer is the cause of more than 600,000 deaths every year in the United States, a mortality rate second only to heart disease (Khalil et al., 2016; Walker et al., 2017). Owing to the seriousness of this situation, scientific approaches to the prevention and control of cancer have become a major public health issue (Gu et al., 2015; Viegas et al., 2017).

It has long been believed that the occurrence and development of tumors are attributable to only genetic abnormalities, which include gene mutations, translocations, and chromatin insertions (Dupont et al., 2009; Li et al., 2018). However, in recent years, the emergence and progress of genome sequencing technology have led to the rapid development of epigenetics and many researchers have determined that epigenetics plays an important role in the regulation of tumors. Epigenetic changes are reversible, heritable changes in gene expression and protein function in which the genomic DNA sequence remains unchanged (Biswas and Rao, 2018). Epigenetic changes can regulate gene expression at multiple levels, for example, at the DNA level through DNA methylation, at the RNA level through non-coding RNA regulation, at the protein level through histone modification, and at the chromatin level through chromatin remodeling. The continuous presence of these mechanisms in cell division allows cells to retain their respective characteristics, respond to intrinsic cellular signals, and participate in cell evolution and adaptation to environmental changes. Many research studies have confirmed that epigenetic mechanisms are implicated in tumorigenesis through the regulation of oncogene activation and tumor suppressor gene inactivation. For example, DNA methylation can inactivate tumor suppressor genes, abnormal histone acetylation can change tumor-associated gene expression, and non-coding microRNAs can result in dysregulation of tumor suppressor genes (Blandino et al., 2014; Wong and Chim, 2015). It is of note that different epigenetic modifications in cells often interact with each other in a synergistic manner to maintain body's homeostasis through the regulation of the expression of key genes, and that when abnormal changes occur, they may cause a variety of diseases, including tumors (Vijayaraghavalu et al., 2013). Recent evidence has suggested that epigenetic modifications may be involved in the processes tumor cells use to shape a microenvironment suitable for their own growth (Honda et al., 2006). There are a large number of active substances, such as growth factors, inflammatory factors, and proteases, in the tumor microenvironment and these participate in the various processes of tumorigenesis through their own functional properties or mediated signaling pathways (Booth and Gutierrez-Hartmann, 2015). Epigenetic modifications are involved in the regulation of the secretory processes of these biomolecules or their mediated signaling pathways (Li et al., 2018). From the perspective of the tumor development process, the regulation of epigenetic modification in the tumor microenvironment occurs at various stages of tumorigenesis, progression, and metastasis, and is one of the important tools for diversifying between tumor cells and the tumor microenvironment. That is to say, tumors may have specific epigenetic modification characteristics that may lead to changes in cell biological characteristics and malignant transformation. Therefore, an exploration the mechanism of tumor biology from the perspective of epigenetics is of great significance.

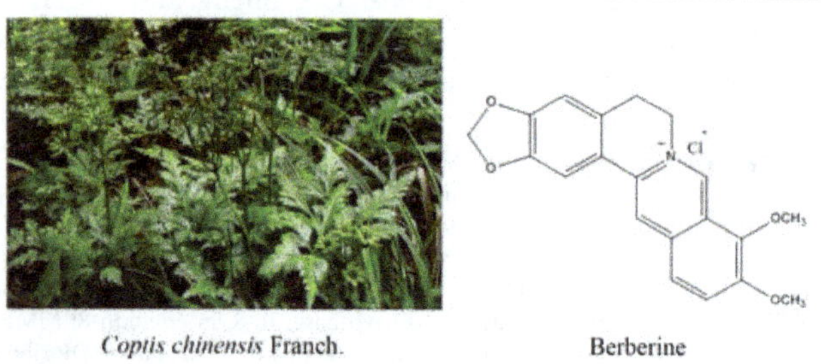

FIGURE 1 | *Coptis chinensis* Franch. and chemical structure of berberine.

THE BIOLOGICAL EFFICACY OF BERBERINE

Berberine Inhibits the Migration and Invasion of Tumor Cells

Migration and invasion are the basic characteristics of tumor cells. Therefore, it is valuable to study whether berberine can affect the migration and invasion ability of tumor cells. It is well known that E-cadherin and *N*-Cadherin proteins are closely related to cell migration and invasion. Moreover, E-cadherin is not only an important mediator that regulates cell-cell adhesion, but also an important molecule in the maintenance of the morphology and structural integrity of epithelial cells (Qi et al., 2014; Shi et al., 2017). There is a large amount of experimental evidence suggesting that berberine can inhibit the migration and invasion of tumor cells. In human lung cancer A549 cells, berberine increased the expression of E-cadherin protein in a concentration- and time-dependent manner (Li et al., 2018), and significantly downregulated the expression of *N*-cadherin; these changes inhibited invasion and metastasis. MMPs are a class of important proteins that are involved in that the degradation of the extracellular matrix barrier, which is the first step in tumor cell metastasis (Hao et al., 2017). Studies have shown that berberine inhibits the expression of MMP2 and MMP9 in a time- and concentration-dependent manner. Simultaneously, berberine also regulates the expression of MMPs through the inhibition of the transfer of p-STAT3 to the nucleus, which affects its activity. Wang X et al. found that berberine was an effective inhibitor of the invasion and migration of HCC cells. Berberine treatment of HCC cells downregulated the expression of cox-2, NF-κB, uPA, and MMP9 in a dose-dependent manner (Sengupta et al., 2017). In summary, the data strongly suggest that berberine has an important role in the regulation of cadherin- and MMP-mediated pathways, which leads to inhibitory effects on cancer migration and invasion (**Table 1**).

Furthermore, Jin Y. et al. (2017) showed that the effect of berberine on the metastatic potential of cancer cells may be mediated by the activation of the AMPK signaling pathway, which reduces the activity of ERK and the expression of COX-2, thereby inhibiting the adhesion, migration, and invasion of tumor cells. Moreover, berberine inhibited tumor cells through signaling pathways, including the NF-κB and AMPK pathways. Studies have demonstrated that berberine prevents tumor cells from producing IL-8 and blocks NF-κb signaling pathway, ultimately inhibiting endometrial cancer metastasis, and that colon cancer cell migration was inhibited by targeting AMPK signaling (Li et al., 2014).

Vascular endothelial growth factor, the most important angiogenic factor secreted from tumor cells, stimulates tumor neovascularization through an increase in the mitogenic and survival properties of vascular endothelial cells. Berberine not only reduces the expression of SC-M1 cells with normal oxygen content and low oxygen content. VEGF also directly inhibits the proliferation and migration of umbilical vein epithelial cells. Berberine treatment in B16F-10 melanoma cells reduced the expression of VEGF mRNA and inhibited angiogenesis. Inflammation plays an important role in tumor angiogenesis, which is mainly manifested through the activation of NF-κB to regulate VEGF, and results have shown that berberine treatment of tumor cells significantly inhibited NF-κB and ultimately decreased the expression of VEGF and IL-8 in tumor cells (Hamsa and Kuttan, 2011; Siveen and Kuttan, 2011). In addition, berberine significantly inhibited the VEGF-induced migration and invasion of human umbilical vein endothelial cells HUVEC in a dose-dependent manner, and significantly reduced the expression of COX-2, Inos, and VEGF mRNA and downregulated pro-angiogenic factors to inhibit angiogenesis (Naveen et al., 2016; Wang et al., 2018). These results indicated the critical effects of berberine on the HIF1α/VEGF pathway.

Angiogenesis plays an important role in tumor growth, as progression and metastasis are prerequisites for solid tumor growth. The angiogenic process is therefore a target for the inhibition of tumor growth and metastasis (Ma et al., 2008) Studies have shown that berberine can reduce the levels of IL-1β, IL-6, TNF, and GMCSF in the serum of tumor-inoculated animals and inhibit the elevation of NO and TNF-α, inflammatory mediators involved in angiogenesis. Wang Y et al. inferred that berberine suppressed the growth and metastasis of endometrial cancer cells via miR-101/COX2, and berberine is also known to inhibit tumors via the COX-2/PGE2 signaling pathway. The transcription of miR-101 is up-regulated by berberine through AP-1 to regulate the transcription of COX-2 in EC cells (Wu et al., 2012). The high expression of p-STAT3 in malignant tumor cells and the expression level of p-STAT3 in tumor tissues, the more obvious the proliferation and metastasis of tumor cells (Munir et al., 2000).

Berberine Inhibits Tumor Cell Proliferation (Autophagy, Apoptosis)

Apoptosis is an ideal form of cell death in cancer therapy because it generally does not cause an inflammatory response. Thus, the induction of apoptosis is one of the various mechanisms that inhibit the growth of tumor cells (Yakata et al., 2007). It has also been reported that berberine significantly inhibited the proliferation of human prostate cancer PC3 cells (Huang et al., 2015). In recent years, studies have shown that the proliferation of renal cell cancer cells can be effectively inhibited by berberine; when a certain concentration of berberine is treated to renal cell cancer cells, the effects continue for some time. The inhibitory effect of berberine on the tumor cells gradually increased, and it was found that the effect of inhibitory effect was greatest for treatment times of up to 48 h. In addition, the total apoptotic rate of renal tumor cells detected by a double staining method showed that after treatment of renal cell cancer cell lines A498 and 786-0 with different concentrations of berberine, the rate of total apoptosis in cells gradually increased as the concentration of the drug increased (Wang et al., 2015a; Liu et al., 2017a,b, 2018).

Berberine induces apoptosis in tumor cells, mainly through upregulation of pro-apoptotic genes and downregulation of apoptosis-inhibiting genes. For example, berberine can upregulate the expression of the pro-apoptotic protein BAD in HL-60 cells and downregulate the expression of anti-apoptotic protein Bcl-2 to achieve regulation of tumor cell apoptosis. In addition, apoptosis can be induced by the mitochondrial/caspase pathway, DNA cleavage induces tumor cell apoptosis, tumor cell apoptosis is induced by inflammatory factors, and tumor cell apoptosis is induced by cyclooxygenase. For example, berberine treatment of liver cancer cells revealed that DNA fragments, caspase-3, and caspase-8 were activated, which was followed by the activation of PARP, and the release of cytochrome c to inhibit tumor metastasis (Mistry et al., 2017).

Studies have showed that berberine can regulate apoptosis-associated proteins. Caspase cleavage is a typical phenomenon in apoptosis cells. Thus, numerous reports have used the detection of this cleavage to clarify the role of berberine in the induction of apoptosis. For example, berberine decreased the expression of Bcl-2 and survivin and, conversely, increased the expression of the pro-apoptotic genes Bax and cleaved caspase-3 in a dose-dependent manner in human ovarian cancer SKOV3 cells (Su et al., 2015). Moreover, the treatment of berberine to treat human colorectal adenocarcinoma (HCT-15) cells significantly increased the expression of spliced caspase-3 and the mitochondrial apoptosis-related protein Bax, and significantly decreased the expression of Bcl-2 and survivin, finally inducing apoptosis (Agnarelli et al., 2018). Berberine inhibited the proliferation of human cervical cancer Ca Ski cells through alteration of the ratio of p53 and Bax/Bcl-2 proteins, upregulation of ROS, and enhancement of caspase-3 activity to induce apoptosis (Kalaiarasi et al., 2016). In addition, berberine induced the proliferation of BIU-87 and T24 cells through the inhibition of protein expression, the induction of G1 cell cycle arrest, and the induction of apoptosis via the caspase-3 and caspase-9 pathways (Lu et al., 2015). Agnarelli A et al. treated U343 cells and MIA PaCa-2 cells with 50 μM berberine for 48 h, and found that the activity of caspase-3 was decreased in U343 cells and increased in MIA PaCa-2 cells. Therefore, they concluded that berberine promoted the apoptosis of tumor cells (Katona et al., 2014). It has been reported that berberine induces Bax activation in human lung cancer A549 cells, enables p53 pathway-mediated cytochrome c release, and leads to the activation of caspase signaling ultimately causing apoptosis (Shi et al., 2013). The reported data also showed that berberine induced cancer cell apoptosis mainly through the regulation of the expression of caspases and Bcl-2; this results in the release of cytochrome c and the activation of the mitochondria-dependent apoptotic pathway to promote apoptosis in PC3 cells (Wang et al., 2017).

Autophagy is one type of cellular self-protection mechanism, consisting mainly of the degradation of macromolecular material and damaged organelles in cytoplasm after autophagosome formation with lysosomes. The products of degradation are used to restore cell homeostasis. There are three forms of cell autophagy: macro-autophagy, micro-autophagy, and autophagy, which are mediated by different molecular chaperones. Autophagy is involved in many of the physiological and pathological processes of cells, and there is a close relationship between autophagy and tumorigenesis. The effects of autophagy vary in different cell lines and maybe inhibitory or stimulatory. In addition, the occurrence of autophagy is regulated by various signal pathways. Recent experimental studies have shown that berberine inhibits the proliferation of colon cancer cells through the downregulation of the expression of EGFR and that it activates autophagy and apoptosis through the p38 signaling pathway to inhibit the proliferation of HCT-15 cells. Similarly, in berberine-treated HCT-15 cells, the autophagy marker proteins ATG5 and LC3 were upregulated in a time-dependent manner (Zhang L. et al., 2017), indicating that berberine induced autophagy in HCT-15 cells. These data demostrate a role of Berberin in regulating cancer cell proliferation (**Tables 1, 2**).

Berberine Arrests Tumor Cell Cycle

Many studies have shown that low concentrations of berberine arrest human osteosarcoma U20S cells in the G1 phase through the induction of DNA double-strand breaks that activate the p53-p21 pathway. In contrast to low concentrations of berberine, high concentrations induce arrest in the G2/M phase, but do not depend on the p53-p21 pathway (Yang et al., 2015; Li et al., 2017). Other studies demonstrated that berberine significantly inhibited human ovarian cancer cells (HEY and SKOV3 cells) in a time- and dose-dependent manner. It is demonstrated that that berberine exerts a significant inhibitory effect on human gastric cancer MGC 80 3 cells in a dose-dependent manner. Using laser confocal microscopy, the nucleus condenses, and apoptotic bodies are seen, which indicate that berberine can inhibit the proliferation of MGC 80 3 cells and arrest cells in the G0/G1 phase to inhibit the proliferation of tumor cells *in vitro*.

B-cell translocation gene 2 is a transient early-response gene induced by p53. It is a member of the gene family that regulates cell proliferation and is an important bridge molecule that links

TABLE 1 | Inhibitory effects of berberine on tumor migration and invasion.

Cell lines	Mechanism	Reference
Human non-small cell lung cancer (A549)	N-Cadherin↓ E-cadherin↑	Li et al., 2018
Hepatocellular carcinoma (HCC) cells	COX-2↓,NF-κB↓ UPA,MMP-9↓	Sengupta et al., 2017
Endothelial canjcer colon cells	IL-8↓, NF-κB↓ AMPK↑	Li et al., 2014
Mouse melanoma cell (B16F-10)	VEGF mRNA↓	Siveen and Kuttan, 2011; Hamsa and Kuttan, 2011
Human umbilical vein endothelial cells (HUVEC)	COX-2↓, iNOS↓, VEGF mRNA↓	Ma et al., 2008
Human endometrial cancer cell lines(AN3 CA and HEC-1-A)	COX-2↓ PEG-2↓	Wu et al., 2012

TABLE 2 | Inhibitory effects of berberine on tumor cell proliferation.

Cell Lines	Mechanism	Reference
Liver cancer cells	Caspase-3↑, Caspase-8↑,PARP↑	Mistry et al., 2017
Human ovarian cancer cell (SKOV3)	Bcl-2↓ Bax↑, Cleaved-Caspase-3↑,	Su et al., 2015
Colorectal adenocarcinoma cell line (HCT-15)	EGFR↓, Bcl-2↓, Survivin↓ ATG5↑, Bax↑, LC3↑	Agnarelli et al., 2018
Human cervical cancer cell (CaSki)	p53↑, Bax/Bcl-2↑ ROS↑, Caspase-3↑	Kalaiarasi et al., 2016
Human bladder cancer cell (BIU-87, T24)	Caspase-3↑, Caspase-9↑	Lu et al., 2015
Human pancreatic carcinoma cell (MIA PaCa-2)	Caspase-3↑ P53↓	Katona et al., 2014

p53, pRB, the cell cycle, cell proliferation, and differentiation. The current body of evidence indicates that berberine can promote the cell cycle arrest of human hepatoma HEPG2 cells in the G1 phase through the upregulation of BTG2 and the downregulation of cyclin D1, consequently inhibiting the proliferation of hepatoma cells and inducing apoptosis.

Cyclin is one of the target proteins that regulate the G1 phase. As a proto-oncogene, it is involved in the regulation of the cell cycle, and its overexpression is closely related to the occurrence and development of tumors. Berberine has a variety of effects on the cell cycle; for example, it can arrest the G2/M phase in the cell growth cycle through a reduction in the expression of cyclin B1 and increase in the expression of Weel, which stops the tumor cells in the early stage of DNA synthesis (G1) and late DNA synthesis (G2). The induction of tumor cell apoptosis through the downregulation of cyclin E expression and upregulation of p21 expression, which causes G1 arrest in HEY and SKOV3 cells and downregulates Bcl-2 protein expression and upregulates Bax protein expression. Berberine treatment of MDA-MB-231 and MCF-7 human breast cancer cells dose-dependently caused G0/G1 arrest, which was possibly associated with a decrease in the cell cycle regulation protein cyclin B1. Furthermore, it increased the expression of CDC4 and cyclin B1 through an increase in the expression of CDC2 and caspase-3 in human hepatoma HepG2 cells, causing arrest in the S and G2/M phases, and activating the AMPK signaling pathway to induce the apoptosis of HepG2 cells (Chidambaram et al., 2012; Murthy et al., 2012; Balestrieri et al., 2018). Li et al. demonstrated that berberine regulates the PI3K-AKT and MAPK signaling pathways in PTC (the most common subtype) and ATC (the most malignant and aggressive subtype), leading to mitochondrial apoptosis, G0/G1 cell cycle arrest, increased Bax/Bcl-2, cleaved caspase-3, p21, and decreased cyclin E1, CDK2, and vimentin were verified by western blotting (Waterbeemd et al., 2013). The combination of drugs upregulated the expression of the cell cycle-dependent kinase inhibitory proteins p27 and p21, and downregulated the expression of cyclin D1, CDK2, and CDK4-cyclin.

In addition, studies have reported that berberine can bind to topoisomerase (TOP1), which hinders the synthesis of S phase cells and prevents cell proliferation.

Effects of Berberine in Compatibility

With the identification of numerous anti-tumor drugs, research of cancer therapy has gradually shifted from a focus on monotherapy to combined therapy. More and more reports have demonstrated that berberine combined with radio-therapy or chemotherapy drugs can achieve better anti-tumor effect. For instance, berberine combined with gamma-radiation enhance the anti-cancer effects, including inducing apoptosis and ROS generation (Jung-Mu et al., 2009). Also, berberine sensitizes lung cancer cells to radiation via autophagy both *in vitro* and *in vivo* (Peng et al., 2008). Indicated an adjuvant role in radio-therapy of cancer. Another major anti-cancer therapy is chemotherapy, several novel chemotherapy drugs such like doxorubicin, rapamycin were texted combined with berberine, and showed a more effective result. It is reported that berberine sensitizes mutliple human cancer cells to the anticancer effects of doxorubicin (Tong et al., 2012). More details and drugs were summarized in **Table 3**, which clarified that berberine synergistic work with chemotherapy drugs in anti-tumor proliferation through inducing cell cycle arrest, apoptosis, as well as autophagy. These data have laid theoretical foundation for the combined therapy in clinic trial.

EPIGENETIC EFFECTS OF BERBERINE ON TUMORS

For many years, researchers have been studying and developing drugs for cancer prevention and treatment. Chinese medicines, such as berberine, are commonly used as drugs. As an active ingredient of Coptis, berberine is inevitably closely related to the occurrence and development of tumors (Wang-Johanning et al., 2008; Coward et al., 2014; Delga-docruzata et al., 2015; Dkhil et al., 2015). Extensive research has led scholars to conclude that, ultimately, the antitumor effect of berberine may be related to epigenetic effects. The following is a brief description of the methods through which berberine regulates tumor cells, including migration, proliferation, and apoptosis, through epigenetic mechanisms.

DNA Methylation

DNA methylation refers to the covalent attachment of the fifth carbon atom of cytosine on the CpG dinucleotide to the methyl group through the action of DNMT, which is modified to 5-methylcytosine. DNA methylation is a potential epigenetic mechanism involving a variety of biological processes. The DNMT family consists of three main members: DNMT1, DNMT3A, and DNMT3B. DNMT1 mainly maintains DNA methylation status and DNMT3A and DNMT3B catalyze new DNA methylations (Kalinkova et al., 2018; Li et al., 2018; Puneet et al., 2018). Human CpG exists mainly in two forms: one is dispersed in genomic DNA; the other is highly aggregated to form CpG islands, which are present in the promoter region or the first exon region of various genes. In the human genome, the CpG site is usually in an unmethylated state in the CpG islands, but in a methylated outside the CpG islands. When tumors occur, the degree of unmethylation of CpG sites outside CpG islands increases, whereas the CpG sites in CpG islands are highly methylated, causing a decrease in the overall methylation level of the genome, as well as certain gene CpG islands. Local methylation levels are abnormally elevated, leading to genomic instabilities, such as chromosomal instability, the activation of proto-oncogenes, and the silencing of tumor suppressor genes (Qing et al., 2014; Crawford et al., 2018; Lee and Gang, 2018; Sanna et al., 2018). DNA methylation abnormalities are mainly divided into the hypomethylation state of proto-oncogenes and the hypermethylation state of tumor suppressor genes. The most studied of these is the hypermethylation of tumor suppressor genes. It is of interest that berberine has been found to inhibit the expression of human DNA methyltransferases DNMT1 and DNMT3B in multiple myeloma U266 cells. For example, berberine can alter the CpG methylation of p53

TABLE 3 | Berberine combined with chemotherapy drugs.

Combined With	Cells	Mechnisms/Effect	Reference
2-deoxy-D-glucose	Human lymphoblastoid TK6 cells	BBR combined with the glucose analog 2-deoxy-D-glucose (2-dG) synergistic inducing the apoptosis of human lymphoblastoid TK6 cells	Halicka et al., 2017
5-Fluorouracil	Gastric cancer cells AGS	BBR sensitized gastric cancer cells to 5-FU, the combination shows a synergistic inhibition of surviving and STAT3 level	Pandey et al., 2015
Cinnamaldehyde	Lung carcinogenesis A549 cell	BBR combined with cinnamaldehyde prevented A549 cell substance permeability via AMPK-reduced AQP-1 expression	Meng et al., 2017
Cisplatin	Breast cancer MCF-7	BBR sensitized MCF-7 cells to cisplatin through inducing DNA breaks and caspase-3-dependent apoptosis	Zhao et al., 2016
D-limonene	Human gastric carcinoma cell line MGC803	BBR in combination with d-limonene showed synergistic anticancer effects on MGC803 cells through inducing cell-cycle arrest, ROS production, and apoptosis via the mitochondria-mediated intrinsic pathway	Zhang et al., 2014
Doxorubicin	Murine melanoma B16F10 cells	BBR combined with Doxorubicin inhibit melanoma tumor growth through casepase-3 dependent apoptosis	Mittal et al., 2014
	Lung cancer cell lines	BBR sensitizes lung cancer cells to Doxorubicin by promoting STAT3 degradation, inhibiting doxorubicin mediated STAT3 activation.	Zhu et al., 2015
Evodiamine	Breast cancer MCF-7	BBR in combination with evodiamine inducing cell cycle arrest and apoptosis, further inhibit MCF-7 prolieration	Du et al., 2017
Hsp90 inhibitor NVP-AUY922	Colorectal cancer	BBR combined with NVP-AUY922 inhibit proliferation of colorectal cancer via mutiple pathways	Su et al., 2015
Metformin	NSCLC	BBR combined with metformin synergistic induced cell cycle arrest, as well as reduced migration and invasion of NSCLC cells	Zheng et al., 2018
Rapamycin	Human hepatoma cell SMMC7721 cells	BBR combined with rapamycin can improve HCC therapy through inhibiting the mTOR signaling pathway	Guo et al., 2014
S-allyl-cysteine (SAC)	Human liver cancer HepG2 cells	BBR combined with SAC effectively reduced Rb-phosphorylation resulting insignificant nuclear E2F presence, further inhibiting cancer cell proliferation	Sengupta et al., 2017
	DEN+CCl4 induced hepatocarcinoma	BBR in combination with SAC inhibited Akt mediated cell proliferation, and inducing PP2A/JNK mediated apoptosis.	Sengupta et al., 2014
Sorafenib	Human liver cancer SMMC-7721 and HepG2 cells	berberine combined with sorafenib inhibited the proliferation of liver cancer cells by inducing cancer cell apoptosis.	Huang Y. et al., 2018
Tamoxifen	Breast cancer MCF-7	BBR sensitized MCF-7 cells to tamoxifen via inducing the G1 phase arrest and activating apoptosis.	Wen et al., 2016
Tetrahydropalmatine	MDA-MB-231 breast cancer cells	BBR combined with tetrahydropalmatine synergistic inhibited the proliferation of MDA-MB-231	Zhao et al., 2014
TPD7	T-cell acute lymphoblastic leukemia cell	BBR combined with TPD7 induced G1 -phase cell-cycle arrest of T-cell acute lymphoblastic leukemia cell.	Ma et al., 2017

DNA, affect the mRNA expression of key apoptosis-related proteins, and increases apoptosis in U266 cells, and thereby leads to cell cycle arrest. Although the hypomethylation of the p53 promoter can regulate apoptosis-related genes, such as GADD45, Bax, PMAIP1, BBC3, CCNB1, CCND3, and CCNE1. Specifically, in the p53 pathway, CDKN1A, GADD45B, Bax, PMAIP1, and BBC3 were upregulated, and CCNB1, CCND3, and CCNE1 were downregulated, which suggested that berberine activated the p53 signaling pathway through the impairment of U266 cells. In addition, results have shown that treatment of colorectal cancer cells with berberine results in a significant increase in the expression of DNMT1 and DNMT3A in the presence of TGF-β1; this hypermethylation in the promoter CpG island leads to further silencing of TSG, which results in tumor cell proliferation (Riaz et al., 2015; Asadi et al., 2018; Nardi et al., 2018).

Histone Modification

Histones play an important role in gene expression and tumorigenesis and development. The nucleosome is the basic constituent unit of chromatin. A nucleosome is an octamer composed of histones H2A, H2B, H3, and H4 and DNA entangled on the outside of the 147 base pairs. Histones not only protect the DNA structure and genetic information, but also participate in the regulation of gene expression. The extracellular amino terminus of histones can be modified by a variety of

TABLE 4 | Epigenetic regulation of berberine on tumor.

Type of Regulation	Cell Lines	Mechanism	Reference
DNA methylation	Multiple myeloma	DNMT1↓, DNMT3B↓ CDKN1A↑, GADD45B↑ Bax↑, PMAIP1↑	Asadi et al., 2018; Riaz et al., 2015; Nardi et al., 2018
	U266 cells	CCNB1↓, CCND3↓, CCNE1↓	
Histone Modification	Human non small cell lung cancer A549	HDAC↓MMP2↓ MMP9↓	Huang et al., 2017
	U266 cells	CBP/P300↑ SIRT3↑	Sun et al., 2017
MicroRNA	Human U266 multiple myeloma cells	miRNA21, Bcl-2↓	Hashiguchi et al., 2017
	Colon cancer	miR-152↓; miR-429↓ miR-29a↓	Hu et al., 2013

enzymes to form specific "histone codes" that alter the "open" or "closed" state of the local chromatin structure, or determine which proteins bind to specific DNA regions. Consequently, they regulate the various functions of DNA, including transcription and damage repair. Histone acetylation is highly dynamic and is coordinated by HATs and HDACs, and occurs at the amino-specific lysine residues of histones (Stevens et al., 1984; Yan et al., 2001; Bhat et al., 2018; Georgoff et al., 2018; Liu et al., 2018; Rahnamoun et al., 2018). Histone modification is a major determinant of the epigenetic silencing of genes and the regulation of cellular processes. Histone modifications often occur at the amino terminus of histones, and modifications of various chemical groups are acceptable due to exposure to chromatin (Oliver et al., 2013; Bennetzen and Wang, 2014; Hoen and Bureau, 2015; Yamada et al., 2015; Zhang et al., 2015; Li and Zhao, 2016; Rayan et al., 2016; Jiang et al., 2018; Salimian et al., 2018; Shang et al., 2018; Yan et al., 2018; Sahebi et al., 2018; Zhang L. et al., 2018; Zhang S. et al., 2018). The most widely studied are the acetylation and methylation of lysine K on histone H3 and H4. Histone acetylation plays an important role in the epigenetic theory proposed in recent years. Histone acetylation can affect the chromatin structure in cells, and thus participate in the transcriptional regulation of genes at specific sites, playing an important role in cell growth and differentiation. With a deeper understanding of the mechanism of histone acetylation in gene transcriptional regulation, the role of HDAC inhibitors in tumor therapy has received increasing attention (Sun et al., 2017).

CBP and p300 proteins with acetylase activity are transcriptional coactivators and hematopoietic tumor suppressors. Studies have shown that berberine can upregulate the expression of CBP/P300 and SIRT3 in U266 cells, and downregulate the expression of HDAC8; however, in HL-60/ADR and KG1-α cells, CBP/P300 and SIRT3 were also upregulated, but HDAC8 did not change significantly. Histone acetylation maintains its balance through HAT and HDAC. Berberine downregulated HDAC in human lung cancer A549 cells, which resulted in decreased expression of the metalloproteinases MMP-2 and MMP-9 mRNA and protein, inhibiting cell migration and invasion (Huang et al., 2017). Simultaneously, another study has shown that berberine treatment of A549 cells significantly reduced the expression of class I, II-a, II-b, and IV mRNA, histone H3, and H4 hyperacetylation.

MicroRNA

MicroRNAs (miRNAs) are short-chain non-coding RNAs of 19–22 nucleotides in length that bind to the 3′UTR in target mRNAs, thereby degrading or blocking the translation of target mRNAs. It plays an important role in the growth, differentiation, apoptosis, and tumor cell development. miRNAs can regulate the expression of multiple tumor-associated genes. In accordance with the function of miRNAs, they can be divided into two types: oncogenes or tumor suppressor genes (Hu et al., 2013). Not only can it act directly as a proto-oncogene or a tumor suppressor gene, but also regulate the expression of other proto-oncogenes or tumor suppressor genes. miRNAs play a central role in many cellular biology processes, and their dysregulation is a ubiquitous feature in tumors. Epigenetic effects have been shown to be a major cause of miRNA dysregulation in tumors (Hashiguchi et al., 2017). In the TGF-β1-induced colorectal cancer model, berberine significantly decreased the expression of miR-152

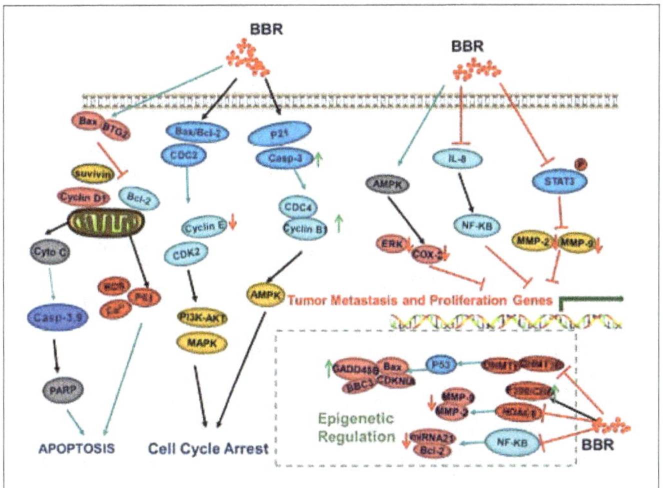

FIGURE 2 | Signaling pathways regulated by berberine.

(targeting DNMT1), miR-429 (targeting DNMT3A), and miR-29a (targeting DNMT3A/3B), which suggested that berberine inactivates some tumor suppressor factors, including DNMT1 and DNMT3A/3B, through the regulation of the expression of the above miRNAs during colon cancer development. Furthermore, other evidence has suggested that berberine treatment of human U266 multiple myeloma cells led to the inhibition of NF-κB nuclear translocation via Set9-mediated lysine methylation, which resulted in decreased miRNA21 and Bcl-2 expression, inducing the cells to produce ROS and promoting cell apoptosis. Berberine treatment of colorectal cancer cells increased the expression of miR-200a-5p and decreased the expression of miR-429. These epigenetic regulation affected by Berberine was briefly summarized in **Table 4**.

SUMMARY AND FUTURE PERSPECTIVES

The importance of epigenetic regulation in the occurrence and development of tumors is now an established fact. An increasing body of research has been devoted to the exploration of epigenetic molecular markers for the early diagnosis, treatment, and prognosis of tumors. Simultaneously, epigenetic drugs provide a new direction for the treatment of tumors owing to the reversibility and ease of regulation of epigenetics. At present, the anticancer drugs that inhibit the proliferation of malignant tumor cells via induction of apoptosis or that regulate signal transduction are mostly multi-targeted (He et al., 2010). Berberine is a natural isoquinoline alkaloid that significantly contributed to the development of anticancer drugs (**Figure 2**). Given the continuous development in the field of medicine and the extension of research and development in the field of medicine, berberine has gained attention of researchers owing to the combination of multiple effects. Berberine is not irreplaceable with respect to its traditional pharmacological activities, such as antibacterial, anti-inflammatory, and antiviral effects (Huang S.X. et al., 2018). Moreover, the efficacy of the antihypertensive, antitumor, and hypolipidemic effects has also become a "hot topic" in contemporary research. Berberine regulates the molecular mechanisms that cause tumor cells through a variety of signaling pathways, confirming the potential therapeutic effects in a variety of tumor cells. However, there are few reports on the effects of berberine on the epigenetic functions of tumors. Epigenetics is also the main controlling factor of oncogenes in the development of cancer. Therefore, the application of epigenetic properties of berberine in the treatment of malignant tumors offers broad prospects for drug development. At the same time, extended research into epigenetics has provided a new strategy to understand the various characteristics of tumors, optimize the early diagnosis of tumors, and improve the prognosis of patients. In future, basic research and clinical transformations in the epigenetics of cancer will provide new strategies for the precise diagnosis and treatment of cancer.

AUTHOR CONTRIBUTIONS

DL contributed significantly to analysis and manuscript preparation. XM contributed significantly to manuscript preparation. DW helped to writing the manuscript. ZQ and HL contributed to the conception of the study.

FUNDING

This work was supported by the National Natural Science Foundation of China (Grant No. 81803680). Jilin Province Science and Technology Development Project in China (Grant Nos. 20170307031 and YY20180520050JH).

REFERENCES

1. Agnarelli, A., Natali, M., Garciagil, M., Pesi, R., Tozzi, M. G., Ippolito, C., et al. (2018). Cell-specific pattern of berberine pleiotropic effects on different human cell lines. *Sci. Rep.* 8:10599. doi: 10.1038/s41598-018-28952-3
2. Asadi, R., Omrani, M. D., Ghaedi, H., Mirfakhraie, R., Azargashb, E., Habibi, M., et al. (2018). Premutations of fmr1 cgg repeats are not related to idiopathic premature ovarian failure in iranian patients: a case control study. *Gene* 676, 189–194. doi: 10.1016/j.gene.2018.07.034
3. Balestrieri, E., Argaw-Denboba, A., Gambacurta, A., Cipriani, C., Bei, R., Serafino, A., et al. (2018). Human endogenous retrovirus k in the crosstalk between cancer cells microenvironment and plasticity: a new perspective for combination therapy. *Front. Microbiol.* 9:1448. doi: 10.3389/fmicb.2018.01448
4. Bennetzen, J. L., and Wang, H. (2014). The contributions of transposable elements to the structure, function, and evolution of plant genomes. *Annu. Rev. Plant Biol.* 65:505. doi: 10.1146/annurev-arplant-050213-035811
5. Bhat, A. V., Hora, S., Pal, A., Jha, S., and Taneja, R. (2018). Stressing the (epi) genome: dealing with reactive oxygen species in cancer. *Antioxid. Redox Signal.* 29, 1273–1292. doi: 10.1089/ars.2017.7158
6. Biswas, S., and Rao, C. M. (2018). Epigenetic tools (The Writers, the readers and the erasers) and their implications in cancer therapy. *Eur. J. Pharmacol.* 837, 8–24. doi: 10.1016/j.ejphar.2018.08.021
7. Blandino, G., Fazi, F., Donzelli, S., Kedmi, M., Saschen, A., Muti, P., et al. (2014). Tumor suppressor micrornas: a novel non-coding alliance against cancer. *FEBS Lett.* 588, 2639–2652. doi: 10.1016/j.febslet.2014.03.033
8. Booth, A. K., and Gutierrez-Hartmann, A. (2015). Signaling pathways regulating pituitary lactotrope homeostasis and tumorigenesis. *Adv. Exp. Med. Biol.* 846, 37–59. doi: 10.1007/978-3-319-12114-7_2
9. Chidambaram, A., Fillmore, H. L., Van Meter, T. E., Dumur, C. I., Band roaddus, W. C., (2012). Novel report of expression and function of CD97 in malignant gliomas: correlation with Wilms tumor 1 expression and glioma cell invasiveness. *J. Neurosurg.* 116, 843–853. doi: 10.3171/2011.11.JNS111455
10. Cicero, A. F., and Baggioni, A. (2016). Berberine and its role in chronic disease. *Adv. Exp. Med. Biol.* 928:27. doi: 10.1007/978-3-319-41334-1_2
11. Coward, W. R., Feghalibostwick, C. A., Jenkins, G., Knox, A. J., and Pang, L. (2014). A central role for g9a and ezh2 in the epigenetic silencing of cyclooxygenase-2 in idiopathic pulmonary fibrosis. *FASEB J.* 28, 3183–3196. doi: 10.1096/fj.13-241760
12. Crawford, B., Craig, Z., Mansell, G., White, I., Spaull, S., Imm, J., et al. (2018). DNA methylation and inflammation marker profiles associated with a history of depression. *Hum. Mol. Genet.* 27, 2840–2850. doi: 10.1093/hmg/ddy199
13. Delga-docruzata, L., Zhang, W., Mcdonald, J. A., Tsai, W. Y., Valdovinos, C., Falci, L., et al. (2015). Dietary modifications, weight loss, and

changes in metabolic markers affect global dna methylation in hispanic, african american, and afro-caribbean breast cancer survivors. *J. Nutr.* 145:783. doi: 10.3945/jn. 114.202853

14. Dkhil, M. A., Metwaly, M. S., Saleh, A. Q., Sherif, N. E., Denis, D., Omar, S. Y. A., et al. (2015). Anti-eimeria activity of berberine and identification of associated gene expression changes in the mouse jejunum infected with eimeria papillata. *Parasitol. Res.* 114, 1–13. doi: 10.1007/s00436-015-4344-z
15. Du, J., Sun, Y., Lu, Y. Y., Lau, E., Zhao, M., Zhou, Q. M., et al. (2017). Berberine and evodiamine act synergistically against human breast cancer mcf-7 cells by inducing cell cycle arrest and apoptosis. *Anticancer Res.* 37, 6141–6151.
16. Dupont, C., Armant, D. R., and Brenner, C. A. (2009). Epigenetics: definition, mechanisms and clinical perspective. *Semin. Reprod. Med.* 27, 351–357. doi: 10.1055/s-0029-1237423
17. Foroutan, F., Alba, A. C., Stein, M., Krakovsky, J., Chien, K. G. W., Chih, S., et al., (2018). Validation of the International Society for Heart and Lung Transplantation primary graft dysfunction instrument in heart transplantation. *J. Heart Lung Transplant.* doi: 10.1016/j.healun.2018.12.007 [Epub ahead of print].
18. Foroutan, T., Farhadi, A., Abroun, S., and Mohammad Soltani, B. (2018). Adipose derived stem cells affect miR-145 and p53 expressions of co-cultured hematopoietic stem cells. *Cell J.* 19, 654–659. doi: 10.22074/cellj.2018.4393
19. Georgoff, P. E., Nikolian, V. C., Higgins, G., Chtraklin, K., Eidy, H., Ghandour, M. H., et al. (2018). Valproic acid induces pro-survival transcriptomic changes in swine subjected to traumatic injury and hemorrhagic shock. *J. Trauma Acute Care Surg.* 84:1. doi: 10.1097/TA.0000000000001763
20. Gu, L., Frommel, S. C., Oakes, C. C., Simon, R., Grupp, K., Gerig, C. Y., et al. (2015). Baz2a (tip5) is involved in epigenetic alterations in prostate cancer and its overexpression predicts disease recurrence. *Nat. Genet.* 47:22. doi: 10.1038/ng.3165
21. Guo, N., Yan, A., Gao, X., Chen, Y., He, X., Hu, Z., et al. (2014). Berberine sensitizes rapamycin-mediated human hepatoma cell death in vitro. *Mol. Med. Rep.* 10, 3132–3138. doi: 10.3892/mmr.2014.2608
22. Halicka, H. D., Garcia, J., Li, J., Zhao, H., and Darzynkiewicz, Z. (2017). Synergy of 2-deoxy-d-glucose combined with berberine in inducing the lysosome/autophagy and transglutaminase activation-facilitated apoptosis. *Apoptosis* 22, 229–238. doi: 10.1007/s10495-016-1315-5
23. Hamsa, T. P., and Kuttan, G. (2011). Studies on anti-metastatic and anti-invasive effects of harmine using highly metastatic murine b16f-10 melanoma cells. *J. Environ. Pathol. Toxicol. Oncol.* 30:123. doi: 10.1615/JEnvironPatholToxicolOncol.v30.i2.40
24. Hao, D. C., He, C. N., and Shen, J. (2017). Anticancer chemodiversity of ranunculaceae medicinal plants molecular mechanisms and functions. *Curr. Genomics* 18, 39–59. doi: 10.2174/1389202917666160803151752
25. Hashiguchi, Y., Kawano, S., Goto, Y., Yasuda, K., Kaneko, N., Sakamoto, T., et al. (2017). Tumor-suppressive roles of ⊠np63β-mir-205 axis in epithelial-mesenchymal transition of oral squamous cell carcinoma via targeting zeb1 and zeb2. *J. Cell. Physiol.* 233, 6565–6577. doi: 10.1002/jcp.26267
26. He, X. Y., Chen, J. X., Zhang, Z., Li, C. L., Peng, Q. L., and Peng, H. M. (2010). The let-7a microrna protects from growth of lung carcinoma by suppression of k-ras and c-myc in nude mice. *J. Cancer Res. Clin. Oncol.* 136, 1023–1028. doi: 10.1007/s00432-009-0747-5
27. Hoen, D. R., and Bureau, T. E. (2015). Discovery of novel genes derived from transposable elements using integrative genomic analysis. *Mol. Biol. Evol.* 32, 1487–1506. doi: 10.1093/molbev/msv042
28. Honda, H., Pazin, M. J., Ji, H., Wernyj, R. P., and Morin, P. J. (2006). Crucial roles of sp1 and epigenetic modifications in the regulation of the cldn4 promoter in ovarian cancer cells. *J. Biol. Chem.* 281:21433. doi: 10.1074/jbc.M603767200
29. Liu, H. C., Lämke, J., Lin, S. Y., Hung, M. J., Liu, K. M., Charng, Y. Y., et al. (2018). Distinct heat shock factors and chromatin modifications mediate the organ-autonomous transcriptional memory of heat stress. *Plant J.* 95, 401–413. doi: 10.1111/tpj.13958
30. Hu, H., Li, K., Wang, X., Liu, Y., Lu, Z. G., Dong, R. H., et al. (2013). Set9, NF-κB, and microRNA-21 mediate berberine-induced apoptosis of human multiple myeloma cells. *Acta Pharmacol. Sin.* 34:157. doi: 10.1038/aps.2012.161
31. Huang, C., Liu, H., Gong, X. L., Wu, L. Y., and Wen, B. (2017). Effect of evodiamine and berberine on the interaction between dnmts and target micrornas during malignant transformation of the colon by tgf-β1. *Oncol. Rep.* 37, 1637–1645. doi: 10.3892/or.2017.5379
32. Huang, S. X., Qiu, G., Cheng, F. R., Pei, Z., Yang, Z., Deng, X. H., et al. (2018). Berberine protects secondary injury in mice with traumatic brain injury through anti-oxidative and anti-inflammatory modulation. *Neurochem. Res.* 43, 1–12. doi: 10.1007/s11064-018-2597-5
33. Huang, Y., Wang, K., Gu, C., Yu, G., Zhao, D., Mai, W., et al. (2018). Berberine, a natural plant alkaloid, synergistically sensitizes human liver cancer cells to sorafenib. *Oncol. Rep.* 40, 1525–1532. doi: 10.3892/or.2018.6552
34. Huang, Z. H., Zheng, H. F., Wang, W. L., Wang, Y., Zhong, L. F., Wu, J. L., et al. (2015). Berberine targets epidermal growth factor receptor signaling to suppress prostate cancer proliferation in vitro. *Mol. Med. Rep.* 11:2125. doi: 10.3892/mmr.2014.2929
35. Iizuka, N., Miyamoto, K., Okita, K., Tangoku, A., Hayashi, H., Yosino, S., et al. (2000). Inhibitory effect of coptidis rhizoma and berberine on the proliferation of human esophageal cancer cell lines. *Cancer Lett.* 148, 19–25. doi: 10.1016/S0304-3835(99)00264-5
36. Imenshahidi, M., and Hosseinzadeh, H. (2016). Berberis vulgaris and berberine. *Phytother. Res.* 30, 1745–1764. doi: 10.1002/ptr.5693
37. Jiang, L., Xue, W., and Wang, Y. (2018). Inhibition of miR-31a-5p decreases inflammation by down-regulating IL-25 expression in human dermal fibroblast cells (CC-2511 cells) under hyperthermic stress via Wnt/β-catenin pathway. *Biomed. Pharmacother.* 107, 24–33. doi: 10.1016/j.biopha.2018.07.142
38. Jin, Y., Liu, S., Ma, Q., Xiao, D., and Chen, L. (2017). Berberine enhances the ampk activation and autophagy and mitigates high glucose-induced apoptosis of mouse podocytes. *Eur. J. Pharmacol* 794, 106–114. doi: 10.1016/j.ejphar.2016. 11.037
39. Jung-Mu, H., Mee-Sun, H., Sang-Yong, L., Woo-Yiel, L., and Dongho, K. (2009). The combination of berberine and irradiation enhances anti-cancer effects via activation of p38 mapk pathway and ros generation in human hepatoma cells. *J. Cell. Biochem.* 107, 955–964. doi: 10.1002/jcb.22198
40. Kalaiarasi, A., Anusha, C., Sankar, R., Rajasekaran, S., John, M. J., Muthusamy, K., et al. (2016). Plant isoquinoline alkaloid berberine exhibits chromatin remodeling by modulation of histone deacetylase to induce growth arrest and apoptosis in the a549 cell line. *J. Agric. Food Chem.* 64:9542. doi: 10.1021/acs.jafc.6b04453
41. Kalinkova, L., Zmetakova, I., Smolkova, B., Minarik, G., Sedlackova, T., Kajabova, V. H., et al. (2018). Decreased methylation in the SNAI2 and ADAM23 genes associated with de-differentiation and haematogenous dissemination in breast cancers. *BMC Cancer* 18:875. doi: 10.1186/s12885-018-4783-x
42. Katona, B. W., Liu, Y., Ma, A., Jin, J., and Hua, X. (2014). Ezh2 inhibition enhances the efficacy of an egfr inhibitor in suppressing colon cancer cells. *Cancer Biol. Ther.* 15:11. doi: 10.4161/15384047.2014.972776
43. Khalil, I., Colombara, D. V., Forouzanfar, M. H., Troeger, C., Daoud, F., Moradi-Lakeh, M., et al. (2016). Burden of diarrhea in the eastern mediterranean region, 1990–2013: findings from the global burden of disease study 2013. *Am. J. Trop. Med. Hyg.* 95, 1319–1329. doi: 10.4269/ajtmh.16-0339
44. Kong, W., Wei, J., Abidi, P., Lin, M., Inaba, S., Li, C., et al. (2004). Berberine is a novel cholesterol-lowering drug working through a unique mechanism distinct from statins. *Nat. Med.* 7, 464–464. doi: 10.1016/S1567-5688(06) 81865-9
45. Kumar, A., Ekavali, Chopra, K., Mukherjee, M., Pottabathini, R., and Dhull, D. K. (2015). Current knowledge and pharmacological profile of berberine: an update. *Eur. J. Pharmacol.* 761, 288–297. doi: 10.1016/j.ejphar.2015.05.068
46. Lee, C., and Gang, J. (2018). A label-free detection of ndei endonuclease activity by using dna-templated silver nanoclusters. *J. Nanosci. Nanotechnol.* 18:6339. doi: 10.1166/jnn.2018.15657
47. Li, B., Wang, Z., Wu, H., Xue, M., Lin, P., Wang, S., et al. (2018). Epigenetic regulation of cxcl12 plays a critical role in mediating tumor progression and the immune response in osteosarcoma. *Cancer Res.* 78:3938. doi: 10.1158/0008-5472.can-17-3801
48. Li, C. H., Wu, D. F., Ding, H., Zhao, Y., Zhou, K. Y., and Xu, D. F. (2014). Berberine hydrochloride impact on physiological processes and modulation of twist levels in nasopharyngeal carcinoma cne-1 cells. *Asian Pac. J. Cancer Prev.* 15, 1851–1857. doi: 10.7314/APJCP.2014.15.4.1851
49. Li, J., Liu, F., Jiang, S., Liu, J., Chen, X., Zhang, S., et al. (2018). Berberine hydrochloride inhibits cell proliferation and promotes apoptosis of non-

small cell lung cancer via the suppression of the mmp2 and bcl-2/bax signaling pathways. *Oncol. Lett.* 15:7409. doi: 10.3892/ol.2018.8249

50. Li, L., Wang, X., Sharvan, R., Gao, J., Qu, S., Li, L., et al. (2017). Berberine could inhibit thyroid carcinoma cells by inducing mitochondrial apoptosis, g0/g1 cell cycle arrest and suppressing migration via pi3k-akt and mapk signaling pathways. *Biomed. Pharmacother.* 95, 1225–1231. doi: 10.1016/j.biopha.2017.09.010
51. Li, L., and Zhao, G. (2016). Downregulation of microrna-218 relieves neuropathic pain by regulating suppressor of cytokine signaling 3. *Int. J. Mol. Med.* 37:851. doi: 10.3892/ijmm.2016.2455
52. Li, N., Xu, F., Cheng, J., Zhang, Y., Huang, G., Zhu, J., et al. (2018). Perfluorocarbon nanocapsules improve hypoxic microenvironment for the tumor ultrasound diagnosis and photodynamic therapy. *J. Biomed. Nanotechnol.* 14, 2162–2171. doi: 10.1166/jbn.2018.2656
53. Li, W., Li, Q., Kang, S., Same, M., Zhou, Y., Sun, C., et al. (2018). Cancerdetector: ultrasensitive and non-invasive cancer detection at the resolution of individual reads using cell-free dna methylation sequencing data. *Nucleic Acids Res.* 46:e89.
54. Liu, L., Chen, L., Jiang, C., Guo, J., Xie, Y., Kang, L., et al. (2017a). Berberine inhibits the lps-induced proliferation and inflammatory response of stromal cells of adenomyosis tissues mediated by the lps/tlr4 signaling pathway. *Exp. Therap. Med.* 14:6125. doi: 10.3892/etm.2017.5316
55. Liu, L., Luo, N., Guo, J., Xie, Y., Chen, L., and Cheng, Z. (2017b). Berberine inhibits growth and inflammatory invasive phenotypes of ectopic stromal cells: imply the possible treatment of adenomyosis. *J. Pharmacol. Sci.* 137, 5–11. doi: 10.1016/j.jphs.2017.12.001
56. Lu, W., Du, S., and Wang, J. (2015). Berberine inhibits the proliferation of prostate cancer cells and induces g0/g1 or g2/m phase arrest at different concentrations. *Mol. Med. Rep.* 11, 3920–3924. doi: 10.3892/mmr.2014.3139
57. Ma, C. Y., Shen, S. C., Huang, D. W., Chang, H. M., and Wu, J. S. B. (2008). Growth inhibition and induction of apoptosis in u937 cells by coptis chinensis extract. *J. Food Sci.* 73, H127–H133. doi: 10.1111/j.1750-3841.2008.00837.x
58. Ma, W., Zhu, M., Yang, L., Yang, T., and Zhang, Y., (2017). Synergistic effect of TPD7 and berberine against leukemia jurkat cell growth through regulating ephrin-B2 signaling. *Phytother. Res.* 31, 1392–1399.
59. Meng, F. C., Wu, Z. F., Yin, Z. Q., Lin, L. G., Wang, R., and Zhang, Q. W. (2018).Coptidis rhizoma and its main bioactive components: recent advances in chemical investigation, quality evaluation and pharmacological activity. *Chinese Med.* 13:13. doi: 10.1186/s13020-018-0171-3
60. Meng, M., Geng, S., Du, Z., Yao, J., Zheng, Y., Li, Z., et al. (2017). Berberine and cinnamaldehyde together prevent lung carcinogenesis. *Oncotarget* 8:76385. doi: 10.18632/oncotarget.20059
61. Mirhadi, E., Rezaee, M., and Malaekehnikouei, B. (2018). Nano strategies for berberine delivery, a natural alkaloid of berberis. *Biomed. Chromatogr. BMC* 1060:e4279. doi: 10.1002/bmc.4279
62. Mistry, B. M., Keum, Y. S., Pandurangan, M., Kim, D. H., Moon, S. H., Kadam, A. A., et al. (2017). Synthesis and evaluation of antioxidant and cytotoxicity of the n-mannich base of berberine bearing benzothiazole moieties. *Anti- cancer Agents Med. Chem.* 17, 1652–1660. doi: 10.2174/1871520617666170710180549
63. Mittal, A., Tabasum, S., and Singh, R. P. (2014). Berberine in combination with doxorubicin suppresses growth of murine melanoma b16f10 cells in culture and xenograft. *Phytomedicine* 21, 340–347. doi: 10.1016/j.phymed.2013.09.002
64. Munir, I., Fukunaga, K., Kanasaki, H., Miyazaki, K., Ohba, T., Okamura, H., et al. (2000). Expression of cyclooxygenase 2 by prostaglandin e2 in human endometrial adenocarcinoma cell line hec-1b1. *Biol. Reprod.* 63, 933–941. doi: 10.1095/biolreprod63.3.933
65. Murthy, K. N. C., Kim, J., Vikram, A., and Patil, B. S. (2012). Differential inhibition of human colon cancer cells by structurally similar flavonoids of citrus. *Food Chem.* 132, 27–34. doi: 10.1016/j.foodchem.2011. 10.014
66. Nardi, I., Reno, T., Yun, X., Sztain, T., Wang, J., Dai, H., et al. (2018). Triptolide inhibits Wnt signaling in NSCLC through upregulation of multiple Wnt inhibitory factors via epigenetic modifications to Histone H3. *Int. J. Cancer* 143, 2470–2478. doi: 10.1002/ijc.31756
67. Naveen, C. R., Gaikwad, S., and Agrawalrajput, R. (2016). Berberine induces neuronal differentiation through inhibition of cancer stemness and epithelial-mesenchymal transition in neuroblastoma cells. *Phytomed. Int. J. Phytother. Phytopharmacol.* 23, 736–744. doi: 10.1016/j.phymed.2016.03.013
68. Neag, M. A., Mocan, A., Echeverría, J., Pop, R. M., Bocsan, C. I., Crişan, G., et al. (2018). Berberine: botanical occurrence, traditional uses, extraction methods, and relevance in cardiovascular, metabolic, hepatic, and renal disorders. *Front. Pharmacol.* 9:557. doi: 10.3389/fphar.2018.00557
69. Oliver, K. R., Mccomb, J. A., and Greene, W. K. (2013). Transposable elements: powerful contributors to angiosperm evolution and diversity. *Genome Biol. Evol.* 5, 1886–1901. doi: 10.1093/gbe/evt141
70. Pandey, A., Vishnoi, K., Mahata, S., Tripathi, S. C., Misra, S. P., Misra, V., et al. (2015). Berberine and curcumin target survivin and stat3 in gastric cancer cells and synergize actions of standard chemotherapeutic 5-fluorouracil. *Nutr. Cancer Int. J.* 67, 1293–1304. doi: 10.1080/01635581.2015.1085581
71. Peng, P. L., Kuo, W. H., Tseng, H. C., and Chou, F. P., (2008). Synergistic tumor-killing effect of radiation and berberine combined treatment in lung cancer: the contribution of autophagic cell death. *Int. J. Radiat. Oncol. Biol. Phys.* 70, 529–542. doi: 10.1016/j.ijrobp.2007.08.034
72. Puneet, Kazmi, H. R., Kumari, S., Tiwari, S., Khanna, A., and Narayan, G. (2018). Epigenetic mechanisms and events in gastric cancer-emerging novel biomarkers. *Pathol. Oncol. Res.* 2, 1–14. doi: 10.1007/s12253-018-0410-z
73. Qi, H. W., Xin, L. Y., Xu, X., Ji, X. X., and Fan, L. H. (2014). Epithelial- to-mesenchymal transition markers to predict response of berberine in suppressing lung cancer invasion and metastasis. *J. Trans. Med.* 12:22. doi: 10.1186/1479-5876-12-22
74. Qing, Y., Hu, H., Liu, Y., Feng, T., Meng, W., Jiang, L., et al. (2014). Berberine induces apoptosis in human multiple myeloma cell line u266 through hypomethylation of p53 promoter. *Cell Biol. Int.* 38, 563–570. doi: 10.1002/cbin. 10206
75. Rahnamoun, H., Lee, J., Sun, Z., Lu, H., Ramsey, K. M., Komives, E. A., et al. (2018). RNAs interact with BRD4 to promote enhanced chromatin engagement and transcription activation. *Nat. Struct. Mol. Biol.* 25:687. doi: 10.1038/s41594-018-0102-0
76. Rayan, N. A., Rosario, R. C. H. D., and Prabhakar, S. (2016). Massive contribution of transposable elements to mammalian regulatory sequences. *Semin. Cell Dev. Biol.* 57, 51–56. doi: 10.1016/j.semcdb.2016.05.004
77. Riaz, S. K., Saeed, M., and Malik, M. F. (2015). Clinical and therapeutic implications of histone acetylation in breast cancer. *West Indian Med. J.* 65, 337–344. doi: 10.7727/wimj.2014.297
78. Sahebi, M., Hanafi, M. M., van Wijnen, A. J., Rice, D., Rafii, M. Y., Azizi, P., et al. (2018). Contribution of transposable elements in the plant's genome. *Gene* 665, 155–166. doi: 10.1016/j.gene.2018.04.050
79. Salimian, N., Peymani, M., Ghaedi, K., and Esfahani, M. (2018). Modulation in mir-200a/sirt1axis is associated with apoptosis in mpp+-induced sh-sy5y cells. *Gene* 674, 24–30. doi: 10.1016/j.gene.2018.06.061
80. Sanna, L., Marchesi, I., Melone, M. A. B., and Bagella, L. (2018). The role of enhancer of zeste homolog 2: from viral epigenetics to the carcinogenesis of hepatocellular carcinoma. *J. Cell. Physiol.* 233, 6508–6517. doi: 10.1002/jcp.26545
81. Sengupta, D., Chowdhury, K. D., Chatterjee, S., Sarkar, A., Paul, S., Sur, P. K., et al. (2017). Modulation of adenylate cyclase signaling in association with mkk3/6 stabilization under combination of sac and berberine to reduce hepg2 cell survivability. *Apoptosis* 22, 1–18. doi: 10.1007/s10495-017-1407-x
82. Sengupta, D., Chowdhury, K. D., Sarkar, A., Paul, S., and Sadhukhan, G. C., (2014). Berberine and S allyl cysteine mediated amelioration of DEN+ CCl4 induced hepatocarcinoma. *Biochim. Biophys. Acta (BBA)-Gen. Subjects* 1840, 219–244. doi: 10.1016/j.bbagen.2013.08.020
83. Shang, A., Bylipudi, S., and Bieszczad, K. M. (2018). Inhibition of histone deacetylase 3 via rgfp966 facilitates cortical plasticity underlying unusually accurate auditory associative cue memory for excitatory and inhibitory cue-reward associations. *Behav. Brain Res.* 356, 453–469. doi: 10.1016/j.bbr.2018.05.036
84. Shi, H. L., Wu, X. J., Liu, Y., and Xie, J. Q. (2013). Berberine counteracts enhanced il-8 expression of ags cells induced by evodiamine. *Life Sci.* 93, 830–839. doi: 10.1016/j.lfs.2013.09.010
85. Shi, Y., Zhao, Y., Shao, N., Ye, R., Lin, Y., Zhang, N., et al. (2017). Overexpression of microrna-96-5p inhibits autophagy and apoptosis

and enhances the proliferation, migration and invasiveness of human breast cancer cells. *Oncol. Lett.* 13, 4402–4412. doi: 10.3892/ol.2017.6025

86. Signorelli, C., Odone, A., Ciorba, V., Cella, P., Audisio, R. A., Lombardi, A., et al. (2017). Human papillomavirus 9-valent vaccine for cancer prevention: a systematic review of the available evidence. *Epidemiol. Infect.* 145:21. doi: 10.1017/s0950268817000747
87. Siveen, K. S., and Kuttan, G. (2011). Thujone inhibits lung metastasis induced by b16f-10 melanoma cells in c57bl/6 mice. *Can. J. Physiol. Pharmacol.* 89:691. doi: 10.1139/y11-067
88. Stevens, M. S., Aliabadi, Z., and Moore, M. R. (1984). Associated effects of sodium butyrate on histone acetylation and estrogen receptor in the human breast cancer cell line mcf-7. *Biochem. Biophys. Res. Commun.* 119, 132–138. doi: 10.1016/0006-291X(84)91628-0
89. Su, Y. H., Tang, W. C., Cheng, Y. W., Sia, P., Huang, C. C., Lee, Y. C., et al. (2015). Targeting of multiple oncogenic signaling pathways by hsp90 inhibitor alone or in combination with berberine for treatment of colorectal cancer. *BBA - Mol. Cell Res.* 1853, 2261–2272. doi: 10.1016/j.bbamcr.2015.05.012
90. Sun, W., Zhang, L., and Li, R. (2017). Overexpression of miR-206 ameliorates chronic constriction injury-induced neuropathic pain in rats via the MEK/ERK pathway by targeting brain-derived neurotrophic factor. *Neurosci. Lett.* 646, 68–74. doi: 10.1016/j.neulet.2016.12.047
91. Tabeshpour, J., Imenshahidi, M., and Hosseinzadeh, H. (2017). A review of the effects ofberberis vulgarisand its major component, berberine, in metabolic syndrome. *Iran. J. Basic Med. Sci.* 20, 557–568. doi: 10.22038/IJBMS.2017. 8682
92. Tang, J., and Feng, Y. S. (2009). Berberine and coptidis rhizoma as novel antineoplastic agents: a review of traditional use and biomedical investigations. *J. Ethnopharmacol.* 126, 5–17. doi: 10.1016/j.jep.2009.08.009
93. Tao, Y., Lin, Y., She, Z., Lin, M., Chen, P., and Zhang, J. (2015). Anticancer activity and mechanism investigation of beauvericin isolated from secondary metabolites of the mangrove endophytic fungi. *Anti-Cancer Agents Med. Chem.* 15, 258–266. doi: 10.2174/1871520614666140825112255
94. Tong, N., Zhang, J., Chen, Y., Zhubo, L. I., Luo, Y., Zuo, H., et al. (2012). Berberine sensitizes mutliple human cancer cells to the anticancer effects of doxorubicin in vitro. *Oncol. Lett.* 3, 1263–1267. doi: 10.3892/ol.2012.644
95. Viegas, S., Ladeira, C., Costaveiga, A., Perelman, J., and Gajski, G. (2017). Forgotten public health impacts of cancer - An overview. *Arh. Hig. Rada. Toksikol.* 68:287. doi: 10.1515/aiht-2017-68-3005
96. Vijayaraghavalu, S., Dermawan, J. K., and Cheriyath, V. (2013). Highly synergistic effect of sequential treatment with epigenetic and;anticancer drugs to overcome drug resistance in breast cancer cells is;mediated via activation of p21 gene expression leading to g2/m cycle;arrest. *Mol. Pharm.* 10, 337–352. doi: 10.1021/mp3004622
97. Walker, D. K., Edwards, R. L., Bagcivan, G., and Bakitas, M. A. (2017). Cancer and palliative care in the united states, turkey, and malawi: developing global collaborations. *Asia-Pacific J. Oncol. Nurs.* 4, 209–219. doi: 10.4103/apjon.apjon_31_17
98. Wang, J., Kang, M., Wen, Q., Qin, Y. T., Wei, Z. X., Xiao, J. J., et al. (2017). Berberine sensitizes nasopharyngeal carcinoma cells to radiation through inhibition of sp1 and emt. *Oncol. Rep.* 37, 2425–2432. doi: 10.3892/or.2017.5499
99. Wang, N., Feng, Y., Cheung, F., Wang, X., Zhang, Z., and Feng, Y. (2015a). A chinese medicine formula gegen qinlian decoction suppresses expansion of human renal carcinoma with inhibition of matrix metalloproteinase-2. *Integr. Cancer Ther.* 14:75. doi: 10.1177/1534735414550036
100. Wang, N., Tan, H. Y., Li, L., Yuen, M. F., and Feng, Y. (2015b). Berberine and coptidis rhizoma as potential anticancer agents: recent updates and future perspectives. *J. Ethnopharmacol.* 176, 35–48. doi: 10.1016/j.jep.2015. 10.028
101. Wang, S., Xiao, Z., Hong, Z., Jiao, H., Zhu, S., Zhao, Y., et al. (2018). FOXF1 promotes angiogenesis and accelerates bevacizumab resistance in colorectal cancer by transcriptionally activating VEGFA. *Cancer Lett.* 439, 78–90. doi: 10.1016/j.canlet.2018.09.026
102. Wang-Johanning, F., Radvanyi, L., Rycaj, K., Plummer, J. B., Yan, P., Sastry, K. J., et al. (2008). Human endogenous retrovirus k triggers an antigen-specific immune response in breast cancer patients. *Cancer Res.* 68, 5869–5877. doi: 10.1158/0008-5472.CAN-07-6838
103. Waterbeemd, B. V. D., Mommen, G. P. M., Pennings, J. L. A., Eppink, M. H., Wijffels, R. H., Pol, L. A. V. D., et al. (2013). Quantitative proteomics reveals distinct differences in the protein content of outer membrane vesicle vaccines. *J. Proteome Res.* 12, 1898–1908. doi: 10.1021/pr301 208g
104. Wen, C., Wu, L., Fu, L., Zhang, X., and Zhou, H. (2016). Berberine enhances the anti-tumor activity of tamoxifen in drug-sensitive MCF-7 and drug-resistant MCF-7/TAM cells. *Mol. Med. Rep.* 14, 2250–2256. doi: 10.3892/mmr.2016. 5490
105. Wong, K. Y., and Chim, C. S. (2015). DNA methylation of tumor suppressor protein-coding and non-coding genes in multiple myeloma. *Epigenomics* 7, 985–1001. doi: 10.2217/epi.15.57
106. Wu, Y. Q., Chen, X. S., and Chai, J. B. (2012). The involvement of the cd40-cd40l pathway in activated platelet-induced changes in huvec cox-2 and pparα expression. *Inflammation* 35, 1184–1190. doi: 10.1007/s10753-011- 9427-0
107. Xu, Z., Feng, W., Shen, Q., Yu, N., Yu, K., Wang, S., et al. (2017). Rhizoma coptidis and berberine as a natural drug to combat aging and aging-related diseases via anti-oxidation and ampk activation. *Aging Dis.* 8, 760–777. doi: 10.14336/AD.2016.0620
108. Xue, M., Yang, M. X., Zhang, W., Li, X. M., Gao, D. H., Ou, Z. M., et al. (2013). Characterization, pharmacokinetics, and hypoglycemic effect of berberine loaded solid lipid nanoparticles. *Int. J. Nanomed.* 8(Issue 1), 4677–4687. doi: 10.2147/IJN.S51262
109. Yakata, Y., Nakayama, T., Yoshizaki, A., Kusaba, T., and Sekine, I. (2007). Expression of p-stat3 in human gastric carcinoma: significant correlation in tumour invasion and prognosis. *Int. J. Oncol.* 30, 437–442. doi: 10.3892/ijo.30. 2.437
110. Yamada, K., Mizukoshi, E., Sunagozaka, H., Arai, K., Yamashita, T., Takeshita, Y., et al. (2015). Response to importance of confounding factors in assessing fatty acid compositions in patients with non-alcoholic steatohepatitis. *Liver Int.* 35, 1773–1773. doi: 10.1111/liv.12755
111. Yan, L., Yang, X., and Davidson, N. E. (2001). Role of dna methylation and histone acetylation in steroid receptor expression in breast cancer. *J. Mamm. Gland Biol. Neoplasia* 6, 183–192. doi: 10.1023/a:1011308707512
112. Yan, X. T., Zhao, Y., and Cheng, X. L. (2018). Inhibition of mir-200b/mir-429 contributes to neuropathic pain development through targeting zinc finger e box binding protein-1. *J. Cell Physiol.* 233, 4815–4824. doi: 10.1002/jcp. 26284
113. Yang, M., Yang, Y., Cui, H., Guan, Z., Yang, Y., Zhang, H., et al. (2015). The natural compound gambogic acid radiosensitizes nasopharyngeal carcinoma cells under hypoxic conditions. *Tumori* 102:135. doi: 10.5301/tj.500 0411
114. Zhang, J., Lai, Z., Huang, W., Ling, H., Lin, M., Tang, S., et al. (2017). Apicidin inhibited proliferation and invasion and induced apoptosis via mitochondrial pathway in non-small cell lung cancer glc-82 cells. *Anti-cancer Agents Med. Chem.* 17, 1374–1382. doi: 10.2174/1871520617666170419120044
115. Zhang, J., Yi, T., Liu, J., Zhao, Z., and Chen, H. (2013). Quercetin induces apoptosis via the mitochondrial pathway in kb and kbv200 cells. *J. Agric. Food Chem.* 61, 2188–2195. doi: 10.1021/jf305263r
116. Zhang, J., Zhang, H., and Zi, T. (2015). Overexpression of microrna-141 relieves chronic constriction injury-induced neuropathic pain via targeting high-mobility group box 1. *Int. J. Mol. Med.* 36:1433. doi: 10.3892/ijmm.2015.2342
117. Zhang, J. Y., Huang, W. J., Sun, H. M., Liu, Y., Zhao, X. Q., Tang, S. L., et al. (2017). Structure identification and in vitro anticancer activity of lathyrol-3-phenylacetate-5,15-diacetate. *Molecules* 22:1412. doi: 10.3390/molecules22091412
118. Zhang, J. Y., Lin, M. T., Tung, H. Y., Tang, S. L., Yi, T., Zhang, Y. Z., et al. (2016). Bruceine d induces apoptosis in human chronic myeloid leukemia k562 cells via mitochondrial pathway. *Am. J. Cancer Res.* 6:819.
119. Zhang, J. Y., Lin, M. T., Zhou, M. J., Yi, T., Tang, Y. N., Tang, S. L., et al. (2015). Combinational treatment of curcumin and quercetin against gastric cancer mgc-803 cells in vitro. *Molecules* 20, 11524–11534. doi: 10.3390/molecules200611524
120. Zhang, L., Fang, Y., Xu, X. F., and Jin, D. Y. (2017). Moscatilin induces apoptosis of pancreatic cancer cells via reactive oxygen species and the jnk/sapk pathway. *Mol. Med. Rep.* 15, 1195–1203. doi: 10.3892/mmr.2017.6144
121. Zhang, L., Wang, Y., Wang, L., Yin, G., Li, W., Xian, Y., et al. (2018). miR-23c suppresses tumor growth of human hepatocellular carcinoma by attenuating ERBB2IP. *Biomed. Pharmacother.* 107, 424–432. doi: 10.1016/j.biopha.2018.07.155
122. Zhang, S., Chang, M., Zhou, Z., Dai, X., and Xu, Z. (2018). Pdhs-elm: computational predictor for plant dnase i hypersensitive sites based on extreme

learning machines. *Mol. Genet. Genomics* 293, 1035–1049. doi: 10.1007/s00438-018-1436-3

123. Zhang, X. Z., Wang, L., Liu, D. W., Tang, G. Y., Zhang, H. Y., et al. (2014). Synergistic inhibitory effect of berberine and d-limonene on human gastric carcinoma cell line MGC803. *J. Med. Food* 17, 955–962. doi: 10.1089/jmf.2013.2967

124. Zhao, Y., Gao, J. L., Ji, J. W., Gao, M., Yin, Q. S., Qiu, Q. L., et al. (2014).

125. Cytotoxicity enhancement in MDA-MB-231 cells by the combination treatment of tetrahydropalmatine and berberine derived from *Corydalis yanhusuo* WT Wang. *J. Int. Ethnopharmacol.* 3:68. doi: 10.5455/jice.20140123040224

126. Zhao, Y., Jing, Z., Li, Y., and Mao, W., (2016). Berberine in combination with cisplatin suppresses breast cancer cell growth through induction of dna breaks and caspase-3-dependent apoptosis. *Oncol. Rep.* 36, 567–572. doi: 10.3892/or.2016.4785

127. Zheng, F., Wu, J., Tang, Q., Xiao, Q., Wu, W., Hann, S. S., et al. (2018). The enhancement of combination of berberine and metformin in inhibition of DNMT1 gene expression through interplay of SP1 and PDPK1. *J. Cell Mol. Med.* 22, 600–612. doi: 10.1111/jcmm.13347

128. Zhu, T., Li, L. L., Xiao, G. F., Luo, Q. Z., Liu, Q. Z., Yao, K. T., et al. (2015). Berberine increases doxorubicin sensitivity by suppressing stat3 in lung cancer. *Am. J. Chin. Med.* 43, 1487–1502. doi: 10.1142/S0192415X15500846

2

The CXCL8-CXCR1/2 Axis as a Therapeutic Target in Breast Cancer Stem-Like Cells

*Pier Adelchi Ruffini**

Research and Development Department, Dompé farmaceutici S.p.A., Milan, Italy

Correspondence:
Pier Adelchi Ruffini
pieradelchi.ruffini@dompe.com

Cancer stem-like cells (CSC) have been targeted by different strategies over the last decade. This mini review focuses on preclinical and clinical results obtained by interfering with chemokine receptors CXCR1 and CXCR2 in breast cancer. This strategy is currently being tested in a randomized, double blind phase 2 clinical trial.

Keywords: CXCR1, CXCL8, cancer stem-like cells, reparixin, breast cancer

Cancer stem-like cells (CSC) have been the focus of several clinical investigations testing different strategies for a more effective anticancer treatment through inhibition of this unique cell population (1). Targeting the CXCL8-CXCR1/2 axis is one such strategy that has moved from preclinical models to an ongoing randomized phase 2 clinical trial in breast cancer.

CXCL8 (formerly IL-8) is a chemokine whose biological effects are mediated by two G-protein-coupled receptors: **CXCR1** and **CXCR2** (2). CXCL8 has been reported to play multiple roles in cancer, such as increasing proliferation, angiogenesis, invasion, and metastases (3). In **breast cancer**, recent evidence points to this chemokine as a key regulator of CSC activity (4).

PRECLINICAL EVIDENCE IN BREAST CANCER

In breast cancer, tumor cells capable of forming tumors in immunocompromised mice (i.e., CSC by a functional definition) are identified by the expression of either the enzyme aldehyde dehydrogenase (ALDH) (5) and/or the $CD24^{-}/CD44^{+}$ phenotype (6), representing two largely non-overlapping cell populations. CXCR1 was identified as a druggable target on breast cancer CSC identified by the expression of ALDH, while its expression was almost undetectable on bulk (i.e., non-CSC) tumor cells (7). In keeping, breast cancer CSC were shown to proliferate *in vitro* in response to the addition of exogenous CXCL8 while a small molecular weight antagonist of CXCR1/2 (**reparixin**) (8) or a blocking anti-CXCR1 (but not anti-CXCR2) monoclonal antibody were both able to deplete CSC *in vitro* (9). A FAS-FASL mediated bystander effect killed the vast majority of bulk tumor cells *in vitro*, suggesting the possibility of synergistic effects with chemotherapy (9). In human breast cancer cell lines or breast cancer patient-derived xenografts orthotopically implanted in mice, the combination of weekly docetaxel and reparixin for 4 weeks was more effective than either treatment alone in reducing tumor size (9). However, in tumors recovered from mice that had been treated with reparixin, either alone or in combination with chemotherapy, CSC proportion was far lower than in tumors recovered from mice receiving chemotherapy alone (9). These results were framed in a model where, following administration of chemotherapy, CXCL8 and FASL are released by dying bulk tumor cells. Engagement of CXCR1 on the surface of CSC by CXCL8 shelters CSC from apoptotic signals delivered by FASL. To the contrary, when CXCR1 signaling on CSC is blocked by reparixin these cells undergo FASL-mediated apoptosis. Evidence provided later by independent laboratories supports this model. First, as originally reported by Ginestier and coworkers, tumor cells exposed to taxane *in vitro* release CXCL8 (10). Also, Triple-Negative Breast Cancer (TNBC) tumor cells recovered from immunocompromised mice following two doses of paclitaxel displayed a marked and dose-dependent increase in mammosphere forming efficiency as compared with untreated mice (10). Furthermore, and again in line with the original report by Ginestier, administration of a CXCR1 inhibitor reduced CSC percentage *in vitro*. Consistent findings were later reported by an independent group (11). Second, in breast cancer patients with pleural effusions and/or ascites CXCL8 levels were measured and tumor cells recovered and cultured *in vitro* (4). A direct correlation was observed between CXCL8 levels and CSC activity by means of mammosphere formation (4). Surface CXCR1 was detected on the majority of mammosphere cells, and the effects of exogenous CXCL8 on mammosphere formation were blocked by a CXCR1/2 inhibitor, SCH563705 (4).

The relative contribution of CXCR1 inhibition and paclitaxel in this model were further investigated in CSC-enriched mammospheres from the human TNBC cell line MDA-MB231. The combination treatment displayed a synergistic effect on mammosphere number and an additive effect on mammosphere volume as compared with either treatment alone (12). Different than paclitaxel, which increased the number of dead cells, reparixin increased the number of non-proliferating cells, and the combination treatment exerted both effects (12). In keeping with previous reports (9), also in MDA-MB231-derived tumorspheres reparixin activity was mediated by inhibition of the FAK/AKT pathway which is unaffected by paclitaxel. When the effects on cell cycle were investigated, a shift of tumor cells in S phase or a block in G2 phase were observed upon paclitaxel and combination treatment, respectively. In keeping, cyclin B1, which is responsible for the cell cycle progression from G2 to S phase, was also inhibited by the combination treatment (12). Furthermore, paclitaxel + reparixin treatment induced "cell senescence by decreasing PI3K-Akt activation paralleled by a decrease of the cytosolic p-FOXO3A (inactive) and by an increase of p27" (12). The effects on cell cycle, cyclin B1 and p-FAK levels recorded upon exposure to reparixin were reproduced using neutralizing anti-CXCR1 and anti-CXCL8 monoclonal antibodies, thus providing indirect evidence of the ability of reparixin to downregulate CXCL8-CXCR1signaling pathway (12).

Another set of experiments aimed at testing the hypothesis that inhibition of CSC would reduce metastatic spread. First, it was shown that reparixin administration reduced metastasis formation in mice following injection of luciferase-transfected human breast cancer cells into the bloodstream (9). Second, the suppressive activity of CXCR1 inhibition on the metastatic process was tested in a mouse model of brain metastases by the TNBC cell line MDA-MB231. In the absence of brain metastases, reparixin does not cross the blood brain barrier (BBB). However, in the presence of brain metastases and an allegedly damaged BBB, reparixin can be found in the central nervous system (12). When treatment was started on the same day when tumor cells were injected, a significant decrease of both the number and the volume of brain metastases was observed following single agent (i.e., reparixin or paclitaxel) as well as the combination treatment. When treatment was started at day 7 following tumor cell injection and continued until day 21, a significant reduction of the number of brain metastases was observed only following combination treatment, which also showed a trend toward an inhibitory effect on metastases volume (12).

PRECLINICAL EVIDENCE IN TUMORS OTHER THAN BREAST CANCER

Anti-tumor and anti CSC activity of reparixin has been demonstrated in human epithelial thyroid cancer *in vitro* and *in vivo* (13). Reparixin ability to inhibit stemness (evaluated by stemness marker expression and tumorsphere formation) and epithelial-mesenchymal transition (EMT) (evaluated at both the biochemical and functional level) of thyroid cancer was shown to be dependent, different than in breast cancer (9), on its activity on both CXCR1 and CXCR2 (13).

In malignant melanoma, CXCR1/2 inhibition reduced the percentage of ALDH+ cells in human tumors growing in nude athymic mice (14).

In pancreatic cancer (15) a positive correlation was found between CXCR1 and both CD44 and CD133 stemness marker expression. Exogenous CXCL8 added to pancreatic cancer cells *in vitro* increased their invasion ability, tumorsphere formation, and CSC population and addition of a CXCR1-blocking monoclonal antibody was able to revert all these effects (15).

CLINICAL TRIALS IN BREAST CANCER

In a phase Ib study (NCT02001974) (16), patients with HER-2 negative metastatic breast cancer not known to be refractory to paclitaxel who had received no more than three lines of cytotoxic chemotherapy in the metastatic setting were enrolled in cohorts of 3–6 patients to receive escalating doses of the CXCR1/2 inhibitor reparixin oral tablets three times per day (t.i.d.) from day 1 to 21 in combination with a fixed dose of weekly paclitaxel (80 mg/m^2) on days 1, 8, and 15 of a 28-days cycle, for as long as clinical benefit was observed. Primary objectives were the assessment of the safety of the combination and the pharmacokinetic (PK) profile of oral reparixin. Expansion of the highest dose cohort was foreseen to gain additional PK and safety data. Cohorts 1–3 received reparixin 400, 800, and 1,200 mg t.i.d. respectively. In cycle 1 only, patients received a 3 days course of reparixin alone (day −3 to −1) at the assigned dose for the cohort, for purpose of obtaining single agent PK data.

Thirty-three patients were enrolled in the study. Eighty-three percent of patients had visceral disease, and the majority had two or more sites of metastasis. 20/33 patients had received prior (neo)adjuvant chemotherapy, and 16 of these patients had received a taxane in the (neo)adjuvant setting. 19/33 had received chemotherapy in the metastatic setting, with 11 having one prior metastatic regimen and eight having two or more chemotherapy regimens. Thirty patients were evaluated for safety. There were no dose limiting toxicities in any cohort. Most adverse reactions (ADR) were of grade 1 (79.8%), with only 2.7% grade 3 ADR. There was no apparent dose effect of increasing reparixin dose on the incidence, severity or profile of treatment emergent adverse events (TEAE) experienced by the treatment groups, and there were no clinically significant differences between the treatment groups with regards to laboratory measurements, vital signs, ECG, and physical examination assessments. Twenty-seven patients were evaluated for antitumor activity. In total, 8/27 patients had a confirmed RECIST response. Of responding patients, all but one were from cohort 3. Median time to progression (TTP) (95% C.I.) for the 3 cohorts were 58 days (44-infinity) for cohort 1, 67 days (58–82) for cohort 2 and 162 days (60–229) for cohort 3. Remarkably, there were long term remissions among patients treated (16). In this trial, it was not possible to obtain optional serial biopsies of tumor tissue at study entry and during treatment from any patient. However, blood-based biomarkers of CSC were explored. The circulating biomarkers included Circulating Tumor Cell (CTC) enumeration, evaluation of ALDEFLUOR, and EMT transcription factors in peripheral blood, and serum cytokine measurements. Unfortunately, no clear pattern of change in any of these markers was observed. This is likely related to multiple issues, including but not limited to small sample size, low CTC number in the enrolled patient population leading to limited tumor material for testing, and high baseline heterogeneity in the measurements.

Operable breast cancer is a more suitable clinical setting to evaluate the ability of a novel agent to reduce the number of CSC following treatment, as they can be measured on readily available tumor tissue. Thus, after reviewing safety data from the second cohort of the above trial, a window-of-opportunity, pilot trial (NCT01861054) of single agent reparixin was started (17).

Patients with previously untreated HER-2 negative operable breast cancer not eligible for neo(adjuvant) treatment were divided into two cohorts, i.e., group A: histologically proven ER^+ and/or PgR^+ and group B: ER^-/PgR^- breast cancer (i.e., TNBC). This design allowed potential to identify the cohort of patients who might benefit the most from this treatment in later stage clinical trials. Oral reparixin was administered at 1,000 mg t.i.d. for 21 consecutive days before curative surgery. Core biopsies were taken at baseline (day −14 to 0) and at the completion of therapy (day 21). The primary objectives of this study were to evaluate the effects of orally administered reparixin on CSC in the primary tumor and the tumor microenvironment and to evaluate the safety of oral reparixin. Signal of activity was defined as a ≥20% reduction of CSC (defined by either the $ALDH^+$ or $CD24^-/CD44^+$ phenotype) in tumor tissue from baseline values as measured by flow cytometry accompanied by a consistent reduction of the same cell population by immunohistochemistry (IHC).

A total of 20 patients were enrolled, 18 of whom in group A. Signal of activity was detected by flow cytometry in the majority of patients (18), but the very low numbers of CSC hindered the possibility to confirm flow cytometry results by IHC. However, the later published evidence that the two breast cancer CSC populations (i.e., $ALDH^+$ and $CD24^-/CD44^+$) investigated reside in different areas of primary breast tumors and can transition from one phenotype to the other (19) might affect the reliability of CSC counts in this patient population. More in general, the clinical relevance of a ≥20% reduction of CSC following a single 21-day course of reparixin in this patient population is unknown and was beyond the scope of this trial.

From a safety standpoint, also in this trial reparixin appeared to be well-tolerated with 10/20 patients experiencing one or more ADR, all of which of grade ≤2. Neither TEAE leading to treatment discontinuation nor delays in surgery due to TEAE were recorded.

CONCLUSIONS

Evidence for a CXCL8-CXCR1/2 axis in CSC has been reported by independent laboratories and offers a potential therapeutic target. Clinical trials aimed at testing the effective targeting of CSC through this axis have been conducted in breast cancer, where the most information is available from preclinical research. Reparixin appeared to be well-tolerated, however, such trials were faced with several issues for efficacy evaluation, e.g., the very low numbers of CSC in primary operable breast cancer. To circumvent this limitation, circulating markers for monitoring the effect of anti-CSC agents were explored but these assays turned out to be inadequate.

Future prospects for CSC targeting agents include the development of reliable assays to measure stem cell number and/or activity (20) in serial biopsies from accessible tumors (e.g., window-of-opportunity trials), and alternative endpoints in clinical trials in the metastatic setting. One possible endpoint is the development of metastases at new sites (21), which can have also clinical significance (22). In keeping with preclinical findings (9, 12), it is hypothesized that an effective anti-CSC treatment will impact on development of new metastases while progression of pre-existing metastases is more consistent with proliferation of non-CSC, bulk tumor cells that should be addressed by chemotherapy.

As concerns CXCR1/2 inhibition, a randomized, placebo-controlled clinical trial (NCT02370238) of weekly paclitaxel with and without reparixin in front line treatment of metastatic TNBC has completed enrolment. Identification of clinical (e.g., disease sensitivity to chemotherapy) and/or cellular/molecular biomarkers of patients most likely to benefit from treatment represents a future direction of research, while analysis of time to new metastasis may fuel development of this strategy in the (neo)adjuvant setting, also leveraging on safety data generated in metastatic patients.

AUTHOR CONTRIBUTIONS

The author confirms being the sole contributor of this work and has approved it for publication.

ACKNOWLEDGMENTS

The author is grateful to Sonia Amicarella (Dompé farmaceutici S.p.A.) for assistance with formatting the manuscript.

REFERENCES

1. Ramos EK, Hoffmann AD, Gerson SL, Liu H. New opportunities and challenges to defeat cancer stem cells. *Trends Cancer* (2017) 3:780–96. doi: 10.1016/j.trecan.2017.08.007
2. Zlotnik A, Yoshie O. The chemokine superfamily revisited. *Immunity* (2012) 36:705–16. doi: 10.1016/j.immuni.2012.05.008
3. Waugh DJ, Wilson C. The interleukin-8 pathway in cancer. *Clin Cancer Res.* (2008) 14:6735–41. doi: 10.1158/1078-0432.ccr-07-4843
4. Singh JK, Farnie G, Bundred NJ, Simoes BM, Shergill A, Landberg G, et al. Targeting CXCR1/2 significantly reduces breast cancer stem cell activity and increases the efficacy of inhibiting HER2 via HER2-dependent and -independent mechanisms. *Clin Cancer Res.* (2013) 19:643–56. doi: 10.1158/1078-0432.ccr-12-1063
5. Ginestier C, Hur MH, Charafe-Jauffret E, Monville F, Dutcher J, Brown M, et al. ALDH1 is a marker of normal and malignant human mammary stem cells and a predictor of poor clinical outcome. *Cell Stem Cell* (2007) 1:555–67. doi: 10.1016/j.stem.2007.08.014
6. Al-Hajj M, Wicha MS, Benito-Hernandez A, Morrison SJ, Clarke MF. Prospective identification of tumorigenic breast cancer cells. *Proc Natl Acad Sci USA.* (2003) 100:3983–8. doi: 10.1073/pnas.0530291100
7. Charafe-Jauffret E, Ginestier C, Iovino F, Wicinski J, Cervera N, Finetti P, et al. Breast cancer cell lines contain functional cancer stem cells with metastatic capacity and a distinct molecular signature. *Cancer Res.* (2009) 69:1302–13. doi: 10.1158/0008-5472.can-08-2741
8. Bertini R, Allegretti M, Bizzarri C, Moriconi A, Locati M, Zampella G, et al. Noncompetitive allosteric inhibitors of the inflammatory chemokine receptors CXCR1 and CXCR2: prevention of reperfusion injury. *Proc Natl Acad Sci USA.* (2004) 101:11791–6. doi: 10.1073/pnas.0402090101
9. Ginestier C, Liu S, Diebel ME, Korkaya H, Luo M, Brown M, et al. CXCR1 blockade selectively targets human breast cancer stem cells *in vitro* and in xenografts. *J Clin Invest.* (2010) 120:485–97. doi: 10.1172/jci39397
10. Bhola NE, Balko JM, Dugger TC, Kuba MG, Sanchez V, Sanders M, et al. TGF-beta inhibition enhances chemotherapy action against triple-negative breast cancer. *J Clin Invest.* (2013) 123:1348–58. doi: 10.1172/jci65416
11. Samanta D, Gilkes DM, Chaturvedi P, Xiang L, Semenza GL. Hypoxia-inducible factors are required for chemotherapy resistance of breast cancer stem cells. *Proc Natl Acad Sci USA.* (2014) 111:E5429–38. doi: 10.1073/pnas.1421438111
12. Brandolini L, Cristiano L, Fidoamore A, De Pizzol M, Di Giacomo E, Florio TM, et al. Targeting CXCR1 on breast cancer stem cells: signaling pathways and clinical application modelling. *Oncotarget* (2015) 6:43375–94. doi: 10.18632/oncotarget.6234
13. Liotti F, De Pizzol M, Allegretti M, Prevete N, Melillo RM. Multiple anti-tumor effects of Reparixin on thyroid cancer. *Oncotarget* (2017) 8:35946–61. doi: 10.18632/oncotarget.16412
14. Kemp DM, Pidich A, Larijani M, Jonas R, Lash E, Sato T, et al. Ladarixin, a dual CXCR1/2 inhibitor, attenuates experimental melanomas harboring different molecular defects by affecting malignant cells and tumor microenvironment. *Oncotarget* (2017) 8:14428–42. doi: 10.18632/oncotarget.14803
15. Chen L, Fan J, Chen H, Meng Z, Chen Z, Wang P, et al. The IL-8/CXCR1 axis is associated with cancer stem cell-like properties and correlates with clinical prognosis in human pancreatic cancer cases. *Sci Rep.* (2014) 4:5911. doi: 10.1038/srep05911
16. Schott AF, Goldstein LJ, Cristofanilli M, Ruffini PA, McCanna S, Reuben JM, et al. Phase Ib pilot study to evaluate reparixin in combination with weekly paclitaxel in patients with HER-2-negative metastatic breast cancer. *Clin Cancer Res.* (2017) 23:5358–65. doi: 10.1158/1078-0432.ccr-16-2748
17. Goldstein L, Sparano J, Perez R, Vito C, Reuben J, Landis M, et al. Abstract OT2-6-03: a single arm, preoperative, pilot study to evaluate the safety and biological effects of orally administered reparixin in early breast cancer patients who are candidates for surgery. *Cancer Res.* (2013) 73(24 Suppl.):OT2-6-03-OT02-06-03. doi: 10.1158/0008-5472.sabcs13-ot2-6-03
18. Goldstein LJ, Perez RP, Yardley DA, Han LK, Reuben JM, McCanna S, et al. Abstract CT057: a single-arm, preoperative, pilot study to evaluate the safety and biological effects of orally administered reparixin in early breast cancer patients who are candidates for surgery. *Cancer Res.* (2016) 76(14 Suppl.):CT057-CT057. doi: 10.1158/1538-7445.am2016-ct057
19. Liu S, Cong Y, Wang D, Sun Y, Deng L, Liu Y, et al. Breast cancer stem cells transition between epithelial and mesenchymal states reflective of their normal counterparts. *Stem Cell Rep.* (2014) 2:78–91. doi: 10.1016/j.stemcr.2013.11.009
20. Saygin C, Matei D, Majeti R, Reizes O, Lathia JD. Targeting cancer stemness in the clinic: from hype to hope. *Cell Stem Cell* (2019) 24:25–40. doi: 10.1016/j.stem.2018.11.017
21. Giuliano M, Giordano A, Jackson S, De Giorgi U, Mego M, Cohen EN, et al. Circulating tumor cells as early predictors of metastatic spread in breast cancer patients with limited metastatic dissemination. *Breast Cancer Res.* (2014) 16:440. doi: 10.1186/s13058-014-0440-8
22. Twelves C, Cortes J, Kaufman PA, Yelle L, Awada A, Binder TA, et al. "New" metastases are associated with a poorer prognosis than growth of pre-existing metastases in patients with metastatic breast cancer treated with chemotherapy. *Breast Cancer Res.* (2015) 17:150. doi: 10.1186/s13058-015-0657-1

3

MiR-1-3p Inhibits Lung Adenocarcinoma Cell Tumorigenesis via Targeting Protein Regulator of Cytokinesis 1

*Tao Li, Xiuxiu Wang, Lijun Jing and Yu Li**

Department of Respiratory Diseases, Qilu Hospital of Shandong University, Jinan, China

***Correspondence:**
Yu Li
qlliyures@163.com

Lung adenocarcinoma (LUAD) is one of the most lethal malignancies, posing a threat to human health. However, the molecular mechanisms underlying LUAD development remain largely unknown. In this study, we found that miR-1-3p was significantly downregulated in human LUAD tissues and cell lines and played an inhibitory role in LUAD cell tumorigenesis, as evidenced by the significantly reduced viability, migration, and invasion of LUAD cells in response to miR-1-3p overexpression. Mechanistically, microRNA (miR)-1-3p physically interacted with the 3′-untranslated region (UTR) of protein regulator of cytokinesis 1 (PRC1) mRNA, leading to downregulation of PRC1. Overexpression of PRC1 reversed the inhibitory effects of miR-1-3p on LUAD cell tumorigenesis, suggesting that the miR-1-3p/PRC1 axis is majorly involved in suppressing LUAD development and progression. Consistently, PRC1 was dramatically induced in LUAD tissues and cell lines as well as associated with a poor prognosis in LUAD patients. Taken together, our study identified the miR-1-3p/PRC1 axis as an important regulatory mechanism contributing to LUAD inhibition and provided valuable clues for the future development of therapeutic strategies against LUAD.

Keywords: lung adenocarcinoma, miR-1-3p, protein regulator of cytokinesis 1, malignant behavior, mechanism

INTRODUCTION

Lung adenocarcinoma (LUAD) is the most common subtype of non-small cell lung cancer (NSCLC), accounting for 80–85% of all lung cancers; worldwide, approximately 40% of all lung cancer patients are diagnosed with LUAD (1). Compared to other subtypes of NSCLC, LUAD has a higher incidence and a shorter survival time among patients, with a 5-year survival rate as low as 10–15% (2, 3); thus, LUAD poses a serious threat to human health. Currently, chemotherapy is a relatively effective therapeutic option for NSCLC (4). However, the existence and development of intrinsic or acquired chemoresistance greatly limit the application of chemotherapy in cancer treatment. Therefore, there is still an urgent need to develop novel therapeutic strategies against LUAD that are based on the mechanisms underlying the development and progression of LUAD.

MicroRNAs (miRNAs) are a class of small endogenous non-coding RNA molecules (~22 nucleotides) found in animals and plants that are responsible for the degradation or translation repression of mRNAs by binding to the 3′-untranslated region (UTR) of target mRNAs (5). A variety of miRNAs have been identified as novel biomarkers or promising therapeutic targets of human malignant tumors. Among them, miR-1-3p plays an antitumor role in multiple cancer types, including rhabdomyosarcoma as well as lung, thyroid, prostatic, bladder, colorectal, and hepatocellular carcinomas (6–11). However, the role of miR-1-3p in LUAD has not yet been investigated. In addition, the association between miR-1-3p and its target genes may deepen our understanding of the molecular mechanisms contributing to LUAD development, thus facilitating the discovery of improved therapies for LUAD.

The microtubule-associated protein regulator of cytokinesis 1 (PRC1) has been found to be majorly involved in the organization of antiparallel microtubules in the central spindle during cytokinesis. The human PRC1 gene, located on chromosome 15q26.1, encodes a 620-amino-acid protein with a molecular weight of 71 kDa (3). An abnormally high expression of PRC1 has been observed in breast cancer (12), bladder cancer (13), hepatocellular carcinoma (14), and pancreatic cancer (15), which suggests a promotive role of PRC1 in tumorigenesis. However, it remains largely unknown whether there is a functional association between miR-1-3p and the regulation of PRC1 in LUAD. In this study, we examined the role of miR-1-3p in LUAD growth and metastasis as well as the underlying mechanism.

MATERIALS AND METHODS

Tissue Samples From LUAD Patients

Human LUAD tissues were collected from LUAD patients undergoing pulmonary resection or bronchoscopy biopsy, and normal tissues adjacent to cancer were collected from LUAD patients undergoing pulmonary resection at Qilu Hospital between May and September 2018. None of the patients had received chemotherapy or radiotherapy prior to surgery. All the fresh samples were stored in RNAlater Stabilization Solution (Ambion) at −80°C until use. This study was approved by the Ethics Committee of Shandong University, and written informed consent was obtained from all patients prior to enrollment in the present study. The clinicopathological characteristics of the patients are shown in **Supplementary Table 1**.

Cell Culture

Three LUAD cell lines (A549, H1299, and H1975 cells) and a human alveolar epithelial cell line (HPAEpiC) were purchased from the Cell Bank of the Type Culture Collection of the Chinese Academy of Sciences (Shanghai, China). The cells were maintained in RPMI 1640 medium (Gibco, USA) containing 10% fetal bovine serum (Gibco, USA), 100 U/mL penicillin, and 100 μg/mL streptomycin in a humidified atmosphere of 5% CO_2 at 37°C. Cells in the exponential phase of growth were used for the following experiments.

Construction of the miR-1-3p Overexpression Cell Lines

The pre-miR-1-3p sequences were synthesized by Biosune Biotechnology Company (Shanghai, China) and cloned into the lentiviral vector pGIPZ. Lentivirus was produced in HEK293T cells using the packaging vectors psPAX2 and pMD2.G. The cells were infected with lentivirus for 24 h and then cultured for 1 week in medium containing 2 μg/mL puromycin (Merck Millipore, USA) for screening to acquire cells with stable expression of miR-1-3p.

Transient Transfection

The miR-1-3p mimic and its negative control (NC) were chemically synthesized by GenePharma Co., Ltd. (Shanghai, China). The cells were transiently transfected with 50 nM miR-1-3p mimic or 50 nM NC (Boshang, Inc., China) using Lipofectamine 2000 (Invitrogen; Thermo Fisher Scientific, Inc.), according to the manufacturer's protocol. The cells were harvested at 24 or 48 h after the transfection. The NC was a scrambled oligonucleotide that does not encode any known miRNA. The transfection efficiency was confirmed by detecting the miR-1-3p expression level using the SYBR green (Takara)-based real-time quantitative polymerase chain reaction (qPCR) system.

RNA Isolation and qPCR

Total RNA was extracted from the cells using Trizol reagents (Invitrogen; Thermo Fisher Scientific, Inc.), according to the manufacturer's instructions. The cDNA of miRNA was synthesized with the One Step PrimeScript miRNA cDNA Synthesis Kit (Takara Biotechnology, Co., Ltd., Dalian, China). qPCR was performed using the SYBR green Premix Ex Taq II (Takara Biotechnology, Co., Ltd.) with the Step One Plus Real-Time PCR System (Applied Biosystems; Thermo Fisher Scientific, Inc.). The expression of U6 was used as an internal control. The primers for miR-1-3p are indicated in **Supplementary Table 2**.

Western Blot Analysis

The cells were lysed in ice-cold RIPA lysis buffer, and the cell lysates were obtained by centrifugation at 12,000 rpm and 4°C for 10 min. The protein concentration was determined using the bicinchoninic acid method. The protein samples (5–10 μg) were separated by sodium dodecyl sulfate–polyacrylamide gel electrophoresis, followed by transfer to polyvinylidene difluoride membranes, and then immunoblotted with the indicated antibodies. After blocking with 5% nonfat milk, the membranes were incubated with the respective primary antibody overnight at 4°C, followed by incubation with the horseradish peroxidase-coupled secondary antibody for 1 h at room temperature. The protein bands were visualized using enhanced chemiluminescence reagents (PerkinElmer) with an ImageQuant LAS 4000 system (GE Healthcare Life Sciences). The following antibodies were used: anti-PRC1, anti-fibronectin, anti-N-cadherin, anti-vimentin, and anti-β-actin (Cell Signaling Technology).

3-(4,5-Dimethylthiazol-2-yl)-2,5-Diphenyltetrazolium Bromide (MTT) Assay

The cells were seeded into 96-well plates at a density of 2,000 cells/well and grown for 5 days. After the addition of 100 μL of 5 mg/mL MTT solution, the cells were incubated for an additional 4 h at 37°C, and then the supernatant was removed and dissolved in 100 μL of dimethyl sulfoxide (Sigma-Aldrich).

Cell viability was assessed on the 1st, 2nd, 3rd, 4th, and 5th day. The absorbance of each well was measured in triplicate using an iMark Microplate Absorbance Reader (Bio-Rad).

Luciferase Reporter Assay

Luciferase reporter constructs containing wild-type (WT) or mutant PRC1 3′-UTR (pmirGLO-PRC1-WT or pmirGLO-PRC1-mut, respectively) were generated by GenePharma Inc. (Shanghai, China). The cells were cotransfected with 25 ng of PRC1 3′-UTR reporter constructs and 20 nM miR-1-3p mimic using Lipofectamine 2,000 (Invitrogen) in 24-well plates. At 24 h after transfection, luciferase assays were performed using the Dual-Luciferase reporter assay system (Promega). *Renilla* luciferase activity was used to normalize the luciferase activity of the PRC1 3′-UTR reporter constructs.

In vivo Tumorigenicity Assays

Four-week-old male BALB/c nude mice were purchased from the Shanghai Laboratory Animal Center of the Chinese Academy of Sciences (Shanghai, China). The mice were randomly divided into two groups and injected subcutaneously with A549 cells (2×10^6 cells/mouse, $n = 5$ mice/group) that were infected with either control lentivirus or miR-1-3p-overexpressing lentivirus. Tumor growth was monitored by measuring the tumor diameter. Tumor

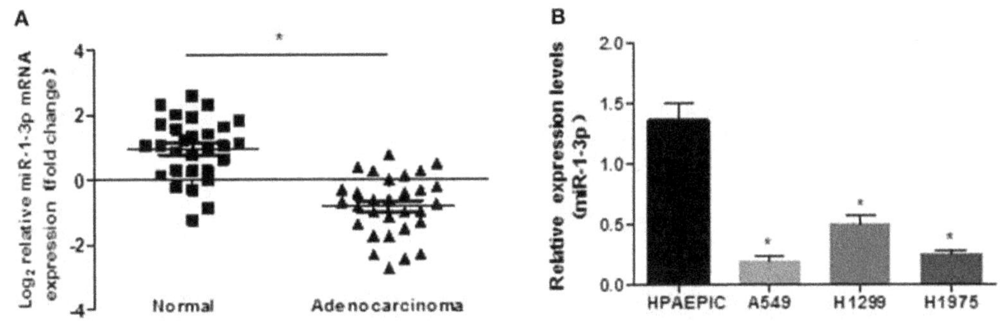

FIGURE 1 | Expression pattern of miR-1-3p in human LUAD tissues and cell lines. qPCR was performed to determine the expression levels of miR-1-3p in human LUAD tissues **(A)** and cell lines **(B)**, as indicated. $^*P < 0.05$ in **(A)** ($n = 30$); $^*P < 0.05$ vs. HPAEpiCs in **(B)** ($n = 3$).

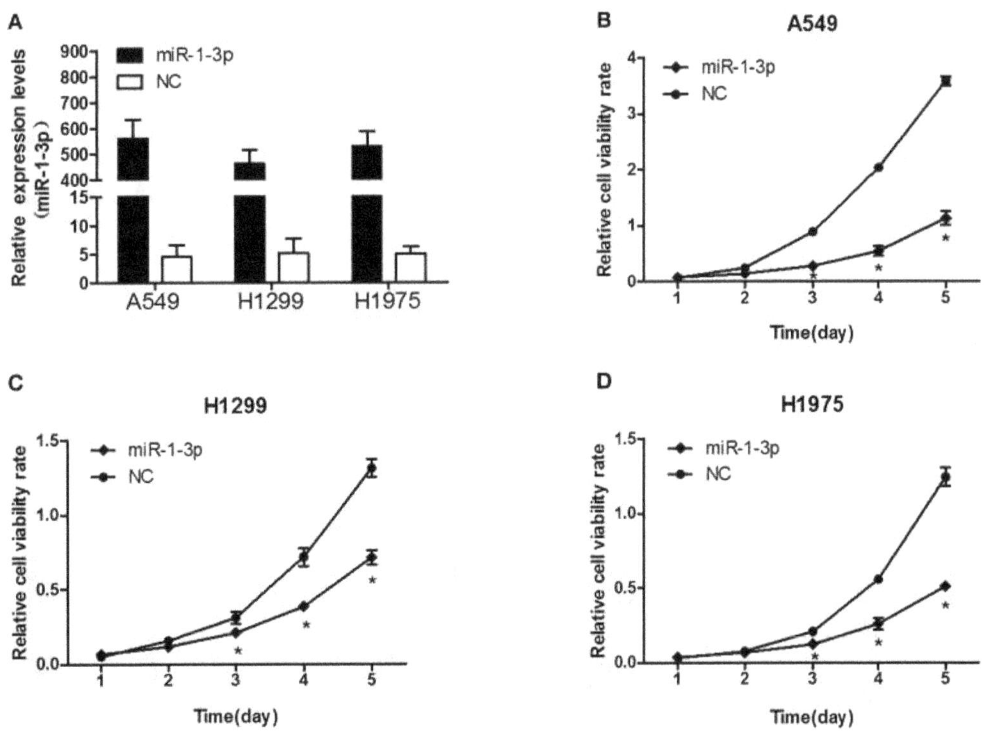

FIGURE 2 | The effect of miR-1-3p overexpression on LUAD cell viability. **(A)** qPCR was performed to validate the overexpression efficiency of miR-1-3p in A549, H1299, and H1975 cells. **(B–D)** The MTT assay was performed to measure the viability of miR-1-3p-overexpressing A549, H1299, and H1975 cells. $^*P < 0.05$ vs. the corresponding negative control (NC) groups ($n = 3$).

volume was calculated according to the formula TV (cm^3) = a × b^2 × π/6, where a is the longest diameter and b is the shortest diameter. The mice were sacrificed after 3 weeks, and then the tumors were excised and weighed. All animal experiments were approved by the Shandong University Animal Care and Use Committee.

Bioinformatics Analyses

PRC1 genetic alterations and copy number variation in LUAD were retrieved from the cBioPortal for Cancer Genomics (http://www.cbioportal.org/) (16, 17). The Cancer Genome Atlas RNA expression data of LUAD tissues were processed and analyzed by the Cancer Genomics Browser (https://xena.ucsc.edu/welcome-to-ucsc-xena/) (18). The PRC1 expression levels and copy number variation were analyzed by Proteinatlas (https://www.proteinatlas.org/), Oncomine (www.oncomine.org) (19), and Gene Expression Profiling Interactive Analysis (http://gepia.cancer-pku.cn/) in LUAD and normal lung tissues via immunohistochemistry. Kaplan–Meier plots (http://kmplot.com/analysis/) (20) were used to analyze the overall survival of the LUAD patients.

Statistical Analysis

Statistical analysis was performed using GraphPad Prism 6.0 (GraphPad Software, La Jolla, CA, USA). Data are expressed as the mean ± standard deviation. Comparison between two groups was performed using the Student's *t*-test or the Mann-Whitney *U*-test. The correlation between the expression levels of miR-1 and PRC1 was analyzed using Pearson's correlation analysis. LUAD tissues with lower miR-1 and PRC1 expression than the median expression were assigned to the low-expression group, whereas those with higher miR-1 and PRC1 expression than the median expression were assigned to the high-expression group. Associations between the clinicopathological features and the expression levels of miR-1 and PRC1 were analyzed using the χ^2 test. Overall survival curves were determined according to the Kaplan–Meier method. A $p < 0.05$ was considered statistically significant.

RESULTS

MiR-1-3p Is Downregulated in Human LUAD Tissues and Cell Lines

To investigate the possible role of miR-1-3p in LUAD development, we first examined the expression levels of miR-1-3p in human LUAD tissues and cell lines. As shown in **Figure 1A**, miR-1-3p expression was significantly decreased in LUAD tissues, compared with the matched adjacent normal lung tissues. Similarly, marked downregulation of miR-1-3p was also observed in the human LUAD cell lines A549, H1299, and H1975,

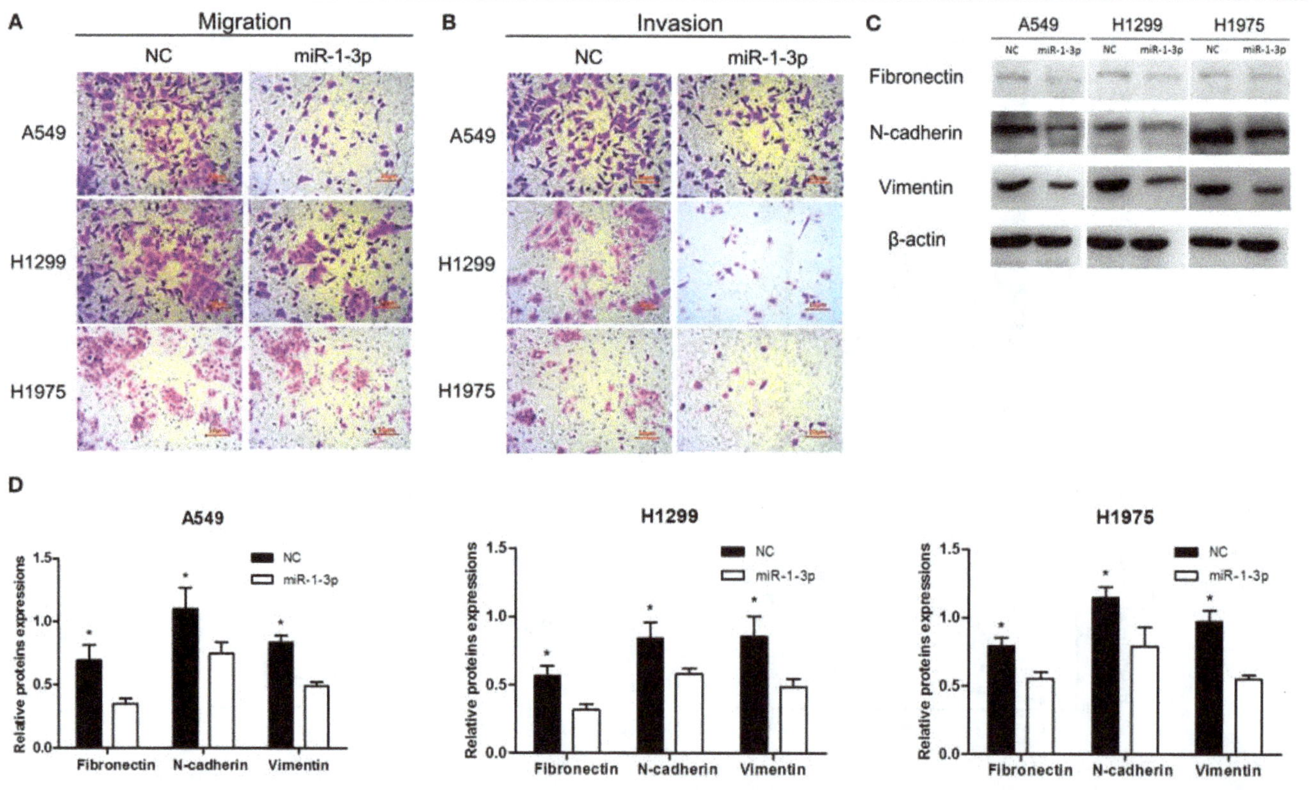

FIGURE 3 | The effect of miR-1-3p overexpression on LUAD cell migration and invasion as well as epithelial-mesenchymal transition. Transwell assays for migration **(A)** and invasion **(B)** of miR-1-3p-overexpressing LUAD cells. **(C)** Western blot assay for the expression of the indicated mesenchymal markers. β-Actin was used as an internal control. **(D)** Quantification of the western blot assay results shown in **(C)**. *$P < 0.05$ vs. miR-1-3p groups in **(C)** ($n = 3$).

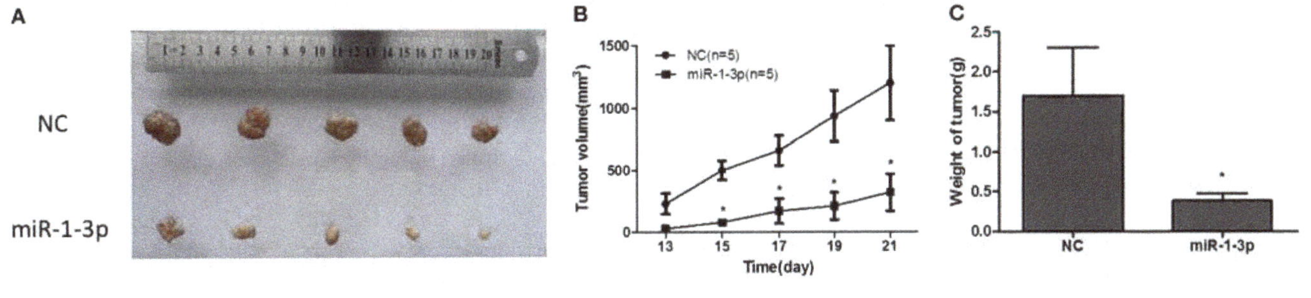

FIGURE 4 | The effect of miR-1-3p overexpression on tumorigenesis *in vivo*. **(A)** Overexpression of miR-1-3p reduced LUAD cell-derived tumor growth in a xenograft model. **(B)** Summary of the tumor growth data; the error bars indicate the standard deviation. **(C)** miR-1-3p overexpression results in a decline of tumor weight. $^*P < 0.05$.

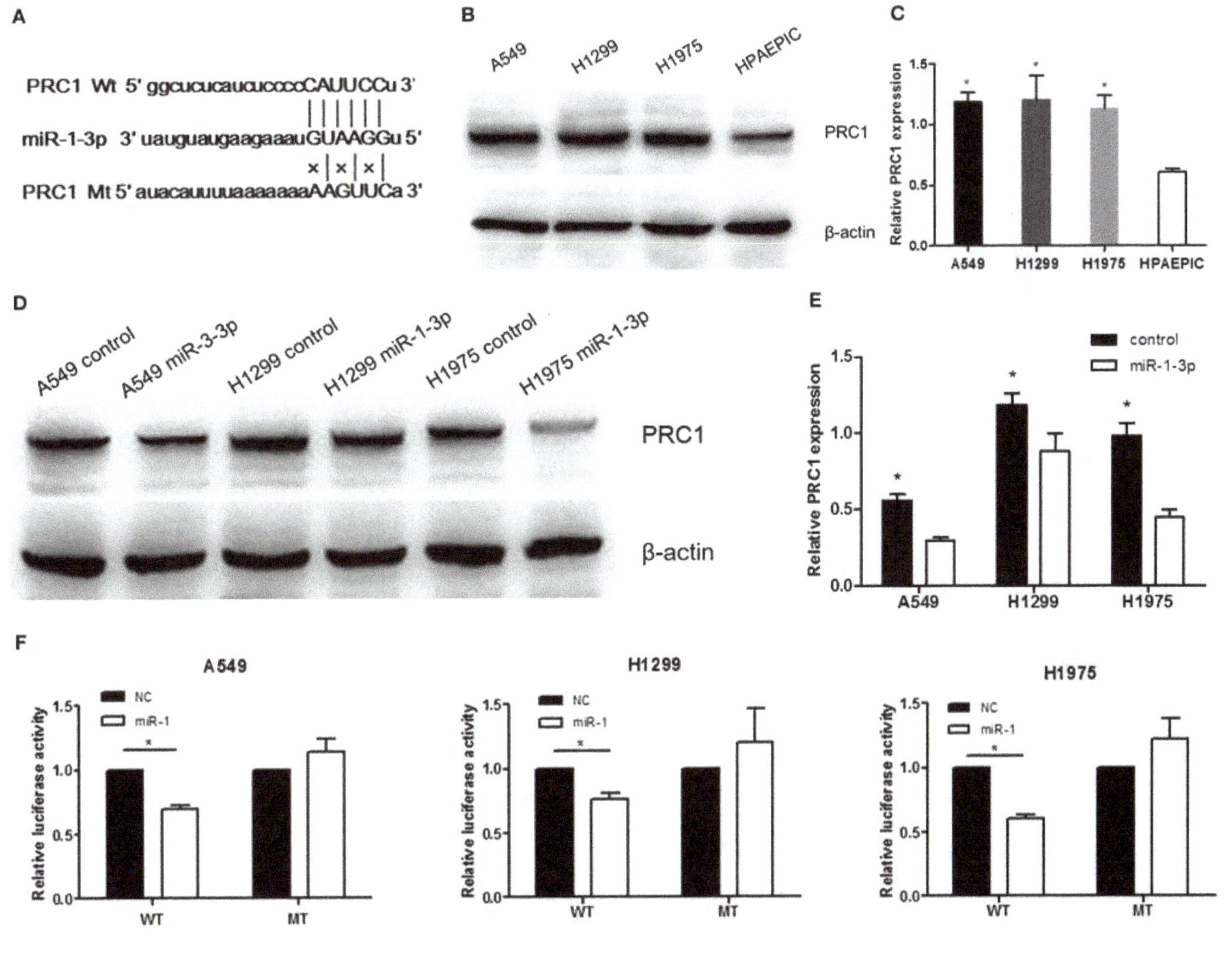

FIGURE 5 | PRC1 is a direct target of miR-1-3p in LUAD cells. **(A)** The putative miR-1-3p-binding sites in PRC1 3′-UTR and the mutated binding sites are shown. **(B,D)** Western blot analysis of PRC1 expression in the nontransfected negative control (NC)- or miR-1-3p-transfected LUAD cells. β-Actin was used as an internal control. **(C)** Quantification of the western blot assay results shown in **(B)**. $^*P < 0.05$ vs. HPAEpiCs ($n = 3$). **(E)** Quantification of the western blot assay results shown in **(D)**. $^*P < 0.05$ vs. the miR-1-3p groups ($n = 3$). **(F)** Luciferase reporter assay for LUAD cells transfected with wild-type (WT) or mutated (MT) pGL3-3′-UTR. The luciferase activity was normalized to *Renilla* luciferase activity. $^*P < 0.05$ ($n = 3$).

compared with the normal HPAEpiCs (**Figure 1B**). These *in vivo* and *in vitro* results suggest that miR-1-3p may play an inhibitory role in LUAD development.

Overexpression of miR-1-3p Suppresses LUAD Cell Viability *in vitro*

Next, we sought to investigate whether miR-1-3p indeed plays a role in suppressing LUAD development using a gain-of-function assay. As shown in **Figure 2A**, transfection of the miR-1-3p mimic led to a dramatic increase in miR-1-3p expression in the LUAD cell lines A549, H1299, and H1975. Importantly, overexpression of miR-1-3p significantly inhibited the viability of these three cell lines in a time-dependent manner, compared with the NC groups (**Figures 2B–D**). These results demonstrate that miR-1-3p is sufficient to suppress LUAD cell growth *in vitro*.

Overexpression of miR-1-3p Inhibits LUAD Cell Migration and Invasion *in vitro*

To further investigate whether miR-1-3p inhibits LUAD progression, Transwell assays were performed to examine the effects of miR-1-3p overexpression on LUAD cell migration and invasion. As shown in **Figures 3A,B**, overexpression of miR-1-3p resulted in a significant decrease in LUAD cell migration and invasion abilities, compared with the NC groups. Consistently, overexpression of miR-1-3p markedly suppressed epithelial-mesenchymal transition (EMT), a process contributing to tumor metastasis, as evidenced by downregulation of the mesenchymal markers fibronectin, N-cadherin, and vimentin (**Figures 3C,D**). These data suggest that miR-1-3p overexpression may suppress LUAD progression through reducing LUAD cell migration and invasion as well as inhibiting EMT in these cells.

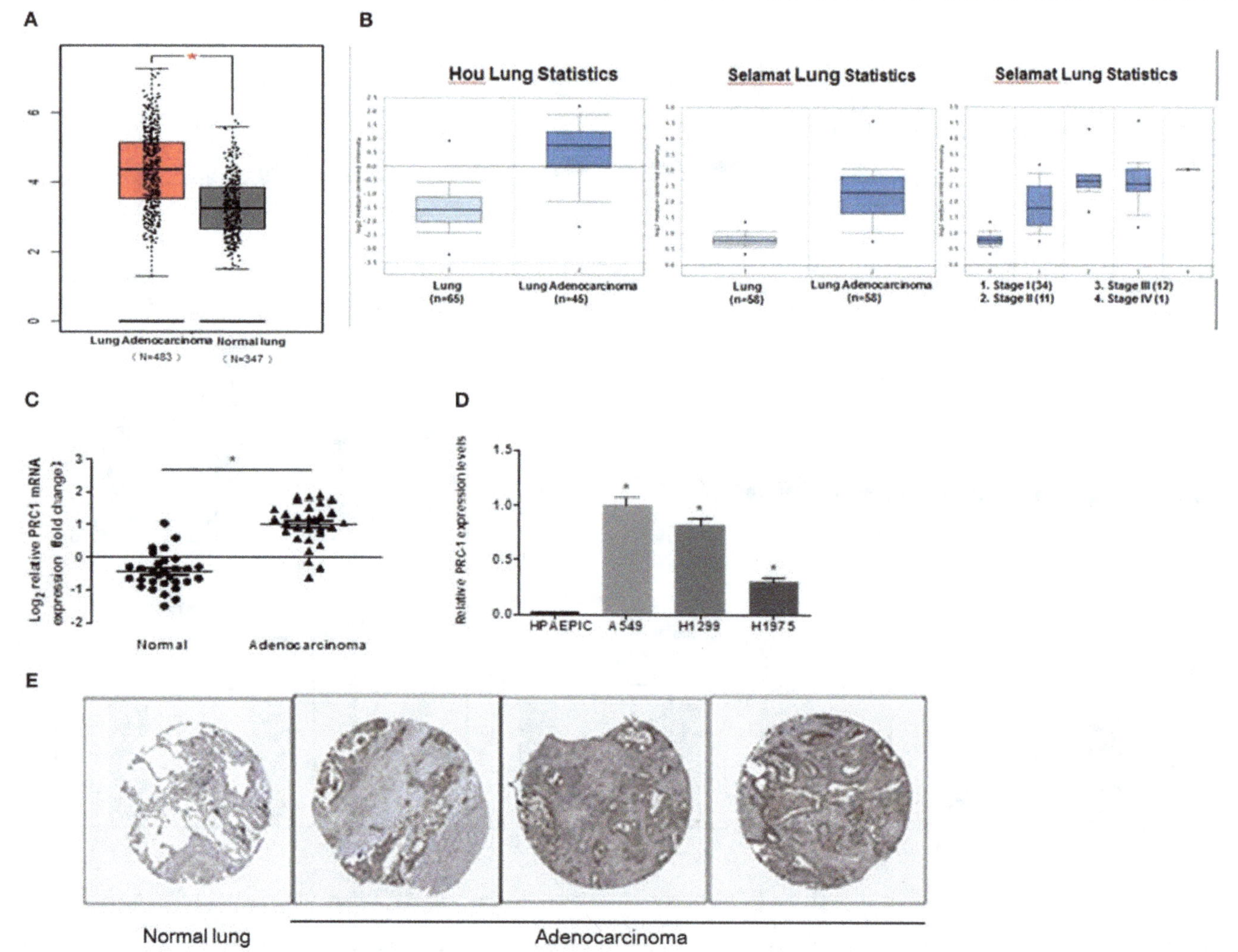

FIGURE 6 | Expression pattern of PRC1 in LUAD tissues and cell lines. **(A)** The data of copy number variation in LUAD from The Cancer Genome Atlas cohort. **(B)** The mRNA expression of PRC1 in different TNM staging groups in Oncomine. **(C)** qPCR analysis of PRC1 expression in LUAD tissues ($n = 30$). **(D)** qPCR analysis of PRC1 expression in LUAD cells and HPAEpiCs. **(E)** Representative images of the immunohistochemical staining of PRC1 from The Human Protein Atlas in LUAD and normal lung tissues. $^{*}P < 0.05$ in **(C)** ($n = 30$); $^{*}P < 0.05$ vs. HPAEpiCs in **(D)** ($n = 3$).

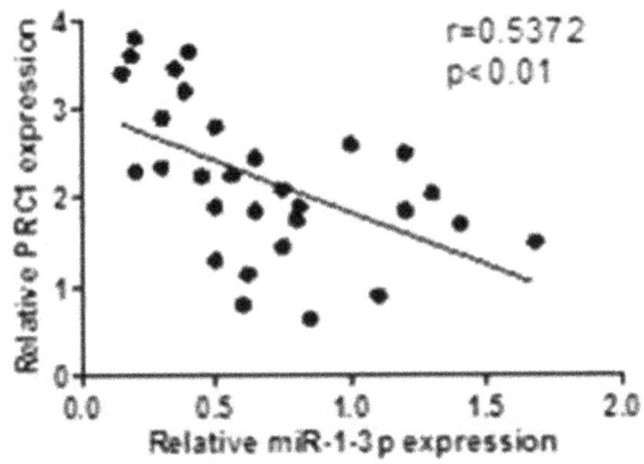

FIGURE 7 | Association between the miR-1-3p and PRC-1 levels in LUAD patients. The PRC1 and miR-1 levels were determined by qPCR in LUAD tissues and matched adjacent normal tissues ($n = 30$).

miR-1-3p Inhibits Xenograft Tumor Growth of LUAD Cells

To further explore whether miR-1-3p overexpression could suppress LUAD growth *in vivo*, human LUAD A549 cells with and without miR-1-3p overexpression were subcutaneously inoculated into nude mice. At 1 week after inoculation, all mice had developed detectable tumors. However, at 3 weeks after inoculation, the mice bearing tumors with miR-1-3p overexpression demonstrated a dramatic decrease in the tumor size and weight (**Figures 4A–C**), compared to the control groups. These results show that overexpression of miR-1-3p inhibits tumorigenesis *in vivo*.

PRC1 Is a Direct Target Gene of miR-1-3p

To further examine the mechanism underlying miR-1-3p-mediated suppression of LUAD development and progression, we employed the TargetScan computational algorithm to predict the target genes of miR-1-3p (21). The results indicated complementary base-pairing between miR-1-3p and the 3′-UTR of PRC1 (**Figure 5A**), suggesting that PRC1 may be a target gene of miR-1-3p. To verify this finding, we detected the expression of PRC1 in LUAD cells. As shown in **Figures 5B,C**, the protein expression of PRC1 was markedly induced in LUAD cells, compared with normal HPAEpiCs, consistent with the expression pattern of miR-1-3p in LUAD tissues and cells. Importantly, miR-1-3p overexpression led to downregulation of PRC1 in LUAD cells (**Figures 5D,E**), confirming that PRC1 is a downstream target of miR-1-3. To determine whether PRC1 is directly targeted by miR-1-3p, we performed a mutation assay through introducing a PRC1 3′-UTR mutation in the pmirGLO vector. The results demonstrated that the PRC1 3′-UTR mutation had no significant effect on the luciferase activity in miR-1-3p-transfected LUAD cells, compared with that in the NC-transfected cells (**Figure 5F**), suggesting that WT PRC1 3′-UTR is essential for the function of miR-1-3p. Taken together, our data show that PRC1 is a direct downstream target gene of miR-1-3p.

PRC1 Is Induced in LUAD Tissues and Cell Lines

To determine whether PRC1 contributes to LUAD development and progression, we examined the expression profile of PRC1 in LUAD tissues using the publicly accessible database Oncomine. As shown in **Figure 6A**, the mRNA expression levels of PRC1 were significantly enhanced in the LUAD tissues, compared with the normal lung tissues. In addition, we also analyzed the mRNA expression of PRC1 in LUAD tissues using two microarray datasets from the Hou and Selamat lung cancer groups, which were downloaded from Oncomine. The results demonstrated that the mRNA expression of PRC1 was significantly induced in the LUAD tissues of these groups and positively correlated with the tumor, lymph node, metastasis (TNM) staging of LUAD (**Figure 6B**). These findings were further confirmed by our mRNA expression data of PRC1 and the immunohistochemical staining of PRC1 in human LUAD tissues and matched adjacent normal lung tissues (**Figures 6C,E**). For the *in vitro* study, the mRNA levels of PRC1 were dramatically increased in the LUAD cell lines A549, H1299, and H1975, compared to those in normal HPAEpiCs (**Figure 6D**). Collectively, these results suggest that PRC1 may be involved in LUAD development and progression.

Correlation of miR-1-3p/PRC1 and Clinicopathological Characteristics of LUAD Patients

To investigate whether the miR-1-3p/PRC1 axis plays a role in LUAD development, we first analyzed the association between the miR-1-3p and PRC1 levels in LUAD tissues. The results revealed that the miR-1-3p levels were negatively correlated with the PRC1 mRNA expression ($r = -0.5858$; $P < 0.01$; **Figure 7**) in the LUAD tissues. Importantly, low levels of miR-1-3p and high levels of PRC1 were strongly associated with the TNM stage, lymph node metastasis, and distant metastasis (**Table 1**). These data suggest that LUAD development may be at least partially attributable to the miR-1-3p/PRC1 axis.

miR-1-3p Inhibits LUAD Cell Metastasis via PRC1

To determine whether miR-1-3p-mediated suppression of PRC1 expression is a major mechanism inhibiting LUAD development and progression, we cotransfected LUAD cells with miR-1-3p and a PRC1-overexpression plasmid for Transwell assays. The plasmid transfection efficacy of miR-1-3p and PRC1 was validated in **Figures 8A,B**. We found that miR-1-3p significantly inhibited the migration and invasion of three LUAD cell lines and that the inhibitory effects of miR-1-3p were markedly reversed by PRC1 overexpression (**Figures 8C–E**), suggesting that miR-1-3p inhibits LUAD cell metastasis in a PRC1-depedent manner and the miR-1-3p/PRC1 axis is majorly involved in LUAD development and progression.

Overexpression of PRC1 Is Associated With a Poor Prognosis in LUAD Patients

MiR-1-3p functions through suppressing PRC1 expression, suggesting a promotive role of PRC1 in LUAD development. To

TABLE 1 | The clinicopathological characteristics of 30 lung adenocarcinoma patients.

Clinicopathological features	*n*	Percent (%)	PRC1 expression		*p*	miR-1-3p expression		*p*
			Low (*n* = 9)	High (*n* = 21)		Low (*n* = 18)	High (*n* = 12)	
GENDER								
Male	19	63.33	7	12	0.419	11	9	0.694
Female	11	36.67	2	9	–	7	3	–
AGE (YEARS)								
≤60	13	43.33	6	7	0.123	8	5	1.000
>60	17	56.67	3	14	–	10	7	–
TUMOR SIZE								
T1 and T2	6	20.00	1	5	0.637	4	2	1.000
T3 and T4	24	80.00	8	16	–	14	10	–
TNM STAGE								
I and II	7	23.33	5	2	0.014	1	6	0.009
III and IV	23	76.67	4	19	–	17	6	–
LYMPHATIC METASTASIS								
Negative	12	40.00	8	4	0.001	2	10	0.000
Positive	18	60.00	1	17	–	16	2	–
DISTANT METASTASIS								
M0	12	40.00	7	5	0.013	3	9	0.002
M1	18	60.00	2	16	–	15	3	–

TNM, tumor, lymph node, metastasis stage.

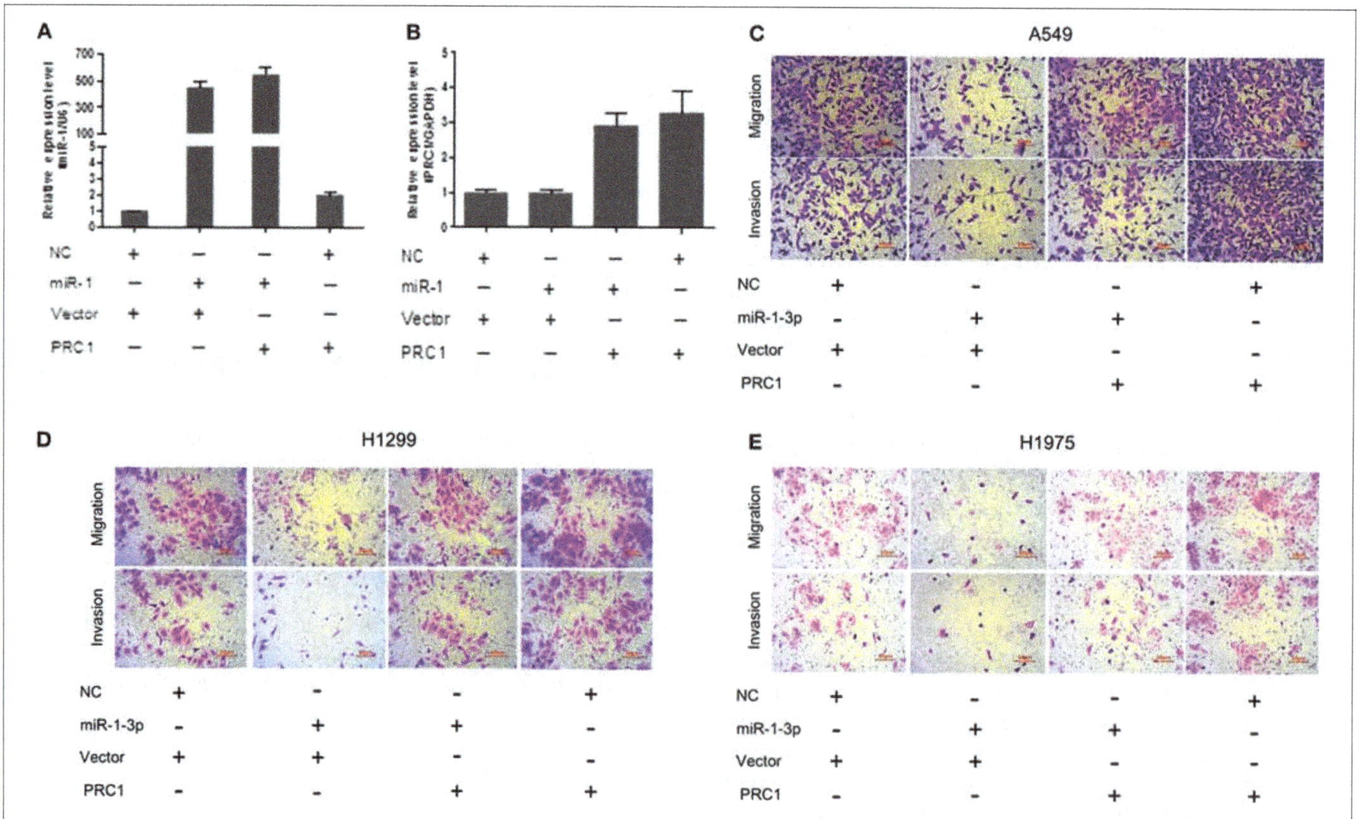

FIGURE 8 | miR-1-3p inhibits LUAD cell migration and invasion via PRC1. **(A,B)** qPCR analysis of the transfection efficiency of the miR-1-3p mimic and the PRC1-overexpression plasmid in LUAD cells. **(C–E)** Transwell assays for migration and invasion of LUAD cells transfected with the miR-1-3p mimic and/or the PRC1-overexpression plasmid.

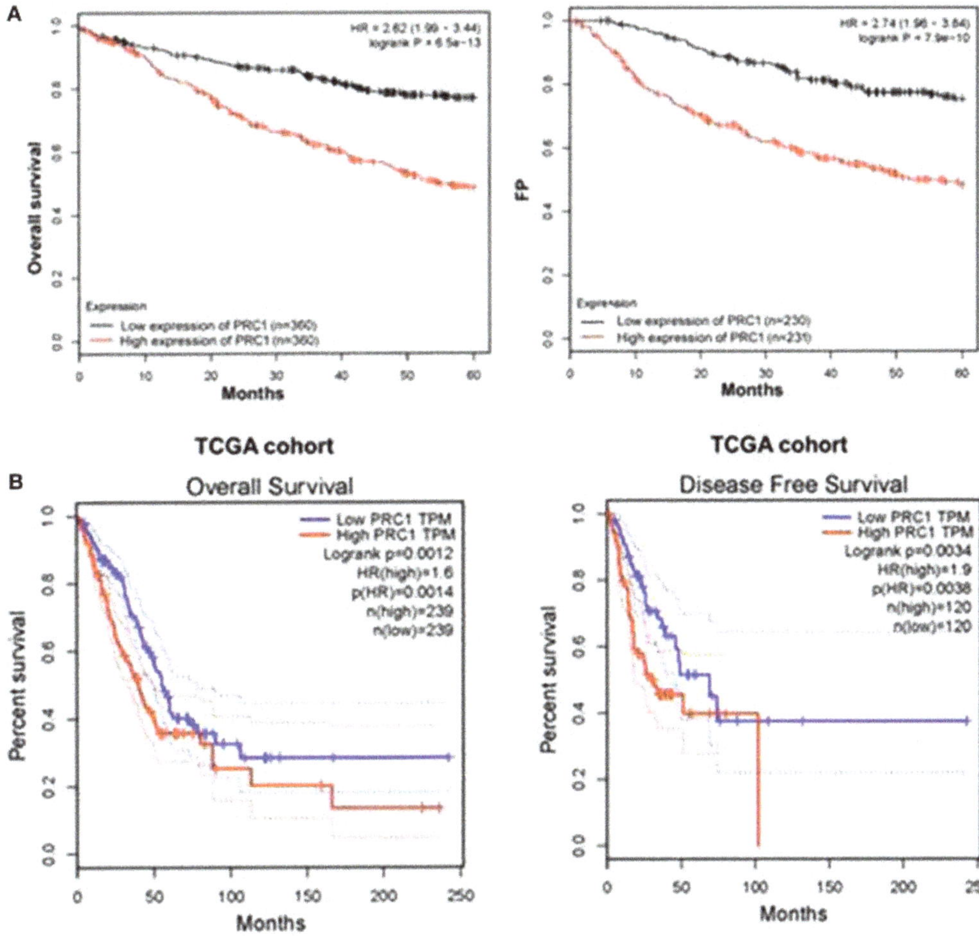

FIGURE 9 | Overexpression of PRC1 is associated with a poor prognosis in LUAD patients. **(A)** The prognostic effect of PRC1 in LUAD patients was evaluated using Kaplan–Meier plots. **(B)** The overall and disease-free survival rates in LUAD patients with different PRC1 expression patterns were evaluated for The Cancer Genome Atlas (TCGA) cohort.

confirm this, we examined the prognostic effect of PRC1 in LUAD patients from a public database by performing Kaplan–Meier analysis (http://www.kmplot.com). The results showed that the LUAD patients with a higher mRNA expression of PRC1 had shorter overall and disease-free survival times than those with a lower mRNA expression of PRC1 (**Figures 9A,B**). These data suggest that PRC1 overexpression may serve as a biomarker of a poor prognosis for LUAD patients, further supporting our findings that miR-1-3p plays a key role in inhibiting LUAD development through targeting PRC1.

DISCUSSION

Carcinogenesis of LUAD is a complex and multistage process involving the regulation of a wide range of genes by miRNAs (22–24). Among them, miR-1-3p, a muscle-specific miRNA, has been shown to play a key role in skeletal muscle differentiation and have inhibitory effects on the growth, migration, and invasion of LUAD (25). The present study revealed that miR-1-3p was significantly downregulated in LUAD tissues and cells. Lower levels of miR-1-3p were strongly associated with a higher TNM stage, earlier lymph node metastasis, and more distant metastasis. Therefore, miR-1-3p is suggested as a tumor suppressor in LUAD. The detection of miR-1-3p expression may be a valuable tool to evaluate the invasion and metastasis of LUAD.

There are hundreds of possible target genes of miR-1-3p, among which PRC1 is a critical protein in cytokinesis and characterized as a mitotic spindle-associated cyclin-dependent kinase substrate (26). Previous studies have provided evidence that PRC1 is involved in different types of cancer (27, 28). Loss of PRC1 leads to the accumulation of bi- and multi-nucleated cells in lung cancer, which further supports its role as the major central spindle organizer in cytokinesis (29). In view of our findings that miR-1-3p overexpression inhibits LUAD cell viability, there is a possibility that the function of PRC1 in apoptosis and senescence is due to induction of miR-1-3p. In this study, we demonstrated that the function of miR-1-3p could be suppressed by dysregulated expression of PRC1. In accordance with the above-mentioned studies, we confirmed that the overexpression of PRC1 significantly promoted the viability, invasion, and migration of LUAD cells. A higher PRC1 expression was also related to a worse outcome in patients with LUAD. Because Wnt/β-catenin signaling is dysregulated in lung cancer (30) and the overexpression of Wnt proteins (Wnt1 and Wnt5a) is significantly associated with adverse outcomes in lung cancer patients (31), we speculate that the miR-1-3p/PRC1 axis participates in dysregulation of Wnt/β-catenin signaling in LUAD development (32); however, this hypothesis requires further investigation. Although our study demonstrated that the miR-1-3p/PRC1 axis is a major mechanism underlying LUAD development, we do not exclude the possibility that other miRNAs or protein regulators besides miR-1-3p/PRC1 are also involved in LUAD pathogenesis. Therefore, more research is needed.

In summary, we identified miR-1-3p as a novel regulator of PRC1 in LUAD. A high PRC1 expression correlates with a poor prognosis in LUAD patients. Thus, targeting miR-1-3p/PRC1 may be a potential therapeutic intervention for the treatment of LUAD.

ETHICS STATEMENT

The Ethics Committee of Qilu Hospital at Shandong University approved this study [KYLL-2018 (KS)-156]. All participants in this study provided informed consent.

AUTHOR CONTRIBUTIONS

TL designed the questionnaire and drafted the manuscript. XW did the statistical analysis. TL and LJ did the relationship analysis and collected the data. YL conceived the study, supervised and reviewed the entire study, and edited the manuscript.

REFERENCES

1. Siegel RL, Miller KD, Jemal A. Cancer statistics. *CA Cancer J Clin.* (2017) 67:7–30. doi: 10.3322/caac.21387
2. Zhang W, Fan J, Chen Q, Lei C, Qiao B, Liu Q. SPP1 and AGER as potential prognostic biomarkers for lung adenocarcinoma. *Oncol Lett.* (2018) 15:7028–36. doi: 10.3892/ol.2018.8235
3. Jiang W, Jimenez G, Wells NJ, Hope TJ, Wahl GM, Hunter T, et al. PRC1: a human mitotic spindle-associated CDK substrate protein required for cytokinesis. *Mol Cell.* (1998) 2:877–85. doi: 10.1016/S1097-2765(00)80302-0
4. Peters S, Popat S, Reinmuth N, De Ruysscher D, Kerr KM, Peters S, et al. Metastatic non-small-cell lung cancer (NSCLC): ESMO clinical practice guidelines for diagnosis, treatment and follow-up. *Ann Oncol.* (2012) 23(Suppl. 7):vii56–64. doi: 10.1093/annonc/mds226
5. Leva GD, Croce CM. The role of microRNAs in the tumorigenesis of ovarian cancer. *Front Oncol.* (2013) 3:153. doi: 10.3389/fonc.2013.00153
6. Han C, Yu Z, Duan Z, Kan Q. Role of microRNA-1 in human cancer and its therapeutic potentials. *Biomed Res Int.* (2014) 2014:428371. doi: 10.1155/2014/428371
7. Li J, Guan J, Long X, Wang Y, Xiang X. mir-1-mediated paracrine effect of cancer-associated fibroblasts on lung cancer cell proliferation and chemoresistance. *Oncol Rep.* (2016) 35:3523–31. doi: 10.3892/or.2016.4714
8. Li SM, Wu HL, Yu X, Tang K, Wang SG, Ye ZQ, et al. The putative tumour suppressor miR-1-3p modulates prostate cancer cell aggressiveness by repressing E2F5 and PFTK1. *J Exp Clin Cancer Res.* (2018) 37:219. doi: 10.1186/s13046-018-0895-z
9. Diniz GP, Lino CA, Moreno CR, Senger N, Barreto-Chaves MLM. MicroRNA-1 overexpression blunts cardiomyocyte hypertrophy elicited by thyroid hormone. *J Cell Physiol.* (2017) 232:3360–8. doi: 10.1002/jcp.25781
10. Gao L, Yan P, Guo FF, Liu HJ, Zhao ZF. MiR-1-3p inhibits cell proliferation and invasion by regulating BDNF-TrkB signaling pathway in bladder cancer. *Neoplasma.* (2018) 65:89–96. doi: 10.4149/neo_2018_161128N594
11. Zhu D, Sun Y, Zhang D, Dong M, Jiang G, Zhang X, et al. miR1 inhibits the progression of colon cancer by regulating the expression of vascular endothelial growth factor. *Oncol Rep.* (2018) 40:589–98. doi: 10.3892/or.2018.6463
12. Shimo A, Nishidate T, Ohta T, Fukuda M, Nakamura Y, Katagiri T. Elevated expression of protein regulator of cytokinesis 1, involved in the growth of breast cancer cells. *Cancer Sci.* (2007) 98:174–81.doi: 10.1111/j.1349-7006.2006.00381.x
13. Kanehira M, Katagiri T, Shimo A, Takata R, Shuin T, Miki T, et al. Oncogenic role of MPHOSPH1, a cancer-testis antigen specific to human bladder cancer. *Cancer Res.* (2007) 67:3276–85. doi: 10.1158/0008-5472.CAN-06-3748
14. Chen J, Rajasekaran M, Xia H, Zhang X, Kong SN, Sekar K, et al. The microtubule-associated protein PRC1 promotes early recurrence of hepatocellular carcinoma in association with the Wnt/beta-catenin signalling pathway. *Gut.* (2016) 65:1522–34. doi: 10.1136/gutjnl-2015-310625
15. Nakamura T, Furukawa Y, Nakagawa H, Tsunoda T, Ohigashi H, Murata K, et al. Genome-wide cDNA microarray analysis of gene expression profiles in pancreatic cancers using populations of tumor cells and normal ductal epithelial cells selected for purity by laser microdissection. *Oncogene.* (2004) 23:2385–400. doi: 10.1038/sj.onc.1207392
16. Gao J, Aksoy BA, Dogrusoz U, Dresdner G, Gross B, Sumer SO, et al. Integrative analysis of complex cancer genomics and clinical profiles using the cBioPortal. *Sci Signal.* (2013) 6:pl1. doi: 10.1126/scisignal.2004088
17. Cerami E, Gao J, Dogrusoz U, Gross BE, Sumer SO, Aksoy BA, et al. The cBio cancer genomics portal: an open platform for exploring multidimensional cancer genomics data. *Cancer Discov.* (2012) 2:401–4. doi: 10.1158/2159-8290.CD-12-0095
18. Zhu J, Sanborn JZ, Benz S, Szeto C, Hsu F, Kuhn RM, et al. The UCSC cancer genomics browser. *Nat Methods.* (2009) 6:239–40. doi: 10.1038/nmeth0409-239
19. Rhodes DR, Yu J, Shanker K, Deshpande N, Varambally R, Ghosh D, et al. ONCOMINE: a cancer microarray database and integrated data-mining platform. *Neoplasia.* (2004) 6:1–6. doi: 10.1016/S1476-5586(04)80047-2
20. Gyorffy B, Surowiak P, Budczies J, Lánczky A. Online survival analysis software to assess the prognostic value of biomarkers using transcriptomic data in non-small-cell lung cancer. *PLoS ONE.* (2013) 8:e82241. doi: 10.1371/journal.pone.0082241
21. Jiao D, Chen J, Li Y, Tang X, Wang J, Xu W, et al. miR-1-3p and miR-206 sensitizes HGF-induced gefitinib-resistant human lung cancer cells through inhibition of c-Met signalling and EMT. *J Cell Mol Med.* (2018) 22:3526–36. doi: 10.1111/jcmm.13629
22. Nadal E, Chen G, Gallegos M, Lin L, Ferrer-Torres D, Truini A, et al. Epigenetic inactivation of microRNA-34b/c predicts poor disease-free survival in early-stage lung adenocarcinoma. *Clin Cancer Res.* (2013) 19:6842–52. doi: 10.1158/1078-0432.CCR-13-0736
23. Yu QQ, Wu H, Huang X, Shen H, Shu YQ, Zhang B, et al. MiR-1 targets PIK3CA and inhibits tumorigenic properties of A549 cells. *Biomed Pharmacother.* (2014) 68:155–61. doi: 10.1016/j.biopha.2014.01.005
24. Singh A, Happel C, Manna SK, Acquaah-Mensah G, Carrerero J, Kumar S, et al. Transcription factor NRF2 regulates miR-1 and miR-206 to drive tumorigenesis. *J Clin Invest.* (2013) 123:2921–34. doi: 10.1172/JCI 66353
25. Chiu KL, Lin YS, Kuo TT, Lo CC, Huang YK, Chang HF, et al. ADAM9 enhances CDCP1 by inhibiting miR-1 through EGFR signaling

activation in lung cancer metastasis. *Oncotarget.* (2017) 8:47365–78. doi: 10.18632/oncotarget.17648

26. Zhan P, Zhang B, Xi GM, Wu Y, Liu HB, Liu YF, et al. PRC1 contributes to tumorigenesis of lung adenocarcinoma in association with the Wnt/beta-catenin signaling pathway. *Mol Cancer.* (2017) 16:108. doi: 10.1186/s12943-017-0682-z
27. Brynychova V, Ehrlichova M, Hlavac V, Nemcova-Furstova V, Pecha V, Leva J, et al. Genetic and functional analyses do not explain the association of high PRC1 expression with poor survival of breast carcinoma patients. *Biomed Pharmacother.* (2016) 83:857–64. doi: 10.1016/j.biopha.2016.07.047
28. Hanselmann S, Wolter P, Malkmus J, Gaubatz S. The microtubule-associated protein PRC1 is a potential therapeutic target for lung cancer. *Oncotarget.* (2018) 9:4985–97. doi: 10.18632/oncotarget.23577
29. Glotzer M. The 3Ms of central spindle assembly: microtubules, motors and MAPs. *Nat Rev Mol Cell Biol.* (2009) 10:9–20. doi: 10.1038/nrm2609
30. Stewart DJ. Wnt signaling pathway in non-small cell lung cancer. *J Natl Cancer Inst.* (2014) 106:djt356. doi: 10.1093/jnci/djt356
31. Jin J, Zhan P, Qian H, Wang X, Katoh M, Phan K, et al. Prognostic value of wingless-type proteins in non-small cell lung cancer patients: a meta-analysis. *Transl Lung Cancer Res.* (2016) 5:436–42. doi: 10.21037/tlcr.2016.08.08
32. Anton R, Chatterjee SS, Simundza J, Cowin P, Dasgupta R. A systematic screen for micro-RNAs regulating the canonical Wnt pathway. *PLoS ONE.* (2011) 6:e26257. doi: 10.1371/journal.pone.0026257

4

A High-Content Screening Approach to Identify MicroRNAs Against Head and Neck Cancer Cell Survival and EMT in an Inflammatory Microenvironment

Bruno Sangiorgi[1,2], *Felipe Canto de Souza*[1,2], *Ildercílio Mota de Souza Lima*[1,2], *Josiane Lilian dos Santos Schiavinato*[1,2], *Amanda Cristina Corveloni*[1,2], *Carolina Hassibe Thomé*[1,3], *Wilson Araújo Silva Jr.*[1,2], *Vitor Marcel Faça*[1,3], *Dimas Tadeu Covas*[1], *Marco Antônio Zago*[1] *and Rodrigo Alexandre Panepucci*[1,2*]

[1] Center for Cell-Based Therapy (CTC), Regional Blood Center of Ribeirão Preto, Ribeirão Preto, Brazil, [2] Department of Genetics and Internal Medicine, Ribeirão Preto Medical School, University of São Paulo (FMRP-USP), Ribeirão Preto, Brazil, [3] Department of Biochemistry and Immunology, Ribeirão Preto Medical School, University of São Paulo (FMRP-USP), Ribeirão Preto, Brazil

***Correspondence:**
Rodrigo Alexandre Panepucci
panepucci@hemocentro.fmrp.usp.br

Head and neck squamous cell carcinoma (HNSCC) is among the most common cancer types. Metastasis, the main cause of death by cancer, can be promoted by an inflammatory microenvironment, which induces epithelial-mesenchymal transition (EMT) through a NF-κB-mediated stabilization of Snail. Here, we aimed to explore how microRNAs (miRs) can affect cell survival and EMT in HNSCC cells under an inflammatory microenvironment. By using a high-content screening (HCS) approach, we evaluated alterations in morphometric parameters, as well as expression/localization of Snail/Slug, in HNSCC cells primed with TNF-α. Based on those quantitation, we established the optimal experimental conditions of EMT induction driven by TNF-α. Those conditions were applied to cells transfected with distinct miRs ($N = 31$), followed by clusterization of miRs based on alterations related to cell survival and EMT. The signaling pathways enriched with molecular targets from each group of miRs were identified by *in silico* analyses. Finally, cells were transfected with siRNAs against signaling pathways targeted by miRs with anti-survival/EMT effect and evaluated for alterations in cell survival and EMT. Overall, we observed that TNF-α, at 20 ng/ml, induced EMT-related changes in cell morphology, Snail/Slug expression, and cell migration. Predicted targets of miRs with anti-survival/EMT effect were enriched with targets of NF-κB, PI3K/ATK, and Wnt/beta catenin pathways. Strikingly, individual gene silencing of elements from those pathways, namely *RELA* (NF-kB), *AKT1* (PI3K/AKT), and *CTNNB1* (Wnt/beta catenin) reduced cell survival and/or expression of Snail/Slug in cells stimulated with TNF-α. As a whole, our HCS approach allowed for the identification of miRs capable of inhibiting cell survival and EMT considering the presence of an inflammatory microenvironment, also indicating the common signaling pathways and molecular targets most likely to underlie those alterations. These findings may contribute to the development of targeted therapies against HNSCC.

Keywords: head and neck squamous cell carcinoma, high-content screening, microRNAs, epithelial-mesenchymal-transition, inflammation, NF-κB

INTRODUCTION

Head and neck squamous cell carcinoma (HNSCC) comprises a group of upper aerodigestive tract neoplasia and is among the ten types of cancer with the highest incidence and mortality in the world (1). Over the past decades, despite advances in treatment strategies of HNSCC, it was observed a growth in mortality associated with distant metastases (2). Studies to date demonstrated that metastasis initiation is promoted by tumor cells that undergoes epithelial-mesenchymal transition (EMT), a transformation process which cells acquire a mesenchymal-like phenotype and dislodges from the tumor bulk, invading adjacent vessels and entering in the circulation (3).

EMT events are coordinated by transcription factors known as "EMT master regulators," including members of the Snail family: SNAI1 (Snail) and SNAI2 (Slug), which are capable of both silencing and promoting the expression of genes related to epithelial and mesenchymal phenotypes, respectively (4). As a consequence of the "EMT master regulators" activity, cancer cells undergo drastic phenotypic changes in cell morphology: from polygonal to elongated, expression of cell adhesion proteins: downregulation of E-Cadherin and upregulation of N-Cadherin and integrins, expression of structural proteins: upregulation of Vimentin, among others that lead to the formation of mesenchymal cancer cells with migratory/invasive capacities (5).

Increasing literature data have established that, for several types of cancer including HNSCC, the presence of an inflamed tumor microenvironment is associated with tumor progression, the acquisition of EMT-like features by cancer cells and the formation of metastasis (6). In different types of cancer, multiple lines of evidence have supported that inflammatory cytokines secreted by tumor-associated macrophages (which can represent half of the tumor mass), including tumor necrosis factor alpha (TNF-α), are capable of inducing EMT events in cancer cells (7). TNF-α activates the nuclear factor kappa b (NF-κB) signaling pathway, which the main effector p50/p65 (RelA) promotes the nuclear translocation of Snail, thereby inducing EMT (8). Additionally, NF-κB crosstalk with other oncogenic signaling pathways in HNSCC including Ras/MAPK, PI3K/AKT, and Wnt/beta catenin, that collectively promotes cancer cell survival, evasion from apoptosis and therapy resistance (9, 10). Due to the complexity of intracellular signaling pathways and tumor microenvironment in cancer, including HNSCC, a multi-target therapy (targeting multiple signaling pathways) may be an interesting therapeutic approach (11).

MicroRNAs (miRs) are a class of small non-coding RNAs that act predominantly through the destabilization and degradation of multiple targeted messenger RNAs (mRNAs) thereby affecting several biological processes independently (12, 13). In HNSCC, as in other types of cancer, there is mounting evidence that miRs are capable of interfering in multiple cellular processes, such as cancer cell proliferation, invasion, and apoptosis, thereby promoting (oncomiRs) or inhibiting (tumor suppressor miRs) the progression from normal tissue to carcinoma and subsequently metastasis (14, 15). Importantly, the HNSCC oncomiR: miR-21 and tumor suppressor miR: miR-29, are both involved in transcriptional networks that regulates the activity of the NF-κB signaling pathway (14, 16), highlighting the importance of NF-κB as a regulator of both inflammation and tumor progression in HNSCC.

Since its discovery, miRs have been drawing attention due to their capacity to be used either as prognostic biomarkers or in miR-based targeted therapies against cancer (17, 18). Currently, miR-based targeted therapeutic strategies comprehends the delivery of either mimetics of miRs with tumor suppressor activity (microRNA replacement or restoration therapy) or molecules capable of inactivating oncomiRs (microRNA reduction or inhibition therapy) (19). Importantly, a functional study conducted by Lindenbergh-van der Plas and coworkers provided a proof-of-concept that miRs can be used to selectively kill HNSCC cancer cells (20). However, despite the potential use of miRs in drug discovery and therapeutic applications, it is a current challenge to identify, among the several signaling pathways regulated by a given miR, those that has an effective therapeutic value (21).

In the last decade, advances in the High-Content Screening (HCS) approach (cell-based functional screens based on automated microscopy and image analysis) allowed for the quantitative measurement of a broad spectrum of phenotypic alterations at a cellular level (22). Noteworthy, the advantage of the HCS approach to measure the phenotype in a multiparametric fashion makes it especially suited to investigate the pleiotropic effects exerted by miRs (23). In addition, target-prediction tools can also be utilized for the identification of the molecular targets shared by groups of miRs and thereby indicating the ones that are most likely responsible for the observed effects (24). In the present work, through an HCS approach and *in-silico* analysis, we investigated the capacity of miRs to alter the phenotypic features related to tumor progression (e.g., cell survival) and metastasis (e.g., EMT) in HNSCC cells considering the presence of an inflammatory microenvironment. Overall, we have identified miRs capable of inhibiting cell survival and EMT as well as potential targets and signaling pathways involved in the observed effects.

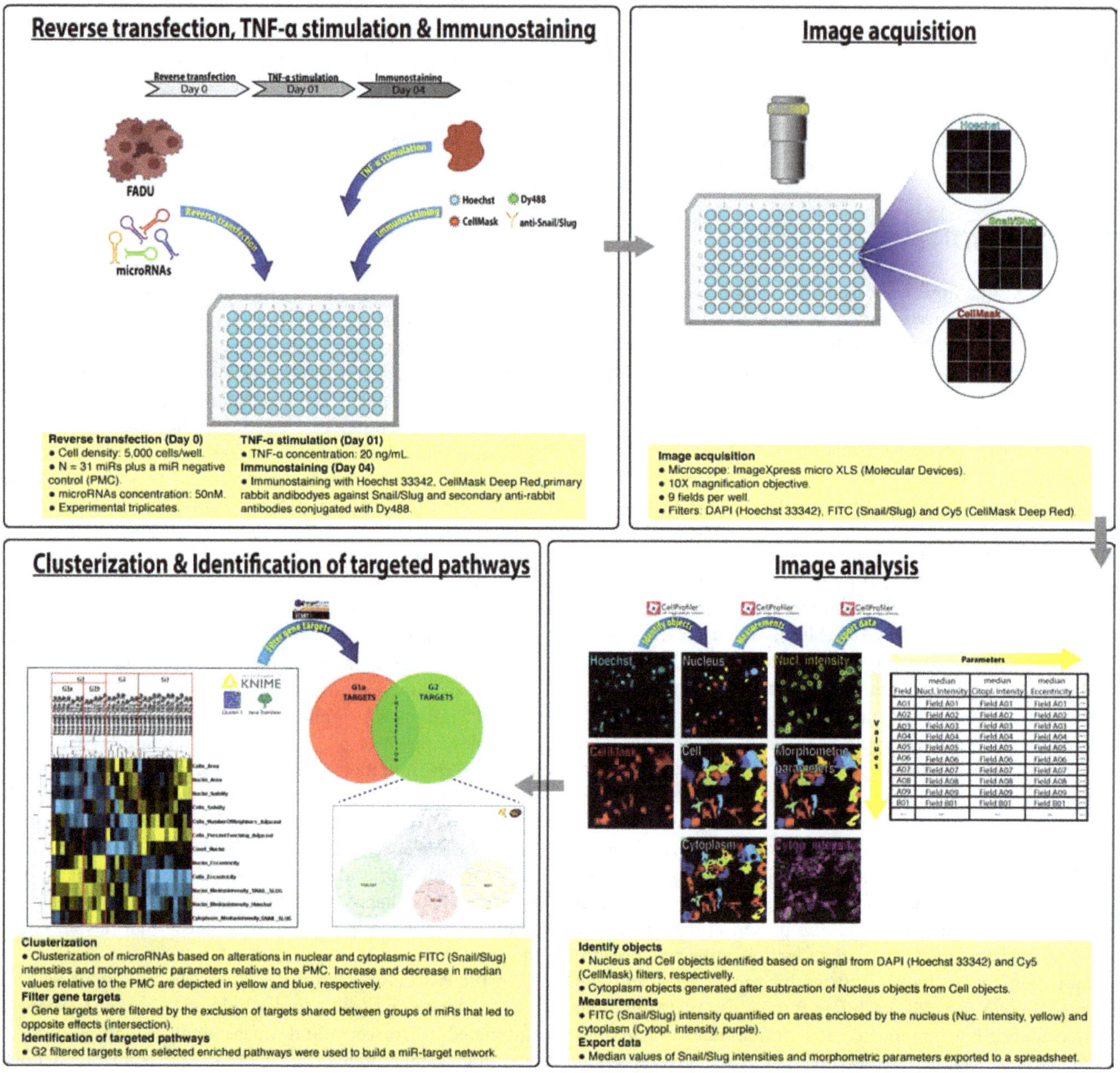

FIGURE 1 | Study design. Reverse transfection, TNF-α stimulation and Immunostaining: Cells from the FADU cell line were transfected (day 0) with microRNAs ($N = 31$), followed by stimulation with TNF-α (20 ng/mL, Day 01) and immunostaining with primary rabbit antibodies against Snail/Slug, secondary anti-rabbit antibodies conjugated with Dy488, nuclear (Hoechst) and cytoplasmic (CellMask) fluorescent dyes (Day 04). Image acquisition: Images (9 fields per well) were acquired using a 10X objective and excitation/emission filters DAPI (Hoechst), FITC (Snail/Slug), and Cy5 (CellMask), using an ImageXpress Micro XLS HCS system (Molecular Devices). Image analysis: Nuclei and corresponding cytoplasm objects were identified and segmented based on images from DAPI (Hoechst) and Cy5 (CellMask) channels, respectively. FITC (Snail/Slug) intensity on nuclei and cytoplasm, as well as morphometric parameters were then quantified. Median values per field were exported into a spreadsheet. Clusterization and Identification of targeted pathways: Based on alterations in median values per well relative to the PMC, microRNAs were subjected to an unsupervised hierarchical clustering. After the exclusion of genes commonly targeted by miRs from G1a (pro-survival/EMT) and G2 (anti-survival/EMT), genes from signaling pathways targeted by G2 miRs were used to generate a microRNA regulatory network.

MATERIALS AND METHODS

Study Design

The design of this study is illustrated in **Figure 1**. Cells from the FADU cell line were transfected (reverse transfection) into 96 well plates with miR mimetics ($N = 31$ plus a miR negative control) in experimental triplicates, followed by stimulation with TNF-α (20 ng/mL) for 72 h and immunostaining with primary rabbit antibodies against Snail/Slug, secondary anti-rabbit antibodies conjugated with Dy488, nuclear (Hoechst) and cytoplasmic (CellMask) fluorescent dyes. Images (nine fields per well) were acquired using a 10X objective and excitation/emission filters

DAPI (Hoechst), FITC (Snail/Slug), and Cy5 (CellMask), using an ImageXpress Micro XLS HCS system (Molecular Devices). With aid of CellProfiler, images from filters DAPI (Hoechst) and Cy5 (CellMask) were used to identify nuclear, cell and cytoplasm objects, followed by quantification of nuclear and cytoplasmic median FITC (Snail/Slug) intensity, as well as morphometric parameters. Median values per field were exported into spreadsheets and with help of KNIME software, we obtained the percentage change of the median values per well relative to the miR negative control (PMC). By using Cluster3 and Java TreeView software, we performed a unsupervised hierarchical clustering of miRs by which the four groups of miRs (G1a, G1b, G2, and G4) were identified. With help of KNIME and Targetscan software, we identified the genes targeted by most (N-2, minimum of 4) of the microRNAs in each group. With help of Venny online tool, genes targeted by groups that led to opposite phenotypic effects were identified and excluded from further analyses. With aid of Database for Annotation, Visualization and Integrated Discovery (DAVID, version 6.7) online tool, we identified signaling pathways enriched with filtered targets. With help of the Kyoto Encyclopedia of Genes and Genomes (KEGG) database, the filtered targets from G2 miRs were assigned to the NF-kB, PI3K/AKT, and Wnt/beta-catenin signaling pathways, which were used to generate a microRNA regulatory network with help of Cytoscape software. Based on information from those analyses, secondary functional assays using siRNAs were designed to evaluate the effect, in cell survival and EMT, of interferences in NF-kB, PI3K/AKT, and Wnt/beta-catenin signaling pathways.

Cell Lines

Cells derived from the HNSCC cell lines FADU (oropharynx), HN30 (pharynx), and UMSCC1 (floor of mouth) were cultured in Dulbecco's modified Eagle's medium (DMEM) supplemented with 10% fetal bovine serum (FBS), 50 U/mL penicillin and 50 μg/mL streptomycin. Cells were passaged by using a 10% trypsin solution.

Reagents

Throughout this work, cells were treated with TNF-α (300-01A, PrepoTech, USA) or mitomycin C (MMC, M4287, sigma-aldrich, USA). For immunostaining, we used the nuclear dye Hoechst 33342 (10 μg/mL; H1399, Thermo Scientific, USA) and cytoplasmic dye HCS CellMask Deep Red (5 μg/mL, H10294, Thermo Scientific, USA), primary antibodies: Anti-N-Cadherin mouse IgG2ab mAb (SC-271386, Santa Cruz Biotechnology, USA), Rabbit anti-Snail/Slug (ab180714, abcam, USA), Goat anti-Vimentin (sc-7558, Santa Cruz Biotechnology) and Mouse-anti-Caspase-7 (cleaved caspase-7 p10, clone h207, sc-22179, Santa Cruz Biotechnology, USA), as well as secondary antibodies: Goat anti-Rabbit DyLight 488 (dy488, 35553, Thermo Scientific, USA), Goat anti-Rabbit DyLight 594 (35561, Thermo Scientific, USA) DyLight 488 mouse (35503, Thermo Scientific, USA) and Donkey anti-Goat DyLight 594 (SA5-1088, Thermo Scientific, USA). For western blot, we used the antibodies rabbit anti-snail (#3879, Cell Signaling, USA), rabbit anti-slug (#9585, Cell Signaling, USA), rabbit anti-vimentin (#5741, Cell Signaling, USA), rabbit anti N-cadherin (#13116, Cell Signaling, USA), rabbit anti-β-catenin (#8480, Cell Signaling, USA) and mouse anti-β-actin (sc-81178, Santa Cruz, CA).

Western Blot

For protein extraction and quantification, cells were washed with PBS and disrupted in lyses buffer (20 mM Tris-HCl, 150 mM NaCl, 1 mM Na2EDTA, 1 mM EGTA, 1% Triton X-100, 2.5 mM sodium pyrophosphate, 1 mM β-glycerophosphate, 1 mM Na3VO4 and 1 μg/ml leupeptin). After three sonication cycles at 45 W for 5 min each in a sonicator bath, the samples were centrifuged at 20,000 × g for 30 min at 4°C. The protein concentration was determined by the Bradford method (Bio-Rad, Hercules, CA).

Proteins were submitted to SDS–PAGE and electrotransferred to PVDF membranes (GE Lifesciences, Pittsburgh, PA, USA). Membranes were blocked with 5% non-fat dry milk in 0.1% Tween-TBS and incubated with the primary antibody. After 1 h of incubation with horseradish peroxidase-conjugated goat anti-rabbit IgG (#7074, Cell Signaling) or horse anti-mouse IgG (#7076, Cell Signaling) secondary antibodies The antibody-protein complex was detected using ECL Western Blotting Detection Reagents (GE Lifesciences) using a CCD-Camera (Image QuantLAS 4000 mini, Uppsala, Sweden). Densitometric analysis was performed using the ImageJ software, and bands were normalized to the constitutive protein β-actin.

MicroRNA Mimics and siRNAs

Transfection assays were carried out with human microRNA mimetic molecules (50 nM, Thermo Scientific) or synthetic siRNA molecules (10 nM; **Supplementary File 1**).

Reverse Transfection

Reverse transfection assays were performed using lipofectamine LTX transfection reagent (15338100, Thermo Scientific) and synthetic miRs/siRNAs according to manufacturer's instructions. Transfection efficiency was calculated by evaluating the percentage reduction in cell numbers following transfection with a cytotoxic siRNA against Ubiquitin (siUBC) as compared to cells transfected with a control miR (PMC) or siRNA (siCTR).

Immunostaining

Cells were fixed and permeabilized with a 2% formaldehyde solution in methanol for 20 min at −20°C. Quenching of formaldehyde was achieved by incubation for 15 min with a 0.1 M glycine solution and blocking with a 1% FBS solution for 30 min. Afterwards, cells were incubated for 1 h at room temperature with primary antibodies, followed by incubation for 45 min with a solution containing secondary antibodies and nuclear/cytoplasmic dyes.

Image Analysis

Image analyses were performed with aid of MetaXpress software (Molecular Devices, USA) or CellProfiler (version 2.2.0, Broad Institute, USA). Briefly, images from functional assays that aimed to evaluate only the presence/absence of fluorescent dyes or markers were analyzed using MetaXpress software, whereas CellProfiler was used to analyze images from functional assays aiming both the evaluation of morphometric parameters and the presence and subcellular localization of fluorescent markers. Data from image analyses were processed with the aid of KNIME software (version 3.2.0).

HCS-Based Functional Assays

Alterations in cell morphology and expression/localization of proteins were assessed through HCS-based functional assays, which comprises of:

i) MiR/siRNA reverse transfection of FADU cells into 96-well culture plates (CLS3603, Corning, USA);
ii) Stimulation or not with TNF-α, 24 h after reverse transfection;
iii) Immunostaining using antibodies, nuclear and cytoplasmic dyes;
iv) Image acquisition (9 fields per well) with aid of an ImageXpress® Micro XLS High-Content Screening (HCS) system (Molecular Devices, USA), using a 10X magnification objective and excitation/emission filters DAPI, FITC, Cy3, Texas Red, and Cy5;
v) Image analysis with aid of MetaXpress (Molecular Devices, USA) or CellProfiler (version 2.2.0, Broad Institute, USA) software.

Migration Assay

Cells were seeded on culture plates specific for migration assays Oris Pro Cell Migration Assay, 96 wells (PROCMA5, Platypus Technologies, USA). After 24 h, cells were treated with 0.2 μg/mL of mitomycin C for 2 h (to suppress proliferation), followed or not by incubation with TNF-a at 20 or 50 ng/mL for 72 h (experimental triplicates). Images were acquired using a 4X phase-contrast objective after cell seeding and at the endpoint using the ImageXpress HCS system. The area occupied by cells was quantified after cell seeding and at the endpoint, which were used to measure cell migration using $M = (Ae/As * 100)\text{-}100$, in which M = migration, Ae = Area occupied by cells at the endpoint, As = Area occupied by cells 24 h after seeding.

Clusterization of miRs

A unsupervised hierarchical clustering of miRs was performed with aid of Cluster 3 software (25) and visualized with help of Java TreeView software (26). Groups of miRs were classified as of pro/anti survival/EMT properties based on alterations in the following phenotypic parameters: "count nuclei (cell survival)," "cells eccentricity (EMT)," "Nuclei Median Intensity Snail/Slug (EMT)," and "Cytoplasm Median Intensity Snail/Slug (EMT)."

Identification of Genes and Signaling Pathways Targeted by Groups of miRs

Using the KNIME software (version 3.7) and TargetScan database of predicted miR targets (version 7.1) (27), we created a pipeline to identify the transcripts commonly targeted by most of the miRs contained in each of the identified groups (N-2, minimum of 4). Venn diagrams were generated using Venny 2.1 online tool (bioinfogp.cnb.csic.es/tools/venny) by comparing the identified targets from groups of miRs with opposite phenotypic effects, followed by the exclusion (filtering) of the shared targets. Afterwards, with help of the Database for Annotation, Visualization and Integrated Discovery (DAVID, version 6.7) (28), we identified signaling pathways that were enriched with the filtered targets from each group of miRs.

The filtered targets were assigned to their given signaling pathways according to information available on the Kyoto Encyclopedia of Genes and Genomes (KEGG) database about the following signaling pathways: NF-κB (hsa04064), PI3K/AKT (hsa04151), and Wnt (hsa04310) (29). The miRs and targets from the selected pathways were used to generate a microRNA regulatory network with aid of Cytoscape software (30).

Quantitative PCR (qPCR)

RNA extraction was performed using TRIZOL reagent (Invitrogen Life Technologies, Grand Island, NY, USA) and total RNA was reverse transcribed using the High Capacity cDNA Reverse Transcription Kit (Applied Biosystems, Foster City, CA, USA), according to the manufacturer's instructions. Gene expression qPCR reactions were carried in duplicates with Power SYBR Green Master Mix (Applied Biosystems) and primers for AKT2 (Forward: AAGGATGAAGTCGCTCACAC; Reverse: ACTCCATCACAAAGCACAGG), CCND1 (Forward: CCCGCACGATTTCATTGAAC; Reverse: GGCGGATTGGAAATGAACTTC), GAPDH (Forward: GAAGGTGAAGGTCGGAGTC; Reverse: GAAGATGGTGATGGGATTTC); IL6 (Forward: ATGCAATAACCACCCCTGAC; Reverse: GAGGTGCCCATGCTACATTT); MYC (Forward: CAGATCAGCAACAACCGAAA; Reverse: GGCCTTTTCATTGTTTTCCA) and RELA (Forward: TGACAAGGTGCAGAAAGAGG; Reverse: CACATCAGCTTGCGAAAAGG) using a CFX96 Real-Time PCR system (Bio-Rad). Relative gene expression levels were assessed using the $2^{-\Delta\Delta Ct}$ strategy (31).

Statistics

All statistical analyses were performed with aid of GraphPad Prism software version 5.0. Comparisons between multiple experimental conditions were performed using either unpaired *t*-test or univariate "ONE-WAY Anova" test. Statistical significance was considered at $p < 0.05$.

RESULTS

Stimulation With Tumor Necrosis Factor Alpha Leads to EMT-Related Morphometric Alterations

We performed an HCS-based functional assay in cells primed with TNF-α at different concentrations and time points followed by quantification of morphometric features. Stimulation for 48 h with TNF-α, at all concentrations used (5–50 ng/mL), reduced the percentage of intercellular contact by around 15% while not changing cell eccentricity (elongation). On this same endpoint, we found a trend for increase and decrease in cell area and number of neighboring cells, respectively, in a concentration-dependent manner, attaining significance at 20 and 50 ng/mL. On the other hand, stimulation for 72 h with all TNF-α concentrations used, led to a significant increase in cell

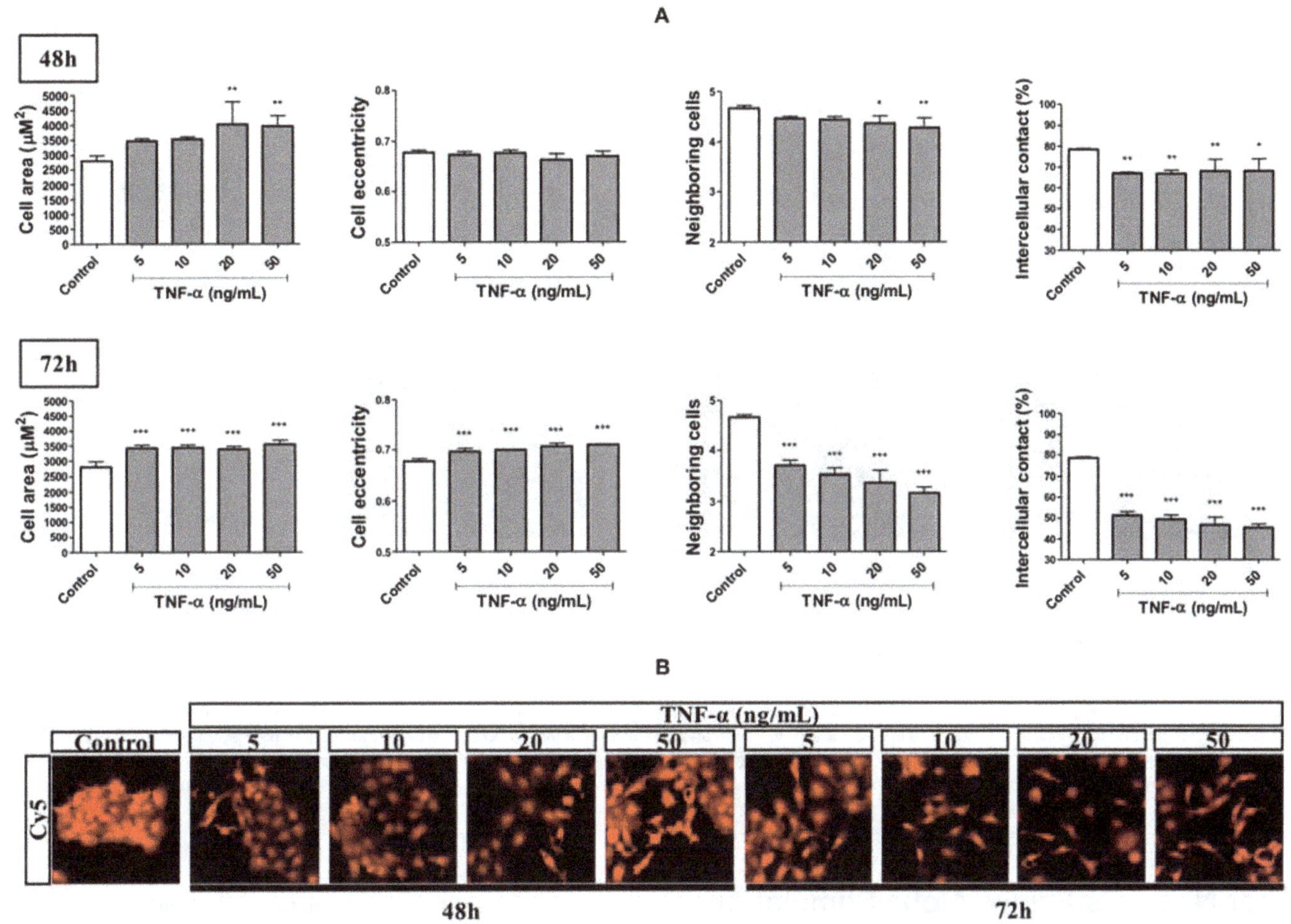

FIGURE 2 | Effects of TNF-α in EMT-related morphometric parameters. The FADU cell line was stimulated or not (Control) with TNF-α (5 to 50 ng/mL), for 48 or 72 h (squares). At the endpoint, the cells were stained with nuclear (Hoechst) and cytoplasmic (CellMask) fluorescent dyes. Images (nine fields per well) were acquired using a 10X objective and excitation/emission filters DAPI (Hoechst) and Cy5 (CellMask), using an ImageXpress Micro XLS HCS system (Molecular Devices). Images were analyzed using CellProfiler, in order to quantify the following parameters: cell area, cell eccentricity, number of neighboring cells and percentage of intercellular contact. **(A)** Quantitative changes (Mean +-SD) in morphometric parameters due to TNF-α stimulation for 48 and 72 h. **(B)** Representative images of cells stimulated with TNF-α for 48 and 72 h. Statistically significant differences (ONE-WAY Anova with Tukey post-test), in comparison to the control condition: $^{*}p < 0.05$; $^{**}p < 0.01$; $^{***}p < 0.001$.

area (around 1,000 μm^2) and cell eccentricity. These changes were accompanied by significant reductions in both the number of neighboring cells (by around 1.5) and the percentage of intercellular contact (by around 30%; **Figure 2**).

Stimulation With Tumor Necrosis Factor Alpha Leads to the Expression of EMT-Related Proteins

An HCS-based functional assay was done in cells primed with TNF-α for 72 h and at different concentrations, with further quantification of changes in the percentage of cells positive for markers of EMT. Generally, we observed that stimulation with TNF-α led to a concentration-dependent increase in the percentage of cells positive for all markers evaluated. More specifically, the higher concentration of 50 ng/mL led to a significant increase in the percentage of cells expressing N-Cadherin in the cytoplasm (from 30 to 50%, approximately). Moreover, the percentage of cells expressing cytoplasmic Vimentin significantly increased by 25% after treatment with TNF-α at 20 and 50 ng/mL. Finally, the percentage of cells expressing Snail/Slug in the nucleus significantly increased at all concentrations of TNF-α, ranging from below 20% (in untreated cells) up to above 60% ate the highest TNF-α concentration.

By western blot, we observed that after 72 h of treatment with TNF-α at 20 ng/mL, the protein levels of Snail and N-Cadherin increased by 2.2- and 5.4- fold in comparison to the untreated control group, respectively. Moreover, the levels of Slug and Vimentin were increased by around 1.1-fold, whereas the protein level of beta-catenin was increased by 1.2-fold (**Figure 3**).

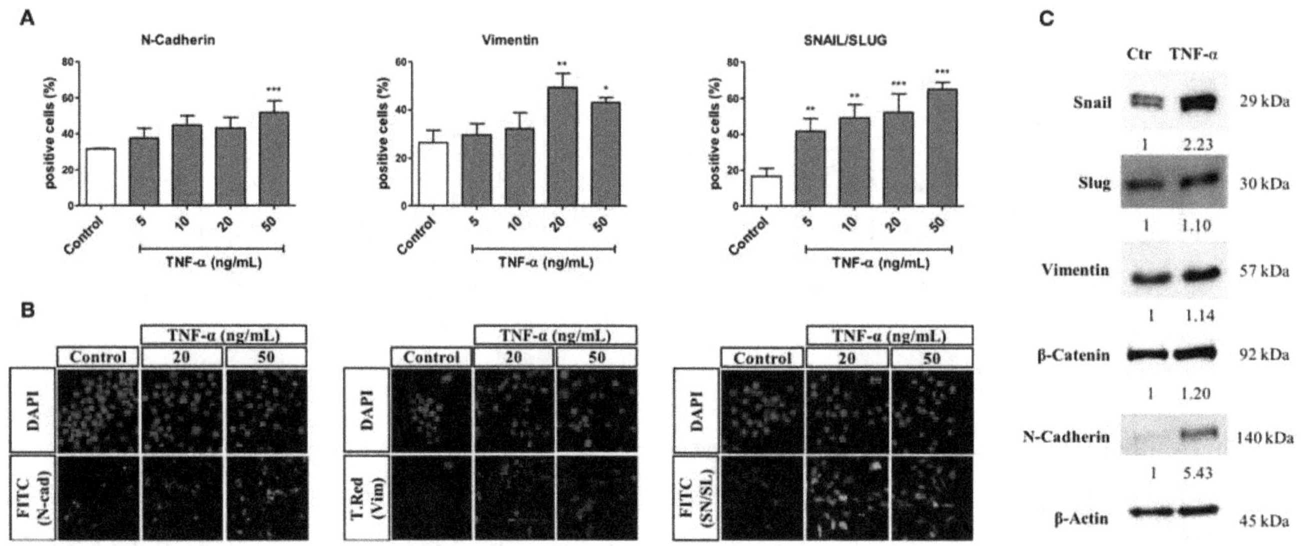

FIGURE 3 | Effects of TNF-α in the expression of EMT-related proteins. The FADU cell line was stimulated or not (Control) with TNF-α (5 to 50 ng/mL), for 72 h, followed by analyses of EMT-related protein levels by immunostaining or western blot. After immunostaining using antibodies against N-cadherin (N-cad), Vimentin (Vim) and Snail/Slug (SN/SL), cells were co-stained with nuclear (Hoechst) and cytoplasmic (CellMask) fluorescent dyes. Images (nine fields per well) were acquired using a 10X objective and excitation/emission filters DAPI (Hoechst), FITC (N-Cadherin and SN/SL), and Texas Red (T.Red; Vimentin), using an ImageXpress Micro XLS HCS system (Molecular Devices). Images were analyzed using MetaXpress, in order to evaluate the percentage of cells positive for each protein in the nucleus or cytoplasm. For western blot, protein detection was achieved using antibodies against Snail, Slug, Vimentin, beta-catenin and N-Cadherin. **(A)** Nuclear or cytoplasmic quantitative changes (Mean +-SD) in protein levels of N-Cadherin, Vimentin and Snail/Slug, as evaluated by immunofluorescence. **(B)** Representative images of stained cells stimulated with TNF-α at 20 and 50 ng/mL. **(C)** Alterations (fold change) in the protein levels of Snail, Slug, Vimentin, beta-catenin and N-Cadherin, as evaluated by western blot after 72 h of TNF-α stimulation (20 ng/mL). Statistically significant differences (ONE-WAY Anova with Tukey post-test), in comparison to the control condition: $^{*}p < 0.05$; $^{**}p < 0.01$; $^{***}p < 0.001$.

Tumor Necrosis Factor Alpha Stimulation Induces Cell Migration

A migration assay was performed in cells treated with mitomycin C and primed with TNF-α at different concentrations, for 72 h. Stimulation with TNF-α at 20 and 50 ng/mL increased the migratory capacity of FADU cells by around 30 and 20%, respectively (**Figure 4**).

HCS-Based miR Screening Identifies miRs With Distinct Effects on Cell Survival and EMT

An HCS-based functional assay was performed in cells transfected with our library of miRs ($N = 31$), followed by priming with TNF-α (20 ng/mL) for 72 h, in order to evaluate changes on morphometric parameters and Snail/Slug levels/localization. We identified miRs that altered cell survival (nuclei count) and EMT-related features including nuclear Snail/Slug levels and morphometric parameters such as cellular/nuclear area, eccentricity and cell distancing relative to the miR negative control. After unsupervised hierarchical clustering, miRs were distributed into three main groups (G1, G2, and G3). Based on distinct alterations in cell survival (nuclei count), G1 was further subdivided into the subgroups G1a and G1b.

MiRs from G3 led to a pro-survival and anti-EMT effect, as seemed by increase in cell survival and epithelial phenotype: tightly packed juxtaposed (higher number of neighboring cells and percentage of touching) round cells (lower eccentricity and higher solidity) with low nuclear Snail/Slug levels. In contrast, the subgroup G1b had the exact opposite phenotypic features (anti-survival and pro-EMT), with low cell counts, high Snail/Slug intensity and interspersed cells with mesenchymal phenotype (high eccentricity and low solidity). Since a higher cell density by itself excerpts a strong inhibitory effect on EMT, while a lower cell density is able to promote it (32), G1b and G3 are hereafter referred as anti-survival and pro-survival miR groups, respectively.

The subgroup G1a promoted cell survival while increasing nuclear Snail/Slug levels and morphological EMT-related features comparable to that of G1b; thus, clearly displaying a pro-survival/EMT effect. Otherwise, miRs from G2 had the strongest negative impact on survival while some of its members were still capable of reducing or preventing the increase of cell eccentricity or nuclear Snail/Slug levels, thereby displaying a anti-survival/EMT effect (**Figure 5**).

Anti-survival/EMT miRs Target Inflammatory-Associated Pathways

After identifying the genes collectively targeted by the miRs from G1a, G1b, G2, and G3, we eliminated targets shared by groups that led to opposite phenotypic effects. Thereby,

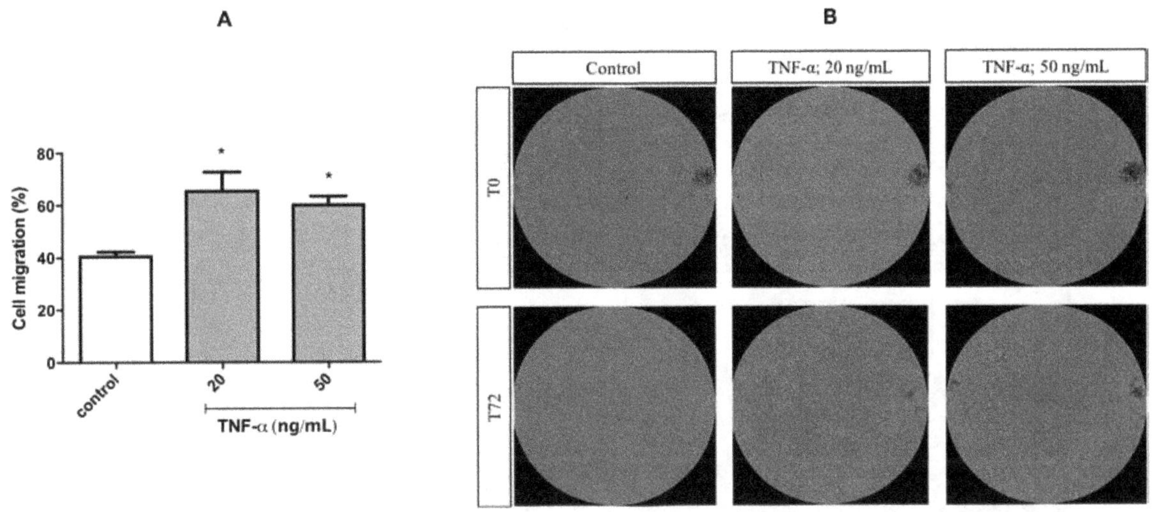

FIGURE 4 | Cell migration of FADU cells following stimulation with TNF-α. The FADU cell line was cultured for 24 h in cell culture plates designed for migration assays, treated with mitomycin for 2 h (to inhibit cell proliferation) and stimulated or not (Control) with TNF-α at 20 or 50 ng/mL for 72 h. Phase-contrast transmitted light images were acquired, with an ImageXpress Micro XLS HCS system (Molecular Devices), using a 4X objective. With aid of CellProfiler, cell migration was quantified based on the percentage of increase in the area occupied by cells. **(A)** Percentage of cell migration after 72 h (Mean +-SD). **(B)** Representative images of different experimental conditions at initial time (T0) and after 72 h (T72). Statistically significant differences (ONE-WAY Anova with Tukey post-test), in comparison to the control condition: $^{*}p < 0.05$.

targets shared between G1a (pro-survival/EMT) and G2 (anti-survival/EMT), as well as G1b (anti-survival) and G3 (pro-survival) were eliminated from further analyses as they were considered not relevant for the phenotypic effects driven by the groups of miRs (**Supplementary File 2**). Then, the filtered targets were used for enrichment analysis on signaling pathways and biological processes (**Supplementary File 3**). Strikingly, we found that miRs from both G1b (anti-survival) and G2 (anti-survival/EMT) targeted inflammatory pathways including "TNF signaling pathway (G1b)" and "Toll-like receptor signaling pathway (G2)" and shared targets from the following pathways: NF-κB *(IKBKG);* PI3K/AKT (*AKT2*), and MAPK (*MAPK9*). Moreover, we found that miRs from G2 also targeted additional genes (not found in G1b) from the NF-κB and PI3K/AKT pathways including *RELA* and *PIK3R3*, respectively. Finally, the Wnt/beta catenin signaling pathway was also found to be enriched with targets from G2. The miRs from G2 (anti-survival/EMT) and its targets from the NF-κB, PI3K/AKT, and Wnt/beta-catenin signaling pathways were used to generate a microRNA regulatory network (**Figure 6**).

Anti-survival/EMT miRs Reduce the Transcript Levels of Their Direct and Indirect Targets

We evaluated the capacity of three miRs with anti-survival/EMT effects (miR-29b-3p, miR-302a-3p, and miR-372-3p) to reduce the transcript levels of direct predicted targets, as well as indirect downstream transcriptional targets. Overall, with the exception of *CCND1* (an indirect target of the miRs), the targets were downregulated by most of the miRs among the cell lines, however a stronger effect and less variability were observed on the FADU cell line. More specifically, we observed a reduction on the expression levels of the direct target *AKT2*, with the exception of miR-372 (on FADU) and miR-302a (on HN30 and UMSCC1). The same was observed for the direct target *RELA*, with the exception of miR-29b (on HN30 and UMSCC1) and miR-372 (on HN30 and UMSCC1). As for the indirect targets, *MYC* was downregulated with the exception of miR-372 (on FADU) and miR-29b (on HN30 and UMSCC1). Finally, *IL6* was also downregulated by the miRs, with the exception of miR-29b (on FADU), and miR-372 (on HN30 and UMSCC1) (**Figure 7**).

Interferences in Signaling Pathways Targeted by Anti-survival/EMT miRs Partially Recapitulate Their Effects

HCS-based functional assays were done in cells transfected with siRNAs against elements of signaling pathways regulated by the anti-survival/EMT miRs: *RELA* (siRELA, NF-κB pathway), *AKT1* (siAKT1, PI3K/AKT pathway), and *CTNNB1* (siCTNNB1, Wnt/beta-catenin signaling pathway), besides a non-targeting control siRNA (siCTR) and cytotoxic siRNA (siUBC), followed or not by stimulation with TNF-α.

After 72 h of TNF-α stimulation, siRNA-mediated knockdown of *RELA* transcripts led to an expressive reduction in cell number (count nuclei) and number of neighboring cells, while increased cell eccentricity. Silencing the expression of *AKT1* (of high homology with *AKT2*, target of G2) led to a discrete reduction in cell number, while increased cell area and significantly reduced nuclear and cytoplasmic levels of Snail/Slug. Finally, knockdown of *CTNNB1* significantly reduced cell number, cytoplasmic levels

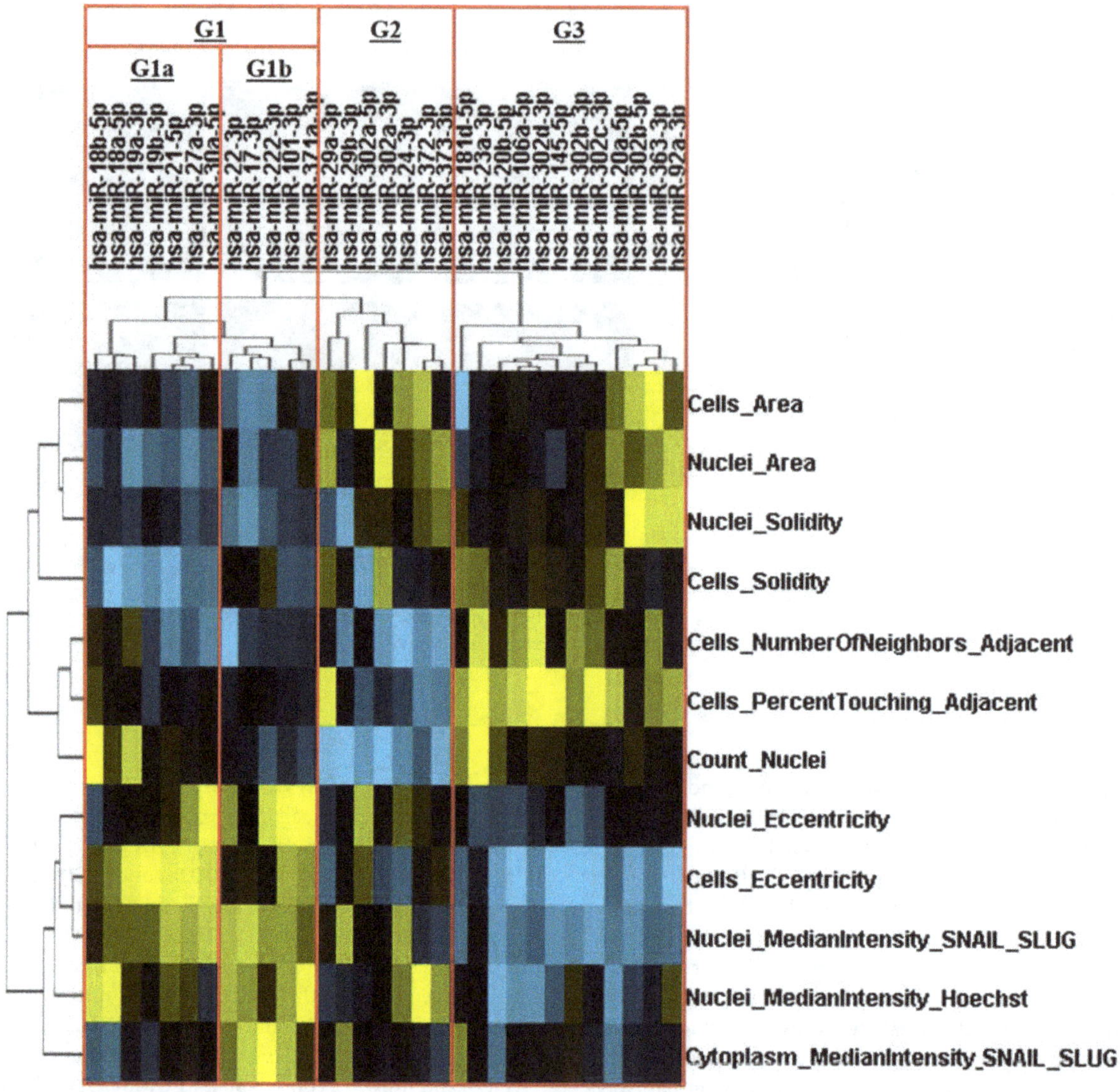

FIGURE 5 | Hierarchical clustering of miRs based on their effects on multiparametric phenotypic alterations. The FADU cell line was transfected with human miRs mimics, for 24 h, followed by stimulation with TNF-α (20 ng/mL) for 72 h. After immunostaining with antibodies against Snail/Slug (SN/SL) and co-staining with nuclear (Hoechst) and cytoplasmic (CellMask) dyes, images were acquired with an ImageXpress Micro XLS HCS system (Molecular Devices), using a 10X objective and excitation/emission filters DAPI (Hoechst), FITC (SN/SL), and Cy5 (CellMask Deep Red). With aid of CellProfiler, we evaluated several morphometric parameters, besides cell quantity (count nuclei) and the presence/location of Snail/Slug. Multiparametric phenotypic profiles, describing the effects of each miR, were obtained and subjected to an unsupervised hierarchical cluster analysis. Heatmap showing the multiparametric phenotypic profiles induced by each miR, and the four groups of miRs identified (G1a, G1b, G2, and G3. Red rectangles). Increase and decrease relative to PMC are depicted in yellow and blue, respectively.

of Snail/Slug and number of neighboring cells, while increased cell area and eccentricity.

Without TNF-α stimulation, the knockdown of the selected targets led to a reduction in cell counts as early as 24 h post-transfection, especially on cells transfected with siRELA, in which the impact was comparable to siUBC (a cytotoxic siRNA). At the same time point, the percentage of apoptotic cells (positive for cleaved caspase-7) transfected with siRELA and siAKT1 was around 25% higher than the control group (10%) but was unaltered on cells transfected with siCTNNB1, which also reduced the cell number. After 48 h of siRNA transfection, in comparison to 24 h after transfection, the number of cells in the control condition had almost doubled (indicating cell proliferation), while only slightly increasing in cells transfected with siAKT1 and siCTNNB1 and further decreasing in cells transfected with siRELA and siUBC. The percentage of apoptotic cells slightly decreased in cells transfected with siAKT1, while increased in cells transfected with siCTNNB1 (although not attaining significance), siRELA and siUBC (**Figure 8**).

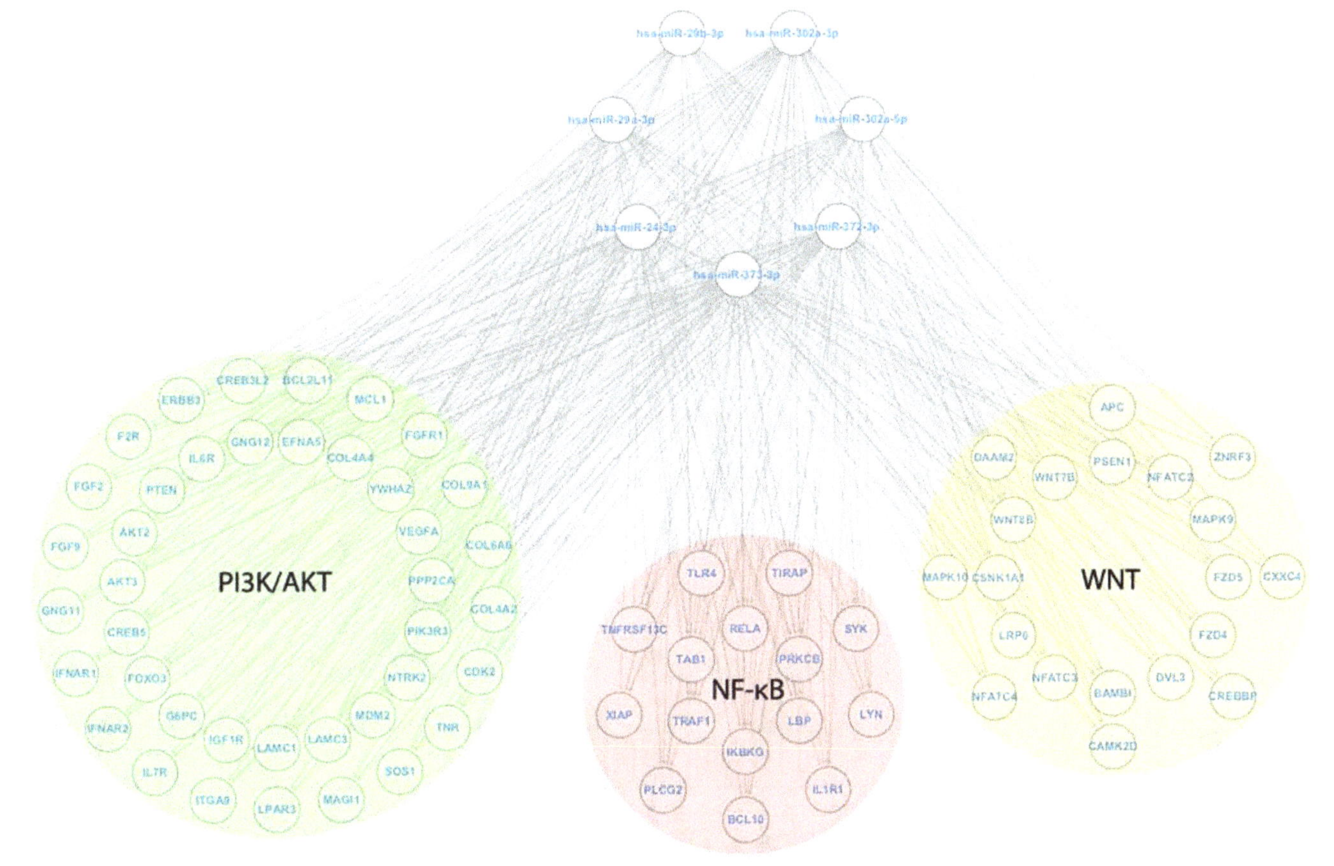

FIGURE 6 | MicroRNA Regulatory network with miRs from the anti-survival/EMT group. A microRNA regulatory network was composed of miRs from the anti-survival/EMT group, along with their targets from the PI3K/AKT (Green circle), NF-κB (Red circle), and Wnt (Yellow circle) signaling pathways. For each pathway, targets from the outer portion of the circle are the ones targeted by no more than 5 miRs, whereas the ones from the inside portion of the circle are the ones targeted by more than 5 miRs (maximum of 7). The following genes are shared between the signaling pathways NF-κB and PI3K/AKT: *IKBKG*, *RELA*, *SYK*, and *TLR4*; NF-κB and WNT: *PRKCB*.

DISCUSSION

Many of the functional studies conducted so far about the impact of small molecules in cancer cell survival disregards the presence of an inflammatory microenvironment, which is known to promote apoptosis resistance, epithelial to mesenchymal transition, among other phenotypic changes that promotes therapy resistance and disease recurrence (7).With that in mind, our study aimed to identify, through functional assays using an HCS approach, miRs and signaling pathways with the potential to suppress both cell survival and EMT features in HNSCC cells considering the presence of an inflammatory microenvironment. This approach should provide evidence if the effect of previously studied miRs translates or not to cancer cells under inflammatory stimuli, as well as to describe the effect of miRs with no known effect in HNSCC cells so far.

Initially, we demonstrated the capacity of TNF-α to promote a broad spectrum of phenotypic changes characterizing EMT, including an increase in nuclear expression of Snail/Slug, mesenchymal markers N-Cadherin and Vimentin, as well as cell eccentricity, inter-cell distancing and cell migration. Interestingly, our results of the western blot assay indicate that Snail, rather than Slug, might be involved in the induction of EMT driven by stimulation with TNF-α. Moreover, the increased levels of beta-catenin after stimulation with TNF-α also indicates a possible role, in our model, for the Wnt/beta-catenin pathway for the induction of EMT. Based on our observations, we concluded that the treatment of cells with TNF-α at 20 ng/mL is the best option to induce FADU cells to EMT, as it promoted strong changes in all parameters evaluated, as well as a superior induction to cell migration in comparison to a higher concentration.

Next, by performing an HCS-based miR screening, we investigated the capacity of 31 human miR mimics to alter phenotypic features related to cell survival and EMT in FADU cells induced to EMT by TNF-α stimulation. Overall, the results from this screening led us to identify four groups of miRs, namely G1a, G1b, G2, and G3, with distinct activity in promoting/inhibiting cell survival and EMT. Among them, two groups had characteristics of oncomiRs: G1a (pro-survival/EMT)

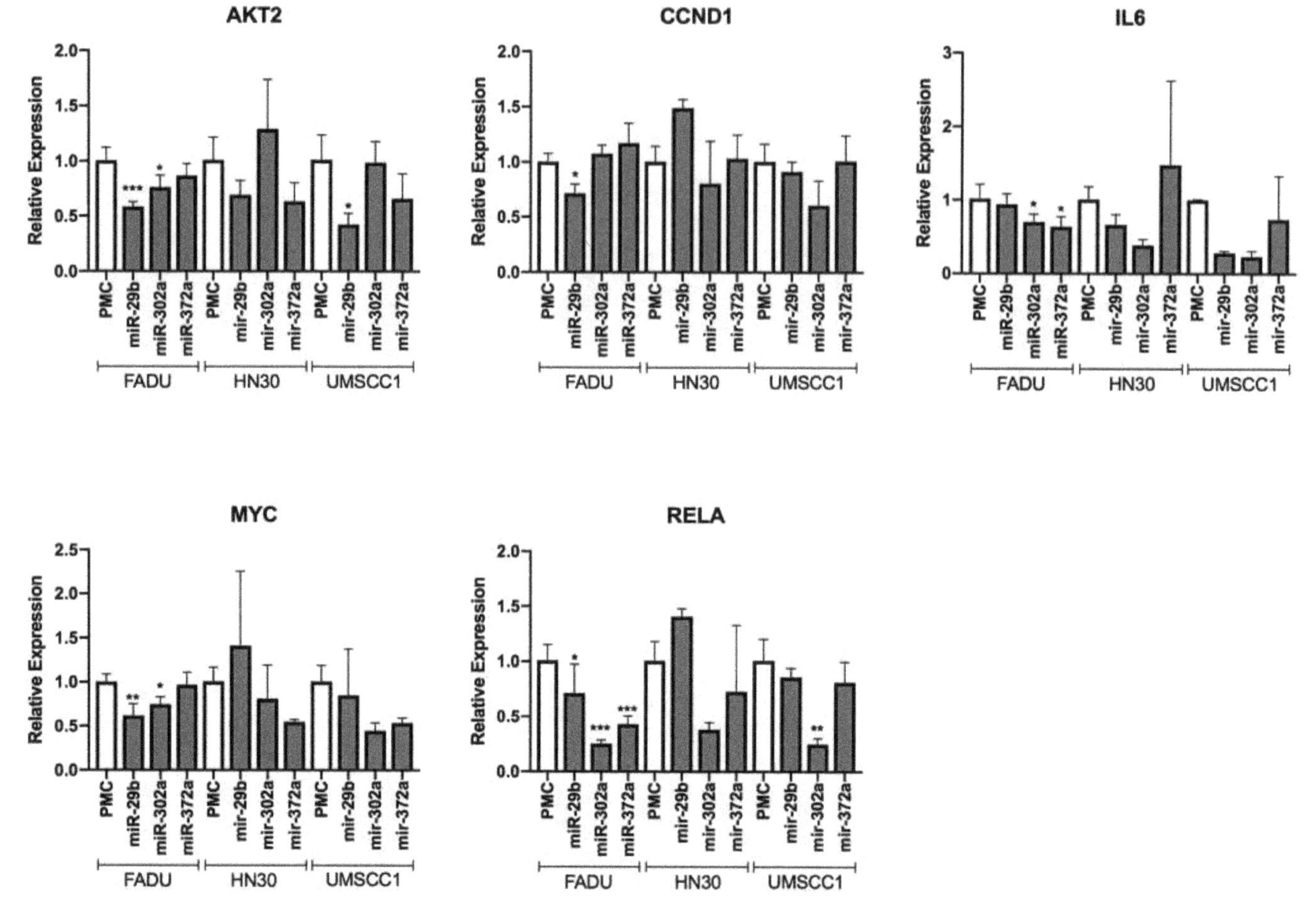

FIGURE 7 | Changes in the transcript levels of direct and indirect targets of anti-survival/EMT miR group following miR transfection. The cell lines FADU, HN30, and UMSCC1 were transfected with PMC (control) or miR mimics from G2 (miR-29b-3p, miR-302a-3p, and miR-372), followed by TNF-α stimulation (20 ng/mL) for 48 h and qPCR with primers for *AKT2*, *CCND1* (cyclin D1), *IL6*, *MYC*, and *RELA*. Alterations in relative gene expression levels, relative to cells transfected with miR-CTR (PMC). Statistically significant differences (*t*-test), in comparison to the reference control group (PMC): $^{*}p < 0.05$; $^{**}p < 0.01$; $^{***}p < 0.001$.

and G3 (pro-survival) whereas the two remaining groups had characteristics of tumor suppressor miRs: G1b (anti-survival) and G2 (anti-survival/EMT). Noteworthy, G1b (anti-survival) also excerpted an pro-EMT effect, while G3 (pro-survival) excerpted a anti-EMT effect, however, as the effects of G1b and G3 in EMT could be a byproduct (i.e., secondary effect) of their alterations in cell survival, those groups were not classified regarding their alterations in EMT (32).

Among the miRs from G1b (anti-survival), it was previously found that miR-101 is downregulated in HNSCC tissues from different anatomical sites, besides having an anti-survival effect on HNSCC cell lines, including FADU (33–35). Additionally, studies conducted with esophageal squamous cell carcinoma (ESCC)-derived cell lines subjected to the ectopic expression of miR-22 (also from G1b) observed a reduction in cell survival and migratory/invasive potential (36, 37). On the other hand, the pro-survival group G3 was mainly composed by miRs from miR-302-367 cluster, which are traditionally associated with pluripotency and malignancy of germ cells tumors (38, 39). In the context of head and neck cancer, overexpression of miR-302a and miR-302b was found in cells derived from HNSCC with characteristics of cancer stem cells including self-renewal and the ability to generate heterogeneous cell populations (40).

The pro-survival/EMT G1a was composed of miRs that are traditionally involved in regulatory mechanisms linking inflammation and tumor progression, including elements of the miR-17-92 cluster, miR-21 (a HNSCC oncomiR) and miR-23a/24/27a cluster (41). Interestingly, Chang and coworkers also observed a pro-survival activity of miR-21, as well as increased expression of miR-21 in primary HNSCC compared to mucosal controls (42). Moreover, in the recent meta-analysis study performed by Lubov et al., it was observed that an increased expression of miR-21 is associated with poor outcome in HNSCC (14). Differently from G1a, G2 (anti-survival/EMT) was composed of miRs from miR-29 family, which displays tumor suppressor activity in several types of cancer, including HNSCC (14, 43). In line with our results, Kinoshita and coworkers observed that the ectopic expression of elements from the mir-29

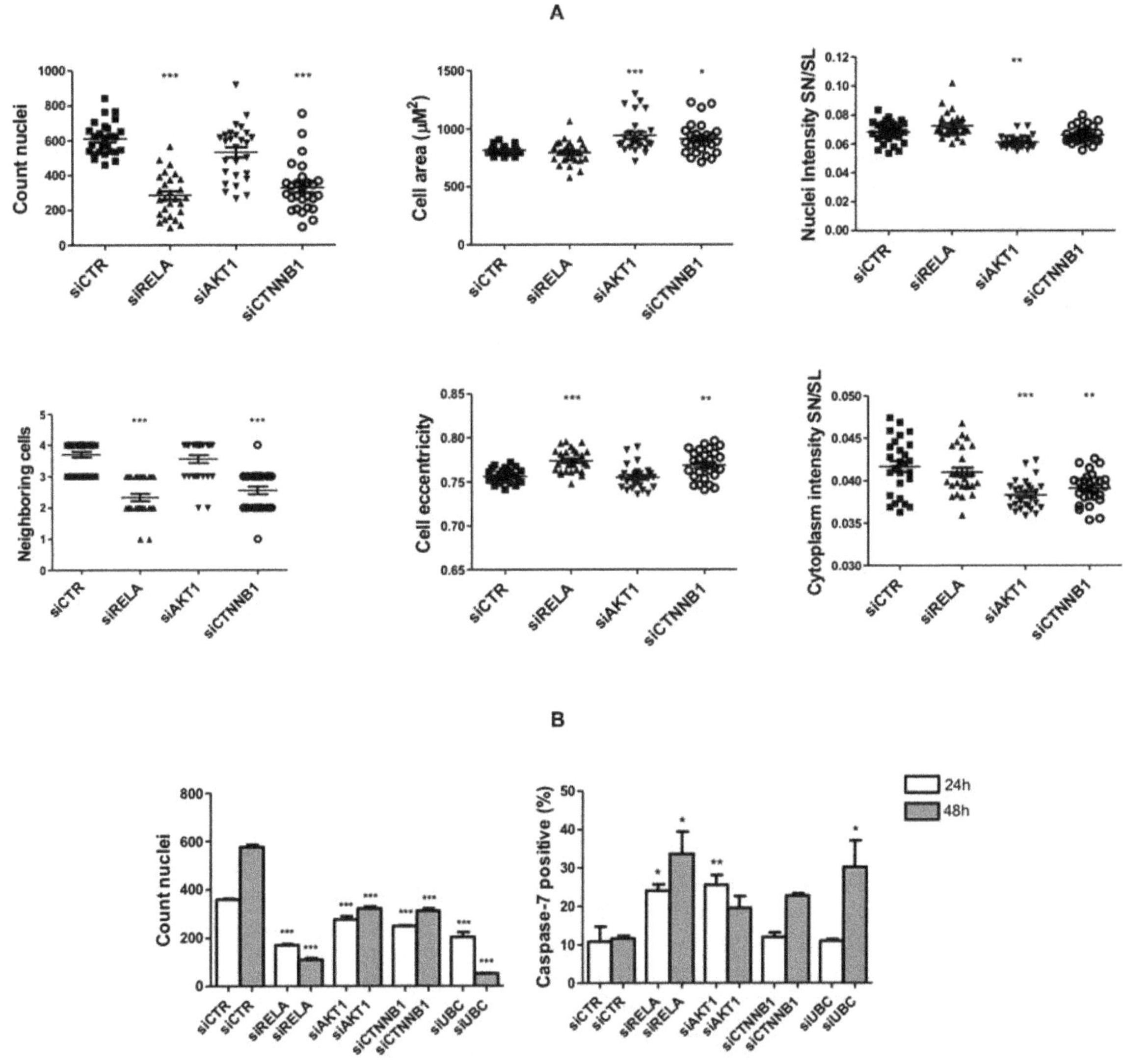

FIGURE 8 | Changes in cell survival and EMT upon interferences in signaling pathways targeted by the anti-survival/EMT group. The FADU cell line was transfected with siRNAs specific for *RELA*, *AKT1*, *CTNNB1*, cytotoxic siUBC, and unspecific siRNA control (siCTR), followed or not by TNF-α stimulation. At the endpoint, images were acquired with an ImageXpress Micro XLS HCS system (Molecular Devices), using a 10X objective and excitation/emission filters DAPI (Hoechst), FITC (SN/SL) and Cy5 (CellMask Deep Red). **(A)** Cells were stimulated for 72 h with TNF-α (20 ng/mL), starting 24 h post-transfection, followed by immunostaining with antibodies against Snail/Slug (SN/SL) and co-staining with nuclear (Hoechst) and cytoplasmic (CellMask) dyes. Alterations in morphometric parameters, cell counts and nuclear/cytoplasmic Snail/Slug due to siRNA transfection as observed after image analysis. **(B)** 24 and 48 h after transfection, cells without TNF-α stimulation were immunostained with antibodies against cleaved Caspase-7 and co-stained with nuclear (Hoechst) and cytoplasmic (CellMask) dyes. Cell counts and percentage of apoptotic cells positive for active caspase-7 as observed after image analysis. Statistically significant differences (ONE-WAY Anova with Tukey post-test), in comparison to the control condition: $^{*}p < 0.05$; $^{**}p < 0.01$; $^{***}p < 0.001$.

family in the FADU cell line resulted in a significant reduction in cell number, as well as in cell migration and invasion (44).

In an effort to identify, among the several targets and signaling pathways regulated by miRs, those that effectively contributed to the observed phenotypic effect, we excluded from further analyses genes that were commonly targeted by groups of miRs that led to opposite phenotypes. Those filtered targets were used in *in silico* enrichment analysis, leading to the identification of specific targets and targeted signaling pathways. Noteworthy, this strategy provided cues on the genes and signaling pathways to be explored to suppress HNSCC tumor growth and metastasis.

By following this strategy, we observed that miRs from G1b (anti-survival) and G2 (anti-survival/EMT) targeted signaling pathways that are associated with the interface between inflammation and tumor initiation/progression, including MAPK, PI3K/AKT and NF-κB pathways (45). However, in comparison to predicted targets from G1b, it was found that miRs from G2 interfered in the PI3K/AKT and NF-κB pathways in a more extensive manner, also targeting a regulatory subunit of PI3K (PIK3R3), a oncogene that regulates AKT activity, as well as *RELA*, which codes for the canonical subunit (p65) of the NF-κB transcription factor (46, 47). Moreover, miRs from G2 also targeted several elements of the Wnt/beta-catenin signaling pathway. Altogether, our results from *in silico* analyses provided evidence that the anti-survival/EMT effects elicited by miRs from G2 likely derives from an extensive perturbation in PI3K/AKT and NF-κB pathways, besides Wnt signaling pathway. Additionally, by evaluating alterations in gene expression levels of cells transfected with miRs from G2 (anti-survival/EMT) group, we confirmed that elements from the following targeted signaling pathways: NF-κB (*RELA* and *IL6*), PI3K/AKT (*AKT2*), as well as Wnt/beta-catenin (*MYC*) were downregulated after the transfection in most cases.

Additional functional assays were performed with siRNAs against genes from the following signaling pathways regulated by anti-survival/EMT group (G2): *AKT1* (PI3K/AKT pathway); *RELA* (NF-κB pathway); and *CTNNB1* (Wnt pathway) followed or not by stimulation with TNF-α. Noteworthy, though *AKT1* and *CTNNB1* are not directly targeted by the miRs from G2, their use is justified by the central role of those genes in regulating the PI3K/AKT and Wnt/beta-catenin pathways, respectively, which were extensively targeted by those miRs. Therefore, results from our functional assays using siRNAs should not be interpreted as direct link between anti-survival/EMT miRs and a specific target, but rather between miRs and targeted signaling pathways. An exception are observations from siRELA transfections, as *RELA* is not only a central gene in the NF-κB pathway but also a direct target of G2.

By stimulating cells with TNF-α after siRNA transfection, we sought to investigate the individual role of NF-κB, PI3K/AKT, and Wnt/beta-catenin signaling pathways on either cell survival or EMT considering the presence of an inflammatory microenvironment. Interestingly, we found that although gene silencing of *RELA* and *CTNNB1* led to an anti-survival effect whereas silencing *AKT1* led to an anti-EMT effect, none of the siRNAs alone impaired both cell survival and EMT, which indicates that the effects of anti-survival/EMT miRs are most likely due to their potential to interfere in multiple signaling pathways simultaneously. This possibility points out to the potential benefits of a multi-target approach to treat HNSCC, especially considering that so far, clinical trials evaluating the capacity of PI3K inhibitors to treat HNSCC have shown disappointing results (48). In line, a recent study by Li et al. demonstrated that co-targeting EGFR (upstream of PI3K/AKT) and NF-κB pathways led to a superior inhibition of cell survival and xenograph tumor growth, when compared to targeting either pathway alone (49).

By not stimulating cells with TNF-α after siRNA transfection, we aimed to evaluate if the effects coming from the interferences in NF-κB, PI3K/AKT, and Wnt/beta-catenin signaling pathways are influenced by the presence of an inflammatory microenvironment. Additionally, we investigated if effects on cell survival are due to alterations in apoptosis by evaluating the percentage of cells positive for cleaved caspase-7. Strikingly, we found that transfection with siRELA not only dramatically reduced the number of cells but also strongly induced cell-death by apoptosis after 24 h and 48 h. This indicates that interferences in the NF-κB pathway is deleterious to HNSCC cells regardless of stimulation with inflammatory factors. Interestingly, transfection with siAKT1 also followed a similar pattern (although not further increasing apoptosis at 48 h) revealing that an inflammatory stimulation exerts a protective effect on HNSCC cells against the deleterious effect of interferences in the PI3K/AKT pathway. Moreover, although transfection with siCTNNB1 reduced cell count, it did not enhance the number of apoptotic cells 24 h post-transfection, indicating a more prominent role of Wnt signaling toward cell proliferation regardless of TNF-α stimulation.

As a whole, our study identified several molecules that may have the potential to be used for prognosis or miR-based targeted therapies against HNSCC considering the presence of an inflammatory microenvironment. By further investigating the miRs with anti-survival/EMT effects, we found that interferences in the signaling pathways: NF-κB and Wnt/beta-catenin were the ones that most likely contributed for the anti-survival effect, whereas interferences in PI3K/AKT signaling pathway was most likely associated with anti-EMT effect. Future studies using *in vivo* models should shed light into the anti-tumor and anti-metastatic activity of the miRs and targets herein identified.

CONCLUSION

The present work characterized the functional role of a set of human miRs in modulating a broad spectrum of phenotypic alterations related to HNSCC cell survival and EMT in cells under an inflammatory stimulation, as well as the potentially involved signaling pathways. More specifically, the following miR mimetics: miR-24-3p, miR-29a-3p, miR-29b-3p, miR-302a-3p, miR-302a-5p, miR-372-3p, and miR-373-3p were identified as the ones with greatest potential use in microRNA replacement therapies, as they displayed an anti-survival/EMT effect. On the other hand, endogenous miRs herein identified as with pro-survival/EMT effects: miR-18a-5p, miR-18b-5p, miR-19a-3p, miR-19b-3p, miR-21-5p, miR-27a-3p, miR-30a-5p, were identified as the ones with greatest potential use in microRNA inhibition therapies. Additionally, we found that together, interferences on NF-κB, PI3K/AKT, and Wnt/beta-catenin signaling pathways are the ones that most likely driven the anti-survival/EMT effects displayed by miRs. Individual gene silencing of components of those pathways, namely *RELA* (NF-κB), *AKT1* (PI3K/AKT), and *CTNNB1* (Wnt/beta-catenin), partially recapitulated the effects displayed by miRs with anti-survival/EMT effects. Our findings revealed miRs and signaling pathways that might be explored to fight HNSCC tumor growth and metastasis considering the presence an inflammatory microenvironment.

AUTHOR CONTRIBUTIONS

BS, WA, VF, DC, MZ, and RP: study concept. BS, FS, and RP: study design. BS, FS, IM, JS, RP, AC, and CT: data acquisition, analysis, and interpretation. BS: statistical analysis. BS and RP:

manuscript preparation and editing. BS, WA, VF, DC, MZ, and RP: manuscript review.

FUNDING

This work was supported by São Paulo Research Foundation (FAPESP), grants #2013/08135-2 (Center for Cell-Based Therapy - CTC) and #2015/08070-3 (Scholarship for Research Abroad - BPE, RP); and by the National Council for Scientific and Technological Development (CNPq).

REFERENCES

1. Torre LA, Bray F, Siegel RL, Ferlay J, Lortet-Tieulent J, Jemal A. Global cancer statistics, 2012. *CA Cancer J Clin.* (2015) 65:87–108. doi: 10.3322/caac.21262
2. Allen CT, Law JH, Dunn GP, Uppaluri R. Emerging insights into head and neck cancer metastasis. *Head Neck.* (2013) 35:1669–78. doi: 10.1002/hed.23202
3. Massague J, Obenauf AC. Metastatic colonization by circulating tumour cells. *Nature.* (2016) 529:298–306. doi: 10.1038/nature17038
4. Lamouille S, Xu J, Derynck R. Molecular mechanisms of epithelial-mesenchymal transition. *Nat Rev Mol Cell Biol.* (2014) 15:178–96. doi: 10.1038/nrm3758
5. Singh M, Yelle N, Venugopal C, Singh SK. EMT: mechanisms and therapeutic implications. *Pharmacol Ther.* (2018) 182:80–94. doi: 10.1016/j.pharmthera.2017.08.009
6. Gao F, Liang B, Reddy ST, Farias-Eisner R, Su X. Role of inflammation-associated microenvironment in tumorigenesis and metastasis. *Curr Cancer Drug Targets.* (2014) 14:30–45. doi: 10.2174/15680096113136660107
7. Suarez-Carmona M, Lesage J, Cataldo D, Gilles C. EMT and inflammation: inseparable actors of cancer progression. *Mol Oncol.* (2017) 11:805–23. doi: 10.1002/1878-0261.12095
8. Wu Y, Zhou BP. TNF-alpha/NF-kappaB/Snail pathway in cancer cell migration and invasion. *Br J Cancer.* (2010) 102:639–44. doi: 10.1038/sj.bjc.6605530
9. Matta A, Ralhan R. Overview of current and future biologically based targeted therapies in head and neck squamous cell carcinoma. *Head Neck Oncol.* (2009) 1:6. doi: 10.1186/1758-3284-1-6
10. Hoesel B, Schmid JA. The complexity of NF-kappaB signaling in inflammation and cancer. *Mol Cancer.* (2013) 12:86. doi: 10.1186/1476-4598-12-86
11. Holohan C, Van Schaeybroeck S, Longley DB, Johnston PG. Cancer drug resistance: an evolving paradigm. *Nat Rev Cancer.* (2013) 13:714–26. doi: 10.1038/nrc3599
12. Bartel DP. MicroRNAs: target recognition and regulatory functions. *Cell.* (2009) 136:215–33. doi: 10.1016/j.cell.2009.01.002
13. Shalgi R, Brosh R, Oren M, Pilpel Y, Rotter V. Coupling transcriptional and post-transcriptional miRNA regulation in the control of cell fate. *Aging.* (2009) 1:762–70. doi: 10.18632/aging.100085
14. Lubov J, Maschietto M, Ibrahim I, Mlynarek A, Hier M, Kowalski LP, et al. Meta-analysis of microRNAs expression in head and neck cancer: uncovering association with outcome and mechanisms. *Oncotarget.* (2017) 8:55511–24. doi: 10.18632/oncotarget.19224
15. Pradhan AK, Emdad L, Das SK, Sarkar D, Fisher PB. The enigma of miRNA regulation in cancer. *Adv Cancer Res.* (2017) 135:25–52. doi: 10.1016/bs.acr.2017.06.001
16. Markopoulos GS, Roupakia E, Tokamani M, Alabasi G, Sandaltzopoulos R, Marcu KB, et al. Roles of NF-kappaB Signaling in the regulation of miRNAs impacting on inflammation in cancer. *Biomedicines.* (2018) 6:E40. doi: 10.3390/biomedicines6020040
17. Castilho RM, Squarize CH, Almeida LO. Epigenetic modifications and head and neck cancer: implications for tumor progression and resistance to therapy. *Int J Mol Sci.* (2017) 18:E1506. doi: 10.3390/ijms18071506
18. Bhome R, Del Vecchio F, Lee GH, Bullock MD, Primrose JN, Sayan AE, et al. Exosomal microRNAs (exomiRs): Small molecules with a big role in cancer. *Cancer Lett.* (2018) 420:228–35. doi: 10.1016/j.canlet.2018.02.002
19. Chakraborty C, Sharma AR, Sharma G, Sarkar BK, Lee SS. The novel strategies for next-generation cancer treatment: miRNA combined with chemotherapeutic agents for the treatment of cancer. *Oncotarget.* (2018) 9:10164–74. doi: 10.18632/oncotarget.24309
20. Lindenbergh-van der Plas M, Martens-de Kemp SR, de Maaker M, van Wieringen WN, Ylstra B, Agami R, et al. Identification of lethal microRNAs specific for head and neck cancer. *Clin Cancer Res.* (2013) 19:5647–57. doi: 10.1158/1078-0432.CCR-12-2295
21. Haefliger B, Prochazka L, Angelici B, Benenson Y. Precision multidimensional assay for high-throughput microRNA drug discovery. *Nat Commun.* (2016) 7:10709. doi: 10.1038/ncomms10709
22. Boutros M, Heigwer F, Laufer C. Microscopy-based high-content screening. *Cell.* (2015) 163:1314–25. doi: 10.1016/j.cell.2015.11.007
23. Serva A, Claas C, Starkuviene V. A potential of microRNAs for high-content screening. *J Nucleic Acids.* (2011) 2011:870903. doi: 10.4061/2011/870903
24. Rupaimoole R, Slack FJ. MicroRNA therapeutics: towards a new era for the management of cancer and other diseases. *Nat Rev Drug Discov.* (2017) 16:203–22. doi: 10.1038/nrd.2016.246
25. de Hoon MJ, Imoto S, Nolan J, Miyano S. Open source clustering software. *Bioinformatics.* (2004) 20:1453–4. doi: 10.1093/bioinformatics/bth078
26. Saldanha AJ. Java Treeview–extensible visualization of microarray data. *Bioinformatics.* (2004) 20:3246–8. doi: 10.1093/bioinformatics/bth349
27. Agarwal V, Bell GW, Nam JW, Bartel DP. Predicting effective microRNA target sites in mammalian mRNAs. *Elife.* (2015) 4:e05005. doi: 10.7554/eLife.05005
28. Huang da W, Sherman BT, Lempicki RA. Systematic and integrative analysis of large gene lists using DAVID bioinformatics resources. *Nat Protoc.* (2009) 4:44–57. doi: 10.1038/nprot.2008.211
29. Kanehisa M, Goto S. KEGG: kyoto encyclopedia of genes and genomes. *Nucleic Acids Res.* (2000) 28:27–30. doi: 10.1093/nar/28.1.27
30. Shannon P, Markiel A, Ozier O, Baliga NS, Wang JT, Ramage D, et al. Cytoscape: a software environment for integrated models of biomolecular interaction networks. *Genome Res.* (2003) 13:2498–504. doi: 10.1101/gr.1239303
31. Livak KJ, Schmittgen TD. Analysis of relative gene expression data using real-time quantitative PCR and the 2(-Delta Delta C(T)) method. *Methods.* (2001) 25:402–8. doi: 10.1006/meth.2001.1262
32. Cichon MA, Nelson CM, Radisky DC. Regulation of epithelial-mesenchymal transition in breast cancer cells by cell contact and adhesion. *Cancer Inform.* (2015) 14:1–13. doi: 10.4137/CIN.S18965
33. Li M, Tian L, Ren H, Chen X, Wang Y, Ge J, et al. MicroRNA-101 is a potential prognostic indicator of laryngeal squamous cell carcinoma and modulates CDK8. *J Transl Med.* (2015) 13:271. doi: 10.1186/s12967-015-0626-6
34. Hui Y, Li Y, Jing Y, Feng JQ, Ding Y. miRNA-101 acts as a tumor suppressor in oral squamous cell carcinoma by targeting CX chemokine receptor 7. *Am J Transl Res.* (2016) 8:4902–11.
35. Wu B, Lei D, Wang L, Yang X, Jia S, Yang Z, et al. MiRNA-101 inhibits oral squamous-cell carcinoma growth and metastasis by targeting zinc finger E-box binding homeobox 1. *Am J Cancer Res.* (2016) 6:1396–407.
36. Yang C, Ning S, Li Z, Qin X, Xu W. miR-22 is down-regulated in esophageal squamous cell carcinoma and inhibits cell migration and invasion. *Cancer Cell Int.* (2014) 14:138. doi: 10.1186/s12935-014-0138-0

37. Qiu K, Huang Z, Huang Z, He Z, You S. miR-22 regulates cell invasion, migration and proliferation *in vitro* through inhibiting CD147 expression in tongue squamous cell carcinoma. *Arch Oral Biol.* (2016) 66:92–7. doi: 10.1016/j.archoralbio.2016.02.013
38. Murray MJ, Nicholson JC, Coleman N. Biology of childhood germ cell tumours, focussing on the significance of microRNAs. *Andrology.* (2015) 3:129–39. doi: 10.1111/andr.277
39. Adlakha YK, Seth P. The expanding horizon of MicroRNAs in cellular reprogramming. *Prog Neurobiol.* (2017) 148:21–39. doi: 10.1016/j.pneurobio.2016.11.003
40. Bourguignon LY, Wong G, Earle C, Chen L. Hyaluronan-CD44v3 interaction with Oct4-Sox2-Nanog promotes miR-302 expression leading to self-renewal, clonal formation, and cisplatin resistance in cancer stem cells from head and neck squamous cell carcinoma. *J Biol Chem.* (2012) 287:32800–24. doi: 10.1074/jbc.M111.308528
41. Tili E, Michaille JJ, Croce CM. MicroRNAs play a central role in molecular dysfunctions linking inflammation with cancer. *Immunol Rev.* (2013) 253:167–84. doi: 10.1111/imr.12050
42. Chang SS, Jiang WW, Smith I, Poeta LM, Begum S, Glazer C, et al. MicroRNA alterations in head and neck squamous cell carcinoma. *Int J Cancer.* (2008) 123:2791–7. doi: 10.1002/ijc.23831
43. Slusarz A, Pulakat L. The two faces of miR-29. *J Cardiovasc Med.* (2015) 16:480–90. doi: 10.2459/JCM.0000000000000246
44. Kinoshita T, Nohata N, Hanazawa T, Kikkawa N, Yamamoto N, Yoshino H, et al. Tumour-suppressive microRNA-29s inhibit cancer cell migration and invasion by targeting laminin-integrin signalling in head and neck squamous cell carcinoma. *Br J Cancer.* (2013) 109:2636–45. doi: 10.1038/bjc.2013.607
45. Raposo TP, Beirao BC, Pang LY, Queiroga FL, Argyle DJ. Inflammation and cancer: till death tears them apart. *Vet J.* (2015) 205:161–74. doi: 10.1016/j.tvjl.2015.04.015
46. Vander Broek R, Mohan S, Eytan DF, Chen Z, Van Waes C. The PI3K/Akt/mTOR axis in head and neck cancer: functions, aberrations, cross-talk, and therapies. *Oral Dis.* (2015) 21:815–25. doi: 10.1111/odi.12206
47. Mitchell S, Vargas J, Hoffmann A. Signaling via the NFkappaB system. *Wiley Interdiscip Rev Syst Biol Med.* (2016) 8:227–41. doi: 10.1002/wsbm.1331
48. Jung K, Kang H, Mehra R. Targeting phosphoinositide 3-kinase (PI3K) in head and neck squamous cell carcinoma (HNSCC). *Cancers Head Neck.* (2018) 3:3. doi: 10.1186/s41199-018-0030-z
49. Li Z, Liao J, Yang Z, Choi EY, Lapidus RG, Liu X, et al. Co-targeting EGFR and IKKbeta/NF-kappaB signalling pathways in head and neck squamous cell carcinoma: a potential novel therapy for head and neck squamous cell cancer. *Br J Cancer.* (2019) 120:306–16. doi: 10.1038/s41416-018-0351-z

5

Nanocarriers of Fe_3O_4 as a Novel Method for Delivery of the Antineoplastic Agent Doxorubicin into HeLa Cells *in vitro*

Kun-kun Xia[1,2†], *Yong Lyu*[2†], *Wei-tang Yuan*[2], *Gui-xian Wang*[2], *Harrison Stratton*[3], *Shui-jun Zhang*[1] *and Jie Wu*[1,3*]

[1] *Department of Hepatobiliary and Pancreatic Surgery, First Affiliated Hospital of Zhengzhou University, Zhengzhou, China,* [2] *Department of Colon and Rectal Surgery, First Affiliated Hospital of Zhengzhou University, Zhengzhou, China,* [3] *Department of Neurobiology, Barrow Neurological Institute, St. Joseph's Hospital and Medical Center, Phoenix, AZ, United States*

***Correspondence:**
Jie Wu
jie.wu@dignityhealth.org;
jiewubni@gmail.com

†*These authors have contributed equally to this work*

Here we report the synthesis and *in vitro* characterization of a redox-sensitive, magnetically inducible nanoparticle carrier system based on the doxorubicin (DOX) drug delivery model. Each quantal nanocarrier unit consists of a magnetite Fe_3O_4 nanoparticle core that is further encapsulated in self-assembled micelles of the redox-responsive polyethylene glycol derivative, DSPE-SS-mPEG. The nanocarrier system was prepared using a combination of ultrasonication and dialysis to produce the microenvironment sensitive delivery system. The final synthesized and DOX-loaded magnetic nanocarriers had an average size of $\sim$150 nm when assembled with a 6.9% DOX payload. The release rate of DOX from these redox-responsive magnetic nanocarriers was shown to be accelerated *in vitro* when in the presence of glutathione (GSH). Furthermore, we demonstrated that more redox-responsive magnetic nanocarriers could be taken up by HeLa cells when a local magnetic field was applied. Once internalized within a cell, the micelles of the outer nanocarrier complex were broken down in the presence of higher concentrations of GSH, which accelerated the release of DOX. This produces a particle with dual operating characteristics that can be controlled via a specific cellular environment coupled with an exogenously applied signal in the form of a magnetic field triggering release.

Keywords: redox-responsive, Fe_3O_4, nanocarriers, drug delivery, HeLa cells

INTRODUCTION

Chemotherapy is the most commonly used approach to treating cancer. Traditionally, the chemotherapeutic agents (doxorubicin, paclitaxel, etc.) are systemically delivered through intravenous injection. While this is often an effective approach and can successfully eliminate malignant cell populations, treatment-associated morbidity is often significant (1). Quite frequently this is a result of unintended action of the therapeutic agent at non-specific cellular targets causing injury to healthy somatic cells in addition to the desired effect on malignant cells (2–6). Despite this large unintended effect on healthy cells of the patient, chemotherapy remains a pillar of cancer treatment due to its efficacy, particularly when used as part of a multimodal treatment plan. At the intersection of the potency of chemotherapy as a curative agent and the extensive side effect profile causing wide-ranging cytotoxicity lays a rationale that suggests transport of the chemotherapeutic agent directly to the tumor site, which avoids systematic exposure, may alleviate unintentional cytotoxic effects on healthy tissue. This concept has existed in the medical literature for quite some time, but only recently has progress in functionalization of mesoscopic carrier particles led to significant progress in realizing this goal. There are now several readily available preparations for a medical oncology approach to cancer treatment that utilizes nanotechnology, in the form of nanoparticle assemblies, to facilitate the transport of highly potent cytotoxic compounds more selectively into tumor sites with restricted systemic circulating concentrations (7–9). These nanoparticles can be constructed such that they resist degradation or internalization except at the target tissue of interest where they are then able to deposit and release their payload at the site of the malignancy and not in healthy tissue (10–12). These particles can also be used to focus energy from external radiative sources into tumor masses acting to physically damage the cancerous cells in addition to the chemical damage affected by the pharmacological agent (13). This is an elegant solution to the problem of how to transport chemotherapeutic drugs to the tumor site without leakage and subsequently release a drug into the tumor-specific microenvironment is an important issue that needs to be solved in the treatment of cancer. The rise of nanotechnology has provided a new set of tools for use in solving this problem of targeted drug delivery (14–17).

The use of nanoparticles as a carrier vehicle for the targeted delivery of chemotherapeutic drugs has the potential to greatly reduce collateral damage to non-cancerous human tissues and organs (18, 19). For example, by modifying the surface of a nanoparticle with intelligent molecules, the nano drug carriers can stimulate drug release in response to the particular micro-environment of pathological tissues to reduce the incidence of healthy cell damage and selectively kill cancer cells (20–22). The study of nano drug carriers provides a new direction for the delivery of care in addition to the traditional cancer treatment approaches already in use and possesses significant potential for future clinical applications (20, 23, 24). In this study, we constructed spherical nanoparticle carriers containing doxorubicin (an antineoplastic drug) with a diameter of about 150 nm. We provide functional data to demonstrate that the entry of the drug carriers into HeLa cells can be enhanced in a magnetic field and the release of the drug can be facilitated by elevating the concentration of glutathione (GSH), resulting in the demise of HeLa cells. As several cancer cells have high intracellular GSH concentrations, using the constructed nanoparticle carriers may achieve satisfying efficacy in killing cancer cells, while causing only minor damage in normal tissue (25–27).

MATERIALS AND METHODS

Materials

The Fe_3O_4 nanoparticles were prepared using a thermal decomposition method described previously (28). DSPE-SS-mPEG 2000 was purchased from Xi'an Ruixi Biotechnology Co. (Xi'an, China), Doxorubicin hydrochloride (DOX·HCl) and GSH were purchased from Sigma-Aldrich (St. Louis, MO, USA), dimethyl sulfoxide (DMSO) and triethylamine (TEA) were obtained from Shanghai Chemical Co. (Shanghai, China) (29).

Human cervical adenocarcinoma (HeLa) cells were purchased from the China Center for Type Culture Collection (Wuhan University) and cultured in Dulbecco's modified Eagle's medium (DMEM, Gibco Life, Grand Island, NY, USA) supplemented with 10% fetal bovine serum (FBS, HyClone, Logan, UT), 2×10^{-3} M L-glutamine and 1% antibiotics mixture (10,000 U of penicillin and 10 mg of streptomycin) (Gibco). The cells were incubated in a humidified atmosphere containing 5% CO_2 at 37°C.

Preparation of Nanocarriers

DOX-loaded redox-responsive magnetic nanocarriers were prepared using an ultrasonication-dialysis method. Briefly, DOX·HCl (10 mg) was stirred in DMSO (5 mL) with twice the number of mole of TEA for 2 h to obtain the DOX base. 80 mg of DSPE-SS-mPEG was added to the solution, which was stirred at room temperature for another 2 h. Meanwhile, the Fe_3O_4 nanoparticles (20 mg) were dissolved in 10 mL of (tetrahydrofuran) THF. The above two solutions were mixed and added to ultrapure water (25 mL) with ultrasonication. The mixed solution was then transferred into a dialysis tube and dialyzed against ultrapure water for 48 h at room temperature. Similarly, DOX-free nanocarriers were prepared using the above mentioned protocol without the addition of DOX.

Characterization of Nanocarriers

The size of the nanocarriers in aqueous solution was measured using a Zetasizer analyzer (Malvern Zetasizer Nano, Zen 3690+MPT2, Malvern, UK). Ultrastructural features and surface geometry of the synthesized nanocarriers was observed by transmission electron microscopy (TEM) (Tecnai G2 F20 S-TWIN electron microscope, FEI company. the USA) at an accelerating voltage of 200 kV.

DOX-loaded nanocarriers were dissolved in DMSO to determine the total content of loaded drug. The DOX content in DMSO was determined by high-performance liquid chromatography (HPLC, Agilent) using a calibration curve obtained from DOX/DMSO solutions containing a known concentration of DOX.

For Fe_3O_4 content measurement, the weighed, freeze-dried nanocarriers were digested in a 1 M HCl solution. The resulting digestion product was then analyzed for atomic species using inductively coupled plasma-atomic emission spectroscopy (TCP-AES, Thermo Electron, USA).

Redox-Triggered Disassembly of Nanocarriers

The change in the size of redox-responsive magnetic nanocarriers in response to 20 mM GSH in PBS (0.01 M, pH 7.4) was measured using dynamic light scattering (DLS). Briefly, 20 mM GSH was added to 1.5 mL of PBS containing nanocarriers within a glass cell. The solution was then placed in a shaking water bath at 37°C, oscillating at 150 rpm. At varying intervals following agitation, the size of nanocarrier particles contained in solution was assessed using DLS.

In vitro Redox-Triggered Release of DOX From DOX-Loaded Nanocarriers

The *in vitro* release profile of nanocarriers was investigated using dialysis of DOX-loaded nanocarriers in two different media: PBS or PBS supplemented with 20 mM GSH. Each solution was diluted to 1.5 mg/mL and 5 mL of the solution was transferred into a membrane tubing. The tubing with the solution was immersed in a tube containing 50 mL of the buffer solution in a shaking water bath at 37°C to acquire the "sink" condition. At predetermined intervals, 20 mL of the external buffer was withdrawn and replaced with a fresh solution of the corresponding buffer. The amount of DOX released was determined using HPLC.

Cell TEM Imaging

For TEM imaging, HeLa cells were incubated with DOX-loaded nanocarriers at a final DOX concentration of 5 μg/mL in DMEM for 2 h at 37°C in the presence or absence of an externally applied magnetic field. The culture medium was removed and the cells were pre-fixed with 2.5% glutaraldehyde in PBS at 4°C for 2 h and post-fixed with 1% osmium tetroxide in PBS at 4°C for 2 h. The cells were then dehydrated using serially increasing concentrations of ethanol and flat embedded in Epon 812. After polymerization at 60°C for 48 h, ultrathin sections (60–80 nm) were trimmed and further stained with uranyl acetate and lead citrate. Micrographs of the stained samples were collected with an FEI Tecnaio G220 TWIN Transmission Electron Microscope.

Cell Viability Assay

To evaluate the anti-tumor activity of DOX-loaded nanocarriers, the cytotoxicity of DOX-loaded nanocarriers or free DOX against HeLa cells was evaluated *in vitro* using the MTT assay. HeLa cells were seeded into a 96-well plate at a density of 4.0×10^3 cells/well in 100 μL of complete DMEM. The cells were cultured for 24 h at 37°C in a 5% CO_2 atmosphere. Subsequently, the cells were incubated with DOX-loaded nanocarriers or free DOX for 24 h at 37°C with or without the presence of an external magnetic field. DOX-loaded nanocarriers or free DOX were diluted in complete DMEM to a final DOX concentration ranging from 0.4 to 40 μg/mL. After the incubation, 10 μL of MTT solution (5 mg/mL in PBS 7.4) was added to each well and incubated for 4 h. The media with MTT solution was removed and 200 μL of DMSO was added to dissolve the formazan crystals and further incubated for 15 min at 37°C. The absorbance readings were recorded using a microplate spectrophotometer (PowerWave XS2, BioTek Instruments, USA) at a wavelength of 540 nm. The cell viability was normalized to that of cells cultured in complete DMEM. The dose-effect curves were plotted and data are presented as the average ± SD ($n = 4$).

Confocal Laser Scanning Microscopy (CLSM) Observation

CLSM was used to examine the intracellular distribution of DOX. HeLa cells were seeded on coverslips in the wells of a 24-well plate at a density of 4.0×10^4 cells/well in 1 mL of complete DMEM. The cells were incubated for 24 h at 37°C in a 5% CO_2 atmosphere. The cells were incubated with DOX-loaded nanocarriers at a final DOX concentration of 5 μg/mL in DMEM for 2 h at 37°C with or without an external magnetic field. After removal of the medium, the cells were washed three times with cold PBS, fixed with 1 mL of 4% paraformaldehyde for 30 min at 4°C, and stained with 2-(4-amidinophenyl)-6-indolecarbamidine dihydrochloride (DAPI, Roche) for 10 min. Finally, the slides were mounted with 10% glycerol solution and viewed using a LeicaTCS SP8 (Leica Microscopy Systems Ltd., Germany).

TABLE 1 | Properties of DOX-free and DOX-loaded nanocarriers.

DOX-free nanocarriers			DOX-loaded nanocarriers			
Size (nm)	PDI	Fe content (wt%)	Size (nm)	PDI	Fe content (wt%)	PLC (wt%)
131	0.26	14.7	150	0.19	13.3	4.6

RESULTS AND DISCUSSION

Characterization of Nanocarriers

The particle size and polydispersity (PDI) of DOX-free or DOX-loaded nanocarriers were determined by DLS, as shown in **Table 1**. The prepared DOX-free nanocarriers and DOX-loaded nanocarriers (**Figure 1A**) were determined to be 131 or 150 nm respectively, with a narrow size distribution, thereby making them suitable as anticancer drug carriers. The morphology of the redox-responsive magnetic nanocarriers was observed using TEM. **Figure 1B** shows the morphology of the nanocarriers. Because DSPE-SS-mPEG does not significantly attenuate electron scattering under TEM, nanocarriers are largely present as isolated clusters of Fe_3O_4 nanoparticles with a spherical shape. The drug loading content values of DOX-loaded nanocarriers was 4.6% (**Table 1**). Whereas, the Fe content of DOX-free or DOX-loaded nanocarriers was 14.7 and 13.3%, respectively (**Table 1**).

The Redox-Responsive Stability of Nanocarriers

Disulfide linkages are known to be readily reduced into free thiols in the presence of reducing agents. To demonstrate the responsiveness, the size change of redox-responsive magnetic nanocarriers in response to 20 mM GSH in PBS was measured by DLS. **Figure 2** shows that the average size of the nanocarriers gradually increased within the first 15 min after the addition of GSH. The size increased from 131 to 340 nm in 15 min, indicating the detachment of hydrophilic PEG shells from the nanocarriers and the enhanced hydrophobic interaction of the inner core. After 1 h, two populations at 547 nm and 1,038 nm were observed, however, after 3 h, the complete destruction of the nanocarriers was observed, and no nanoparticles were detected in the solution.

In vitro Redox-Responsive DOX Release

The drug release behavior of the DOX-loaded nanocarriers was investigated in PBS at 37°C in the presence or absence of

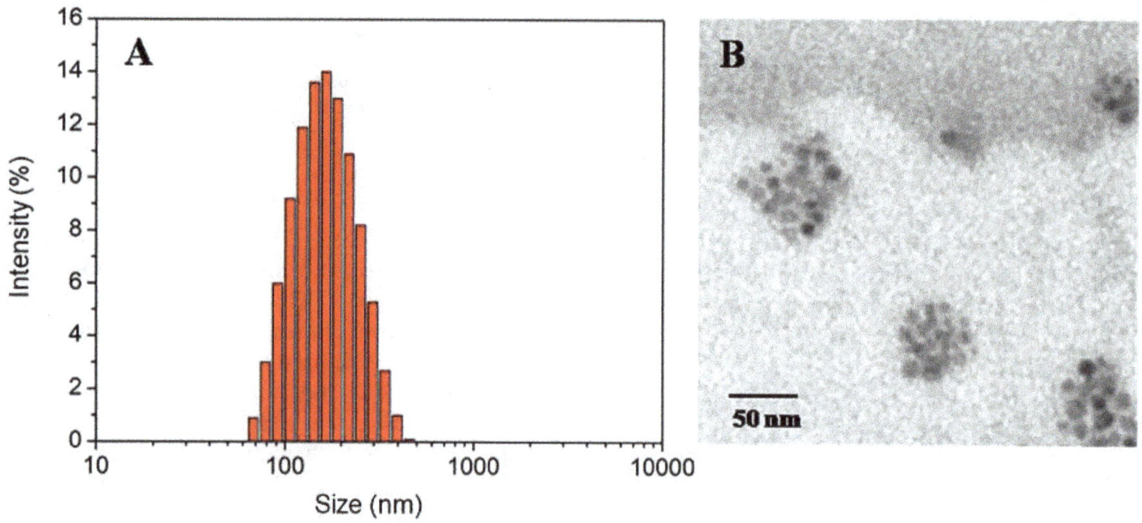

FIGURE 1 | The size distribution by DLS **(A)**, and TEM micrographs **(B)** of redox-responsive magnetic nanocarriers.

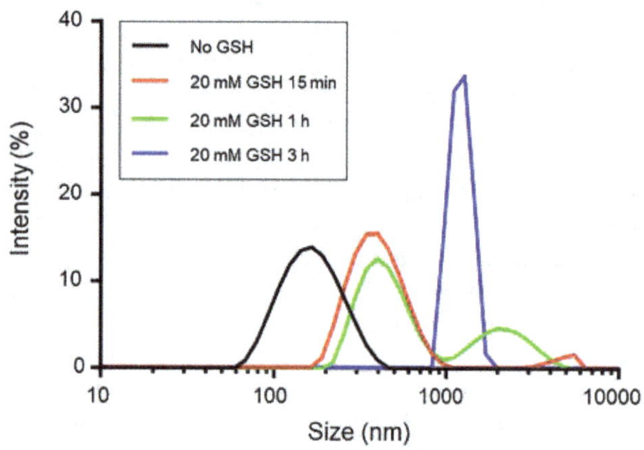

FIGURE 2 | The size change of redox-responsive magnetic nanocarriers in response to 20 mM GSH in PBS determined by DLS measurement.

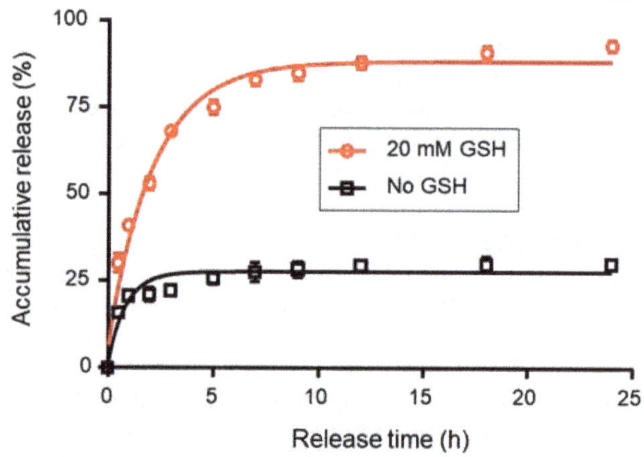

FIGURE 3 | Redox-triggered release of DOX from redox-responsive magnetic nanocarriers in PBS with or without 20 mM GSH. The standard deviation for each data point was averaged over three samples ($n = 3$).

GSH (20 mM). **Figure 3** shows the accumulative drug release profiles as a function of time. **Figure 3** demonstrates that the release of DOX from nanocarriers was markedly correlated with the presence or absence of GSH. The release of DOX from nanocarriers was accelerated by the addition of GSH to the media. In the presence of 20 mM GSH, nanocarriers rapidly released DOX, such that 93.8% of the DOX dose was released within 24 h. However, only 28.7% of DOX was released in the absence of GSH. This difference might be due to cleavage of disulfide bonds, thereby causing the destruction of the nanocarriers and the accelerated release of encapsulated DOX.

Cell TEM Imaging

The rapid accumulation of DOX-loaded nanocarriers was found to be magnetically inducible *in vitro* and was characterized using TEM. When HeLa cells were incubated for 2 h with DOX-loaded nanocarriers in either the presence or absence of a magnetic field, the accumulation of nanocarriers was found to be altered. TEM images demonstrating this observation are shown in **Figure 4**. The heavily electro-dense iron-containing nanoparticles are reproduced in the TEM images as a significantly darker region in contrast to the cellular environment, which facilitated identification of relative particle density between groups. The number of magnetic nanoparticles in cells significantly increased when a magnetic field was applied (**Figure 4B**), suggesting that the presence of a magnetic field enhanced the accumulation of nanocarriers in cells.

Cell Viability Assay

The *in vitro* cytotoxicity of DOX-loaded nanocarriers and free DOX was evaluated using the MTT assay. **Figure 5** shows the

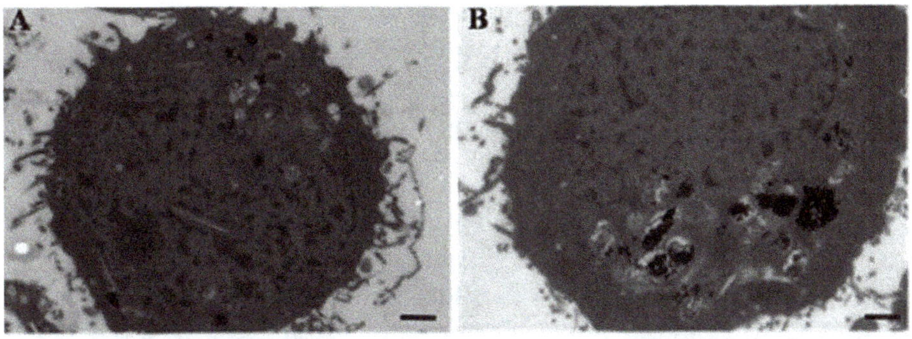

FIGURE 4 | TEM images of HeLa cells incubated with DOX-loaded nanocarriers in the absence **(A)** or presence **(B)** of a magnetic field. Scale bar is 1 μm.

resulting levels of observed cytotoxicity measured as a function of DOX concentration from 0.4 to 40 μg/mL. All test conditions exhibited a dose-dependent cytotoxic effect of the treatment on the population of viable and metabolically active HeLa cells. DOX-loaded nanocarriers exhibited lower cytotoxicity to HeLa cells with or without the magnetic field, as compared to free DOX at the same DOX dose (**Figure 5A**). As a control experiment, we performed a group of experiments using nanocarriers without DOX and examined cytotoxicity under magnetic and non-magnetic conditions, suggesting that the nanocarriers alone did not exhibit cytotoxicity (**Figure 5B**). Given that DOX is a small molecule, it can be quickly transported into cells and enter nuclei by passive diffusion. Furthermore, we found that the presence of a local magnetic field could significantly increase the cytotoxicity of DOX-loaded nanocarriers. This process may be due to the magnetic field increasing cellular uptake of nanocarriers, and once internalized, the redox-responsive nanocarriers are destroyed by high levels of GSH. The DOX is then rapidly released from the destroyed redox-responsive nanocarriers. Taken together these results indicate that the DOX-loaded nanocarriers can achieve both magnetic targeting and reduction-sensitive release simultaneously.

In vitro Cellular Uptake of DOX-Loaded Nanocarriers

The cellular uptake of the nanocarriers and the intracellular location of the encapsulated DOX was monitored by CLSM in HeLa cells. The nuclei of HeLa cells were stained with DAPI, which presented blue fluorescence to distinguish from the red fluorescence of the labeled DOX. **Figure 6** shows CLSM images of HeLa cells incubated with DOX-loaded nanocarriers for 2 h with or without magnet field treatment. As shown in **Figure 6**, we found that cells incubated with DOX-loaded nanocarriers with applied magnetic field demonstrated stronger DOX fluorescence compared to no applied magnetic field. This phenomenon is primarily a result of the magnetic field increase in the cellular uptake of the DOX-loaded nanocarriers. Our results indicate that these nanocarriers are responsive to either magnetic or redox stimulated activation and are therefore suitable for application as anticancer drug carriers.

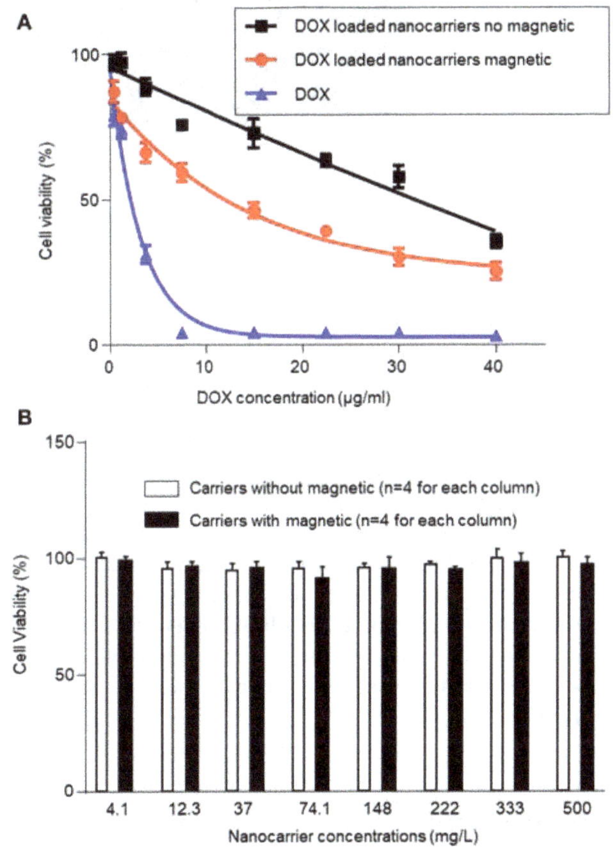

FIGURE 5 | Cytotoxicity of DOX-loaded magnetic nanocarriers and free DOX in HeLa cells with or without magnetic field after incubation for 24 h **(A)**. **(B)** In control experiments, we examined cytotoxicity using magnetic nanocarriers alone with or without magnetic field after incubation for 24 h, and found no cytotoxicity. The standard deviation for each data point was averaged over four samples ($n = 4$) for **(A,B)**.

CONCLUSION

In this article, we use the amphiphilic copolymer DSPE-SS-mPEG, which is connected by disulfide bonds. Afterward, the

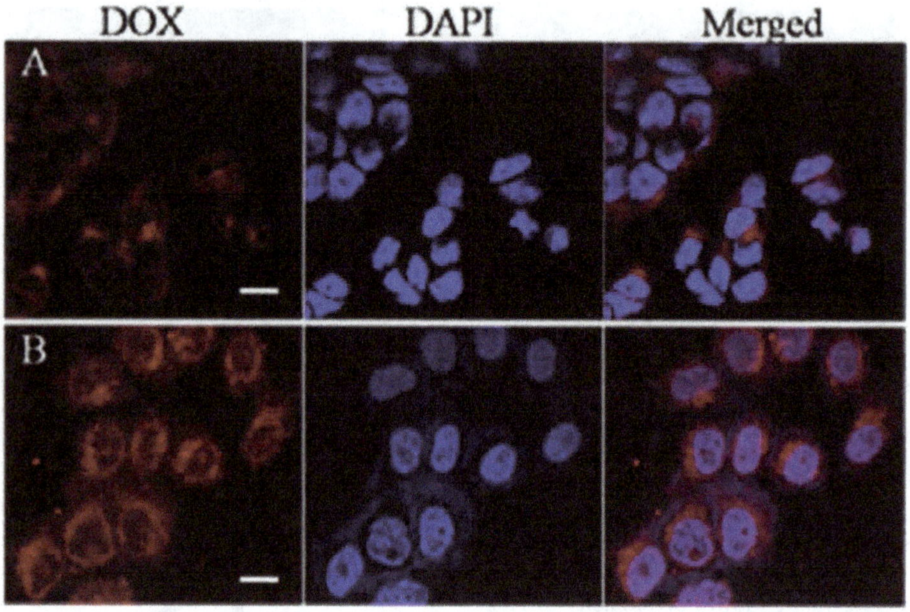

FIGURE 6 | CLSM images of HeLa cells after treatment with DOX-loaded magnetic nanocarriers for 2 h in the absence **(A)** or presence **(B)** of a magnetic field. Scale bar is 15 μm.

magnetic Fe_3O_4 nanoparticles and the hydrophobic drug are made by the self-assembly of the amphiphilic copolymer. DOX is encapsulated in the amphiphilic copolymer to form a magnetic nano drug controlled release system which is sensitive and responds to a reducing environment. This controlled release system can dissociate the disulfide bonds in the presence of dithiothreitol, thereby triggering the release system to disintegrate and expel the drug.

When the DOX-loaded nanocarrier is transported into the cell, intracellular GSH breaks the disulfide bonds, resulting in the disintegration of the transport system and the release of DOX. It is a well-designed enzyme-responsive magnetic-field controlled release system and provides a new foundation for building an efficient and safe nanoscale drug delivery system.

AUTHOR CONTRIBUTIONS

KX and YL equally contributed to this work, conducted the experiments, analyzed data, prepared original figures, and revised the manuscript. WY and GW participated in experimental design, analyzed the data, and revised the manuscript. HS analyzed the data and revised the manuscript. SZ designed the experiments and revised the manuscript. JW designed the experiments and analyzed the data, finalized the figures, and wrote the manuscript.

ACKNOWLEDGMENTS

This work was supported by the Science and Technology Department of Henan Province (Grant # 192102310411) and the Education Department of Henan Province (Grant # 19A320043).

REFERENCES

1. Yasui H. Safe handling of cancer chemotherapy drugs. *Gan to kagaku ryoho Cancer Chemother.* (2016) 43:503–8.
2. Paez JG, Jänne PA, Lee JC, Tracy S, Greulich H, Gabriel S, et al. EGFR mutations in lung cancer: correlation with clinical response to gefitinib therapy. *J Sci.* (2004) 304:1497–500. doi: 10.1126/science.1099314
3. Kerr JF, Winterford CM, Harmon BV. Apoptosis. Its significance in cancer and cancer therapy. *J Cancer.* (1994) 73:2013–26. doi: 10.1002/1097-0142(19940415)73:8<2013::AID-CNCR2820730802>3.0.CO;2-J
4. Wang CY, Mayo MW, Baldwin AS. TNF-and cancer therapy-induced apoptosis: potentiation by inhibition of NF-κB. *J Sci.* (1996) 274:784–7. doi: 10.1126/science.274.5288.784
5. Lowe SW, Bodis S, McClatchey A, Remington L, Ruley HE, Fisher DE, et al. p53 status and the efficacy of cancer therapy *in vivo*. *J Sci.* (1994) 266:807–10. doi: 10.1126/science.7973635
6. Brown JM, Giaccia AJ. The unique physiology of solid tumors: opportunities (and problems) for cancer therapy. *J Cancer Res.* (1998) 58:1408–16.
7. Anselmo AC, Mitragotri S. Nanoparticles in the clinic. *Bioeng Transl Med.* (2016) 1:10–29. doi: 10.1002/btm2.10003
8. Wicki A, Witzigmann D, Balasubramanian V, Huwyler J. Nanomedicine in cancer therapy: challenges, opportunities, and clinical applications. *J Control Release.* (2015) 200:138–57. doi: 10.1016/j.jconrel.2014.12.030
9. Mi Y, Wolfram J, Mu C, Liu X, Blanco E, Shen H, et al. Enzyme-responsive multistage vector for drug delivery to tumor tissue. *Pharmacol Res.* (2016) 113(Pt A):92–9. doi: 10.1016/j.phrs.2016.08.024
10. Bigall NC, Curcio A, Leal MP, Falqui A, Palumberi D, Di Corato R, et al. Magnetic nanocarriers with tunable pH dependence for controlled loading and release of cationic and anionic payloads. *Adv Mater.* (2011) 23:5645–50. doi: 10.1002/adma.201103505
11. Nagaoka H, Sato Y, Xie X, Hata H, Eguchi M, Sakurai N, et al. Coupling stimuli-responsive magnetic nanoparticles with antibody-antigen

detection in immunoassays. *Anal Chem.* (2011) 83:9197–200. doi: 10.1021/ac201814n

12. Ruan G, Vieira G, Henighan T, Chen A, Thakur D, Sooryakumar R, et al. Simultaneous magnetic manipulation and fluorescent tracking of multiple individual hybrid nanostructures. *Nano Lett.* (2010) 10:2220–4. doi: 10.1021/nl1011855
13. Jain S, Hirst DG, O'Sullivan JM. Gold nanoparticles as novel agents for cancer therapy. *Br J Radiol.* (2012) 85:101–13. doi: 10.1259/bjr/59448833
14. Ferrari M. Cancer nanotechnology: opportunities and challenges. *J. Nat Rev Cancer.* (2005) 5:161–71. doi: 10.1038/nrc1566
15. Farokhzad OC, Langer R. Nanomedicine: developing smarter therapeutic and diagnostic modalities. *J Adv Drug Del Rev.* (2006) 58:1456–9. doi: 10.1016/j.addr.2006.09.011
16. Riehemann K, Schneider SW, Luger TA, Godin B, Ferrari M, Fuchs H. Nanomedicine? challenge and perspectives. *J Angewandte Chemie Int Edn.* (2009) 48:872–97. doi: 10.1002/anie.200802585
17. Peer D, Karp JM, Hong S, Farokhzad OC, Margalit R, Langer R. Nanocarriers as an emerging platform for cancer therapy. *J Nat Nanotechnol.* (2007) 2:751–60. doi: 10.1038/nnano.2007.387
18. Xu R, Zhang G, Mai J, Deng X, Segura-Ibarra V, Wu S, et al. An injectable nanoparticle generator enhances delivery of cancer therapeutics. *Nat Biotechnol.* (2016) 34:414–8. doi: 10.1038/nbt.3506
19. Lucky SS, Idris NM, Huang K, Kim J, Li Z, Thong PS, et al. *In vivo* Biocompatibility, biodistribution and therapeutic efficiency of titania coated upconversion nanoparticles for photodynamic therapy of solid oral cancers. *Theranostics.* (2016) 6:1844–65. doi: 10.7150/thno.15088
20. von Maltzahn G, Park JH, Lin KY, Singh N, Schwoppe C, Mesters R, et al. Nanoparticles that communicate *in vivo* to amplify tumour targeting. *Nat Mater.* (2011) 10:545–52. doi: 10.1038/nmat3049
21. Sun S, Murray CB, Weller D, Folks L, Moser A. Monodisperse FePt nanoparticles and ferromagnetic FePt nanocrystal superlattices. *Science.* (2000) 287:1989–92. doi: 10.1126/science.287.5460.1989
22. Gao W, Kagan D, Pak OS, Clawson C, Campuzano S, Chuluun-Erdene E, et al. Cargo-towing fuel-free magnetic nanoswimmers for targeted drug delivery. *Small.* (2012) 8:460–7. doi: 10.1002/smll.201101909
23. Jain RK, Stylianopoulos T. Delivering nanomedicine to solid tumors. *J Nat Rev Clin Oncol.* (2010) 7:653–64. doi: 10.1038/nrclinonc.2010.139
24. Farokhzad OC, Langer R. Impact of nanotechnology on drug delivery. *J ACS Nano.* (2009) 3:16–20. doi: 10.1021/nn900002m
25. Hong R, Han G, Fernandez JM, Kim BJ, Forbes NS, Rotello VM. Glutathione-mediated delivery and release using monolayer protected nanoparticle carriers. *J Am Chem Soc.* (2006) 128:1078–9. doi: 10.1021/ja056726i
26. Chong SF, Chandrawati R, Stadler B, Park J, Cho J, Wang Y, et al. Stabilization of polymer-hydrogel capsules via thiol-disulfide exchange. *Small.* (2009) 5:2601–10. doi: 10.1002/smll.200900906
27. Jones DP, Carlson JL, Samiec PS, Sternberg P, Jr, Mody VC Jr, Reed RL, et al. Glutathione measurement in human plasma. Evaluation of sample collection, storage and derivatization conditions for analysis of dansyl derivatives by HPLC. *Clin Chim Acta.* (1998) 275:175–84.
28. Park J, An K, Hwang Y, Park JG, Noh HJ, Kim JY, et al. Ultra-large-scale syntheses of monodisperse nanocrystals. *J Nat Mater.* (2004) 3:891–5. doi: 10.1038/nmat1251
29. Xu ZC, Shen CM, Hou YL, Gao HJ, Sun SH. Oleylamine as both reducing agent and stabilizer in a facile synthesis of magnetite nanoparticles. *Chem Mater.* (2009) 21:1778–80. doi: 10.1021/cm802978z

6

Schistosoma japonicum MiRNA-7-5p Inhibits the Growth and Migration of Hepatoma Cells via Cross-Species Regulation of S-Phase Kinase-Associated Protein 2

Chao Hu[1], *Shanli Zhu*[1], *Jing Wang*[1], *Yu Lin*[1], *Li Ma*[1], *Liufang Zhu*[1], *Pengyue Jiang*[1], *Zhengli Li*[1] and *Weiqing Pan*[1,2*]

[1] *Institute for Infectious Diseases and Vaccine Development, Tongji University School of Medicine, Shanghai, China,*
[2] *Department of Tropical Diseases, Second Military Medical University, Shanghai, China*

Correspondence:
Weiqing Pan
wqpan0912@aliyun.com

MicroRNAs (miRNAs) play important roles in human diseases, such as cancer. Human miRNA-7-5p is a tumor suppressor miRNA that inhibits tumor growth by regulating multiple oncogenic signal pathways. Recently, studies revealed that plant miRNAs could regulate mammalian gene expression in a cross-kingdom manner. *Schistosoma japonicum* miRNA-7-5p (designated as sja-miR-7-5p) is conserved between the parasites and mammals. Thus, we investigated whether sja-miR-7-5p has similar antitumor activity to its mammalian counterpart. We first showed that sja-miR-7-5p was detected in host hepatocytes during *S. japonicum* infection. The sja-miR-7-5p mimics significantly inhibited the growth, migration, and colony formation of mouse and human hepatoma cell lines *in vitro*, and induced G1/G0 cell cycle arrest. In a xenograft animal model, the tumor volume and weight were significantly reduced in mice inoculated with hepatoma cells transfected with sja-miR-7-5p mimics compared with those transfected with NC miRNAs. Furthermore, the antitumor activity of sja-miR-7-5p was suggested by cross-species downregulation of the S-phase kinase-associated protein 2 gene in the host. Thus, sja-miR-7-5p is translocated into hepatocytes and exerts its anti-cancer activities in mammals, implying that sja-miR-7-5p might strengthen host resistance to hepatocellular carcinoma during schistosome infection.

Keywords: *Schistosoma japonicum*, microRNA, hepatoma cell, SKP2, cross-species regulation

INTRODUCTION

The primary pathology of schistosomiasis caused by *S. japonicum* is egg-induced granuloma and fibrosis. The female adult worms living in the host mesenteric veins lay numerous eggs, and most of them are trapped in the liver tissues via the portal venous system, causing a granulomatous reaction and fibrosis. The parasite eggs in the granuloma are surrounded by host cells, including immunocytes, hepatic mesenchymal cells, and hepatocytes (1). Our previous studies indicated that *S. japonicum* secretes many microRNAs (miRNAs), including *Schistosoma*-specific and conserved miRNAs (2), and parasite miRNA-containing exosomes (2).

MiRNAs are a class of highly conserved, small non-coding RNAs, with a length of about 20–24 nucleotides (nt) that post-transcriptionally regulate gene expression through complete or incomplete binding to their target mRNAs (3). MiRNAs have extensive effects on not only physiological processes, but also on the progression of many human diseases, such as cancers (4, 5). Aberrant miRNA expression promotes the occurrence and development of various cancers (6–8); however, some miRNAs can exert therapeutic effects on multiple cancers through regulation of tumor-related genes, including those that control tumor cell growth or apoptosis (9, 10). Interestingly, miRNAs derived from plants can regulate the expression of their target genes in mammals in a cross-kingdom manner (11–13). For example, miR-159 derived from plants was detectable in human sera and inhibited breast cancer growth by targeting the human transcription factor 7 (*TCF7*) gene (13). Accumulating evidence indicates that heterogeneous miRNAs can modulate cell functions in mammals. However, it remains unclear how the plant miRNAs can survive the passage through the gastrointestinal tract following ingestion.

Unlike plant miRNAs, which need to pass through the gastrointestinal tract before release into the host serum or entering host cells, schistosomal miRNAs from eggs trapped in liver tissue may be directly transferred to the neighboring host cells. Thus, we hypothesized that parasite miRNAs from the eggs might be translocated into neighboring hepatocytes to exert various biological effects, including some that are beneficial to the host, for example, strengthening the resistance of the host to diseases such as cancer, as do plant-derived miRNAs (13). Human miRNA-7-5p (designated as hsa-miR-7-5p) is a tumor suppressor miRNA that regulates multiple oncogenic signal pathways and reverses drug resistance in certain cancers (14–17). Our previous study identified a *S. japonicum* miRNA-7-5p (designated as sja-miR-7-5p) that is conserved between the parasite and mammals, i.e., there is an identical seed sequence (2–8 nt at the 5′ region) in both parasites and mammalian miRNA-7-5p, despite there being 6 nt differences in the rest of the sequence. Thus, it would be interesting to investigate if sja-miR-7-5 secreted by *S. japonicum* has a similar antitumor activity to hsa-miR-7-5p. In the present study, we demonstrated that sja-miR-7-5p is present in hepatocytes during the *S. japonicum* infection and the sja-miR-7-5p exerts anticancer effects on multiple hepatoma cells (assessed using *in vitro* and *in vivo* models) by targeting the S-phase kinase-associated protein 2(*SKP2*) gene, which is a component of the SCF (Skp1-Cullin 1-F-box) E3 ubiquitin-ligase complex. Previous studies have shown that overexpression of the *SKP2* gene was observed in many cancers, such as in liver cancer (18), prostate cancer (19), lymphoma (20), melanoma (21), and breast cancer (22), which plays an important role in regulating cellular proliferation and cancer progression, mainly by targeting cell cycle regulators in an ubiquitin-dependent manner, followed by 26S proteasome degradation (23). In addition, the *SKP2* overexpression also enhanced tumor cell invasion (24), metastasis (25), and resistance to apoptosis (26), and was associated with tumor aggressiveness (27) and poor prognosis (28).

Abbreviations: *S. japonicum, Schistosoma japonicum*; HCC, hepatocellular cancer; SKP2, S-phase kinase associated protein 2; P27(also known as CDKN1B), cyclin dependent kinase inhibitor 1B; MMP9, matrix metallopeptidase 9; miRNA, microRNA; siRNA, small interfering RNA; NC, negative control; Mock, mock control.

MATERIALS AND METHODS

Infection of Mice With *S. japonicum* Cercariae

Animal experiments were performed in accordance with the Guide for the Care and Use of Laboratory Animals of the National Institutes of Health, and approved by the Internal Review Board of Tongji University School of Medicine. The animal surgeries were undertaken under sodium pentobarbital anesthesia. Cercariae of *S. japonicum* were provided by National Institute of Parasitic Disease, Chinese Center for Disease Control and Prevention (CDC). 36 six-week-old male C57BL/6J mice (18–20 g, 3 mice per group), purchased from experimental animal center of the Second Military Medical University and housed under specific pathogen-free conditions, were percutaneously infected with 50 or 100 cercariae of *S. japonicum* per mouse (50 for collection of infected hepatocytes and 100 for collection of early stage parasites). For collection of parasites, the hepatic schistosomula were isolated from the portal system and mesenteric veins of infected mice at 7, 14, and 42 days post-infection (dpi). In addition, 42 days male and female adult worms were manually separated under a light microscope. The eggs were isolated with a traditional method, as described by Cai et al. (29). All the freshly isolated parasites were washed three times with PBS (pH 7.4) and were immediately used for extraction of total RNA or frozen at −80°C until being subjected to further analysis.

Isolation of Primary Mouse Hepatocytes

The primary mouse hepatocytes were isolated by a two-step collagenase perfusion procedure, as described by He et al. (30) with minor modifications. Briefly, after infection, livers of the infected mice collected at various time points of 7, 9, 11, 14, 28, and 42 dpi ($n = 5$) along with the livers of uninfected mice were initially *in situ* digested with 0.03% collagenase type IV and then further digested with 0.08% collagenase type IV at 37°C in a shaking bath for 30 min. The single cell suspensions were harvested by filtration through 400-mesh sieves for removal of the remaining tissue debris and parasite eggs. Next, hepatocytes were isolated by centrifugation of the resulting cell suspensions at 50×g for 4 min and further purified by centrifugation at 50 × g for 4 min. Purified hepatocytes were resuspend in DMEM containing 20 μg/ml Ribonuclease A (Sigma-Aldrich, USA) at 37°C for 30 min to eliminate any miRNA that might be released by schistosome eggs. After washing with PBS for three times, the cell pellet was immediately used for extraction of total RNA or frozen at −80°C until used.

Cell Proliferation Assay

Cells (2×10^5) were seeded in a 6-well plate overnight, respectively. Then cells were transfected with sja-miR-7-5p mimics or NC mimics, respectively, four replicates per group. And 24 h later, cells were digested and seeded in a 96-well plate (2 × 10^3) for 1, 2, 3, and 4 d. At each indicated time, 10 μL Cell Counting Kit-8(CCK-8, Dojindo, Japan) was added to each well and cells were incubated for 1 h at 37 °C, then, using the Microplate reader (Bio-Tek, USA) to measure the abosorbance at 450 nm.

Cell Cycle Analysis

Cells (1 × 10^5) were seeded in a 12-well plate overnight, respectively. Then, cells were transfected with sja-miR-7-5p mimics or NC mimics, respectively, three replicates per group. And 48 h later, cells were collected and fixed with ice-cold 75%(v/v) ethanol and stored at 4°C overnight, then, cells were washed and resuspended in 200 μL phosphate-buffered saline (PBS) contained with 0.05 mg/mL RNase A (Beyotime, China) and 25 mg/mL propidium iodide (PI) (Beyotime, China), cell cycle was determined by the FACSverse flow cytometer (BD Biosciences, USA).

Colony Formation Assay

Cells (2 × 10^5) were seeded in a 6-well plate overnight, then cells were transfected with sja-miR-7-5p mimics or NC mimics, respectively. And 24 h later, cells were digested and 200 cells in 500 μL complete medium were seeded in 24-well plate, three replicates per group. After incubation for 8 days, then cells were

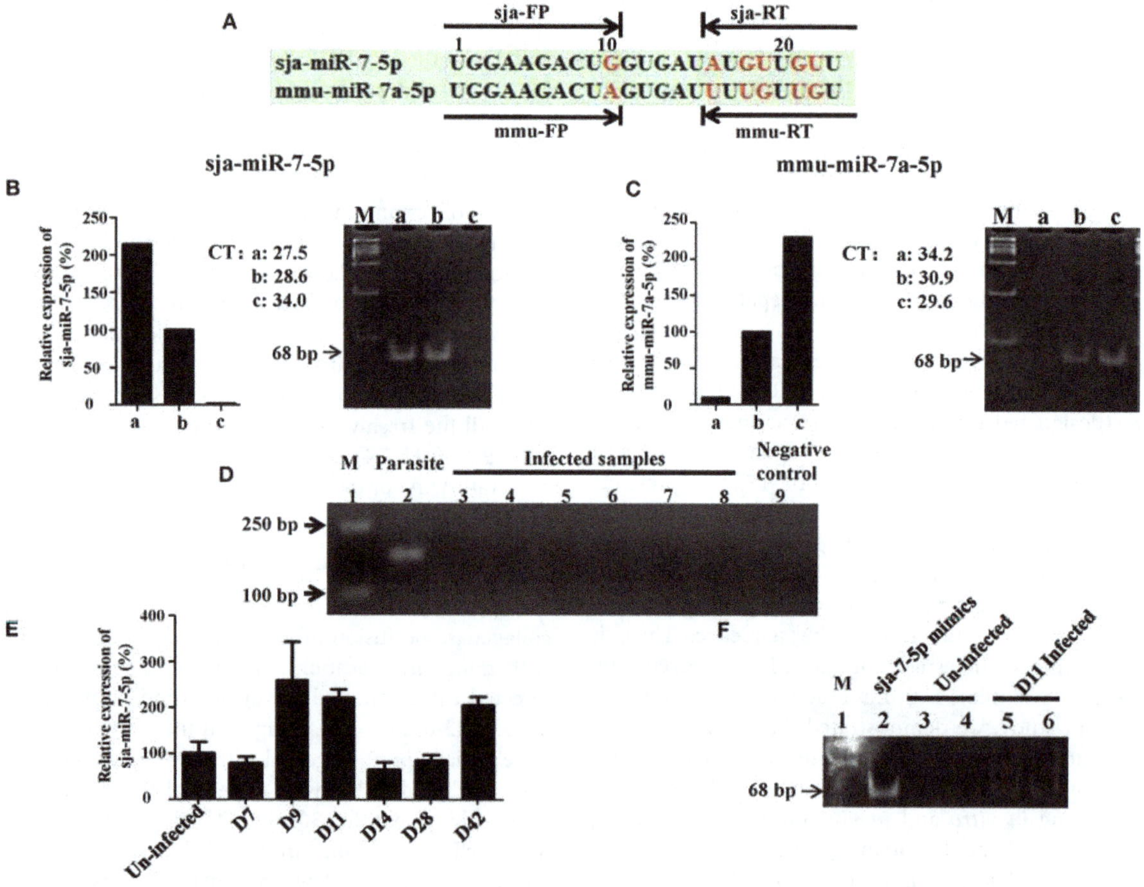

FIGURE 1 | Detection of sja-miR-7-5p in infected hepatocytes. **(A)** A schematic diagram represents two sets of primers of reverse transcription stem-loop primer (RT) and forward primer (FP) for sja-miR-7-5p or mmu-miR-7a-5p, respectively. **(B,C)** Preparation of RNA samples: a. 200 ng *Schistosoma japonicum* egg RNA; b. mixture of equal amount of *Schistosoma japonicum* egg RNA (100 ng) and Hepa1-6 cell RNA (100 ng); c. 200 ng Hepa1-6 cell RNA. The three RNA templates were transcribed into cDNA using the corresponding reverse transcription stem-loop primer, respectively, which were used for qRT-PCR by the corresponding forward primer and common reverse primer, respectively. The PCR products were separated by polyacrylamide gel electrophoresis (PAGE). As shown in B and C, the two sets of primers can effectively distinguished the sja-miR-7-5p and mmu-miR-7a-5p, e.g., the set of sja-miR-7-5p RT and forward primer FP amplified the sja-miR-7-5p [**(B)**, lane a and b] but not mmu-miR-7a-5p (lane c), while the set of mmu-miR-7a-5p RT and forward primer FP generated the mmu-miR-7a-5p but not the sja-miR-7-5p **(C)**. **(D)** Analysis of the RNA samples to ensure no contamination with parasite RNA: the RNA samples used for the above analysis were detected as described in Method by PCR for presence of the NADH gene of *S. japonicum*. Lane 1: marker. Lane 2: parasite positive control: RNA samples of *S. japonicum* eggs as described above. Lane 3–8: six samples of infected hepatocytes with RNase pre-incubation. Lane 9: negative control without the template. **(E)** qRT-PCR analysis of sja-miR-7-5p in the infected hepatocytes at various days after infection; **(F)** 12% PAGE analysis showing sja-miR-7-5p PCR product (68 bp) from the infected hepatocytes: Lane 1: marker; Lane 2: sja-miR-7-5p mimics positive control; Lanes 3 and 4: two uninfected hepatocyte samples with pre-incubation with RNase; Lanes 5 and 6: two infected hepatocyte samples at day 11 post-infection with the pre-incubation. Data are presented as the mean ± SD, $n = 3$.

fixed in methanol for 30 min, followed by staining in crystal violet for 15 min. The number of colonies containing > 50 cells was counted under a light microscope.

Tumor Xenograft Animal Model

Male athymic nude mice were housed and manipulated according to the protocols approved by the Shanghai Medical Experimental Animal Care Commission. Hepa1-6 cells or HepG2 cells were transfected with sja-miR-7-5p mimics or NC mimics, respectively. And 24 h later, for each mouse, 1×10^6 cells in 100 μL PBS after treated with sja-miR-7-5p mimics were injected subcutaneously to the left scapula, while cells after treated with NC mimics were injected subcutaneously to the right scapula, respectively. Tumor volume was measured at 2, 4, 6, and 7 d after injection, At day 7, the mice were sacrificed and tumors were separated to measure their weight and volume. Tumor volume was measured using the formula: $0.5 \times L \times S^2$, where L is the longest diameter of tumor and S is the shortest diameter of tumor. The content of sja-miR-7-5p mimics transfected into the tumor cells measured by quantitative real-time reverse transcription PCR (qRT-PCR), the protein level of SKP2 was determined by Western blotting. And also the expression of Ki67 in the tumor was measured by immunohistochemistry (IHC) as described under this section.

Immunohistochemistry

To determine Ki67 expression in xenograft tumor tissues from the athymic nude mice, immunohistochemistry (IHC) was performed as described previously (31), Antibody against Ki67 was used (1:50 dilution).

Statistical Analysis

All experiments were performed in triplicate and the results were presented as mean ± standard deviation (mean ± SD). All data were analyzed by one-way ANOVA using the software GraphPad Prism 5.0(GraphPad Software, Inc. La Jolla, CA, USA). A value of $P < 0.05$ was considered statistically significant.

RESULTS

Presence of sja-miR-7-5p in Infected Hepatocytes

We first investigated whether sja-miR-7-5p was present in the host liver cells during schistosome infection. For this purpose, we designed a set of two sets primers that could distinguish the sja-miR-7-5p from corresponding miRNA derived from mouse (mmu-miR-7-5p) and human (hsa-miR-7-5p). The sja-miR-7-5p has an identical seed sequence (2–8 nt at the 5' region), but

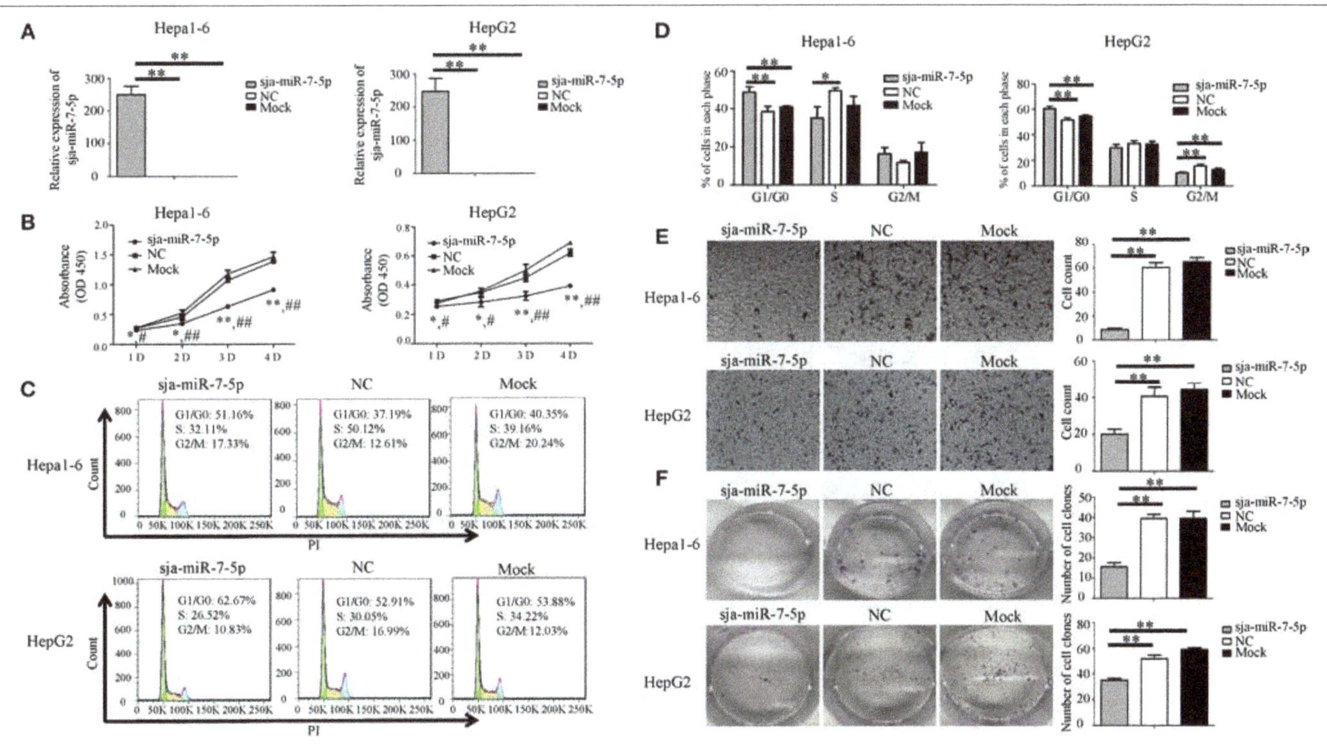

FIGURE 2 | Sja-miR-7-5p inhibits cell proliferation and migration of Hepa1-6 and HepG2 cells *in vitro*. **(A–F)** Hepa1-6 and HepG2 cells were transfected with sja-miR-7-5p mimics and NC (negative control) mimics, respectively, and 48 h later [except for the cell counting kit-8(CCK-8) assay, which was 24 h later], the expression of sja-miR-7-5p was determined using qRT-PCR (A). Cell proliferation was evaluated by CCK-8 assay at 1, 2, 3, and 4 days **(B)**, data are presented as the mean ± SD, $n = 3$, $^*p < 0.05$ or $^{**}p < 0.01$ indicates the comparison between the two groups of sja-miR-7-5p and NC; $\#p < 0.05$ or $\#\#p < 0.01$ indicates the comparison between the groups of sja-miR-7-5p and Mock. Cell cycle was determined by flow cytometry analysis **(C,D)**. Cell migration was evaluated using Transwell inserts without matrigel coating **(E)**. The ability to form cell clones was determined using a colony formation assay **(F)**. Data are presented as the mean ± SD, $n = 3$, $^*p < 0.05$, $^{**}p < 0.01$.

there are 6 nt differences in the rest of the sequence among the species (**Figure 1A**, and **Figure S1**), which allowed us to design sets of specific primers for the mmu-miR-7a-5p (mmu-FP/RT) and the sja-miR-7-5(sja- FP/RT). We first tested specificity of the primers using the RNA samples derived from *S. japonicum* eggs (a), mouse Hepa1-6 cell line (c), and mixture of equal amount of a and c (b). As shown in **Figures 1B,C**, the sja-FP/RT pair primers successfully generated the sja-miR-7a-5p from the samples of a and b, but not c (**Figure 1B**), while the mmu-FP/RT pair primers generated the mmu-miR-7a-5p from the sample b and c, but not a (**Figure 1C**). These data indicated that the two sets of primers can effectively distinguish the sja-miR-7-5p and mmu-miR-7a-5p, and no cross reaction between the mmu-FP/RT and sja-FP/RT primers. All the primers are listed in **Table S1**.

We next used the sja-FP/RT primers for detection of presence of sja-miR-7-5p in the liver cells of infected mice with *S. japonicum*. We prepared RNA samples from the infected liver cells, and carefully analyzed the samples to ensure no contamination with parasite RNA (**Figure 1D**). We showed that sja-miR-7-5p was detected by using qRT-PCR in the hepatocytes from infected mice at the early stage (i.e., days 9 and 11 post infection) and the late stage of infection (day 42) (**Figure 1E**). The presence of this parasite miRNA was further verified by PCR (**Figure 1F**) and cloning and sequencing of the PCR product showed identical sequence of sja-miR-7-5p (**Figure S2A**). In addition, we showed that sja-miR-7-5p was expressed at all these stages, and higher expression of sja-miR-7-5p was detected in adult males compared with that in adult females (**Figure S2B**). These findings indicated that this sja-miR-7-5p is present in the host liver cells during schistosome infection.

Inhibition of Proliferation and Migration of Hepatoma Cells by Sja-miR-7-5p

To investigated the effects of sja-miR-7-5p on the growth of hepatoma cells *in vitro,* both mouse and human hepatoma cells (e.g., Hepa1-6 cells and HepG2 cells) were transfected with the sja-miR-7-5p mimics, NC (a negative control mimics that has no target gene in mice and human) and Mock (transfection reagents only). As shown in **Figure 2A**, the sja-miR-7-5p mimics were effectively transfected into both cell lines. The schistosomal miRNA significantly suppressed the proliferation of both cell lines, as measured by the CCK-8 assay (**Figure 2B**), and substantially arrested the cell cycle at G1/G0 phase, as detected by flow cytometry (**Figures 2C,D**). We also showed that transfection of the sja-miR-7-5p mimics significantly suppressed cell migration, as assessed using the Transwell inserts without matrigel coating (**Figure 2E**) and by the wound-healing assay (**Figures S3B,C**) compared with the NC or Mock control cells. Colony formation assays showed that sja-miR-7-5p inhibited colony formation of hepatoma cells to a greater extent that those in the NC group or Mock group (**Figure 2F**). In addition, the Hepa1-6 cells transfected with sja-miR-7-5p mimics grew bigger and rounder compared with those in the NC or Mock control cells (**Figure S3A**). These data indicated that sja-miR-7-5p inhibited growth, migration, and colony formation of both mouse and human hepatoma cells and arrested their cell cycle

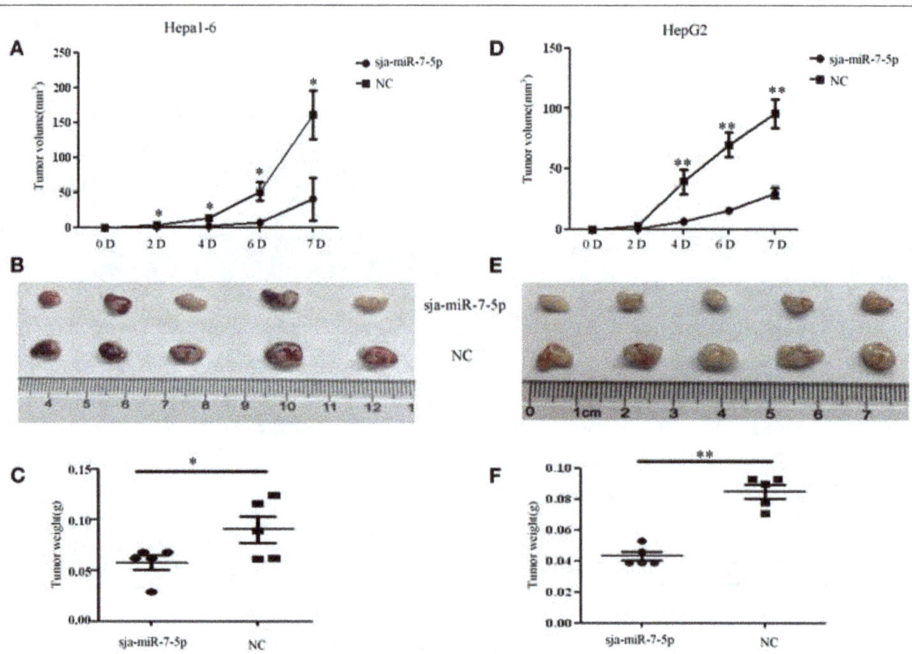

FIGURE 3 | Sja-miR-7-5p inhibits hepatoma cell growth *in vivo*. **(A–F)** Hepa1-6 and HepG2 cells were transfected with sja-miR-7-5p mimics or NC mimics, respectively, and then the sja-miR-7-5p-treated cells (1 × 10^6) were injected subcutaneously to the left scapula of athymic nude mice, and the NC-treated cells were injected subcutaneously into the right scapula ($n = 5$), respectively. Tumor volumes were measured at days 2, 4, 6, and 7 after injection. At day 7, the mice were sacrificed and tumors were separated to measure their weight and volume, **(A–C)** for Hepa1-6 cells, **(D–F)** for HepG2 cells. Data are presented as the mean ± SD, $n = 5$, $^*p < 0.05$, $^{**}p < 0.01$.

at G1/G0 phase *in vitro*, indicating that the schistosomal miRNA is also a tumor suppressor.

Sja-miR-7-5p-Mediated Inhibition of Hepatoma Cell Growth *in vivo*

To further investigate whether sja-miR-7-5p inhibits growth of liver cancer cells *in vivo*, both Hepa1-6 and HepG2 cells were transfected with sja-miR-7-5p mimics or NC mimics, and then injected subcutaneously to the left and right scapula of athymic nude mice to generate subcutaneous tumors. The tumor volume was measured at days 2, 4, 6, and 7 after injection. At day 7, mice were sacrificed and tumors were excised to measure their weight and volume. The results showed that both the tumor volume and weight were significantly reduced in the mice inoculated with Hepa1-6 cells transfected with sja-miR-7-5p mimics compared with those in mice receiving cells transfected with NC miRNAs (**Figures 3A–C**). Similar results were obtained with the human cell line of HepG2 (**Figures 3D–F**). These data indicated that sja-miR-7-5p suppressed tumor growth *in vivo*.

SKP2 Is a Direct Target of Sja-miR-7-5p

To determine the molecular mechanisms by which sja-miR-7-5p inhibits hepatoma cell growth, we used the online software miRDB (32) (http://www.mirdb.org/miRDB/index.html), MR-microT (33) (http://diana.imis.athena-innovation.gr/DianaTools/index.php?r=mrmicrot/index) and RNAhybrid (34) (http://bibiserv.techfak.uni-bielefeld.de/rnahybrid?id=rnahybrid_view_submission).

To search for potential targets of sja-miR-7-5p. We identified the gene encoding S-phase kinase-associated protein 2(*SKP2*) as a potential target for sja-miR-7-5p, because a binding site was located at the 3' UTR of the both murine and human *SKP2* gene that perfectly matched the seed sequence of sja-miR-7-5p. In addition, the *SKP2* gene in human has been characterized as an oncogene during tumorigenesis (21, 35–38).

To investigate the relationship between sja-miR-7-5p and *SKP2* gene in both human and mouse, first, we constructed two plasmids that contain the luciferase reporter gene: One was the pmirGLO-*SKP2*-WT construct in which the firefly luciferase gene is fused to the 3' UTR of *SKP2* gene; the other was the pmirGLO-*SKP2*-MT in which the seven nucleotides in the miRNA binding site were mutated (**Figure 4A**). The constructs were simultaneously transfected with sja-miR-7-5p mimics or NC mimics into both Hepa1-6 cells and HepG2 cells. As shown in **Figure 4B**, the luciferase activity was significantly decreased in the cells transfected with the pmirGLO-*SKP2*-WT but not with the pmirGLO-*SKP2*-MT, indicating that sja-miR-7-5p mimics could directly bind to the site in the 3′ UTR of the *SKP2* gene, while the mutations in the seed sequence abrogated the inhibitory effect.

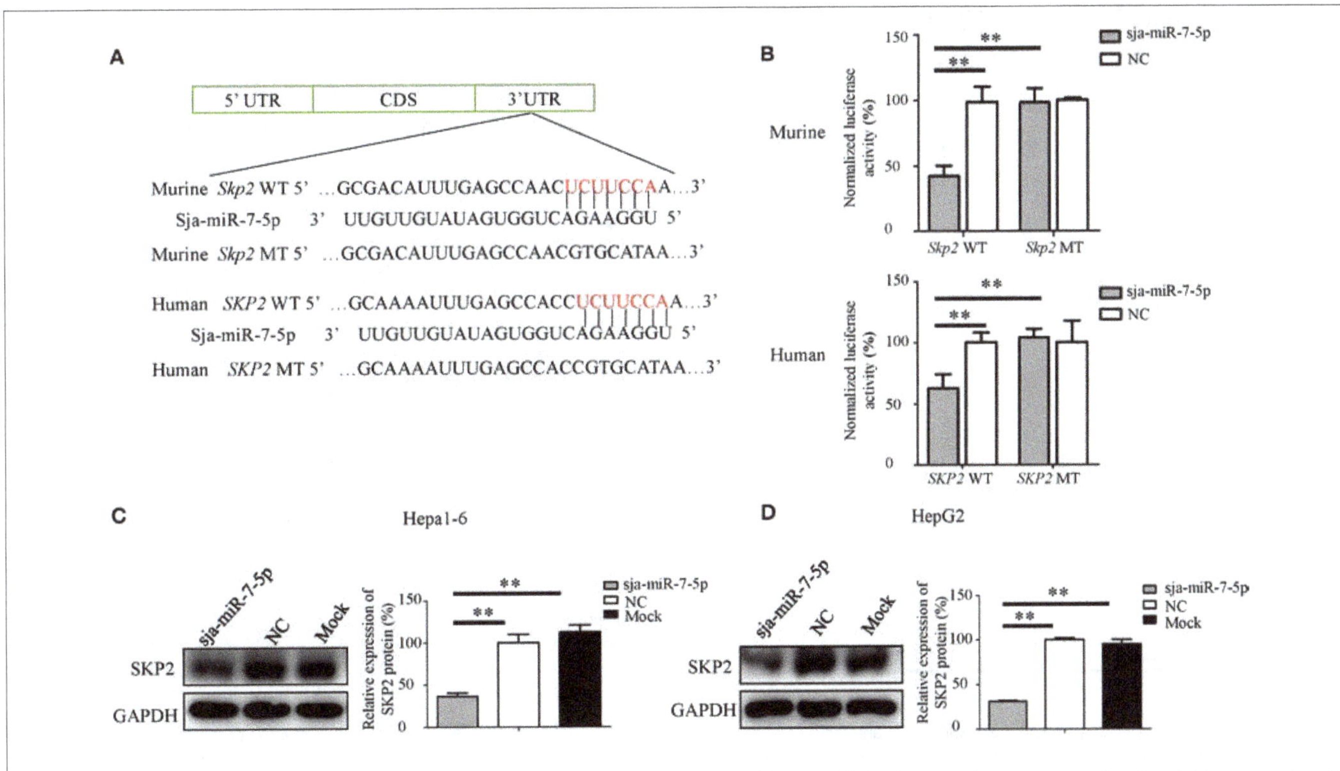

FIGURE 4 | *SKP2* (encoding S-phase kinase-associated protein 2) is a direct target of sja-miR-7-5p. **(A)** A schematic diagram representing the wild-type or mutant 3' untranslated region (UTR) sites of murine *Skp2* and human *SKP2* genes targeted by sja-miR-7-5p. **(B)** A dual-luciferase reporter assay was used to measure the activity of the reporter gene, and the firefly luciferase activity was normalized to renilla luciferase activity. **(C,D)** The protein levels of murine SKP2 **(C)** and human SKP2 **(D)** were measured using western blotting after transfection with sja-miR-7-5p mimics or NC mimics, respectively. Data are presented as the mean ± SD, $n = 3$, $^{**}p < 0.01$.

We then detected the level of the SKP2 protein in both Hepa1-6 or HepG2 cells transfected with sja-miR-7-5p mimics using Western blotting. We found that sja-miR-7-5p downregulated the levels of SKP2 in both Hepa1-6 cells and HepG2 cells compared with that in cells transfected with NC or Mock controls (**Figures 4C,D**).

Sja-miR-7-5p-Mediated Suppression of the Hepatoma Cell Growth Through Downregulation of SKP2 Expression

To investigate whether sja-miR-7-5p inhibits the growth of hepatoma cells through inhibition of SKP2 expression, both Hepa1-6 cells and HepG2 cells were transfected with the *SKP2* small interfering RNAs (siRNAs). We showed that both murine *Skp2* siRNA (SKP2-786) and human *SKP2* siRNA (SKP2-1291) significantly reduced the SKP2 expression in Hepa1-6 cells and HepG2 cells, respectively, at both transcriptional and translational levels detected by qRT-PCR and Western blotting (**Figure 5A**). Importantly, similar to the observations in the sja-miR-7-5p mimics-treated cells, the transfected Hepa1-6 cells and HepG2 cells with the siRNA showed cell cycle arrest at the G0/G1 phase (**Figures 5C,D**), and inhibition of cell proliferation (**Figure 5B**), cell migration (**Figure 5E**), and colony formation (**Figure 5F**), whereas these inhibitory effects were not observed in the cells treated with the NC siRNA. The phenotypes of the cells treated with *SKP2* siRNA were similar to those of sja-miR-7-5p mimics-treated cells, which suggested that the inhibitory effects of the schistosome miRNA on hepatoma cells function by downregulating SKP2 expression.

We also detected the expression of *SKP2* gene in the subcutaneous tumors generated by Hepa1-6 or HepG2 cells transfected with sja-miR-7-5p or NC mimics, respectively. As shown in **Figures 6A,B**, the transfected sja-miR-7-5p was detectable in the tumors on day 7 after injection. We then detected the SKP2 protein level using Western blotting, which showed that the level of SKP2 was significantly decreased in the tumors of both Hepa1-6 and HepG2 cells receiving sja-miR-7-5p compared with that in tumors from cells transfected with the NC control (**Figures 6C,D**). Meanwhile, we evaluated the proliferation of the tumor cells using immunohistochemistry (IHC) for Ki67, which showed that the protein level of Ki67 was also significantly decreased in tumor cells transfected with sja-miR-7-5p compared with that in cells transfected with the NC control (**Figure 6E**). These data further suggested that sja-miR-7-5p inhibited proliferation

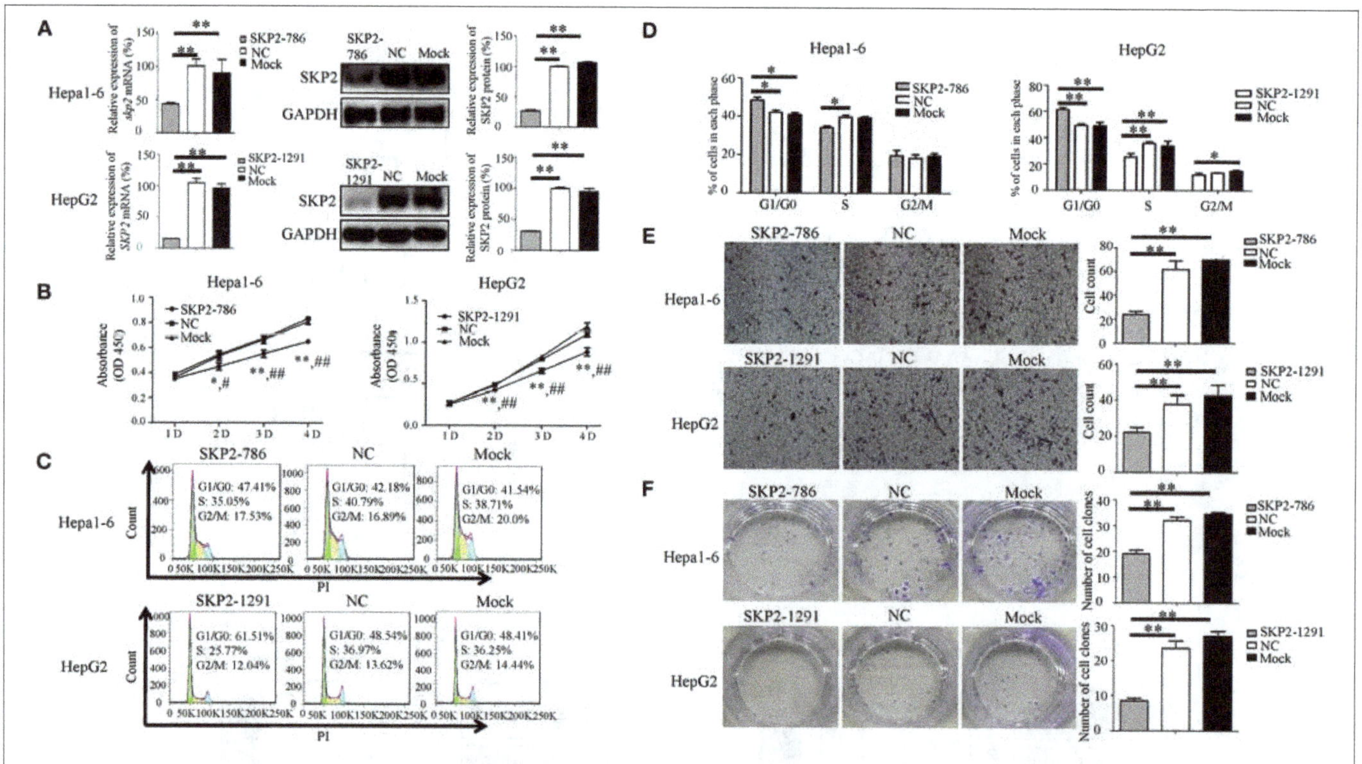

FIGURE 5 | Knockdown of *SKP2* inhibits cell proliferation and migration of Hepa1-6 and HepG2 cells *in vitro*. **(A–F)** Hepa1-6 and HepG2 cells were transfected with *SKP2* siRNA and negative control (NC) siRNA, respectively, and 48 h later (except for the cell counting kit-8(CCK-8) assay, which was 24 h later), the expression of *SKP2* was determined using qRT-PCR and western blotting **(A)**. Cell proliferation was evaluated using the CCK-8 assay at 1, 2, 3, and 4 d **(B)**, data are presented as the mean ± SD, $n = 3$, *$p < 0.05$ or **$p < 0.01$ indicates the comparison between the two groups of sja-miR-7-5p and NC; #$p < 0.05$ or ##$p < 0.01$ indicates the comparison between the two groups of sja-miR-7-5p and Mock. Cell cycle was determined using flow cytometry analysis **(C,D)**. Cell migration was evaluated by using Transwell inserts without matrigel coating **(E)**. The ability to form cell clones was determined using a colony formation assay **(F)**. Data are presented as the mean ± SD, $n = 3$, *$p < 0.05$, **$p < 0.01$.

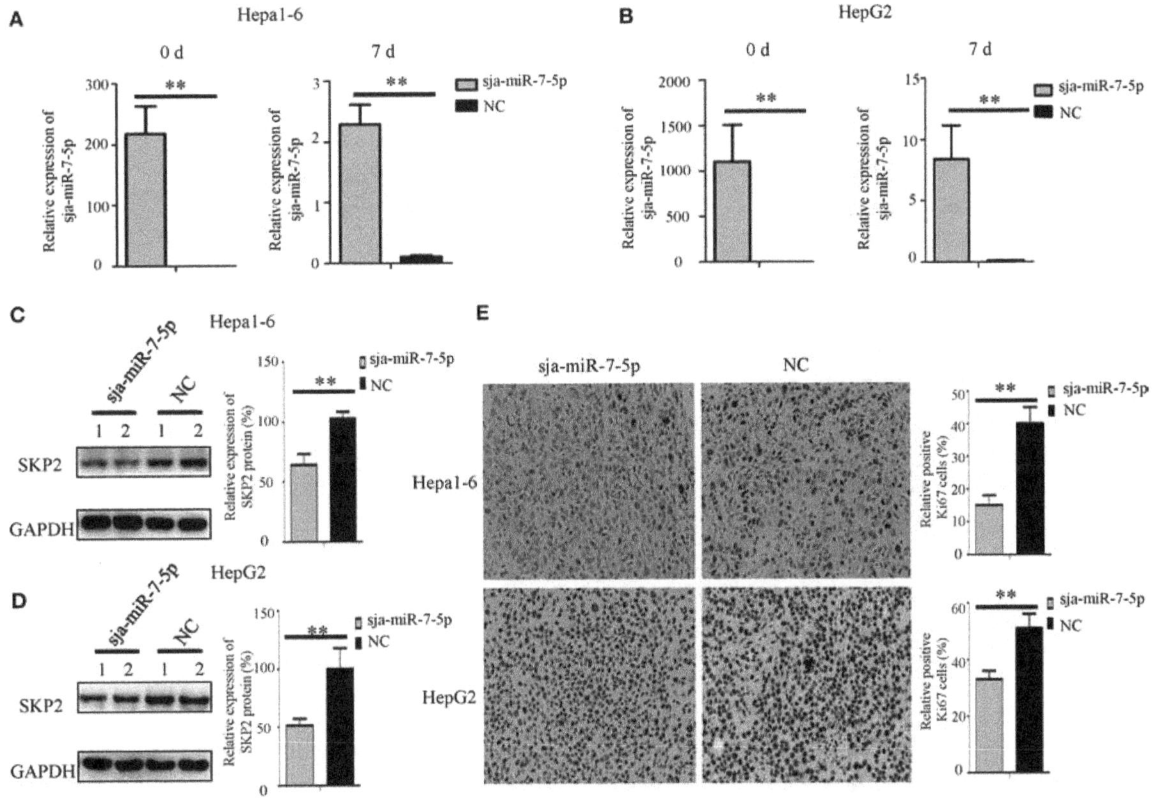

FIGURE 6 | Sja-miR-7-5p inhibits the expression of SKP2 and Ki67 within hepatoma cell tumors. **(A,B)**The content of sja-miR-7-5p mimics after transfection into tumor cells was measured using qRT-PCR before inoculation (0 d) and after sacrifice (7 d), with U6 as the internal control, **(A)** for Hepa1-6 cells, **(B)** for HepG2 cells. Data are presented as the mean ± SD, $n = 5$, $^{**}p < 0.01$. **(C,D)** The protein level of SKP2 was determined by Western blotting, with glyceraldehyde-3-phosphate (GAPDH) as the internal control, **(C)** for Hepa1-6 cells, **(D)** for HepG2 cells. **(E)** The level of Ki67 in tumors was determined using immunohistochemistry.

of both Hepal-6 cells and HepG2 cells via downregulation of SKP2 expression.

To further explore the molecular mechanism by which sja-miR-7-5p exerts its antitumor activities, we detected the expression of two downstream nodes of SKP2, e.g., P27 [also known as cyclin dependent kinase inhibitor 1B (CDKN1B)] and matrix metalloproteinase 9(MMP9), using Western blotting. We found that sja-miR-7-5p downregulated the level of SKP2, which led to significantly increased levels of P27 and reduced levels of MMP9 in the cells receiving sja-miR-7-5p mimics compared with those in the cells receiving the NC mimics (**Figure 7A**). In addition, transfection of the hepatoma cells with the murine *Skp2* siRNA generated a similar outcome to that in cells transfected with sja-miR-7-5p mimics (**Figure 7B**). These data suggested that sja-miR-7-5p exerts its antitumor activity by targeting *SKP2* to elevate P27 levels, which led to suppression of tumor cell growth, and reducing MMP9 levels, resulting in inhibition of cell migration.

DISCUSSION

Hsa-miR-7-5p is well-characterized as a tumor suppressor miRNA that suppresses survival, proliferation, invasion, and migration of multiple cancer cells, as well as increasing the sensitivity of resistant tumor cells to therapeutics. The molecular mechanism underpinning its anticancer activities involves regulation of multiple signaling related genes such as *PI3K/Akt*, *FAK*, *KLF4*, and *REGγ* (10, 39–41). This miRNA has therapeutic potential for human cancers (42). Our previous studies identified a conserved miR-7-5p from *S. japonicum*, sja-miR-7-5p, that has an identical seed sequence to those of hsa-miR-7-5p and mouse mmu-miR-7-5p, although there are 6 nt differences in the rest of the sequence of the miRNA among species. In this study, we have demonstrated that the schistosome miRNA, sja-miR-7-5p, is present in host hepatocytes during schistosome infection, and the *in vitro* transfection of sja-miR-7-5p mimics into hepatoma cells led to cell cycle arrest and inhibition of cell proliferation, colony formation, and cell migration. Furthermore, we showed that sja-miR-7-5p suppressed the growth of both human and mouse hepatoma cells in a xenograft animal model. Analysis of the molecular mechanisms revealed that sja-miR-7-5p exerts its activities by targeting the *SKP2* gene, which is involved in regulation of cell viability and migration. Thus, the present data indicated that the schistosome sja-miR-7-5p is also a tumor suppressor miRNA that may have therapeutic potential for human cancers. In addition, both the presence of

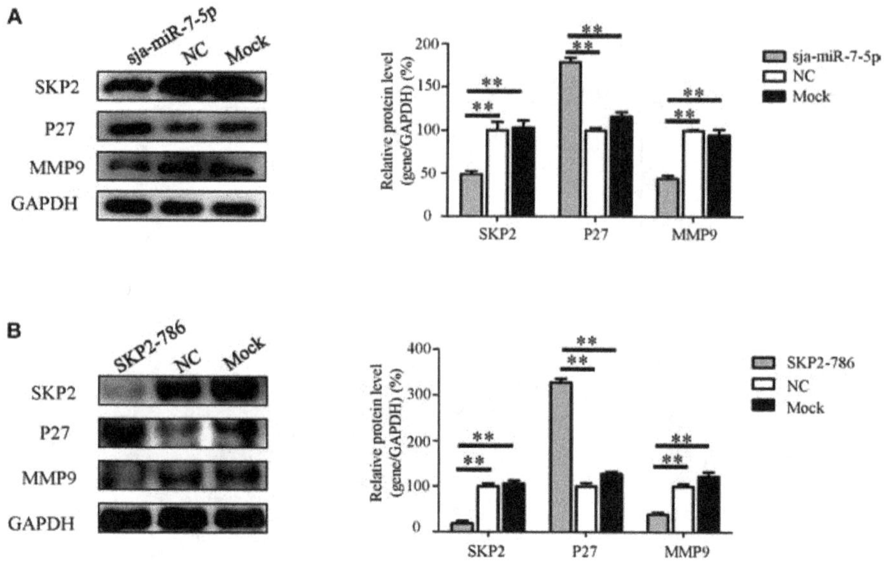

FIGURE 7 | The molecular mechanism whereby sja-miR-7-5p exerts its antitumor activity in hepatoma cells. **(A,B)** In Hepa1-6 cells, the protein levels of SKP2, P27, and MMP9 were measured by Western blotting after transfection with sja-miR-7-5p mimics **(A)** or *Skp2* siRNA **(B)** and their corresponding negative controls, with glyceraldehyde-3-phosphate (GAPDH) as the internal control. Data are presented as the mean ± SD, $n = 3$, $^{**}p < 0.01$.

this miRNA in host hepatocytes and its antitumor effects on human hepatoma cells suggest that schistosome non-small RNA-mediated anticarcinogenic effects might exist in the host liver during schistosome infection.

Infection with several parasites, such as *Opisthorchis viverrini* and *Clonorchis sinensis,* has been reported to be associated with cancer (43, 44). Schistosomiasis is a neglected tropical parasitic disease, affecting approximately 210 million people worldwide. Infection with *Schistosoma haematobium* is associated with bladder cancer (43, 44). However, for infection with *S. japonicum*, the association with hepatocellular carcinoma (HCC) is less evident, although a potential association with colorectal cancer was reported (45). The large retrospective epidemiological surveys conducted in highly endemic areas for schistosomiasis in China showed no correlation between HCC and *S. japonicum* infection (46). Although several other epidemiological and case–control studies proposed a potential association between HCC and *S. japonicum* infection, the evidences for the association remain a matter of debate because the schistosomiasis patients are highly associated with HBV and HCV infections, which are hepatic carcinogens (47). However, accumulating evidence indicates that chronic inflammation plays an important role in carcinogenesis (48). For *S. japonicum* infection, the liver-trapped eggs induce severe hepatic chronic inflammation and fibrosis that could be risk factors for HCC (49). These factors derived from *S. japonicum* infection should contribute to HCC, but this does not seem to happen in *S. japonicum* schistosomiasis. Therefore, we speculated that the *S. japonicum* eggs trapped in the liver might play a dual role in the HCC occurrence and development, i.e., carcinogenic and anticancer activities, similar to those reported for the protozoan *Trypanosoma cruzi*, which has carcinogenic and anticancer activities during infection (50). This study demonstrated that a non-coding small RNA secreted by *S. japonicum*, sja-miR-7-5p, perhaps together with other miRNAs derived from the parasite, could be translocated into liver cells during parasitic infection, and exerts anticancer activity, implying that the *S. japonicum*-producing non-coding small RNAs may, in part, contribute to the anticancer activities in the infected host.

As described above, mammalian miR-7-5p exerts its anticancer activities through regulation of multiple target genes such as *PI3K/Akt*, *FAK* and *KLF4.* To identify the target gene of the parasite sja-miR-7-5p, we first used three online software to search for its potential target genes. We found 5 target gene candidates (*Skp2, Psme3, Pik3cd, Klf4, and Hoxb5*) that were consistently predicted by the three software and involved in tumor-related signaling pathway. Three of them (i.e., *Pik3cd, Klf4, Hoxb5*) were excluded through analysis of their expression in hepatoma cells transfected with the sja-miR-7-5p mimics. Although both *Skp2* and *Psme3* genes were validated as target gene by luciferase reporter assay, our experimental data with *Skp2* and *Psme3* siRNA showed that only the hepatoma cell transfected with the *Skp2* siRNA produced similar phenotype to that of sja-miR-7-5p mimics-treated cells. Thus, *Skp2* gene has been identified as the target gene of sja-miR-7-5p.

SKP2, also known as P45, FBL1, FLB1, and FBXL1, is a component of the SCF (Skp1-Cullin 1-F-box) E3 ubiquitin-ligase complex. Many studies have reported that SKP2 is overexpressed in various cancers of different organs, including the liver (18), colon (51), breast (52), prostate (53), and stomach (54). *SKP2* is characterized as an oncogene, and is involved in modulation of the cell cycle, cell growth, and survival by regulation of its downstream node molecules, such as P27, P16, P21, P57, E2F-1, and c-MYC in an ubiquitin-dependent manner, followed by 26S proteasome degradation (23). Previous studies showed that loss of *SKP2* reduced the migration and invasion abilities of oral squamous cell carcinoma cells by downregulating the expression of MMP2 and MMP9 (55). The best-known substrate of SKP2 is the cyclin dependent kinase (CDK) inhibitor, P27. Overexpression of SKP2 leads to reduction of P27, which is strongly associated with aggressive tumor behavior and poor clinical outcome (19, 36, 56), while knockdown of *SKP2* resulted in the accumulation of P27, causing cell cycle arrest at G1/G0 phase (57). However, the relationship between miR-7-5p and *SKP2* has not yet been reported in HCC. In the present study, we found that in liver cancer cells, including Hepa1-6 cells and HepG2 cells, sja-miR-7-5p inhibited the growth and migration of both mouse and human hepatoma cells by targeting *SKP2* to elevate the expression of P27 and decrease the expression of MMP9. These data were consistent with the results of experiments using the *SKP2* siRNA, and with the outcome of a study in which miRNA-7-5p could suppress cell proliferation of CHO cells partly by targeting *skp2* (58). Therefore, our data demonstrated that sja-miR-7-5p suppresses hepatoma cell growth and migration by downregulating *SKP2*.

The present study demonstrated that sja-miR-7-5p is present in infected hepatocytes, selectively affects the growth and migration of human and mouse tumor cells by targeting the *SKP2* gene, implying that sja-miR-7-5p might strengthen resistance of host to cancer during schistosome infection.

AUTHOR CONTRIBUTIONS

CH and WP conceived and designed the study. CH, SZ, JW, YL, LM, LZ, PJ, and ZL performed the experiments. CH, SZ, and WP analyzed the data. CH and WP wrote the manuscript. All authors read and approved the final manuscript.

FUNDING

This study was supported by the National Natural Science Foundation of China (81430051).

ACKNOWLEDGMENTS

We thank the staff of the National Institute of Parasitic Disease, Chinese Center for Disease Control and Prevention for their help with parasite infections.

REFERENCES

1. Colley DG, Bustinduy AL, Secor WE, King CH. Human schistosomiasis. *Lancet.* (2014) 383:2253–64. doi: 10.1016/S0140-6736(13)61949-2
2. Zhu SL, Wang S, Lin Y, Jiang PY, Cui XB, Wang XY, et al. Release of extracellular vesicles containing small RNAs from the eggs of *Schistosoma japonicum. Parasit Vectors.* (2016) 9:574. doi: 10.1186/s13071-016-1845-2
3. Bartel DP. MicroRNAs: Genomics, biogenesis, mechanism, and function. *Cell.* (2004) 116:281–97. doi: 10.1016/S0092-8674(04)00045-5
4. Calin GA, Croce CM. MicroRNA signatures in human cancers. *Nat Rev Cancer.* (2006) 6:857–66. doi: 10.1038/nrc1997
5. Berindan-Neagoe I, Monroig PD, Pasculli B, Calin GA. MicroRNAome genome: a treasure for cancer diagnosis and therapy. *Ca-a Cancer J Clini.* (2014) 64:311–36. doi: 10.3322/caac.21244
6. Mi Y, Zhang D, Jiang W, Weng J, Zhou C, Huang K, et al. miR-181a-5p promotes the progression of gastric cancer via RASSF6-mediated MAPK signalling activation. *Cancer Lett.* (2017) 389:11–22. doi: 10.1016/j.canlet.2016.12.033
7. Xue X, Fei X, Hou W, Zhang Y, Liu L, Hu R. miR-342-3p suppresses cell proliferation and migration by targeting AGR2 in non-small cell lung cancer. *Cancer Lett.* (2018) 412:170–8. doi: 10.1016/j.canlet.2017.10.024
8. Zhu Y, Gu J, Li Y, Peng C, Shi M, Wang X, et al. MiR-17-5p enhances pancreatic cancer proliferation by altering cell cycle profiles via disruption of RBL2/E2F4-repressing complexes. *Cancer Lett.* (2018) 412:59–68. doi: 10.1016/j.canlet.2017.09.044
9. Hatziapostolou M, Polytarchou C, Aggelidou E, Drakaki A, Poultsides GA, Jaeger SA, et al. An HNF4 alpha-miRNA inflammatory feedback circuit regulates hepatocellular oncogenesis. *Cell.* (2011) 147:1233–47. doi: 10.1016/j.cell.2011.10.043
10. Fang YX, Xue JL, Shen Q, Chen JZ, Tian L. MicroRNA-7 inhibits tumor growth and metastasis by targeting the phosphoinositide 3-kinase/Akt pathway in hepatocellular carcinoma. *Hepatology.* (2012) 55:1852–62. doi: 10.1002/hep.25576
11. Zhang L, Hou DX, Chen X, Li DH, Zhu LY, Zhang YJ, et al. Exogenous plant MIR168a specifically targets mammalian LDLRAP1: evidence of cross-kingdom regulation by microRNA. *Cell Res.* (2012) 22:107–26. doi: 10.1038/cr.2011.158
12. Zhou Z, Li XH, Liu JX, Dong L, Chen Q, Liu JL, et al. Honeysuckle-encoded atypical microRNA2911 directly targets influenza A viruses. *Cell Res.* (2015) 25:39–49. doi: 10.1038/cr.2014.130
13. Chin AR, Fong MY, Somlo G, Wu J, Swiderski P, Wu XW, et al. Cross-kingdom inhibition of breast cancer growth by plant miR159. *Cell Res.* (2016) 26:217–28. doi: 10.1038/cr.2016.13
14. Liu HX, Huang J, Peng J, Wu XX, Zhang Y, Zhu WL, et al. Upregulation of the inwardly rectifying potassium channel Kir2.1 (KCNJ2) modulates multidrug resistance of small-cell lung cancer under the regulation of miR-7 and the Ras/MAPK pathway. *Mol Cancer.* (2015) 14:59. doi: 10.1186/s12943-015-0298-0
15. Liu HX, Wu XX, Huang J, Peng J, Guo LL. miR-7 modulates chemoresistance of small cell lung cancer by repressing MRP1/ABCC1. *Int J Exp Pathol.* (2015) 96:240–7. doi: 10.1111/iep.12131
16. Suto T, Yokobori T, Yajima R, Morita H, Fujii T, Yamaguchi S, et al. MicroRNA-7 expression in colorectal cancer is associated with poor prognosis and regulates cetuximab sensitivity via EGFR regulation. *Carcinogenesis.* (2015) 36:338–45. doi: 10.1093/carcin/bgu242
17. Cheng MW, Shen ZT, Hu GY, Luo LG. Prognostic significance of microRNA-7 and its roles in the regulation of cisplatin resistance in lung

adenocarcinoma. *Cell Physiol Biochem.* (2017) 42:660–72. doi: 10.1159/000477884

18. Lee SW, Li CF, Jin G, Cai Z, Han F, Chan CH, et al. Skp2-dependent ubiquitination and activation of LKB1 is essential for cancer cell survival under energy stress. *Mol Cell.* (2015) 57:1022–33. doi: 10.1016/j.molcel.2015.01.015
19. Wang Z, Gao D, Fukushima H, Inuzuka H, Liu P, Wan L, et al. Skp2: a novel potential therapeutic target for prostate cancer. *Biochim Biophys Acta.* (2012) 1825:11–7. doi: 10.1016/j.bbcan.2011.09.002
20. Seki R, Okamura T, Koga H, Yakushiji K, Hashiguchi M, Yoshimoto K, et al. Prognostic significance of the F-box protein Skp2 expression in diffuse large B-cell lymphoma. *Am J Hematol.* (2003) 73:230–5. doi: 10.1002/ajh.10379
21. Rose AE, Wang G, Hanniford D, Monni S, Tu T, Shapiro RL, et al. Clinical relevance of SKP2 alterations in metastatic melanoma. *Pigment Cell Melanoma Res.* (2011) 24:197–206. doi: 10.1111/j.1755-148X.2010.00784.x
22. Radke S, Pirkmaier A, Germain D. Differential expression of the F-box proteins Skp2 and Skp2B in breast cancer. *Oncogene.* (2005) 24:3448–58. doi: 10.1038/sj.onc.1208328
23. Bochis OV, Irimie A, Pichler M, Berindan-Neagoe I. The Role of Skp2 and its Substrate CDKN1B (p27) in colorectal cancer. *J Gastrointes Liver Dis.* (2015) 24:225–34. doi: 10.15403/jgld.2014.1121.242.skp2
24. Hung WC, Tseng WL, Shiea J, Chang HC. Skp2 overexpression increases the expression of MMP-2 and MMP-9 and invasion of lung cancer cells. *Cancer Lett.* (2010) 288:156–61. doi: 10.1016/j.canlet.2009.06.032
25. Yokoi S, Yasui K, Mori M, Iizasa T, Fujisawa T, Inazawa J. Amplification and overexpression of SKP2 are associated with metastasis of non-small-cell lung cancers to lymph nodes. *Am J Pathol.* (2004) 165:175–80. doi: 10.1016/S0002-9440(10)63286-5
26. Shi C, Pan BQ, Shi F, Xie ZH, Jiang YY, Shang L, et al. Sequestosome 1 protects esophageal squamous carcinoma cells from apoptosis via stabilizing SKP2 under serum starvation condition. *Oncogene.* (2018) 37:3260–74. doi: 10.1038/s41388-018-0217-0
27. Osoegawa A, Yoshino I, Tanaka S, Sugio K, Kameyama T, Yamaguchi M, et al. Regulation of p27 by S-phase kinase-associated protein 2 is associated with aggressiveness in non-small-cell lung cancer. *J Clin Oncol.* (2004) 22:4165–73. doi: 10.1200/JCO.2004.01.035
28. Zhu CQ, Blackhall FH, Pintilie M, Iyengar P, Liu N, Ho J, et al. Skp2 gene copy number aberrations are common in non-small cell lung carcinoma, and its overexpression in tumors with ras mutation is a poor prognostic marker. *Clin Cancer Res.* (2004) 10:1984–91. doi: 10.1158/1078-0432.CCR-03-0470
29. Cai PF, Piao XY, Hao LL, Liu S, Hou N, Wang H, et al. A deep analysis of the small non-coding RNA population in *Schistosoma japonicum* eggs. *PLoS ONE.* (2013) 8:64003. doi: 10.1371/journal.pone.0064003
30. He X, Xie J, Zhang DM, Su Q, Sai X, Bai RP, et al. Recombinant adeno-associated virus-mediated inhibition of microRNA-21 protects mice against the lethal schistosome infection by repressing both IL-13 and transforming growth factor beta 1 pathways. *Hepatology.* (2015) 61:2008–17. doi: 10.1002/hep.27671
31. Yin XD, Xiang TX, Li LL, Su XW, Shu XS, Luo XR, et al. DACT1, an antagonist to Wnt/beta-catenin signaling, suppresses tumor cell growth and is frequently silenced in breast cancer. *Breast Cancer Res.* (2013) 15:R23. doi: 10.1186/bcr3399
32. Wong N, Wang XW. miRDB: an online resource for microRNA target prediction and functional annotations. *Nucl Acids Res.* (2015) 43:D146–52. doi: 10.1093/nar/gku1104
33. Reczko M, Maragkakis M, Alexiou P, Grosse I, Hatzigeorgiou AG. Functional microRNA targets in protein coding sequences. *Bioinformatics.* (2012) 28:771–6. doi: 10.1093/bioinformatics/bts043
34. Kruger J, Rehmsmeier M. RNAhybrid: microRNA target prediction easy, fast and flexible. *Nucl Acids Res.* (2006) 34:W451–4. doi: 10.1093/nar/gkl243
35. Lim MS, Adamson A, Lin ZS, Perez-Ordonez B, Jordan RCK, Tripp S, et al. Expression of Skp2, a p27(Kip1) ubliquitin ligase, in malignant lymphoma: correlation with p27(Kip1) and proliferation index. *Blood.* (2002) 100:2950–6. doi: 10.1182/blood.V100.8.2950
36. Shapira M, Ben-Izhak O, Linn S, Futerman B, Minkov I, Hershko DD. The prognostic impact of the ubiquitin ligase subunits Skp2 and Cks1 in colorectal carcinoma. *Cancer.* (2005) 103:1336–46. doi: 10.1002/cncr.20917
37. Hershko DD. Oncogenic properties and prognostic implications of the ubiquitin ligase Skp2 in cancer. *Cancer.* (2008) 112:1415–24. doi: 10.1002/cncr.23317
38. Schuler S, Diersch S, Hamacher R, Schmid RM, Saur D, Schneider G. SKP2 confers resistance of pancreatic cancer cells towards TRAIL-induced apoptosis. *Int J Oncol.* (2011) 38:219–25. doi: 10.3892/ijo_00000841
39. Kong XJ, Li GP, Yuan Y, He Y, Wu XL, Zhang WJ, et al. MicroRNA-7 Inhibits Epithelial-to-mesenchymal transition and metastasis of breast cancer cells via targeting FAK expression. *PLoS ONE.* (2012) 7:e41523. doi: 10.1371/journal.pone.0041523
40. Okuda H, Xing F, Pandey PR, Sharma S, Watabe M, Pai SK, et al. miR-7 suppresses brain metastasis of breast cancer stem-like cells by modulating KLF4. *Cancer Res.* (2013) 73:1434–44. doi: 10.1158/0008-5472.CAN-12-2037
41. Shi Y, Luo XR, Li P, Tan JX, Wang XY, Xiang TXS, et al. miR-7-5p suppresses cell proliferation and induces apoptosis of breast cancer cells mainly by targeting REG gamma. *Cancer Lett.* (2015) 358:27–36. doi: 10.1016/j.canlet.2014.12.014
42. Kalinowski FC, Brown RAM, Ganda C, Giles KM, Epis MR, Horsham J, et al. microRNA-7: a tumor suppressor miRNA with therapeutic potential. *Int J Biochem Cell Biol.* (2014) 54:312–7. doi: 10.1016/j.biocel.2014.05.040
43. Bouvard V, Baan R, Straif K, Grosse Y, Secretan B, El Ghissassi F, et al. A review of human carcinogens–Part B: biological agents. *Lancet Oncol.* (2009) 10:321–2. doi: 10.1016/S1470-2045(09)70096-8
44. IARC Working Group on the Evaluation of Carcinogenic Risks to Humans. Biological agents. Volume 100 B. A review of human carcinogens. *IARC Monogr Eval Carcinog Risks Hum.* (2012) 100:1–441.
45. Chen MG. Assessment of morbidity due to Schistosoma japonicum infection in China. *Infect Dis Poverty.* (2014) 3:6. doi: 10.1186/2049-9957-3-6
46. Liu BQ, Rong ZP, Sun XT, Wu YP, Gao RQ. Geographical correlation between colorectal cancer and schistosomiasis in China. *Zhongguo Yi Xue Ke Xue Yuan Xue Bao.* (1983) 5:173–7.
47. Arzumanyan A, Reis HM, Feitelson MA. Pathogenic mechanisms in HBV- and HCV-associated hepatocellular carcinoma. *Nat Rev Cancer.* (2013) 13:123–35. doi: 10.1038/nrc3449
48. Zhang R, Takahashi S, Orita S, Yoshida A, Maruyama H, Shirai T, et al. p53 gene mutations in rectal cancer associated with schistosomiasis japonica in Chinese patients. *Cancer Lett.* (1998) 131:215–21. doi: 10.1016/S0304-3835(98)00154-2
49. Takemura Y, Kikuchi S, Inaba Y. Epidemiologic study of the relationship between schistosomiasis due to *Schistosoma japonicum* and liver cancer/cirrhosis. *Am Journal Tropi Med Hygiene.* (1998) 59:551–6. doi: 10.4269/ajtmh.1998.59.551
50. van Tong H, Brindley PJ, Meyer CG, Velavan TP. Parasite infection, carcinogenesis and human malignancy. *EBioMedicine.* (2017) 15:12–23. doi: 10.1016/j.ebiom.2016.11.034
51. Fujita T, Liu WJ, Doihara H, Wan Y. Regulation of Skp2-p27 axis by the Cdh1/anaphase-promoting complex pathway in colorectal tumorigenesis. *Am J Pathol.* (2008) 173:217–28. doi: 10.2353/ajpath.2008.070957
52. Liu J, Wei XL, Huang WH, Chen CF, Bai JW, Zhang GJ. Cytoplasmic Skp2 expression is associated with p-Akt1 and predicts poor prognosis in human breast carcinomas. *PLoS ONE.* (2012) 7:e52675. doi: 10.1371/journal.pone.0052675
53. Moro L, Arbini AA, Marra E, Greco M. Up-regulation of Skp2 after prostate cancer cell adhesion to basement membranes results in BRCA2 degradation and cell proliferation. *J Biol Chem.* (2006) 281:22100–7. doi: 10.1074/jbc.M604636200
54. Ma XM, Liu Y, Guo JW, Liu JH, Zuo LF. Relation of overexpression of S phase kinase-associated protein 2 with reduced expression of p27 and PTEN in human gastric carcinoma. *World J Gastroenterol.* (2005) 11:6716–21. doi: 10.3748/wjg.v11.i42.6716
55. Yamada SI, Yanamoto S, Naruse T, Matsushita Y, Takahashi H, Umeda M, et al. Skp2 Regulates the Expression of MMP-2 and MMP-9, and enhances the invasion potential of oral squamous cell carcinoma. *Pathol Oncol Res.* (2016) 22:625–32. doi: 10.1007/s12253-016-0049-6

56. Wang Z, Fukushima H, Inuzuka H, Wan L, Liu P, Gao D, et al. Skp2 is a promising therapeutic target in breast cancer. *Front Oncol.* (2012) 1:18702. doi: 10.3389/fonc.2011.00057
57. Ding L, Li R, Han X, Zhou Y, Zhang H, Cui Y, et al. Inhibition of Skp2 suppresses the proliferation and invasion of osteosarcoma cells. *Oncol Rep.* (2017) 38:933–40. doi: 10.3892/or.2017.5713
58. Sanchez N, Gallagher M, Lao N, Gallagher C, Clarke C, Doolan P, et al. MiR-7 Triggers Cell Cycle Arrest at the G1/S Transition by Targeting Multiple Genes Including Skp2 and Psme3. *PLoS ONE.* (2013) 8:e65671. doi: 10.1371/journal.pone.0065671

7

Regulation of Wnt Signaling Pathway by Poly (ADP-Ribose) Glycohydrolase (PARG) Silencing Suppresses Lung Cancer in Mice Induced by Benzo(a)pyrene Inhalation Exposure

Wenjuan Dai[1,2†], Yingbin Fu[1†], Yanxia Deng[1†], Zhuoying Zeng[1], Pan Gu[1], Hailong Liu[1], Jianjun Liu[1], Xinyun Xu[1], Desheng Wu[1], Xianru Luo[1], Linqing Yang[1], Jinzhou Zhang[1], Kai Lin[1], Gonghua Hu[2,3] and Haiyan Huang[1]**

[1] *Shenzhen Center for Disease Control and Prevention, Shenzhen, China,* [2] *Jiangxi Provincial Key Laboratory of Preventive Medicine, School of Public Health, Nanchang University, Nanchang, China,* [3] *Department of Preventive Medicine, Gannan Medical University, Ganzhou, China*

***Correspondence:**
Gonghua Hu
hgh0129@163.com
Haiyan Huang
hhy424@126.com

† These authors have contributed equally to this work

Benzo(a)pyrene (BaP) is a polycyclic aromatic hydrocarbon that specifically causes cancer and is widely distributed in the environment. Poly (ADP-ribosylation), as a key post-translational modification in BaP-induced carcinogenesis, is mainly catalyzed by poly (ADP-ribose) glycohydrolase (PARG) in eukaryotic organisms. Previously, it is found that PARG silencing can counteract BaP-induced carcinogenesis *in vitro*, but the mechanism remained unclear. In this study, we further examined this process *in vivo* by using heterozygous PARG knockout mice ($PARG^{+/-}$). Wild-type and $PARG^{+/-}$ mice were individually treated with 0 or 10 $\mu g/m^3$ BaP for 90 or 180 days by dynamic inhalation exposure. Pathological analysis of lung tissues showed that, with extended exposure time, carcinogenesis and injury in the lungs of WT mice was progressively worse; however, the injury was minimal and carcinogenesis was not detected in the lungs of $PARG^{+/-}$ mice. These results indicate that PARG gene silencing protects mice against lung cancer induced by BaP inhalation exposure. Furthermore, as the exposure time was extended, the protein phosphorylation level was down-regulated in WT mice, but up-regulated in $PARG^{+/-}$ mice. The relative expression of Wnt2b and Wnt5b mRNA in WT mice were significantly higher than those in the control group, but there was no significant difference in $PARG^{+/-}$ mice. Meanwhile, the relative expression of Wnt2b and Wnt5b proteins, as assessed by immunohistochemistry and Western blot analysis, was significantly up-regulated by BaP in WT mice; while in $PARG^{+/-}$ mice it was not statistically affected. Our work provides initial evidence that PARG silencing suppresses BaP induced lung cancer and stabilizes the expression of Wnt ligands, PARG gene and Wnt ligands may provide new options for the diagnosis and treatment of lung cancer.

Keywords: benzo(a)pyrene, ADP-ribosylation, poly (ADP-ribose) glycohydrolase, Wnt signaling pathway, lung cancer

INTRODUCTION

Benzo(a)pyrene (BaP) is a polycyclic aromatic hydrocarbon that is known to be carcinogenic. It is mainly produced by pyrolysis and incomplete combustion of carbonaceous materials and is widely distributed in both the working and living environment (Liu et al., 2008). A large number of experiments have shown that BaP can induce cancer in various animals (IARC Working Group on the Evaluation of Carcinogenic Risks to Humans, 2010; Kasala et al., 2016). Furthermore, epidemiological studies suggest that BaP is closely associated with human lung cancer (Rojas et al., 2004; Alexandrov et al., 2010; Widziewicz et al., 2018). On the basis of these studies, BaP was classified as a human class I carcinogen by the International Agency for Research on Cancer in 2006 (IARC Working Group on the Evaluation of Carcinogenic Risks to Humans, 2012).

Lung cancer is the most common malignant tumor in the human respiratory system and is extremely harmful to human health. Globally, the morbidity and mortality of lung cancer are among the highest (Ferlay et al., 2015). According to the American Cancer Society, lung cancer leads to the highest number of deaths in both men and women. Recent evidence suggests that the incidence of lung cancer in China is the highest and the mortality is increasing at a rate of 4.5% per year (Chen et al., 2016).

The occurrence of lung cancer is the result of a combination of both environmental and genetic factors, including epigenetic changes which have been proved to contribute to lung cancer development (Hagood, 2014). ADP-ribosylation, as an epigenetic modification, plays a critical role in cell survival and disease development, including cancers (D'Amours et al., 1999; Min et al., 2010; Huang et al., 2012). Poly-ADP-ribosylation can convert nuclear chromatin to a loose state, allowing accessibility of DNA damage repair enzymes to the injury site, thereby promoting DNA damage repair against cytotoxicity and genetic damage. Poly-ADP-ribose glycohydrolase (PARG) can hydrolyze poly (ADP-ribose) on poly (ADP-ribose) polymerase-1 (PARP-1), which promotes the degradation of intracellular poly (ADP-ribose) (PAR) (Rouleau et al., 2004). It is the only known enzyme that can hydrolyze poly (ADP-ribose) in the nucleus (Meyer et al., 2007). Recent studies have shown that PARG gene silencing can increase intracellular poly-ADP-ribosylation to protect cells against cytotoxicity. Li et al. (Li et al., 2016) found that BaP can induce chromosomal aberrations, micronucleus formation, chromatin structure changes and malignant transformation of normal 16HBE cells, but PARG gene silencing can inhibit these abnormalities. Studies have shown that PARG also is associated with tumorigenesis (Miwa and Masutani, 2007), but the exact mechanism of PARG on tumor promotion has not been fully clarified.

In our previous study, 16HBE cells and PARG-deficient cells were treated with 40 μmol/L BaP for a period of time to induce malignant transformation, and by using MeDIP-sequence analysis, it is found that the methylation levels of Wnt2b and Wnt5b genes in the two cells were significantly different. Wnt2b and Wnt5b are key players in the Wnt/β-Catenin signaling pathway (Klaus and Birchmeier, 2008), which has been highly conserved in evolution and is known to control cell growth, differentiation, apoptosis, and self-renewal. This pathway is activated by binding of Wnt ligands to receptors, which increases the stability of β-catenin in the cytoplasm and promotes its translocation to the nucleus, where it modulates the expression of target genes that lead to tumorigenesis (Klaus and Birchmeier, 2008). Studies have shown that this pathway is abnormally activated during the development of lung cancer and may coordinate or antagonize other signaling pathways to regulate proliferation, migration, and invasion in lung cancer (Reya and Clevers, 2005; Berndt and Moon, 2013). Recently, 30–40% of cells in tumor tissues have been shown to express Wnt ligands, which create a microenvironment that is suitable for tumor cells. In a human lung adenocarcinoma model, 70% of cells have abnormal activation of the Wnt pathway, and 80% of cells may be involved in the formation of the tumor microenvironment, which is critical for the progression of lung cancer (Tammela et al., 2017).

Given the decisive role of the Wnt signaling pathway in the development of lung cancer, inhibition of Wnt ligands provides a viable approach for reducing the expansion of lung cancer cell lines. The purpose of this study was to investigate whether PARG gene silencing can inhibit lung cancer development induced by BaP and whether it can regulate the Wnt ligands to inhibit the development of lung cancer. On the basis of our findings, PARG gene and Wnt ligands may constitute a new option for the diagnosis and treatment of lung cancer.

MATERIALS AND METHODS

Materials

BaP (CAS50-32-8, purity ≥96%) was purchased from American Sigma Company, and dissolved in dimethylsulfoxide (DMSO). Other chemicals were purchased from Sigma–Aldrich (St Louis, MO, United States) or Thermo Fisher Scientific (Shanghai, China), unless otherwise stated.

Animals and Treatment

The PARG knockout mice [B6N (Cg)-Parg$^{tm2b(KOMP)Mbp}$/J]were purchased from the Jackson Laboratory, and WT mice (C57BL/6J) were purchased from Guangdong Medical Lab Animal Center. PARG knockout mice were generated by the targeted mutation 2b of the Parg gene resulting in deletion of the full-length isoform of PARG protein (PARG$_{110}$). The strategy of gene targeting is Cre-mediated excision of the parental Parg$^{tm2b(KOMP)Mbp}$ allele resulted in the removal of the promoter-driven neomycin selection cassette and critical exon(s) leaving behind the inserted lacZ reporter sequence. We screened for heterozygous PARG knockout mice (PARG$^{+/-}$) in our study since death of homozygous PARG knockout mice (PARG$^{-/-}$) occurring before the normal life span of an organism, occurring during pregnancy, parturition or lactation. The mice were maintained under semi-specific-pathogen-free conditions with the temperature controlled at 23 ± 2°C and a 12-h light/dark cycle. We selected 2-month-old $PARG^{+/-}$ and WT mice for this study. The mice were randomly divided into two groups with 6 per group referring to the principles of experimental animal selection and references. And then, they were treated with 0 or 10 $\mu g/m^3$ aerosols through respiratory tract by a dynamic inhalation cabinet (Jiufang Company, Guangzhou) for 90 or 180 days. The dynamic inhalation device makes liquids into aerosols with a diameter of only a few micrometers, which is in line with the actual human exposure to BaP in the air. At the end of the experiment, mice were anesthetized with ether and blood was collected by eyeball sampling. The mice were then euthanized and the lungs were excised rapidly. Half of each lung was stored in 4% paraformaldehyde, and the other half was stored at −80°C. All animal experiments and procedures were approved by the Shenzhen Center for Disease Control and Prevention. Efforts were made to minimize animal suffering and reduce the number of mice used in the experiments.

Genotyping of PARG Knockout Mice

Genomic DNA was purified from mouse tails using TianAMP genomic DNA kits (Tiangen, Beijing, China). The concentration and the quality of DNA were assessed by ultraviolet (UV) absorbance using a NanoDrop ND-2000 spectrophotometer (Thermo Fisher Scientific). The DNA was then amplified by PCR (94°C for 2 min; 10 cycles of 94°C for 20 s, 65°C for 15 s, and 68°C for 10 s; 10 cycles of 94°C for 15 s, 60°C for 15 s, and 72°C for 10 s; 72°C for 2 min, 10°C hold) using primers provided by the Jackson Laboratory (Wild-type Forward: 5′-GAG ATA TCT AAG TCA GAG AAA GGT GGT-3′, Wild-type Reverse: 5′-CCT CCT CTG GTG TGT CTG AAG-3′, Mutant Forward: 5′-CGG TCG CTA CCA TTA CCA GT-3′, Mutant Reverse: 5′-GGT ATC AGC GAT GGT TGT TC-3′). The PCR products were 279 bp for the WT sample, and 279 and 507 bp for the heterozygous PARG knockout ($PARG^{+/-}$) sample.

Hematoxylin and Eosin Staining

Mouse lung tissues were fixed in 4% paraformaldehyde for 48 h, dehydrated in ethanol and embedded in paraffin by using a TissueWave™ 2 Microwave Processor (Thermo Fisher Scientific). Paraffin-fixed tissues were sliced into 5 μm sections, mounted on glass slides, and dried for 1 h. After dewaxing and rehydration, sections were stained with hematoxylin and eosin (Sigma-Aldrich) and examined by light microscopy. The pathology was evaluated by a blinded observer to detect the degree of malignancy.

Real-Time Quantitative PCR

Total RNA was extracted from frozen lung samples with miRNeasy mini kits (Qiagen, China) according to the manufacturer's instructions. Complementary DNA (cDNA) was synthesized from 500 ng of total lung RNA (n = 3 per group) using the PrimeScript™ RT reagent kit (Takara, China). Quantitative PCR (qPCR) was performed on the ABI Prism 7500 system (Applied Biosystems, Foster City, CA, United States) using SYBR select master mix. The mRNA primers were purchased from Sangon Biotech (Shanghai, China) and are listed in **Supplementary Table S1**. Experiments were repeated at least 3 times. The relative level of mRNA for each gene was determined using the $2^{-\Delta\Delta Ct}$ method (Schmittgen and Livak, 2008), and P-values were calculated using the Student's t-test on replicate $2^{-\Delta Ct}$ values for each gene in each treatment group compared to the control group.

Immunohistochemistry

Mouse lung tissues were fixed in 4% paraformaldehyde for 48 h, dehydrated in ethanol and embedded in paraffin by using a TissueWave™ Microwave Processor (Thermo Fisher Scientific). After dewaxing and rehydration, 5 μm-thick coronal sections were incubated in 0.01 M citrate buffer (pH 6.0) with 0.1% Tween-20 at 95–100°C for 10 min for antigen retrieval. For immunochemistry of Wnt2b and Wnt5b (n = 3 per group), the sections were incubated at 4°C overnight with primary antibody (Wnt2b at 1:200 or Wnt5b at 1:50). After being washed with PBST, the sections were stained using the mouse and rabbit-specific HRP/DAB (ABC) detection IHC kit (Abcam, ab64264) and analyzed using an Olympus BX60 compound microscope (Tokyo, Japan).

Western Blot Analysis

Lung proteins (n = 3 per group) were extracted from 30 mg lung tissue with 600 μL lysis buffer (Beyotime, China) and 6 μL protease and phosphatase inhibitor cocktail (Thermo Fisher Scientific, United States) on ice, and then centrifuged and collected. The protein concentration was measured with a BCA protein assay kit (Thermo Fisher Scientific, United States). Each protein sample was combined with loading buffer and heated for 8 min at 100°C. Protein samples were separated on 10% PAGE gels with 5% stacking gels and transferred to PVDF membranes. The membranes were incubated in TBST buffer containing 5% milk at room temperature for 2 h. Subsequently, they were incubated with anti-PARG (mouse monoclonal antibody, 1:100), anti-phosphotyrosine (PY20, mouse monoclonal antibody,1:1000), anti-Wnt2b (rabbit monoclonal antibody, 1:3000), anti-Wnt5b (mouse monoclonal antibody,1:500), or anti-α-tubulin (mouse monoclonal antibody, 1:3000) in TBST buffer for 1.5 h at room temperature. After washing with TBST three times, the membranes were incubated with homologous secondary antibody (anti-rabbit or anti-mouse IgG HRPs) in TBST buffer for 60 min. The membranes were then repeatedly washed with TBST buffer, developed using chemiluminescence reagents from an ECL kit (Pierce ECL, Santa Cruz, CA, United States) and detected on a phosphorimager. The images of the membranes were analyzed by ImageJ software.

Statistical Analysis

The histograms and statistical analyses of the relative expression of each group were completed using Graph-Pad prism 7.0 software (GraphPad Software, Inc.). Data are presented as mean ± SD. Comparisons between two groups were conducted with the Student's t-test. $P < 0.05$ was considered statistically significant.

RESULTS

Genotyping of PARG Knockout Mice

The heterozygous PARG knockout mice were used to characterize the role of PARG in protecting mice from BaP-induced lung cancer. According to the law of Mendelian inheritance, the genotype of the progeny mice may be WT (PARG$^{+/+}$), heterozygous (PARG$^{+/-}$), or homozygous (PARG$^{-/-}$). Based on genomic DNA purified from mouse tails, PARG$^{+/-}$ mice were screened for our study as PARG$^{-/-}$ mice cannot survive to maturity. The PCR product from WT mice was 279 bp, and the PCR products from PARG knockout heteroygotes (PARG$^{+/-}$) were 279 and 507 bp, as shown in **Figure 1A**. After BaP exposure, proteins from the lung tissues were extracted and Western blotting were performed to verify the expression of full-length isoform (PARG$_{110}$). As expected, the expression of PARG$_{110}$ was significantly greater in WT mice than in PARG$^{+/-}$ mice (**Figure 1B**). The results confirm that heterozygous PARG knockout mice were successfully bred in our experiments.

PARG$^{+/-}$ Mice Are Protected From Pathological Changes in Lung Tissues Induced by BaP

To establish a lung cancer model for assessing the effects of heterozygous PARG silencing, we exposed mice to long-term inhalation of BaP and then prepared paraffin sections of lung tissues. Hematoxylin and eosin staining were used to analyze the pathological changes that were observed under light microscopy. As shown in **Figure 2A**, in the lungs of WT mice exposed for 90 days, alveolar diffuse interstitialization occurred, though the alveolar structure was visible; in contrast, the degree of injury in PARG$^{+/-}$ mice was mild with no obvious pathological damage. The results were similar in both male and female mice. After 180-day exposure to BaP, the lungs of the WT mice treated with BaP showed severe alveolar diffuse interstitialization, and the alveolar structure was severely damaged with obvious inflammatory infiltration and abnormal nodules (**Figure 2B**). Comparison between the 90- and 180-d pathology suggests that the degree of lung injury in WT mice treated with BaP was positively correlated with the time of exposure. In PARG$^{+/-}$ mice after 180 days, however, some alveolar interstitial thickening appeared while the alveolar structure was still visible. This suggests that PARG$^{+/-}$ mice were protected from the effects of BaP on lung pathology. A higher magnification was used to examine tumor formation. In WT mice, the number of cells increased abnormally and tumorigenesis could be observed (**Figure 2C**); however, no tumor tissue was found in PARG$^{+/-}$ mice. These results demonstrate that heterozygous PARG gene silencing can inhibit the induction of lung cancer by BaP in mice.

PARG$^{+/-}$ Mice Express Elevated Levels of Phosphorylated Proteins in Lung Tissues After BaP Inhalation Exposure

To determine whether heterozygous PARG silencing affects the overall protein phosphorylation level, we performed Western blot assays using the universal anti-tyrosine phosphorylation monoclonal antibody PY20 with protein extracted from lung tissues. As shown in **Figure 3A**, the levels of total phosphorylated proteins in WT and heterozygous PARG knockout mice were not significantly different from that of the control group after exposure to BaP for 90 days ($P > 0.05$). After 180-d exposure, however, the level of phosphorylated proteins was significantly down-regulated in WT mice ($^{*}P < 0.05$), but was significantly up-regulated in PARG$^{+/-}$ mice compared with the control group ($^{*}P < 0.05$). These results indicate that, at an extended BaP exposure time, PARG affects phosphorylation of proteins, which could potentially be associated with the ability of PARG$^{+/-}$ mice to resist tumorigenesis.

PARG Silencing Inhibits the Relative Expression of Wnt2b and Wnt5b mRNA in Lung Tissues After BaP Inhalation Exposure

To further elucidate whether ADP-ribosylation affects the Wnt pathway in PARG$^{+/-}$ mice, we first performed real-time qPCR to detect the relative expression of the Wnt2b and Wnt5b genes. The relative expression of Wnt2b and Wnt5b mRNA was significantly higher in WT mice than in control mice at 90 and 180 days

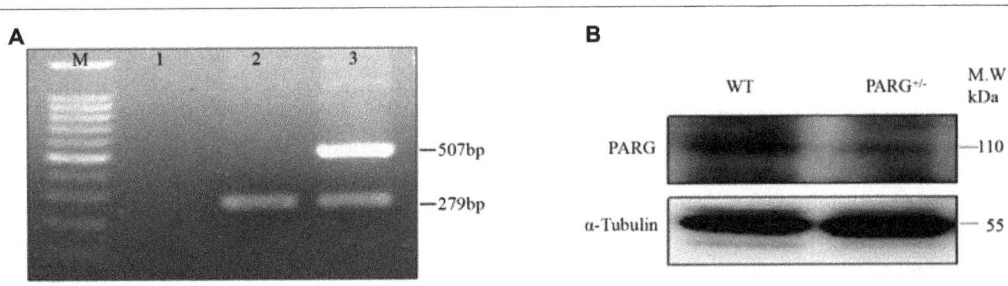

FIGURE 1 | Genotyping of poly (ADP-Ribose) glycohydrolase (PARG) knockout mice. Genotyping of PARG$^{+/-}$ mice. **(A)** Genotyping by PCR. Lane M, 100 bp DNA Marker; Lane 1, blank control; Lane 2, WT mice; and Lane 3, PARG$^{+/-}$ mice. **(B)** Genotyping by Western blotting. The expression of PARG$_{110}$ protein was assessed in lungs from WT and PARG$^{+/-}$ mice.

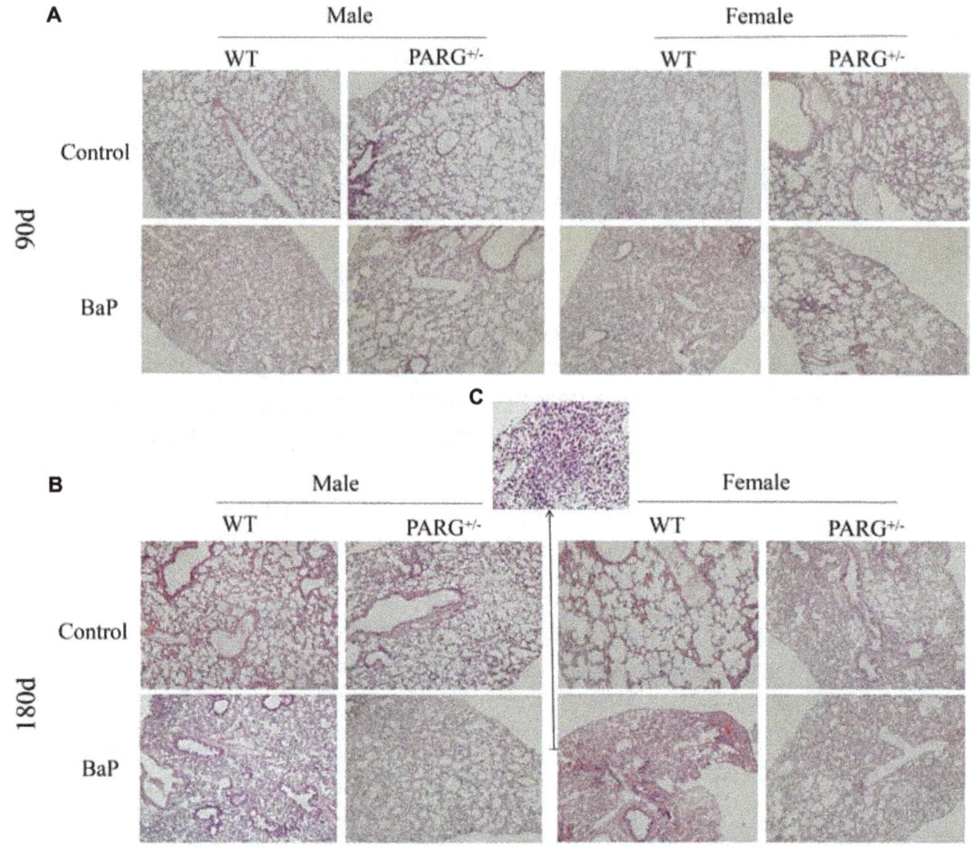

FIGURE 2 | PARG$^{+/-}$ mice are protected from pathological changes in lung tissues induced by BaP inhalation exposure. Pathological changes in lung tissues of WT and PARG$^{+/-}$ mice after benzo(a)pyrene inhalation exposure **(A)** 90-day exposure (×100). **(B)** 180-day exposure to BaP (×100). The red arrows show abnormally increased numbers of cells. **(C)** The magnification of the place pointed by the red arrow in **B**, pathological signs of tumorigenesis (×200). Results are representative of 3 mice from each group.

(***P < 0.001), but there were no significant differences in the PARG$^{+/-}$ mice (P > 0.05) (**Figure 4**).

PARG Silencing Inhibits the Expression of Wnt2b and Wnt5b Protein in Lung Tissues After BaP Inhalation Exposure

The expression of Wnt2b and Wnt5b at the level of the protein were further confirmed by performing Western blotting and immunohistochemistry. The expression of Wnt2b protein was up-regulated in lungs from WT mice that were treated with BaP for 90 and 180 days (*P < 0.05, compared with the control group); however, for PARG$^{+/-}$ mice, no statistically significant differences were observed (P > 0.05) (**Figure 5A**). In immunohistochemistry assays, Wnt2b protein (brownish yellow staining) was localized to the cytoplasm, and after 90 and 180 days of BaP inhalation exposure, the expression levels in WT male and female mice were higher for treated vs. control mice; however, for PARG$^{+/-}$ mice, there were no significant differences (**Figure 5B**). Similar results were observed for Wnt5b, though the effect on Wnt5b expression was more obvious at 180 days than at 90 days (**Figures 5C,D**). These findings suggest that PARG gene silencing stabilizes the expression of Wnt2b and Wnt5b after BaP exposure, possibly inhibiting the progression of lung cancer.

DISCUSSION

Metabolically activated BaP is known to cause cytotoxic, teratogenic, genotoxic, mutagenic and carcinogenic effects in many different tissues and cell types from numerous mammalian studies (Miller and Ramos, 2001; van Delft et al., 2010). BaP in cigarette smoking is implicated as one of the main factors in lung cancer (Rubin, 2001). The occurrence of cancer includes three stages: initiation, promoting and progressing. Epigenetic modification, as a bridge between these stages, can involve DNA methylation, microRNA, chromatin remodeling, and histone modification (Bird, 2007). ADP-ribosylation is one of the most important post-translational modifications in tumorigenesis (Klaus and Birchmeier, 2008). Studies showed that the use of PARG inhibitor to suppress PARG activity facilitates oxidative damage-induced PARylation as well as DNA damage repair (Zhang et al., 2015). PARG gene silencing increases the level of poly (ADP-ribosylation) to regulate DNA

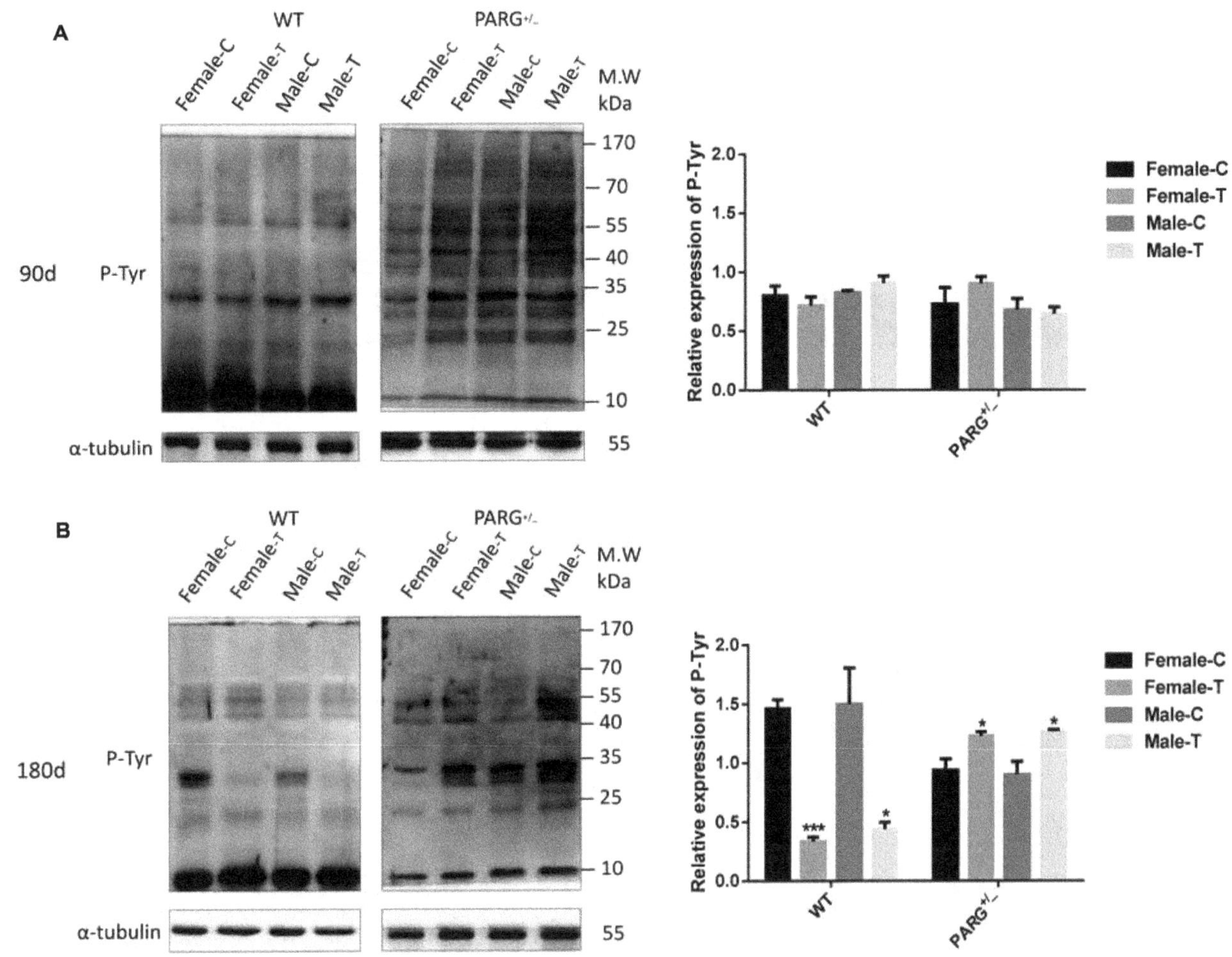

FIGURE 3 | PARG$^{+/-}$ mice express elevated levels of phosphorylated proteins in lung tissues after BaP inhalation exposure. Expression of phosphorylated proteins in lung tissues of mice after BaP inhalation exposure. **(A)** The overall phosphorylation level of proteins in WT and PARG$^{+/-}$ mice that were untreated or were treated with exposure to BaP for 90 days. **(B)** Expression of phosphorylated proteins after 180-day exposure to BaP. Female-C, control untreated female mice; Female-T, treated female mice; Male-C, control untreated male mice; Male-T, treated male mice. $^*P < 0.05$, $^{***}P < 0.001$, significant difference in treated compared to untreated mice. Results represent the mean ± SD of 3 mice from each group. Quantification of the phosphorylation levels was performed using ImageJ software.

damage repair and genome stability (Koh et al., 2004). In our previous study, it is determined that *in vitro* PARG silencing inhibits tumorigenesis by dramatically reducing DNA damage, chromosome abnormalities, micronuclei formations, and malignant transformation. To further investigate the possible *in vivo* role of PARG gene silencing, heterozygous PARG knockout mice were utilized. We exposed WT and PARG$^{+/-}$ mice to BaP by dynamic inhalation for 90 and 180 days. Pathological analysis showed that carcinogenesis appeared in the lungs of WT mice and the injury was progressive for 180-day vs. 90-day treatment, while PARG$^{+/-}$ mice showed no carcinogenesis and minimal signs of lung injury. These results suggest that PARG gene silencing can inhibit lung cancer induced by BaP in mice, which is consistent with our *in vitro* results.

In our previous vitro study, we identified two distinct Wnt ligands (Wnt5b and Wnt2b) that are modulated by PARG by using the MeDIP-sequence techniques. This raises the possibility that ADP-ribosylation may affect the carcinogenesis of BaP by regulating the activation of the Wnt signaling pathway after PARG gene silencing. The Wnt pathway consists of three components: the Wnt/β-catenin canonical pathway, the Wnt/Ca^{2+} pathway and the Wnt/polarity pathway (Wodarz and Nusse, 1998). After activation of the canonical pathway, Wnt ligands bind to Frzzled and LRP5/6 on the cell surface to form a trimer, which weakens the stability of a destruction complex composed by β-catenin, Axin, GSK-3β, and APC to prevent the phosphorylated degradation of β-catenin. The concentration of β-catenin increases in the cytoplasm and then is transferred into the nucleus which ultimately activate the expression of downstream target genes (Veeman et al., 2003). During this process, protein phosphorylation, especially tyrosine phosphorylation (P-Tyr), as a major mode of cell signal transduction and regulation of enzyme activity, plays an vital role in the regulation of β-catenin (Ikeda et al., 1998). ADP-ribosylation can promote phosphorylated proteins

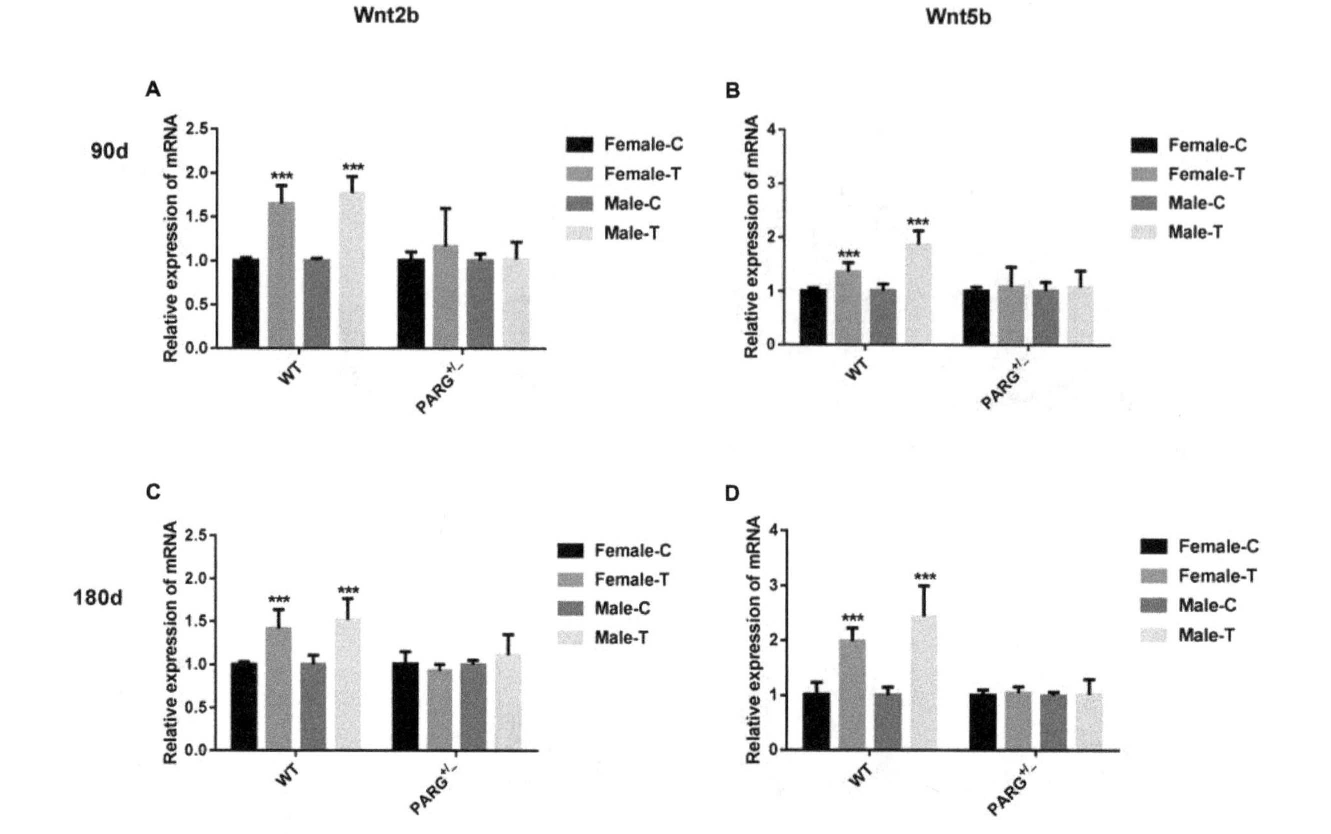

FIGURE 4 | PARG silencing inhibits the relative expression of Wnt2b and Wnt5b mRNA in lung tissues after BaP inhalation exposure. Relative expression of Wnt2b and Wnt5b mRNA in lung tissues of WT and PARG$^{+/-}$ mice after BaP inhalation exposure. The mRNA expression in lungs from WT and PARG$^{+/-}$ mice was measured by real-time quantitative PCR after 90 days (panels **A,B**) or 180 days (panels **C,D**) of BaP inhalation exposure. Female-C, control untreated female mice; Female-T, treated female mice; Male-C, control untreated male mice; Male-T, treated male mice. ***$P < 0.001$, significant difference was found in treated compared to untreated mice. Results represent the mean ± SD of 3 mice from each group.

to bind to Axin scaffolding proteins, affecting the stability of the key protein β-catenin and regulating the activation of the Wnt pathway (Yang et al., 2016). In the current study, the level of total phosphorylated protein in WT mice and PARG$^{+/-}$ mice was not significantly different after 90-day exposure to BaP. However, after 180 d, phosphorylated protein was significantly reduced in WT mice but was up-regulated in PARG$^{+/-}$ mice compared with the control group. These findings are consistent with the possibility that, as the exposure time of BaP extended, loss of PARG promotes phosphorylation of proteins, which possibly leads to phosphorylated degradation of key proteins in the Wnt pathway; supported by the following studies (Zeng et al., 2005; Kim et al., 2013; Yang et al., 2016). We will try to explore how does PARG regulates protein tyrosine phosphorylation to regulate the Wnt signaling against the progression of lung cancer in our next study.

Wnt ligands play a vital role in the development of lung cancer, and inhibition of Wnt ligands may reduce the expansion of lung cancer cell lines (Tammela et al., 2017). Our results demonstrate that the relative expression of Wnt2b and Wnt5b mRNA was up-regulated in lung tissues of WT mice compared with the control group after 90- and 180-day exposure to BaP. Furthermore, the expression of Wnt2b and Wnt5b protein was up-regulated, though there were no significant differences in Wnt2b and Wnt5b mRNA and protein expression in PARG$^{+/-}$ mice. It suggested that loss of PARG stabilized the expression of Wnt ligands, probably suppressing the activation of the Wnt pathway against the progression of lung cancer.

Wnt2b and Wnt5b are two ligands of the Wnt signaling pathway. Wnt2b mainly acts through the canonical Wnt pathway and binds to receptors on the cell membrane to increase the stability of β-catenin in the cytoplasm and promote its translocation to the nucleus to activate downstream target genes that lead to tumorigenesis (Roelink et al., 1992). Studies have shown that Wnt2b is overexpressed in various cancers (Katoh, 2001; Huang et al., 2015). Wnt5b, on the other hand, is a non-canonical Wnt pathway factor that activates the Wnt/Ca^{2+} pathway or blocks the down-regulation of β-catenin by GSK-3β to prevent the classical Wnt pathway (Kohn and Moon, 2005). Studies have shown that Wnt5b plays different roles in different types of cancers. In some cancers, such as lung cancer, it promotes tumorigenesis, and

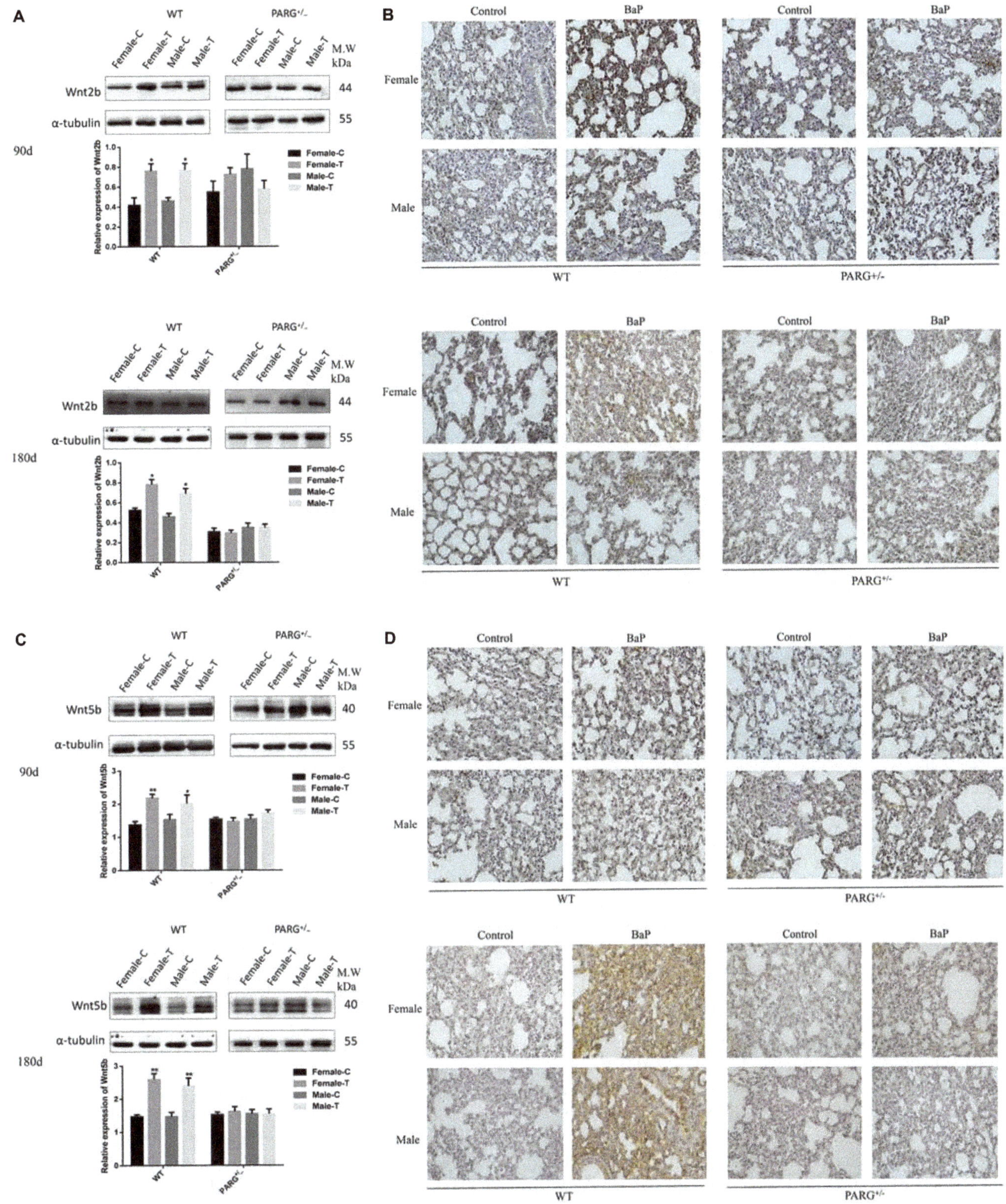

FIGURE 5 | PARG silencing inhibits the expression of Wnt2b and Wnt5b protein in lung tissues after BaP inhalation exposure. Expression of Wnt2b and Wnt5b protein in lung tissues detected by Western blotting and immunohistochemistry. **(A)** Western blotting of Wnt2b expression. **(B)** Immunohistochemical staining of Wnt2b (×200). Protein expression levels are reflected by the area and depth of brownish yellow. **(C)** Western blotting of Wnt5b expression. **(D)** Immunohistochemical staining of Wnt5b (×200). Red arrows indicate Wnt2b and Wnt5b localization in the cytoplasm. Female-C, control untreated female mice; Female-T, treated female mice; Male-C, control untreated male mice; Male-T, treated male mice. *$P < 0.05$, **$P < 0.01$, significant up-regulation in treated vs. control mice.

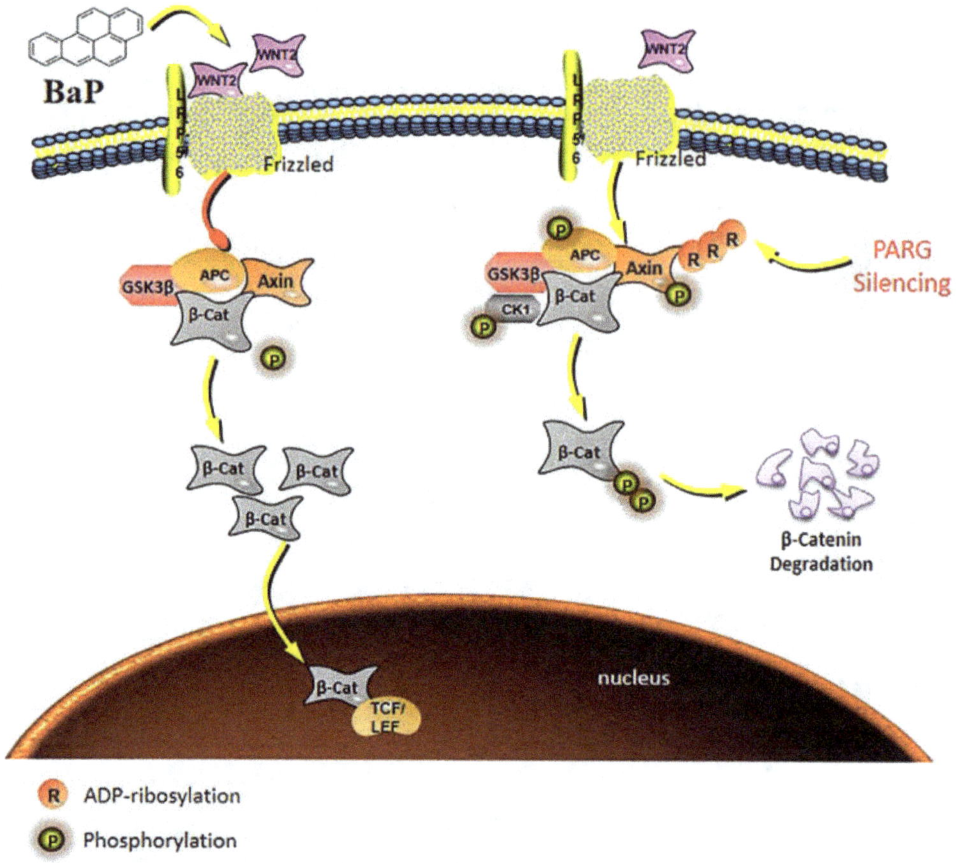

FIGURE 6 | Schematic model of the Wnt/β-catenin signaling pathway regulated by PARG gene silencing during BaP-induced lung cancer. After activation of the canonical pathway, Wnt ligands bind to Frzzled and LRP5/6 on the cell surface to form a trimer, which weakens the stability of a destruction complex composed by β-catenin, Axin, GSK-3β, and APC to prevent the phosphorylated degradation of β-catenin. The concentration of β-catenin increases in the cytoplasm, and then transfers into the nucleus to ultimately activate the expression of downstream target genes. PARG gene silencing may promote binding of phosphorylated proteins to the Axin scaffolding proteins, affecting the stability of the key protein β-catenin, and then suppressing the activation of the Wnt/β-catenin pathway to stabilize the expression of Wnt2b against the progression of lung cancer.

in other cancers, it suppresses tumorigenesis (Kikuchi and Yamamoto, 2008; Harada et al., 2017). On the basis of its different roles in different cancers, Wnt5b may constitute a specific marker for lung cancer screening. In our study, it is found that the up-regulation of Wnt2b was similar at 90 and 180 days, while the up-regulation times of Wnt5b was more obvious at 180 days than at 90 days. These findings may suggest that the Wnt non-canonical pathway increased with extended exposure times, while the classical pathway remains activated at both 90 and 180 days. Specific mechanisms of interaction between the two pathways remains to be further studied.

In conclusion, in the development of lung cancer induced by BaP, the expression of Wnt ligands are up-regulated, which is consistent with current understanding of the role of this pathway. Additionally, PARG gene silencing may regulate the phosphorylation level of proteins to stabilize the expression of Wnt2b, possibly inhibiting the ability of Wnt/β-catenin pathway to drive lung cancer progression as shown in the schematic model in **Figure 6**. The mechanism how PARG gene silencing affects the expression of Wnt5 remains to be futher explored. Understanding of the unresolved issue will contribute to the development of applications of PARG for cancer therapy. Lung cancer is one of the world's most serious threats to human health and has become a global public health problem (Siegel et al., 2018). Therefore, studying the mechanisms of lung cancer provides increased understanding that is relevant to its diagnosis and treatment. Though epigenetic modification is extensive, basic and reversible, its theory and results are gradually being applied to the diagnosis and treatment of cancer (Dawson and Kouzarides, 2012). In this study, it is shown that PARG gene silencing can prevent the occurrence of lung cancer induced by BaP. Our results demonstrate that PARG may be a target for the diagnosis and treatment of lung cancer. Furthermore, the inhibition of Wnt ligands may inhibit lung cancer. These results provide a new potential approach for the treatment of lung cancer. In concludsion, the use of Wnt ligands in the diagnosis of lung cancer and the use of PARG inhibitors as a potential therapeutic against lung cancer is supported.

ETHICS STATEMENT

This study was carried out in accordance with the Principles of Laboratory Animal Care (NIH publication No. 80-23, revised 1985). The protocol was approved by the Regulations for Animal Care and Use Committee of Experimental Animal Center at Shenzhen University.

AUTHOR CONTRIBUTIONS

HH, WD, and JL conceived the project. WD, YF, and YD performed the experiments. WD, YD, DW, XL, LY, and KL analyzed the results. WD, ZZ, PG, HL, JZ, and XX wrote the first draft. All authors revised the manuscript. HH and GH edited and approved the manuscript.

FUNDING

This study was funded by NSFC China (No. 81370080), the Shenzhen Science and Technology Development Fund Project (Nos. JCYJ20170306160932340, JCYJ20170413101713324, JCYJ20160428143634086, and JCYJ20160428142316603) and Sanming Project of Medicine in Shenzhen (SZSM201611090).

REFERENCES

1. Alexandrov, K., Rojas, M., and Satarug, S. (2010). The critical DNA damage by benzo(a)pyrene in lung tissues of smokers and approaches to preventing its formation. *Toxicol. Lett.* 198, 63–68. doi: 10.1016/j.toxlet.2010.04.009
2. Berndt, J. D., and Moon, R. T. (2013). Cell biology. Making a point with Wnt signals. *Science* 339, 1388–1389. doi: 10.1126/science.1236641
3. Bird, A. (2007). Perceptions of epigenetics. *Nature* 447, 396–398. doi: 10.1038/nature05913
4. Chen, W., Zheng, R., Baade, P. D., Zhang, S., Zeng, H., Bray, F., et al. (2016). Cancer statistics in China, 2015. *CA Cancer J. Clin.* 66, 115–132. doi: 10.3322/caac.21338
5. D'Amours, D., Desnoyers, S., D'Silva, I., and Poirier, G. G. (1999). Poly(ADP-ribosyl)ation reactions in the regulation of nuclear functions. *Biochem. J.* 342(Pt 2), 249–268.
6. Dawson, M. A., and Kouzarides, T. (2012). Cancer epigenetics: from mechanism to therapy. *Cell* 150, 12–27. doi: 10.1016/j.cell.2012.06.013
7. Ferlay, J., Soerjomataram, I., Dikshit, R., Eser, S., Mathers, C., Rebelo, M., et al. (2015). Cancer incidence and mortality worldwide: sources, methods and major patterns in GLOBOCAN 2012. *Int. J. Cancer* 136, E359–E386. doi: 10.1002/ijc. 29210
8. Hagood, J. S. (2014). Beyond the genome: epigenetic mechanisms in lung remodeling. *Physiology* 29, 177–185. doi: 10.1152/physiol.00048.2013
9. Harada, T., Yamamoto, H., Kishida, S., Kishida, M., Awada, C., Takao, T., et al. (2017). Wnt5b-associated exosomes promote cancer cell migration and proliferation. *Cancer Sci.* 108, 42–52. doi: 10.1111/cas.13109
10. Huang, C., Ma, R., Xu, Y., Li, N., Li, Z., Yue, J., et al. (2015). Wnt2 promotes non- small cell lung cancer progression by activating WNT/beta-catenin pathway. *Am. J. Cancer Res.* 5, 1032–1046.
11. Huang, H. Y., Cai, J. F., Liu, Q. C., Hu, G. H., Xia, B., Mao, J. Y., et al. (2012). Role of poly(ADP-ribose) glycohydrolase in the regulation of cell fate in response to benzo(a)pyrene. *Exp. Cell Res.* 318, 682–690. doi: 10.1016/j.yexcr.2012.01.007
12. IARC Working Group on the Evaluation of Carcinogenic Risks to Humans (2010). IARC monographs on the evaluation of carcinogenic risks to humans. Ingested nitrate and nitrite, and cyanobacterial peptide toxins. *IARC Monogr. Eval. Carcinog. Risks Hum.* 94, 1–412.
13. IARC Working Group on the Evaluation of Carcinogenic Risks to Humans (2012). Chemical agents and related occupations. *IARC Monogr. Eval. Carcinog. Risks Hum.* 100(Pt F), 9–562.
14. Ikeda, S., Kishida, S., Yamamoto, H., Murai, H., Koyama, S., and Kikuchi, A. (1998). Axin, a negative regulator of the Wnt signaling pathway, forms a complex with GSK-3beta and beta-catenin and promotes GSK-3beta-dependent phosphorylation of beta-catenin. *EMBO J.* 17, 1371–1384. doi: 10.1093/emboj/17.5.1371
15. Kasala, E. R., Bodduluru, L. N., Barua, C. C., Madhana, R. M., Dahiya, V., Budhani, M. K., et al. (2016). Chemopreventive effect of chrysin, a dietary flavone against benzo(a)pyrene induced lung carcinogenesis in Swiss albino mice. *Pharmacol. Rep.* 68, 310–318. doi: 10.1016/j.pharep.2015.08.014
16. Katoh, M. (2001). Differential regulation of WNT2 and WNT2B expression in human cancer. *Int. J. Mol. Med.* 8, 657–660. doi: 10.3892/ijmm.8.6.657
17. Kikuchi, A., and Yamamoto, H. (2008). Tumor formation due to abnormalities in the beta-catenin-independent pathway of Wnt signaling. *Cancer Sci.* 99, 202–208. doi: 10.1111/j.1349-7006.2007.00675.x
18. Kim, W., Kim, S. Y., Kim, T., Kim, M., Bae, D. J., Choi, H. I., et al. (2013). ADP-ribosylation factors 1 and 6 regulate Wnt/beta-catenin signaling via control of LRP6 phosphorylation. *Oncogene* 32, 3390–3396. doi: 10.1038/onc.2012.373
19. Klaus, A., and Birchmeier, W. (2008). Wnt signalling and its impact on development and cancer. *Nat. Rev. Cancer* 8, 387–398. doi: 10.1038/nrc2389
20. Koh, D. W., Lawler, A. M., Poitras, M. F., Sasaki, M., Wattler, S., Nehls, M. C., et al. (2004). Failure to degrade poly(ADP-ribose) causes increased sensitivity to cytotoxicity and early embryonic lethality. *Proc. Natl. Acad. Sci. U.S.A.* 101, 17699–17704. doi: 10.1073/pnas.0406182101
21. Kohn, A. D., and Moon, R. T. (2005). Wnt and calcium signaling: beta-catenin-independent pathways. *Cell Calcium* 38, 439–446. doi: 10.1016/j.ceca.2005.06.022
22. Li, X., Li, X., Zhu, Z., Huang, P., Zhuang, Z., Liu, J., et al. (2016). Poly(ADP-Ribose) glycohydrolase (PARG) silencing suppresses benzo(a)pyrene induced cell transformation. *PLoS One* 11:e0151172. doi: 10.1371/journal.pone.0151172
23. Liu, G., Niu, Z., Van Niekerk, D., Xue, J., and Zheng, L. (2008). Polycyclic aromatic hydrocarbons (PAHs) from coal combustion: emissions, analysis, and toxicology. *Rev. Environ. Contam. Toxicol.* 192, 1–28. doi: 10.1007/978-0-387-71724-1_1
24. Meyer, R. G., Meyer-Ficca, M. L., Whatcott, C. J., Jacobson, E. L., and Jacobson,M. K. (2007). Two small enzyme isoforms mediate mammalian mitochondrial poly(ADP-ribose) glycohydrolase (PARG) activity. *Exp. Cell Res.* 313, 2920–2936. doi: 10.1016/j.yexcr.2007.03.043
25. Miller, K. P., and Ramos, K. S. (2001). Impact of cellular metabolism on the biological effects of benzo[a]pyrene and related hydrocarbons. *Drug Metab. Rev.* 33, 1–35. doi: 10.1081/DMR-100000138
26. Min, W., Cortes, U., Herceg, Z., Tong, W. M., and Wang, Z. Q. (2010). Deletion of the nuclear isoform of poly(ADP-ribose) glycohydrolase (PARG) reveals its function in DNA repair, genomic stability and tumorigenesis. *Carcinogenesis* 31, 2058–2065. doi: 10.1093/carcin/bgq205
27. Miwa, M., and Masutani, M. (2007). PolyADP-ribosylation and cancer. *Cancer Sci.* 98, 1528–1535. doi: 10.1111/j.1349-7006.2007.00567.x
28. Reya, T., and Clevers, H. (2005). Wnt signalling in stem cells and cancer. *Nature* 434, 843–850. doi: 10.1038/nature03319
29. Roelink, H., Wagenaar, E., and Nusse, R. (1992). Amplification and proviral activation of several Wnt genes during progression and clonal variation of mouse mammary tumors. *Oncogene* 7, 487–492.
30. Rojas, M., Marie, B., Vignaud, J. M., Martinet, N., Siat, J., Grosdidier, G., et al. (2004). High DNA damage by benzo[a]pyrene 7,8-diol-9,10-epoxide

in bronchial epithelial cells from patients with lung cancer: comparison with lung parenchyma. *Cancer Lett.* 207, 157–163. doi: 10.1016/j.canlet.2003.11.016
31. Rouleau, M., Aubin, R. A., and Poirier, G. G. (2004). Poly(ADP-ribosyl) ated chromatin domains: access granted. *J. Cell Sci.* 117(Pt 6), 815–825. doi: 10.1242/jcs.01080
32. Rubin, H. (2001). Synergistic mechanisms in carcinogenesis by polycyclic aromatic hydrocarbons and by tobacco smoke: a bio-historical perspective with updates. *Carcinogenesis* 22, 1903–1930. doi: 10.1093/carcin/22.12.1903
33. Schmittgen, T. D., and Livak, K. J. (2008). Analyzing real-time PCR data by the comparative C(T) method. *Nat. Protoc.* 3, 1101–1108. doi: 10.1038/nprot.2008.73
34. Siegel, R. L., Miller, K. D., and Jemal, A. (2018). Cancer statistics, 2018. *CA Cancer J. Clin.* 68, 7–30. doi: 10.3322/caac.21442
35. Tammela, T., Sanchez-Rivera, F. J., Cetinbas, N. M., Wu, K., Joshi, N. S., Helenius, K., et al. (2017). A Wnt-producing niche drives proliferative potential and progression in lung adenocarcinoma. *Nature* 545, 355–359. doi: 10.1038/nature22334
36. van Delft, J. H., Mathijs, K., Staal, Y. C., van Herwijnen, M. H., Brauers, K. J., Boorsma, A., et al. (2010). Time series analysis of benzo[A]pyrene-induced transcriptome changes suggests that a network of transcription factors regulates the effects on functional gene sets. *Toxicol. Sci.* 117, 381–392. doi: 10.1093/ toxsci/kfq214
37. Veeman, M. T., Axelrod, J. D., and Moon, R. T. (2003). A second canon. Functions and mechanisms of beta-catenin-independent Wnt signaling. *Dev. Cell* 5, 367–377. doi: 10.1016/S1534-5807(03)00266-1
38. Widziewicz, K., Rogula-Kozlowska, W., Loska, K., Kociszewska, K., and Majewski, G. (2018). Health risk impacts of exposure to airborne metals and benzo(a)pyrene during episodes of high PM10 concentrations in Poland. *Biomed. Environ. Sci.* 31, 23–36. doi: 10.3967/bes2018.003
39. Wodarz, A., and Nusse, R. (1998). Mechanisms of Wnt signaling in development. *Annu. Rev. Cell Dev. Biol.* 14, 59–88. doi: 10.1146/annurev.cellbio. 14.1.59
40. Yang, E., Tacchelly-Benites, O., Wang, Z., Randall, M. P., Tian, A., Benchabane, H., et al. (2016). Wnt pathway activation by ADP-ribosylation. *Nat. Commun.* 7:11430. doi: 10.1038/ncomms11430
41. Zeng, X., Tamai, K., Doble, B., Li, S., Huang, H., Habas, R., et al. (2005). A dual-kinase mechanism for Wnt co-receptor phosphorylation and activation. *Nature* 438, 873–877. doi: 10.1038/nature04185
42. Zhang, C., Luo, T., Cui, S., Gu, Y., Bian, C., Chen, Y., et al. (2015). Poly(ADP-ribose) protects vascular smooth muscle cells from oxidative DNA damage. *BMB Rep.* 48, 354–359. doi: 10.5483/BMBRep.2015.48.6.012

8

Copper Chaperone for Superoxide Dismutase Promotes Breast Cancer Cell Proliferation and Migration *via* ROS-Mediated MAPK/ERK Signaling

Yanping Li[1†], Ronghui Liang[1†], Xiaoya Zhang[1], Jiyan Wang[2], Changliang Shan[1,2], Shuangping Liu[3*], Leilei Li[1*] and Shuai Zhang[4*]*

[1]Biomedical Translational Research Institute, Jinan University, Guangzhou, China, [2]State Key Laboratory of Medicinal Chemical Biology, College of Pharmacy and Tianjin Key Laboratory of Molecular Drug Research, Nankai University, Tianjin, China, [3]Department of Pathology, Medical School, Dalian University, Dalian, China, [4]School of Integrative Medicine, Tianjin University of Traditional Chinese Medicine, Tianjin, China

***Correspondence:**
Changliang Shan
changliangshan@nankai.edu.cn
Shuangping Liu
liushuangping@dlu.edu.cn
Leilei Li
89509306@qq.com
Shuai Zhang
shuaizhang@tjutcm.edu.cn

†These authors have contributed equally to this work

Copper chaperone for superoxide dismutase (CCS) is a critical component of oxidation–reduction system and functions as a potential tumor promoter in several cancers. However, the function and clinical significance of CCS in breast cancer remain unclear. Here, we found CCS was highly expressed in breast cancer, where it promoted breast cancer cell proliferation and migration. Suppression of CCS expression was sufficient to attenuate the phosphorylation level of ERK1/2 and increase the accumulation of reactive oxygen species (ROS). Mechanistically, we found that knockdown of CCS decreases the activity of ERK1/2 mediated by the accumulation of ROS, which leads to the inhibition of cell proliferation and migration. In summary, these results indicated that CCS promotes the growth and migration of breast cancer cells *via* regulating the ERK1/2 activity mediated by ROS.

Keywords: breast cancer, CCS, ROS, MAPK/ERK, proliferation, migration

INTRODUCTION

Breast cancer is the leading cause of cancer-related deaths in women worldwide (Christofori, 2006; Bray et al., 2018). Breast cancer patients with metastases have an extremely poor prognosis (Gupta et al., 2005; Bacac and Stamenkovic, 2008; Thiery, 2009; Chaffer and Weinberg, 2011; Valastyan and Weinberg, 2011). Thus, exploring new targets for breast cancer treatment is important.

Copper, a redox-active transition metal essential for most living organisms, serves as a catalytic cofactor for enzymes that function in antioxidant defense, iron homeostasis, cellular respiration, and a variety of biochemical processes (Mandinov et al., 2003; Lowndes and Harris, 2005; Ashino et al., 2010; Xu et al., 2016; Sciegienka et al., 2017). The uncontrolled accumulation of copper could lead to increased oxidative stress and inappropriate binding to macromolecules. Copper chaperone for superoxide dismutase (CCS) delivers copper to specific cellular destinations and to superoxide dismutase (SOD1) (Kawamata and Manfredi, 2008; Ulloa, 2009). Mounting evidences suggest that CCS plays a crucial role in oxidative metabolism (Kawamata and Manfredi, 2008; Leitch et al., 2009; Suzuki et al., 2013a; Wang et al., 2015). Blockade of the copper-trafficking chaperone CCS contributes to the increased cellular reactive oxygen species (ROS) level due to the overall accumulation of copper inside the cells and the decreased SOD1 activity (Ulloa, 2009). Wang et al reported that inhibiting CCS blocks lung cancer and leukemia cell growth (Wang et al., 2015). In addition, they show that blocking copper trafficking induces cellular oxidative stress and reduces cellular ATP levels. The reduced level of ATP results in activation of the AMP-activated protein kinase that leads to reduced lipogenesis. However, the mechanisms underlying the relationship between CCS and tumorigenesis are still largely unknown, although the positive correlation between CCS and redox homeostasis has been revealed (Wang et al., 2015). Therefore, this study aimed to explore the critical role and molecular mechanism of CCS in migration and proliferation of breast cancer.

In aforementioned study by Wang et al, a CCS inhibitor was developed and shown to have the same effect as knocking down CCS in cancer cells (Wang et al., 2015). However, the precise role of CCS in migration and proliferation of breast cancer cells is unknown. In the present study, we report that CCS is highly expressed in breast cancer tissues and invasive breast cancer cells and promotes cell proliferation and migration. Furthermore, we found that inhibition of CCS by shRNA or an inhibitor blocks breast cancer proliferation and migration by triggering ROS mediated ERK activity. These results suggest that metastasis-prone breast cancer cells reprogram oxidative metabolism to promote cell proliferation and migration. Targeting CCS may represent a promising approach for selectively causing cell proliferation and migration in breast cancer cells.

MATERIALS AND METHODS

Reagents and Antibodies

DC_AC50, a CCS inhibitor, was provided by the Shanghai Institute of Materia Medica of the Chinese Academy of Sciences. U0126-EtOH (catalog number: S1102) was purchased from Selleck. Antibody against phospho-p44/42 MAPK (Erk1/2) (Thr202/Tyr204) (1:1000 times dilution) (catalog number: 4370S), p44/42 MAPK (Erk1/2) (1:1000 times dilution) (catalog number: 4695S), phpspho-MEK1/2 (Ser217/221) (1:1000 times dilution) (catalog number: 9154S), MEK1/2 (1:1000 times dilution) (catalog number: 8727S), β-actin (1:1000 times dilution) (catalog number: 8457S), mouse IgG (1:3000 times dilution) (catalog number: 7076S), and rabbit IgG (1:3000 times dilution) (catalog number: 7074S) were from cell signaling technology. Anti-Superoxide Dismutase 4 (1:500 times dilution) (catalog number: ab167170) was from Abcam. Anti-Flag tag (1:1000 times dilution) (catalog number: 66008) was from proteintech. CCS shRNA was purchased from Open Biosystems, Huntsville, AL. The sequence of targeted CCS shRNA was as follows: 5′-CCGGCTGATTATTGATGAGGGAGAACTCGAGTTCTCCC TCATCAATA ATCAGTTTTTG-3′. Lipofectamine RNA iMAX was purchased from Invitrogen. The sequences of targeted CCS siRNA were as follows: sense: 5′-GUCUUGGUACACACCAC UCUA-3′; Antisense: 5′-UAGAGUGGUGUGUACCAAGAC-3′.

Cell Culture and Cell Lines

The human breast cancer cell lines MDA-MB-231, MCF-7, SUM159, and T47D were obtained from American Type Culture Collection (Manassas, USA). The human normal epithelial lung cell line BEAS-2B was gifted from Dr. Chenglai Xia (Guangzhou Medical University, Guangdong, China). MDA-MB-231, MCF-7, SUM159, and T47D cells were cultured in Dulbecco Modified Eagle Medium (DMEM) with 10% fetal bovine serum (FBS, ExCell Bio). BEAS-2B cells were cultured in RPMI 1640 medium with 10% FBS. For routine passages, cultures were split 1:3 when they reached 80–90% confluences. All experiments were performed on exponentially growing cells.

Plasmid Construction and Lentivirus Packaging

Exogenous human CCS CDS sequence was inserted into pLVX-3FLAG plasmid. Primer sequences were as follows: pLVX-3FLAG-CCS: 5′-CGGGATCCATGGCTTCGGATTCGG-3′ (forward) and 5′-CCCTCGAGTCAAAGGTGGGCAGG-3′ (reverse). Exogenous pCDH-HA-MEK plasmid was gifted from Dr. ShiZhi (JinanUniversity, Guangdong, China). For transient transfections, cells were grown to 80% confluency and transfected with plasmids using PEI Transfection Reagent (Invitrogen, USA) according to the manufacturer's protocol. Stable knockdown of endogenous CCS was achieved by using lentiviral vector harboring shRNA construct. 5′-CCGGCTGATTATTGATGAGG GAGAACTCGAGTTCTCCCTCATCAATAATCAGTTTTTG-3′. We generated CCS stable knockdown cell lines by infected lentiviral shRNA and selected by antibiotic puromycin. The knockdown effective was confirmed by western blot. PLKO.1 is the name of the lentiviral vector as a control.

Small Interference RNA Transfection

MDA-MB-231, MCF-7, and BEAS-2B cells (2×10^5) were seeded into 6-well plates and cultured in a humidified incubator at 37°C and 5% CO_2 for 24 h. Cells were transfected with a negative control siRNA (NC-siRNA) and siRNA targeting CCS by Lipofectamine RNA iMAX (Invitrogen corporation). Transfected cells were cultured for 48°C before being used for further experiments. The sequences of targeted CCS siRNA were 5′-GUCUUGGUACACACCACUCUA-3′. The sequences of negative control siRNA were 5′-UUCUCCGAACGUGUCACGUTT-3′(forward). All siRNA sequences were purchased from the Invitrogen Ribobio corporation of Guangzhou.

Abbreviations: AMP, Adenosine Monophosphate; ATP, Adenosine Triphosphate; CCS, Copper Chaperone for Superoxide Dismutase; ERK, Extracellular Regulated Protein Kinases; MAPK, Mitogen-Activated Protein Kinase; NAC, N-Acetyl-L-cysteine; ROS, Reactive Oxygen Species; PCR, Polymerase Chain Reaction; PEI, Polymine; PVDF, Polyvinylidene Fluoride; qRT-PCR, Real-time Quantitative Reverse Transcription-PCR; SDS-PAGE, Sodium Dodecyl Sulfate Polyacrylamide Gel Electropheresis; ShRNA, Short Hairpin RNA; SiRNA, Small Interfering RNA; SOD1, Superoxide Dismutase; TCGA, The Cancer Genome Atlas.

Real-Time Quantitative Reverse Transcription-PCR

Total cellular RNA was extracted using the Eastep & Super RNA Extract reagent Kit (Promega). cDNA was generated from purified RNA using PrimeSciptTM RT reagent Kit (Takara) according to the manufacturer's instructions. Gene expression levels and PCR efficiency, along with its standard error, were calculated using the Bio-Rad CFX Manager, version 3.1 (Bio-Rad), The efficiencies were nearly 100%, allowing the use of the $2^{-\Delta\Delta Ct}$ method for calculating the relative gene expression levels and reference gene normalization using β-actin. All PCR runs were performed in triplicate, and the data analyzed by CFX Manager software (Bio-Rad). Primer sequences were as following: CCS: 5′-CATCGAGG GAACTATTGACG-3′ (forward) and 5′-ATGCTCCATCAGGGT TAAAG-3′(reverse); β-actin:5′-ACGTGGACATCCGCAAAG-3′ (forward) and 5′-GACTCGTCATACTCCTGCTTG-3′ (reverse).

Cell Proliferation Assay

Cell proliferation assays were performed by seeding 5 × 10^4 cells in 6-well plates and culturing the cells at 37°C. Relative cell proliferation was determined by cell numbers recorded at 4 days after being seeded and normalized to that of each of the cell lines at the starting time (t = 0 h).

Western Blot Analysis

Cells were lysed with lysis buffer (1.5 M NaCl, 1 M HEPES [pH = 7.0], 1% NP40, 0.1 M $Na_4P_2O_7$, 0.1 M NaF, 0.1 M Na_3VO_4, protease inhibitor) on ice 30 min and then centrifuged at 12,000 rpm for 15 min at 4°C. Protein samples were separated by 12%.

SDS-PAGE and transferred onto PVDF membranes (Millipore). The membranes were blocked with 5% non-fat milk for 2 h and then incubated overnight at 4°C with the primary antibody and 1 h at room temperature with secondary antibody. Signals were detected using luminol substrate solution.

Transwell Migration Assay

For the Transwell (24-well insert, 8 mm pore size with polycarbonate membrane; Corning Costar, Lowell, MA, USA) migration assays, 600-mL media supplemented with 10% FBS was added to the lower chamber, and the cells resuspended in serum-free media were added to the upper insert after transfection. Transwell membranes were fixed and stained using crystal violet after specified time. The cells adhering to the lower surface of the membrane were counted under a light microscope (Olympus, Tokyo, Japan) at a magnification of 200.

Wound Healing Assay

To determine cell motility, cells were seeded into 6-well plates and grown to 90% confluence. A monolayer of the cells was then scratched with a sterile micropipette tip, followed by washing with PBS to remove cellular debris. The cell migration was observed and counted under a light microscope (Olympus, Tokyo, Japan) at a magnification of 200. The cells that migrated across the black lines were counted in three randomly chosen fields from each triplicate treatment.

Intracellular Reactive Oxygen Species (ROS) Production

The amount of intracellular ROS was measured by detecting dichlorodihydrofluorescein, which is the cleavage product of carboxy-H_2DCFDA (Invitrogen) by ROS. A total of 200,000 cells were seeded in 6-well plate. Twenty-four hours after seeding, cells were washed with PBS and loaded with 12.5 μM carboxy-H_2DCFDA for 60 min. The cells were harvested, resuspended in PBS, and analyzed using a FACS (BD Biosciences; excitation and emission at 490 and 530 nm, respectively).

Bioinformatics Analysis

The public Gene Expression Omnibus datasets (GSE9574 and GSE21422) and the TCGA (The Cancer Genome Atlas) dataset were used for bioinformatics analysis.

Statistical Analysis

The concentration of DC_AC50 required to reduce cell proliferation by 50% (IC50) was determined graphically using the Dose-response-Stimulation function in GraphPad Prism7 (San Diego, CA, United States). Statistical analyses of the significance of differences between groups were performed using Student's t-test with GraphPad Prism7. All data were obtained from three independent experiments performed in triplicate and were presented as the mean ± standard error. $p < 0.05$ was considered to indicate a statistically significant difference.

RESULTS

Higher CCS Gene Expression in Breast Cancer Patients

Bioinformatics analysis has been used to discover previously unknown function of genes associated with cancer. To determine the role of CCS in human breast cancer, we first examined the expression of CCS utilizing Gene Expression Omnibus (GEO) profiles; we found that the expression of CCS was higher in breast cancer tissue than in noncancerous tissue (**Figure 1A,** GSE9574). We also confirmed these finding using The Cancer Genome Atlas (TCGA) dataset. CCS expression was also significantly higher in breast cancer tissue than in noncancerous tissue in the Cancer Genome Atlas (TCGA) (**Figure 1B**). In addition, we also found that the expression of CCS was higher in invasive ductal carcinoma (IDC) than in ductal carcinoma (DCIS) (**Figure 1A,** GSE21422). To validate these findings, we checked CCS expression in various breast cancer cells lines. CCS was differentially expressed in several breast cancer cell lines, including MCF-7, T47D, MDA-MB-231, and SUM159. Of note, the expression of CCS was higher in T47D and MDA-MB-231 cell lines compared to MCF-7 and SUM159 cells (**Figure 1D**). All these findings indicate the potential role of CCS in tumor formation and progression.

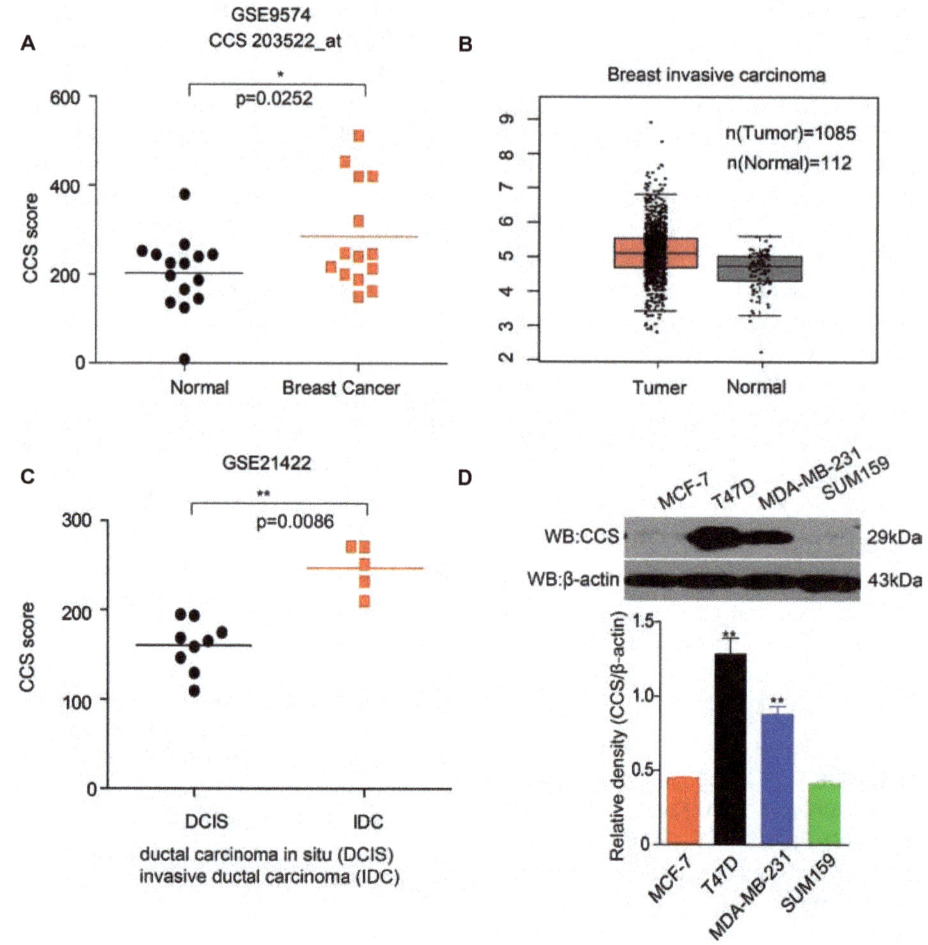

FIGURE 1 | Up-regulation of CCS is associated with cell proliferation and metastasis in human breast cancer. **(A)** CCS expression was analyzed in normal and breast cancer cells using Gene Expression Omnibus (GEO) profiles (GSE9574). **(B)** CCS expression was determined in normal and breast cancer cells in TCGA. **(C)** CCS expression was analyzed in ductal carcinoma in situ (DCIS) and invasion ductal carcinoma (IDC) using Gene Expression Omnibus (GEO) profiles (GSE21422). **(D)** CCS protein levels were analyzed in the majority of a spectrum of diverse human breast cancer cells, including MCF-7, MDA-MB-231, SUM159, and T47D by western blotting. $^{*}p < 0.05$; $^{**}p < 0.01$.

CCS Promotes Breast Cancer Cell Proliferation *in vitro*

We found that the expression of CCS was higher in breast cancer tissue than in noncancerous tissue, suggesting the potential role of CCS in breast cancer cell proliferation. To test our hypothesis, we generated stable cell lines in which CCS was knocked down in MDA-MB-231 cells (**Figure 2A** lower) and exogenously expressed in MCF-7 and SUM159 cells (**Figures 2B,C** lower). Cell number counting assays showed that knockdown of CCS reduced the proliferation of MDA-MB-231 cells (**Figure 2A** upper), while exogenous expression of CCS demonstrated the opposite effect (**Figures 2B,C** upper). To validate these findings, we knocked down the expression of CCS in MDA-MB-231, MCF-7, and BEAS-2B cells using siRNA. Cell number counting assays showed that knockdown of CCS significantly inhibited the proliferation of metastasis-prone breast cancer cell lines MDA-MB-231 but did not have any effect on the proliferation of breast cancer MCF-7 cells or normal BEAS-2B cells (**Figures 2D–F**). Real-time PCR was used to determine the knockdown efficiency of CCS by siRNA (**Figure 2G**). Next, we sought to explore the role DC_AC50, a potent and selective CCS inhibitor, in breast cancer. DC_AC50 has been shown to inhibit the proliferation of acute leukemia cells (Wang et al., 2015). We treated cells with DC_AC50 and found that MCF-7 cells exhibited significantly higher resistance to DC_AC50 than MDA-MB-231 cells (**Figure 2H**). Meanwhile, DC_AC50 treatment resulted in decreased cell proliferation of MDA-MB-231 cells in a time and dose-dependent manner (**Figure 2I**). These results imply that CCS plays an important role in breast cancer cell proliferation and suggests that CCS is a promising anti-cancer target.

CCS Promotes Breast Cancer Cells Migration

We found that the expression of CCS was higher in invasive ductal carcinoma than in ductal carcinoma (**Figure 1C**), suggesting the potential role of CCS in promoting breast cancer migration.

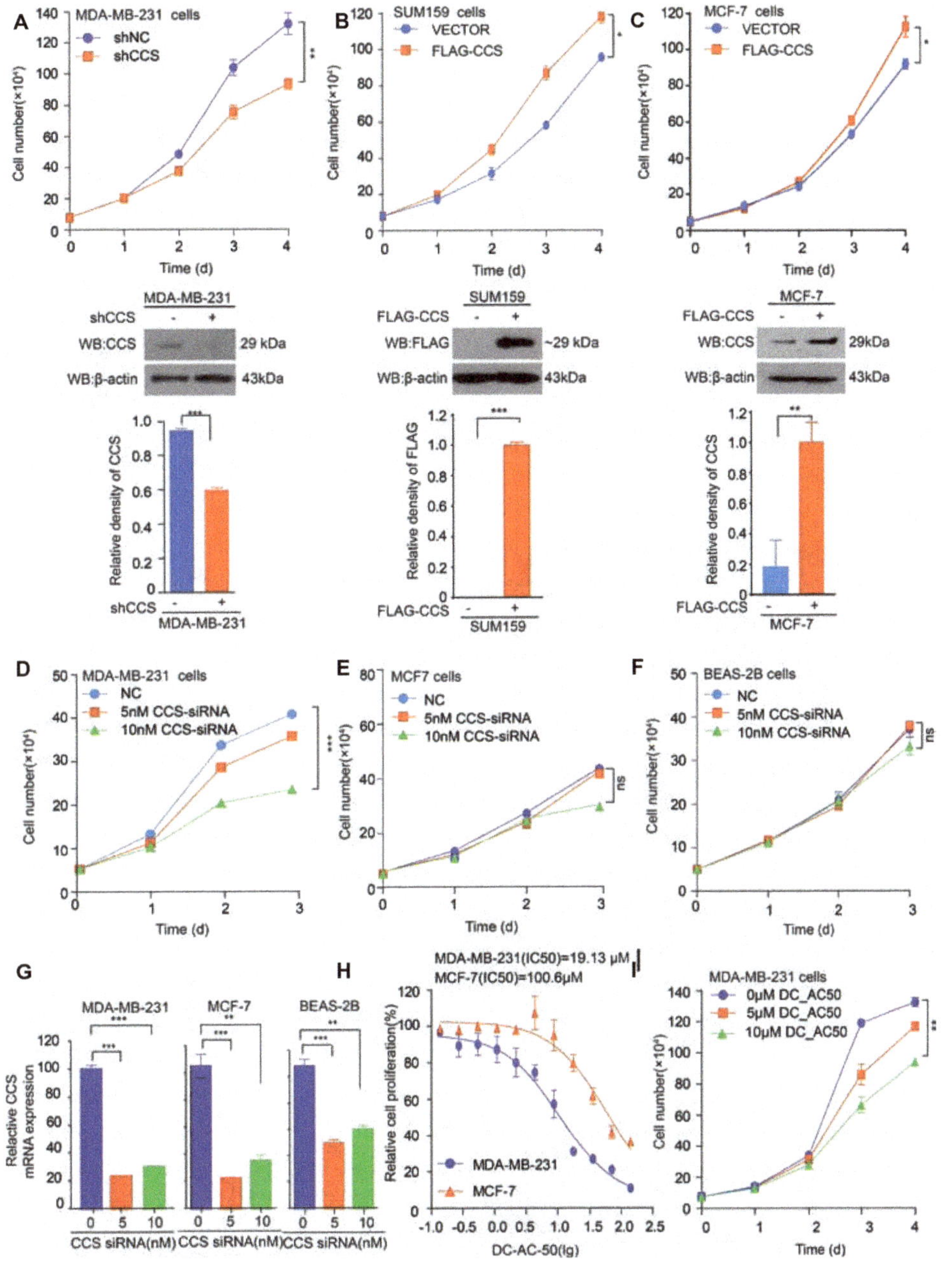

FIGURE 2 | CCS promotes breast cancer cell proliferation. **(A)** Cell proliferation was determined by cell number counting assays in CCS stable knockdown MDA-MB-231 cells, and the knockdown efficiency was determined by western blotting. **(B)** Cell proliferation was determined by cell number counting assays in CCS overexpressing SUM159 cells, and CCS expression was determined by western blotting. **(C)** Cell proliferation was determined by cell number counting assays in CCS overexpressing MCF-7 cells, and CCS expression was determined by western blotting. **(D–F)** Cell proliferation was determined by cell number counting assays in MDA-MB-231 cells **(D)**, MCF-7 cells **(E)**, and normal human BEAS-2B cells **(F)**, which were transiently transfected with increasing concentrations of CCS siRNA and control siRNA. **(G)** The relative CCS mRNA level was determined by q-PCR in MDA-MB-231, MCF-7and BEAS-2B cells, which were transiently transfected with increasing concentrations of CCS siRNA and control siRNA. **(H)** The sensitivities of MDA-MB-231 and MCF-7 cells to DC_AC50 were determined by cell number counting assays when the cells were treated with increasing concentrations of DC_AC50 for 48 h. **(I)** Cell proliferation was determined by cell count assays in MDA-MB-231 cells treated with increasing concentrations of DC_AC50. All results performed above are presented as mean ± SD from three independent experiments. $^{*}p < 0.05$; $^{**}p < 0.01$; $^{***}p < 0.001$, ns: not significant.

Next, we explore the role of CCS in the motility of the breast cancer cells. We performed a transwell migration assay that showed knockdown of CCS significantly inhibited breast cell migratory abilities in MDA-MB-231 (**Figure 3A**), while exogenous express CCS exhibited the opposite effects in MCF-7 and SUM159 cells (**Figures 3B,C**). To validate these finding, we treated MDA-MB-231 with CCS inhibitor, DC_AC50, and performed a transwell migration assay. We found that DC_AC50 blocked MDA-MB-231 cell migration in a dose-dependent manner (**Figure 3D**). In addition, we also assessed migration of MDA-MB-231 in a wound

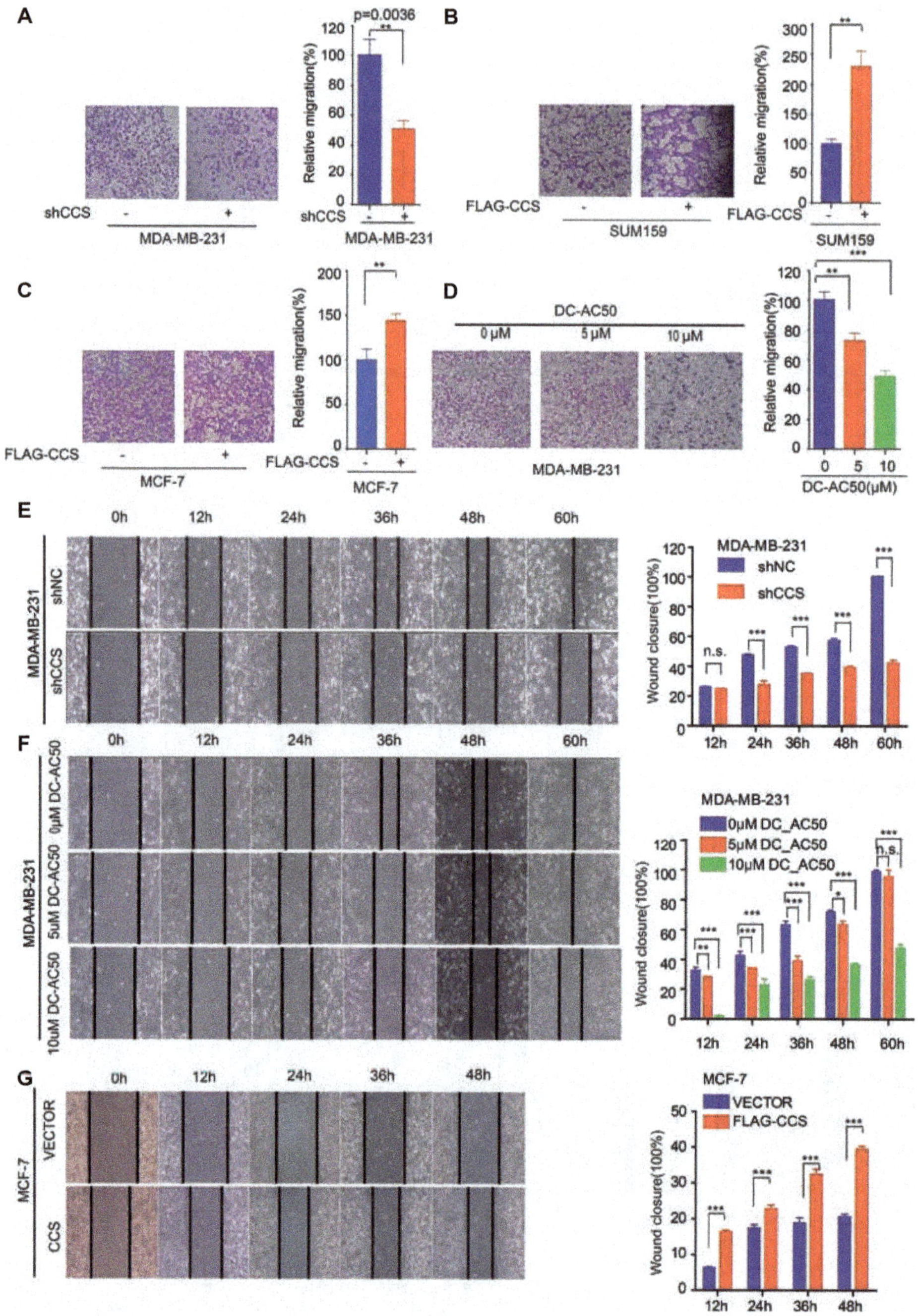

FIGURE 3 | CCS promotes breast cancer cell migration. **(A)** Cell migration in CCS knockdown and control MDA-MB-231 cells was determined by transwell migration assay (Boyden chamber assay). **(B)** Cell migration in CCS overexpressing and control SUM159 cells was determined by transwell migration assay. **(C)** Cell migration in CCS overexpressing and control MCF-7 cells was determined by transwell migration assay. **(D)** Cell migration in CCS overexpressing and control MDA-MB-231 cells with increasing concentrations of DC_AC50 was determined by transwell migration assay. **(E)** Cell migration in CCS knockdown and control MDA-MB-231 cells was also determined by wound healing assay. **(F)** Cell migration in MDA-MB-231 cells treated with increasing concentrations of DC_AC50 was determined by wound healing assay. **(G)** Cell migration in CCS overexpressing and control MCF-7 cells was determined by the wound healing assay. The modified migration assay was evaluated by calculating the ratio of the cell numbers through the chamber or wound closure after the wound healing assay. All results performed above are presented as mean ± SD from three independent experiments. *$p < 0.05$; **$p < 0.01$; ***$p < 0.001$, ns: not significant.

healing assay. We found that knockdown or inhibition of CCS dramatically suppressed MDA-MB-231 cell migratory abilities (**Figures 3E,F**). To consolidate our findings, we overexpressed FLAG tagged CCS in MCF-7 cells. As expected, overexpression of CCS accelerated breast cancer cell migration in a wound healing assay (**Figure 3G**). Taken together, our results suggest that CCS plays an important role in promoting breast cancer cells migration.

CCS Promotes Breast Cancer Migration *via* MAPK/ERK Signaling

Activation of survival signaling has been shown to play an essential role in tumor development (Baud and Karin, 2001). Several studies have demonstrated that the MAPK/ERK signaling pathway is activated in cancer cells to promote cancer cell proliferation, migration, and invasion (Rajalingam et al., 2005; El Touny et al., 2014). Therefore, we examined whether

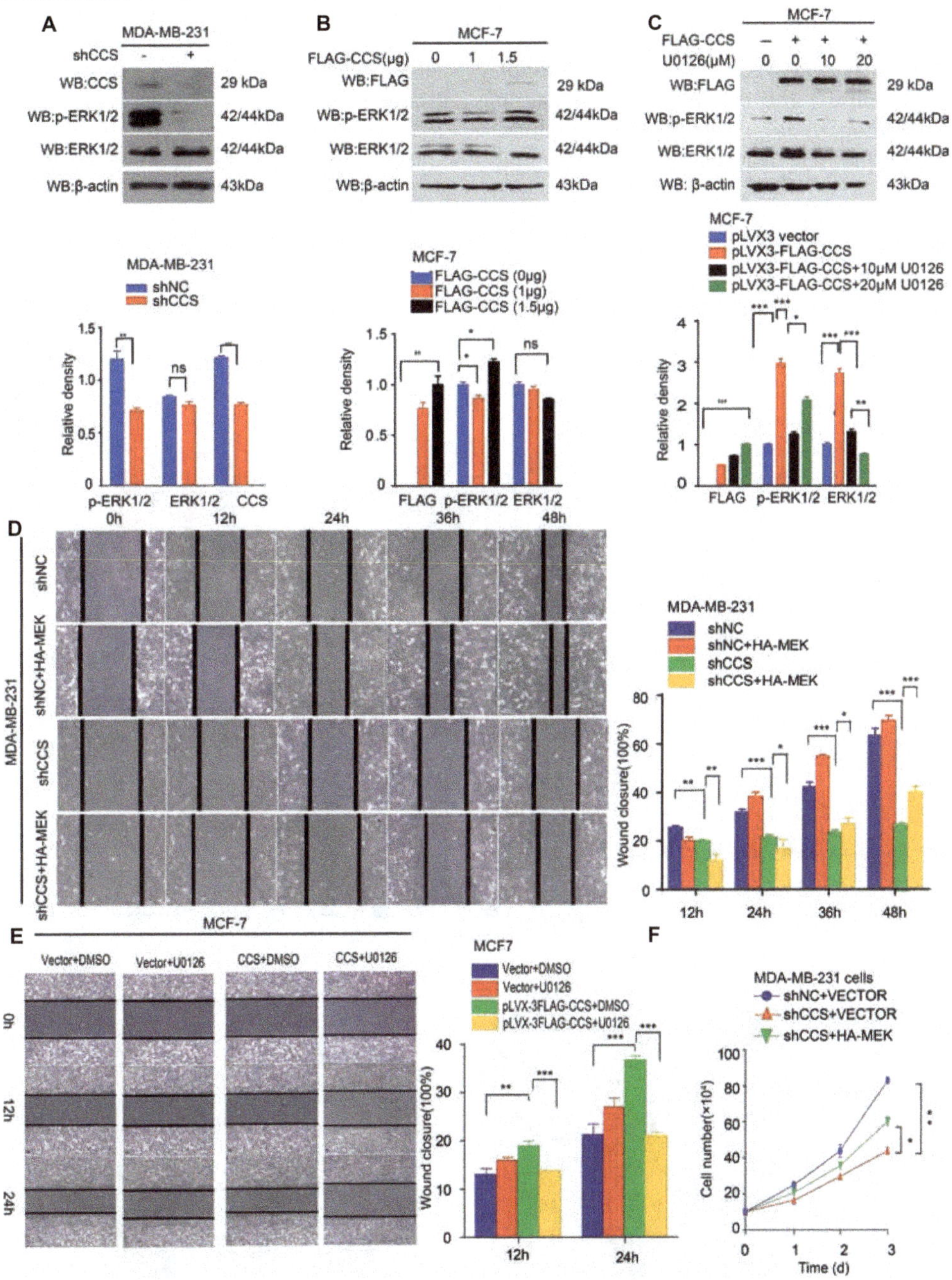

FIGURE 4 | CCS promotes breast cancer cell migration and cell proliferation *via* ERK1/2 activity. **(A)** Phosphorylated ERK1/2 and total ERK1/2 levels were determined in CCS knockdown MDA-MB-231 cells by western blotting. **(B)** Phosphorylated ERK1/2 and total ERK1/2 levels were determined in CCS overexpressing MCF-7 cells by western blotting. **(C)** Phosphorylated ERK1/2 and total ERK1/2 levels were determined in CCS overexpressing MCF-7 cells treated with increasing concentrations of U0126 for 12 h by western blotting. **(D)** Cell migration in CCS knockdown and control MDA-MB-231 cells as determined by wound healing assay when overexpressing exogenous HA-tagged MEK. **(E)** Cell migration in CCS overexpressing and control MCF-7 cells treated with U0126 was determined by wound healing assay. The modified migration assay was evaluated by calculating the ratio of the cell numbers through the chamber or wound closure after the wound healing assay. **(F)** Cell proliferation was determined by cell number counting assays in CCS stable knockdown MDA-MB-231 cells with overexpression of exogenous HA-tagged MEK. All results performed above are presented as mean ± SD from three independent experiments. $^{*}p < 0.05$; $^{**}p < 0.01$; $^{***}p < 0.001$, ns not significant.

MAPK/ERK signaling is involved in CCS mediated cell proliferation and migration. To test this hypothesis, we examined the ERK1/2 and MEK1/2 activity in CCS knockdown MDA-MB-231 cells. Western blotting shows that the activity of ERK1/2 was drastically decreased in CCS knockdown MDA-MB-231 cells (**Figure 4A**). Additionally, overexpression of FLAG tagged CCS increased the activity of ERK1/2 in MCF-7 cells (**Figure 4B**), but the increased activity of ERK1/2 was blocked in MCF-7 with ERK inhibitor U0126 (**Figure 4C**). To validate the role of MAPK signaling in the process of CCS-induced migration and proliferation in breast cancer cells, we first reactivated ERK by transfecting exogenous HA tagged MEK into MDA-MB-CCS-KD cells. As expect, the replenishment of MEK in MDA-MB-231-CCS-KD cells could partially rescue the capability of migration in MDA-MB-231-CCS-KD cells due to the reactivation of ERK1/2 (**Figure 4D**). Secondly, we demonstrated that inhibition of MEK with U0126 treatment inhibited CCS-induced cell migration (**Figure 4E**). Thirdly, overexpression of MEK in MDA-MB-231-CCS-KD cells partially rescues the decreased cell proliferation in CCS knockdown MDA-MB-231 cells (**Figure 4F**). These results suggest that activation of the MAPK/ERK pathway is essential for the CCS-promoted migration abilities and cell proliferation of breast cancer cells.

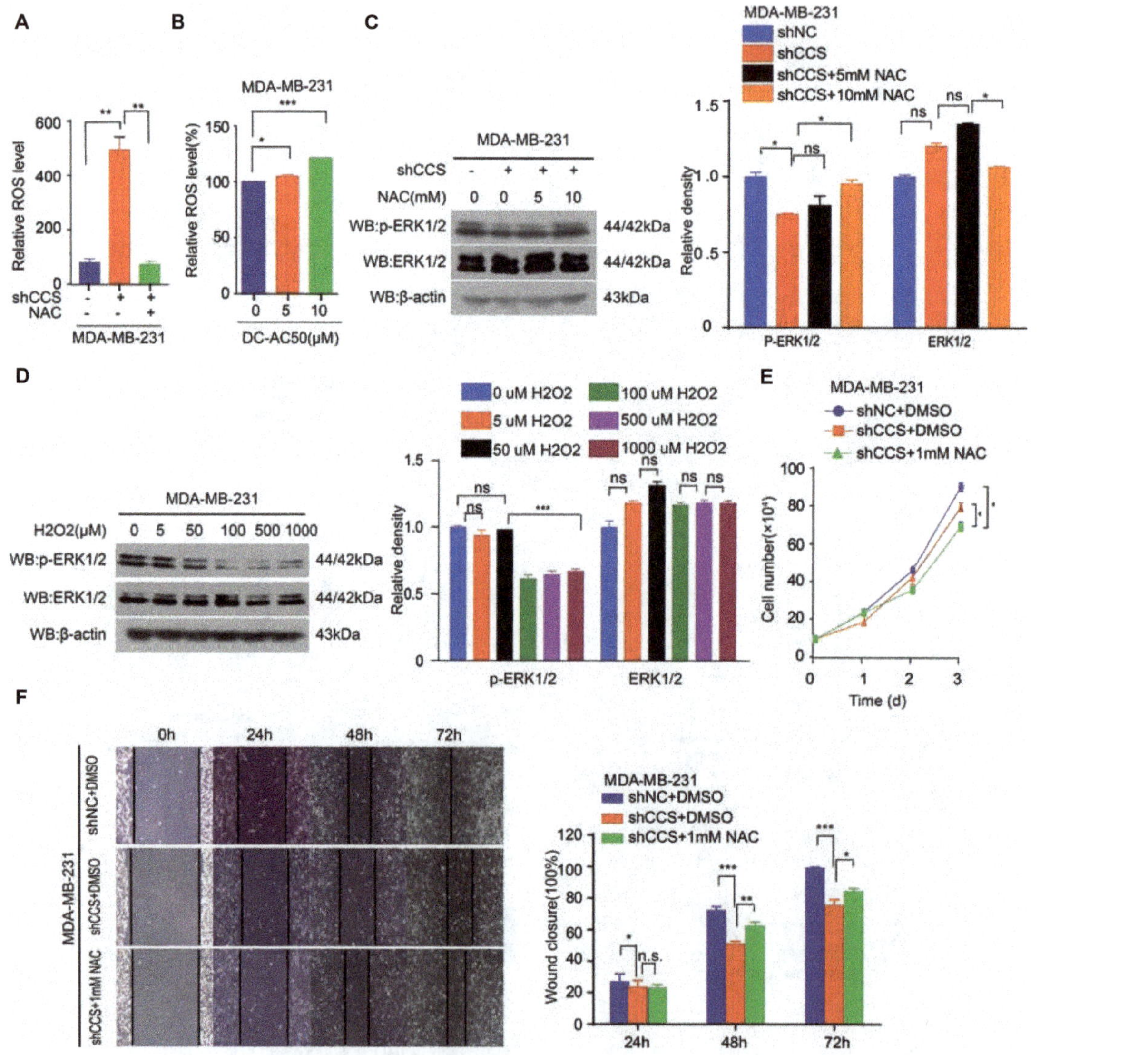

FIGURE 5 | CCS promotes breast cancer cell migration and cell proliferation via ERK1/2 activity mediated by ROS. **(A)** Knockdown of CCS increased ROS level in MDA-MB-231 cells, which was rescued by treatment with 1 mM NAC. **(B)** Treatment with DC_AC50 (5, 10 μM) induced ROS elevation in MDA-MB-231 cells. **(C)** Western blot analysis of total and phosphorylated ERK1/2 levels. β-actin was used as a loading control. Reduced ERK1/2 activity by CCS knockdown was rescued by treatment with NAC (5, 10 mM) for 12 h. **(D)** H_2O_2 significantly abolished ERK1/2 activity in MDA-MB-231cells after 12 h. **(E)** Cell proliferation assays showed that NAC (1 mM) treatment partially rescued the decreased cell proliferation in CCS knockdown MDA-MB-231 cells. **(F)** Wound healing assays showed that NAC (1 mM) treatment partially rescued the decreased cell migration in CCS knockdown MDA-MB-231 cells. All results performed above are presented as mean ± SD from three independent experiments. *$p < 0.05$; **$p < 0.01$; ***$p < 0.001$, ns: not significant.

CCS Activates MAPK/ERK Signaling *via* ROS

The inhibition of CCS leads to increased ROS levels. Thus, we hypothesized that CCS regulates the activity of ERK1/2 through ROS. To test this hypothesis, we examined ROS levels in MDA-MB-231 cells treated with CCS shRNA or DC_AC50. Indeed, we found that knockdown or inhibition of CCS significantly increases the cellular ROS levels (**Figures 5A,B**), while the increased ROS was blocked by treating cells with antioxidant N-Acetyl-L-cysteine (NAC; **Figure 5A**). In addition, we also observed that NAC abrogates the decreased activity of ERK1/2 in CCS knockdown MDA-MB-231 cells (**Figure 5C**). Consistently, we also found that H_2O_2 impaired phosphorylation of ERK1/2 in a dose-dependent manner but did not affect the total expression level of ERK1/2 (**Figure 5D**). Finally, we found that NAC could rescue the decreased cell proliferation and migration of MDA-MB-231 CCS knockdown cells (**Figures 5E,F**). These results further support the idea that inhibition of CCS induces a ROS overload, which impairs MAPK/ERK signaling to attenuate cancer cell proliferation. The combined results presented here also establish CCS as a viable anticancer target and copper trafficking as a new pathway for future therapeutic development.

DISCUSSION

Rapid cellular growth and migratory abilities play a crucial role in tumorigenesis and metastasis, which have been recognized to be associated with ROS levels (Aykin-Burns et al., 2009; Doskey et al., 2016). Those cells that survive oxidative stress stand a good chance to have acquired adaptive mechanisms to counteract the potential toxic effects of elevated ROS and to promote cell-survival pathways (Irmak et al., 2003). CCS, a co-enzyme of SOD1, is a critical component of the oxidation–reduction system in cancer, and its differential expression in different types of breast cancer suggests a relationship between CCS and cancer cell growth and migration (**Figure 6**). However, the link between CCS-activated ROS and the occurrence and development of tumors is still in its infancy.

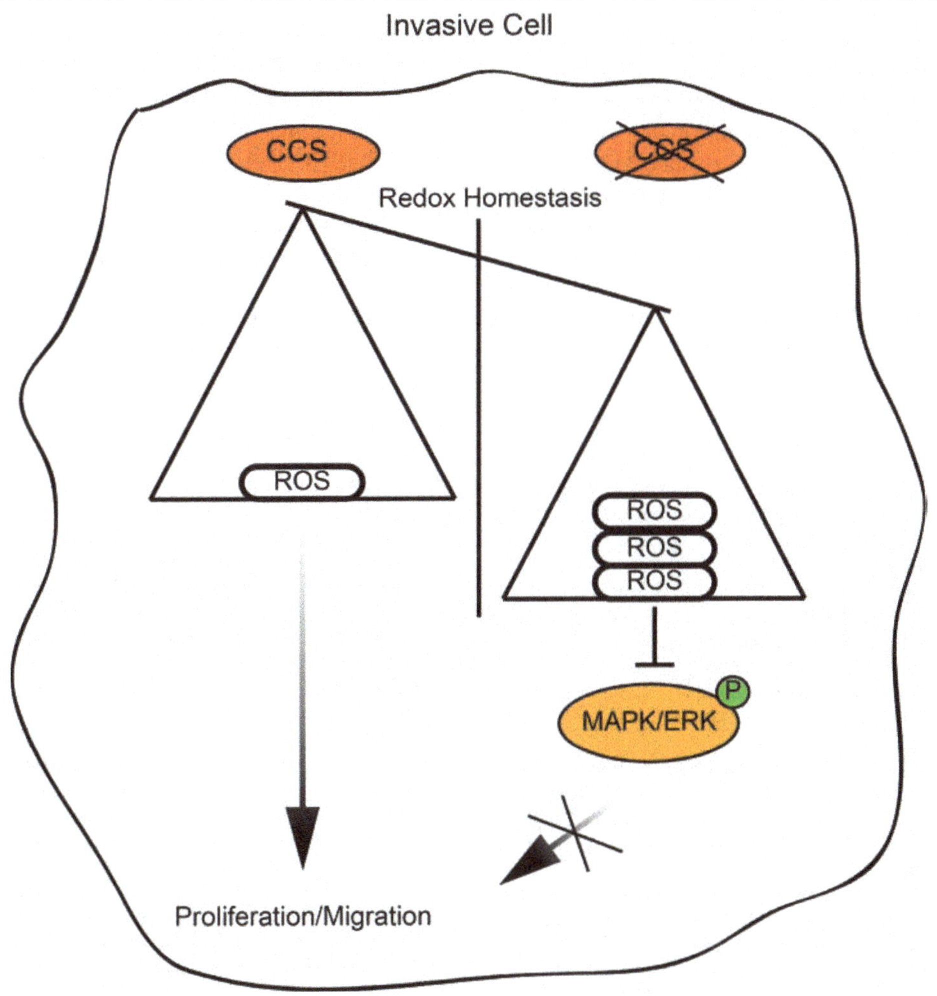

FIGURE 6 | Proposed working model. Schematic model shows that the role and mechanism of CCS in promoting breast cancer cell proliferation and migration.

In this study, we utilized MDA-MB-231 cells (triple-negative breast cancer) and MCF-7 cells (estrogen receptor positive breast cancer) as human cell line models and identified a novel function and mechanism of CCS in facilitating breast cancer cell proliferation and migration. This novel mechanism provides a link between oxidative metabolism and survival signaling. Wang et al. reported that inhibition of CCS leads to a selective suppression of cancer cell proliferation (Wang et al., 2015). Consistent with this, we found that knockdown of CCS significantly reduced cell proliferation in MDA-MB-231 cells but not MCF-7. Interestingly, we revealed a novel function of CCS in regulating migration of breast cancer cells by transwell and wound healing assays. In all, we show that CCS not only plays a vital role in cell proliferation, but it also drives breast cancer migration.

Previous evidence has shown that CCS serves as a co-enzyme of SOD1 to activate its catalytic activity, which is a critical component of oxidation–reduction system (Suzuki et al., 2013b). Since ROS associated oxidative stress has been proven to play important roles in several cancer types and served as promising target for therapy (Perše, 2013; Sosa et al., 2013), we hypothesized that dysregulated ROS levels provide a second signal for CCS-induced proliferation and migration in breast cancer cells. In our study, we showed that knockdown or inhibition of CCS led to increased total ROS levels in MDA-MB-231. ROS overload blocks the activation of the MAPK/ERK pathway, which plays a critical role in tumor formation and progression (Berger et al., 2017; Mayo et al., 2017). By mimicking oxidative stress with H_2O_2 treatment, we were able to suppress the phosphorylation level of ERK1/2, which could be reversed upon treatment with antioxidant NAC. Furthermore, we found that the activation of MAPK/ERK pathways was essential for CCS-induced cell proliferation and migration. Treatment of MCF-7 with U0126-EtOH, a highly selective ERK kinase inhibitor, diminished CCS-induced migration. Conversely, overexpression of MEK enhanced the phosphorylation level of ERK1/2 and partially rescued migration in CCS knockdown MDA-MB-231 cells.

In summary, CCS-mediated ROS decreases the activation of ERK1/2, resulting in attenuation of cell proliferation and migration. Thus, CCS may be a therapeutic strategy to suppress tumor growth and metastasis.

AUTHOR CONTRIBUTIONS

RL and YL performed and analyze all the experiments. XZ and JW drafted the work an provided intellectual content. LL and CS edited the language and figures. CS, SL and SZ designed the study and wrote the manuscript.

FUNDING

This work was supported by the Science and Technology Program of Guangzhou (Grant 201807010003), the Program from the Science and Technology Department of Guangdong Province of China (Grant 2017A030313890), and the National Nature Science Foundation of China (31560312, 81672781 and 81702746). This work was also supported by the China Postdoctoral Science Foundation (2017M612839), the Fundamental Research Funds for the Central Universities (21616323, 21617433), and the Program of Introducing Talents of Discipline to Universities (111 Project, No. B16021).

ACKNOWLEDGMENTS

We thank Dr. Shannon Elf (The University of Chicago) for critical review and edit of the manuscript.

REFERENCES

1. Ashino, T., Sudhahar, V., Urao, N., Oshikawa, J., Chen, G. F., Wang, H., et al. (2010). Unexpected role of the copper transporter ATP7A in PDGF-induced vascular smooth muscle cell migration. *Circ. Res.* 107, 787–799. doi: 10.1161/ CIRCRESAHA.110.225334
2. Aykin-Burns, N., Ahmad, I. M., Zhu, Y., Oberley, L. W., and Spitz, D. R. (2009). Increased levels of superoxide and H2O2 mediate the differential susceptibility of cancer cells versus normal cells to glucose deprivation. *Biochem. J.* 418, 29–37. doi: 10.1042/BJ20081258
3. Bacac, M., and Stamenkovic, I. (2008). Metastatic cancer cell. *Annu. Rev. pathmechdis. Mech. Dis.* 3, 221–247. doi: 10.1146/annurev. pathmechdis.3.121806.151523
4. Baud, V., and Karin, M. (2001). Signal transduction by tumor necrosis factor and its relatives. *Trends Cell Biol.* 11, 372–377. doi: 10.1016/S0962-8924(01)02064-5 Berger, M. D., Stintzing, S., Heinemann, V., Yang, D., Cao, S., Sunakawa, Y., et al. (2017). Impact of genetic variations in the MAPK signaling pathway
5. on outcome in metastatic colorectal cancer patients treated with first-line FOLFIRI and bevacizumab: data from FIRE-3 and TRIBE trials. *Ann. Oncol.* 28, 2780–2785. doi: 10.1093/annonc/mdx412
6. Bray, F., Ferlay, J., Soerjomataram, I., Siegel, R. L., Torre, L. A., and Jemal, A. (2018). Global cancer statistics 2018: GLOBOCAN estimates of incidence and mortality worldwide for 36 cancers in 185 countries. *CA Cancer J. Clin.* 68, 394–424. doi: 10.3322/caac.21492
7. Chaffer, C. L., and Weinberg, R. A. (2011). A perspective on cancer cell metastasis. *Science* 331, 1559–1564. doi: 10.1126/science.1203543
8. Christofori, G. (2006). New signals from the invasive front. *Nature* 441:444. doi: 10.1038/nature04872
9. Doskey, C. M., Buranasudja, V., Wagner, B. A., Wilkes, J. G., Du, J., Cullen, J. J., et al. (2016). Tumor cells have decreased ability to metabolize H2O2: implications for pharmacological ascorbate in cancer therapy. *Redox Biol.* 10, 274–284. doi: 10.1016/j.redox.2016.10.010
10. El Touny, L. H., Vieira, A., Mendoza, A., Khanna, C., Hoenerhoff, M. J., and Green, J. E. (2014). Combined SFK/MEK inhibition prevents metastatic outgrowth of dormant tumor cells. *J. Clin. Invest.* 124, 156–168. doi: 10.1172/ JCI70259
11. Gupta, P. B., Mani, S., Yang, J., Hartwell, K., and Weinberg, R. A. (2005). The evolving portrait of cancer metastasis. *Cold Spring Harbor Symposia on Quantitative Biology* 70, 291–297. doi: 10.1101/sqb.2005.70.033
12. Irmak, M. B., Ince, G., Ozturk, M., and Cetin-Atalay, R. (2003). Acquired tolerance of hepatocellular carcinoma cells to selenium deficiency: a selective survival mechanism? *Cancer Res.* 63, 6707–6715. doi: 10.1016/ S0165-4608(02)00795-1 Kawamata, H., and Manfredi, G. (2008). Different regulation of wild-type and mutant Cu, Zn superoxide dismutase localization in mammalian mitochondria. *Hum. Mol. Genet.* 17, 3303–3317. doi: 10.1093/hmg/ddn226
13. Leitch, J. M., Jensen, L. T., Bouldin, S. D., Outten, C. E., Hart, P. J., and Culotta, V. C. (2009). Activation of Cu, Zn-superoxide dismutase in the

absence of oxygen and the copper chaperone CCS. *J. Biol. Chem.* 284, 21863–21871. doi: 10.1074/jbc.M109.000489

14. Lowndes, S. A., and Harris, A. L. (2005). The role of copper in tumour angiogenesis. *J. Mammary Gland Biol. Neoplasia* 10, 299–310. doi: 10.1007/s10911-006-9003-7
15. Mandinov, L., Mandinova, A., Kyurkchiev, S., Kyurkchiev, D., Kehayov, I., Kolev, V., et al. (2003). Copper chelation represses the vascular response to injury. *Proc. Natl. Acad. Sci.* 100, 6700–6705. doi: 10.1073/pnas.1231994100
16. Mayo, J. C., Hevia, D., Quiros-Gonzalez, I., Rodriguez-Garcia, A., Gonzalez-Menendez, P., Cepas, V., et al. (2017). IGFBP 3 and MAPK/ERK signaling mediates melatonin-induced antitumor activity in prostate cancer. *J. Pineal Res.* 62:e12373. doi: 10.1111/jpi.12373
17. Perše, M. (2013). Oxidative stress in the pathogenesis of colorectal cancer: cause or consequence? *Biomed. Res. Int.* 2013. doi: 10.1155/2013/725710
18. Rajalingam, K., Wunder, C., Brinkmann, V., Churin, Y., Hekman, M., Sievers, C., et al. (2005). Prohibitin is required for Ras-induced Raf–MEK–ERK activation and epithelial cell migration. *Nat. Cell Biol.* 7:837. doi: 10.1038/ncb1283
19. Sciegienka, S. J., Solst, S. R., Falls, K. C., Schoenfeld, J. D., Klinger, A. R., Ross, N. L., et al. (2017). D-penicillamine combined with inhibitors of hydroperoxide metabolism enhances lung and breast cancer cell responses to radiation and carboplatin via H_2O_2-mediated oxidative stress. *Free Radic. Biol. Med.* 108, 354–361. doi: 10.1016/j.freeradbiomed.2017.04.001
20. Sosa, V., Moliné, T., Somoza, R., Paciucci, R., Kondoh, H., and LLeonart, M. E. (2013). Oxidative stress and cancer: an overview. *Ageing Res. Rev.* 12, 376–390. doi: 10.1016/j.arr.2012.10.004
21. Suzuki, Y., Ali, M., Fischer, M., and Riemer, J. (2013a). Human copper chaperone for superoxide dismutase 1 mediates its own oxidation-dependent import into mitochondria. *Nat. Commun.* 4, 1–9. doi: 10.1038/ncomms3430
22. Suzuki, Y., Ali, M., Fischer, M., and Riemer, J. (2013b). Human copper chaperone for superoxide dismutase 1 mediates its own oxidation-dependent import into mitochondria. *Nat. Commun.* 4:2430. doi: 10.1038/ncomms3430
23. Thiery, J. P. (2009). Metastasis: alone or together? *Curr. Biol.* 19, R1121–R1123. doi: 10.1016/j.cub.2009.11.001
24. Ulloa, J. L. (2009). *The copper chaperone as a dual regulator of effects related to oxidative stress and chromatin remodeling.* (ProQuest Dissertations Publishing: The Johns Hopkins University), 3339899.
25. Valastyan, S., and Weinberg, R. A. (2011). Tumor metastasis: molecular insights and evolving paradigms. *Cell* 147, 275–292. doi: 10.1016/j.cell.2011.09.024 Wang, J., Luo, C., Shan, C., You, Q., Lu, J., Elf, S., et al. (2015). Inhibition of human copper trafficking by a small molecule significantly attenuates cancer cell proliferation. *Nat. Chem.* 7, 968–979. doi: 10.1038/nchem.2381
26. Xu, S., Hoshan, L., and Chen, H. (2016). Improving lactate metabolism in an intensified CHO culture process: productivity and product quality considerations. *Bioprocess Biosyst. Eng.* 39, 1689–1702. doi: 10.1007/s00449-016-1644-3

9

Identification of Genetic Mutations in Cancer: Challenge and Opportunity in the New Era of Targeted Therapy

Jing Jin [1†], Xu Wu [2,3†], Jianhua Yin [2,3], Mingxing Li [2,3], Jing Shen [2,3], Jing Li [4], Yueshui Zhao [2,3], Qijie Zhao [2,3], Jingbo Wu [1], Qinglian Wen [1], Chi Hin Cho [2,3], Tao Yi [5], Zhangang Xiao [2*] and Liping Qu [6]*

[1] Department of Oncology, The Affiliated Hospital of Southwest Medical University, Southwest Medical University, Luzhou, China, [2] Laboratory of Molecular Pharmacology, Department of Pharmacology, School of Pharmacy, Southwest Medical University, Luzhou, China, [3] South Sichuan Institute of Translational Medicine, Luzhou, China, [4] Department of Oncology and Hematology, Hospital (T.C.M) Affiliated to Southwest Medical University, Luzhou, China, [5] School of Chinese Medicine, Hong Kong Baptist University, Hong Kong, China, [6] College of Pharmacy, Chengdu University of Traditional Chinese Medicine, Chengdu, China

***Correspondence:**
Tao Yi
yitao@hkbu.edu.hk
Zhangang Xiao
xzg555898@hotmail.com*

† These authors have contributed equally to the work

The introduction of targeted therapy is the biggest success in the treatment of cancer in the past few decades. However, heterogeneous cancer is characterized by diverse molecular alterations as well as multiple clinical profiles. Specific genetic mutations in cancer therapy targets may increase drug sensitivity, or more frequently result in therapeutic resistance. In the past 3 years, several novel targeted therapies have been approved for cancer treatment, including drugs with new targets (i.e., anti-PD1/PDL1 therapies and CDK4/6 inhibitors), mutation targeting drugs (i.e., the EGFR T790M targeting osimertinib), drugs with multiple targets (i.e., the EGFR/HER2 dual inhibitor neratinib) and drug combinations (i.e., encorafenib/binimetinib and dabrafenib/trametinib). In this perspective, we focus on the most up-to-date knowledge of targeted therapy and describe how genetic mutations influence the sensitivity of targeted therapy, highlighting the challenges faced within this era of precision medicine. Moreover, the strategies that deal with mutation-driven resistance are further discussed. Advances in these areas would allow for more targeted and effective therapeutic options for cancer patients.

Keywords: targeted therapy, cyclin-dependent kinases 4/6, somatic mutation, resistance, EGFR, PD-1/PD-L1

INTRODUCTION

Targeted therapies usually present with high selectivity, target precisely to specific gene or protein, and exert a biological function with minimal side effects (1), which has distinguished them from most conventional non-specific chemotherapeutic drugs. Targeted therapy has thus been regarded as the biggest success in the treatment of cancer in the past few decades. Many novel promising agents have been experimentally designed and developed and are increasingly entering clinical evaluation. However, the frequently observed alterations in the drug targets have posed a big challenge to successful cancer treatment. Genetic mutations in cancer are resulted from both inherited and environmental factors. In a recent report, it is demonstrated that a large proportion of cancer-related mutations are due to randomized DNA replication errors (2). Notably, the mutations in cancer therapy targets can greatly affect drug sensitivity. Mutation-driven drug resistance is very common in cancer. The efficacy of targeted therapy is thus largely dependent on the mutation profile of tumors in patients. Accurate molecular and genetic profiling of tumor cells is becoming a routine practice before the introduction of targeted therapy in patients.

In recent years, great progress has been made in targeted therapy discovery. Notably, many new drugs are designed primarily based on specific genetic background. For instance, nearly 40–50% of metastatic cutaneous melanoma possess v-raf murine sarcoma viral oncogene homolog B1 (BRAF) mutations (3), and ~90% of these BRAF mutations are caused by substitution of glutamic acid for valine at codon 600 (V600E) (4). Two selective BRAF inhibitors vemurafenib and dabrafenib were approved for the treatment of patients with BRAF-V600E mutation, showing improved progression-free survival (5). In November 2018, the U.S. Food and Drug Administration (FDA) approved an inhibitor of tropomyosin receptor kinases (TRKs), larotrectinib, for treatment of any type of solid tumors with TRK gene fusion (6). This is the second targeted therapy approved not for specific cancer types but for any cancers with specific mutations. Targeted therapies are becoming more precise.

In this perspective, we focus on the updated knowledge of targeted therapy in the last 3 years and describe how genetic mutations influence sensitivity of targeted therapy, highlighting the challenges faced within this era of precision medicine. Moreover, the strategies dealing with mutation-driven resistance are further discussed.

INFLUENCE OF GENETIC MUTATION ON SENSITIVITY OF TARGETED THERAPY

It is well-acknowledged that mutations in therapeutic targets can increase or decrease drug sensitivity (**Table 1**). The main challenge of targeted therapy today is the identification of particular cancer mutations which affect efficacy of targeted therapies as well as the identification of a specific group of patients most likely or unlikely to respond to certain targeted therapies. Despite the great challenges, in the last 3 years, we have seen significant progress in targeted therapy (**Table 2**), largely owing to the rise of large-scale sequencing technology and big data analysis. Several novel targets, including the programmed death-1/programmed death-ligand 1 (PD1/PDL1) and cyclin-dependent kinases 4 and 6 (CDK4/6), have been validated, with several new targeted drugs being approved. Some newly approved drugs are directly designed to deal with some known activating mutations, such as the T790M mutation in epidermal growth factor receptor (EGFR). Moreover, many new findings have been added to our knowledge of how mutations influence targeted therapies [e.g., the inhibitors of human epidermal growth factor receptor 2 (HER2) and anaplastic lymphoma kinase (ALK)]. Here, based on the most updated research in the last 3 years, we summarize the recent advances of several targeted therapies.

Anti-PD1/PDL1 Therapies

So far, there are a total of 6 anti-PD1/PDL1 therapies that have been approved by the FDA. Notably, in 2017, a PD1 antibody pembrolizumab was approved for the treatment of any solid tumor with a mismatch repair deficiency or a microsatellite instability. Monotherapy of PD1/PDL1 blockade has received great success in many types of cancers (21, 22). However, there are certain patients that are gradually developing resistance after an initial response (23). Mutation-driven resistance of anti-PD1/PDL1 therapies has recently been studied in a small number of cancer patients. Zaretsky et al. reported that mutations of JAK1/JAK2 led to the desensitization of cancer cells to IFN-γ and contributed to an acquired resistance of pembrolizumab in patients with melanoma (23). Moreover, in one resistant patient, a frame-shift deletion in exon 1 of the β-2-microglobulin was detected, which may result in the loss of expression of surface the MHC class I (23). More studies are advocated to explore the acquired resistance of immune checkpoint inhibitors.

Resistance of CDK4/6 Inhibitors

Currently, three CDK 4/6 selective targeting inhibitors, palbociclib, ribociclib, and abemaciclib have been approved to treat breast cancer. CDK4/6 inhibitors are increasingly used in clinical settings, but patients eventually show disease progression and the major reasons remain unclear (24). Dysregulation of cyclin D1-CDK4/6-retinoblastoma (Rb) pathway has been implicated in hormone receptor positive (HR^+) breast cancer and in chemotherapeutic drug-resistance. Rb is usually intact in HR^+ breast cancer and is important for the efficacy of CDK4/6-inhibitors in the treatment of breast cancer (25). It is indicated that T47D cells that become resistant to CDK4/6 inhibitors, develop CCNE1 amplification or Rb1 loss (26). Moreover, the acquisition of multiple *de novo* somatic Rb1 mutations in metastatic breast cancer patients may result in the emergence of a resistance to CDK 4/6 inhibitors (24). Until now, there has been no report on CDK4/6 mutations in cancer patients and their effect on efficacy of CDK4/6 inhibitors.

EGFR and Different Generation of Tyrosine Kinase Inhibitors (TKIs)

EGFR is a prevalent target in several human cancers, such as lung, breast, colorectal, thyroid, and melanoma cancer. In lung cancer, several generations of small-molecular inhibitors have been developed to target the EGFR tyrosine kinases (27), such as inhibitors gefitinib, erlotinib, osimertinib, and necitumumab. The EGFR mutation in non-small cell lung cancer (NSCLC) was first identified in 2004, and the major missense and deletion mutation of EGFR in NSCLC occurs in the tyrosine kinase-coding domain in exons 18–21 (28). The L858R mutation in the exon 21 and exon-19 frame deletion are the most commonly detected mutation types of EGFR, representing 50 and 40% of tumor patients, respectively (7). These two types of mutations are sensitive to EGFR tyrosine kinase inhibitors (TKIs) in NSCLC. The first-generation TKIs, gefitinib and erlotinib,

TABLE 1 | Therapeutic response of targeted therapy in mutant cancers.

Drugs	Sensitivity	Target mutations	Cancer types	Reference
Gefitinib	+	EGFR-L858R	Lung cancer	(7)
Erlotinib	+	EGFR-L858R	Lung cancer	(7)
Gefitinib	–	EGFR-T789M	Lung cancer	(8)
Osimertinib	+	EGFR-T790M	Lung cancer	(9)
Osimertinib	–	EGFR-L718Q	Lung cancer	(10)
Trastuzumab	–	HER2-A859T, -G776L	Lung cancer	(11)
Afatinib	+	HER2-p.Tyr772_Ala775dup	Lung cancer	(12)
Neratinib	–	HER2-T798I, -L869R	Breast cancer	(13)
Lapatinib	–	HER2-T798M	Breast cancer	(14)
Trastuzumab	–	HER2-T798M	Breast cancer	(14)
Neratinib	+	HER2-S310, -L755, -V777, -G778_P780dup, and -Y772_A775dup	Breast, cervical and biliary cancers	(15)
Crizotinib	–	ALK-C1156Y, -L1196M	Lung cancer	(16, 17)
Lorlatinib	–	ALK-L1198F	Lung cancer	(18)
2,4-Pyrimidinediamine derivative	–	EML4-ALK-C1156Y, -L1196M	Lung cancer	(19)
TAE684	–	EML4-ALK-L1152R	Lung cancer	(20)
Dabrafenib	+	BRAF-V600E	Melanoma	(5)

TABLE 2 | Cancer targeted therapy approved by FDA in 2017 and 2018.

Drugs	Targets	Cancer types
Pembrolizumab (2017)	PD-1	Solid tumor with mismatch repair deficiency or microsatellite instability
Cemiplimab (2018)	PD-1	Squamous cell carcinoma
Durvalumab (2017)	PD-L1	Urothelial carcinoma
Avelumab (2017)	PD-L1	Merkel cell carcinoma, urothelial carcinoma
Brigatinib (2018)	ALK	ALK-positive NSCLC
Lorlatinib (2018)	ALK	ALK-positive NSCLC
Ribociclib (2017)	CDK4/6	Breast cancer
Abemaciclib (2017)	CDK4/6	Breast cancer
Niraparib (2017)	PARP	Ovarian cancer, peritoneal cancer
Dacomitinib (2018)	EGFR	NSCLC with EGFR exon 19 deletion or exon 21 L858R substitution mutations
Talazoparib (2018)	PARP	Breast cancer with germline BRCA mutations
Duvelisib (2018)	PI3Kδ, PI3Kγ	Chronic lymphocytic leukemia, small lymphocytic lymphoma
Larotrectinib (2018)	TRKs	Solid tumor with TRK gene fusion
Neratinib (2017)	EGFR/HER2	HER2-amplified breast cancer

have a high selective inhibitory activity against both wild-types and these sensitive mutant EGFR (29). Previous studies show that gefitinib and erlotinib are important for the first-line treatment of NSCLC patients with the sensitive EGFR mutations (30, 31). On the other hand, another mutation T790M, a secondary EGFR mutation emerging in NSCLC, can lead to the resistance of more than half of patients' TKIs treatment (32). Very recently, the third-generation TKI inhibitor osimertinib has been approved to effectively target to EGFR T790M mutation with a response rate of 61% in NSCLC, significantly extending the overall survival in patients with the T790M mutation (9). However, the further mutation of a residue in the P-loop (L718Q) has been found to cause resistance to osimertinib (10). Nevertheless, though diverse EGFR mutations are present, the overall survival of lung cancer patients is markedly improved with TKI therapy.

HER2 and Its Inhibitors

In breast cancer, the overall HER2 mutation rate is ~1.6% (25 out of 1,499 patients). In a study by Bose et al., seven HER2 somatic mutations including G309A, D769H, D769Y, V777L, P780ins, V842I, and R896C, have been identified as activating mutations (33). Several patients with HER2 activating mutations are resistant to the reversible HER2 inhibitor lapatinib, but sensitive to the irreversible HER2 inhibitor neratinib. Neratinib as a dual inhibitor of HER2 and EGFR was approved by FDA in 2017. It has been shown that the HER2 L755S mutation results in an acquired resistance to lapatinib in breast cancer, which could be overcome by the neratinib (34). In another study, the HER2-T798I gatekeeper mutation in breast cancer patients with a AHER2-L869R mutation was identified as a mechanism of acquired resistance to neratinib (13). The trial of neratinib has also been conducted in colorectal cancer

(CRC) patients. The HER2 gene amplification and mutation in CRC can lead to the resistance of EGFR-targeted therapies cetuximab and panitumumab (35, 36). A negative effect of neratinib monotherapy has recently been confirmed in 12 CRC patients with different tumors harboring HER2 mutations (15). There were no positive therapeutic response and the median PFS was only 1.8 months, indicating that monotherapy with neratinib is ineffective. The underlying mechanisms still require further investigations.

ALK and Different Generation of ALK Inhibitors

ALK has long been identified as a therapeutic target in cancer. The first ALK inhibitor crizotinib was approved by the FDA in 2011 (37). Although most NSCLC patients respond to this drug, tumors become resistant after 1–2 years of treatment. Around 1/3 of crizotinib-resistant tumors harbor mutations within the ALK kinase domain. The most commonly observed mutations of L1196M and G1269A lead to a decreased affinity for crizotinib (38). Other ALK point mutations, such as L1152R, C1156Y, I1171T, F1174L, G1202R, and S1206Y, are also associated with crizotinib resistance (39). Another oncoprotein of fusion-type tyrosine kinase, the EML4-ALK, results from the inversion within the short arm of the human chromosome 2 in 4–5% of cases of NSCLC (40). Two mutations of EML4-ALK, C1156Y, and L1196M, confer a significant resistance to ALK inhibitors, such as crizotinib and PDD (2,4-pyrimidinediamine derivative) (19). The EML4-ALK C1156Y mutation can contribute to a higher resistance to PDD than those in the L1196M mutant form. It is reported that a candidate ALK inhibitor TAE684 can bind to these mutant kinases, which may have potency in overcoming the mutation-driven resistance (41). The new generation ALK inhibitors lorlatinib and brigatinib were approved in 2018 for the treatment of patients with ALK-rearranged NSCLC. Lorlatinib has been demonstrated to inhibit resistant ALK mutations, including ALK G1202R (16). However, Shaw et al. showed that an ALK L1198F mutation together with the C1156Y mutation results in the resistance of lorlatinib in a patient with metastatic ALK-rearranged NSCLC (18). However, the L1198F mutation re-sensitized crizotinib treatment of a resistant tumor. It was demonstrated that both lorlatinib and brigatinib can overcome crizotinib resistance in NSCLC patients (42, 43). Moreover, when brigatinib was combined with anti-EGFR antibody, it was effective against EGFR triple-mutant cells *in vitro* and *in vivo* (44).

STRATEGIES FOR OVERCOMING MUTATION-DRIVEN RESISTANCE

Mutations in cancer therapy targets usually result in the loss of functions and the accumulation of dysfunctional proteins in tumors (45). Moreover, many mutants have oncogenic gain-of-function (GOF) activities including increased tumor proliferation, metastasis and drug resistance (46). Notably, tumor cells that receive targeted therapy may lead to an overactivation of the by-pass signaling pathways to develop resistance. In most cases, multiple alterations are observed in a resistant tumor.

Recently, many strategies dealing with mutation-driven drug resistance have been proposed and evaluated both experimentally and clinically. The traditional chemotherapy concept of "one ligand to one receptor" for a biological response is inadequate. The treatment of a particular type of cancer with the prescriptive drugs involves many special genes, interacting with their respective targets and triggering a series of biological responses. The concept of using multi-drug therapy and seeking multifunctional compounds that can efficiently interact with various targets might be feasible (47). Currently, to overcome mutation-driven drug resistance, the main strategies include: (1) the design of new mutation-targeted compounds to restore wide-type protein activities, to delete mutants or to influence downstream targets; (2) the application of combinational therapy or new compounds for multiple targeting. Here, we give some examples of how to overcome mutation-driven resistance of targeted therapy.

Dacomitinib, an Irreversible Pan-ERBB Inhibitor, Targeting EGFR Activating Mutants

Recently, dacomitinib was approved to use for metastatic NSCLC with EGFR exon 19 deletion or exon 21 L858R substitution mutations. In a randomized, multicenter, open-label, phase III trial (ARCHER 1050), the patients with newly diagnosed advanced NSCLC and one EGFR mutation (exon 19 deletion or L858R) received a 45 mg/day dose of oral dacomitinib or a 250 mg/day gefitinib for 28 days. In the dacomitinib group, the progression-free survival (14.7 months, 95% CI 11.1–16.6) was significantly longer than that in the gefitinib group (9.2 months, 95% CI 9.1–11.0) (48). This investigation supports the dacomitinib as the first line therapy for EGFR-mutation NSCLC patients.

Dacomitinib is initially designed for irreversible pan-ERBB inhibition. As a small-molecule covalent binding inhibitor of enzymatically active HER family tyrosine kinases EGFR and HER2, it may act as a potent inhibitor of EGFR T790M mutation (49). Additionally, dacomitinib significantly inhibits both wild-type and the gefitinib-resistant ERBB2 mutation in lung cancer. Based on an in-depth investigation, dacomitinib is an effective drug that may treat NSCLC patients with a T790M-related acquired resistance to gefitinib or erlotinib (8). It has been indicated that dacomitinib significantly improves progression-free survival in EGFR-mutation NSCLC patients and is considered as a new treatment option for this population.

Encorafenib/Binimetinib and Dabrafenib/Trametinib for Dual Inhibition of BRAF and MEK

The FDA approved dabrafenib plus trametinib for the anaplastic thyroid cancer (ATC) with BRAF-V600E mutation in May 2018, as well as for the adjuvant treatment of BRAF V600E/K-mutated melanoma in April 2018. Previous studies revealed that dabrafenib plus trametinib have shown substantial antitumor activity in patients with previously treated BRAF-V600E mutated metastatic NSCLC and untreated BRAFV-600E mutated NSCLC (50, 51). Trametinib is an orally administered MEK1/MEK2 inhibitor that suppresses RAF-dependent MEK phosphorylation and persistently inhibits phosphorylated ERK (a substrate of MEK) (52). Dabrafenib is a reversible and high-efficiency ATP-competitive inhibitor of RAF kinases, especially the mutant BRAF (53). Subbiah et al. reported that the overall response rate of dabrafenib plus trametinib applied in BRAF V600E-mutated ATC (complete reaction plus partial reaction to the best overall response) is 69% (54). In contrast to BRAF inhibitor monotherapy, it has longer progression-free survival and overall survival. Overall, the most common adverse events include fatigue, pyrexia and nausea (54), consistent with previous reports in advanced or metastatic melanoma and NSCLC (50). Dabrafenib plus trametinib is the first regimen approved to have significant clinical efficacy in BRAF V600E-mutated ATC.

In June 2018, the FDA approved the combination of BRAF inhibitor encorafenib and the MEK inhibitor binimetinib for treatment of patients with unresectable or metastatic melanoma with a BRAF-V600E or -V600K mutation. It is the third BRAF/MEK inhibitor combination approved following the dabrafenib/trametinib and vemurafenib/cobimetinib combinations (55). The main adverse events for encorafenib plus binimetinib when applied to BRAF-V600 mutant melanoma are gastrointestinal reactions, including nausea, diarrhea and vomiting. Additionally, this combination has a lower calorific value and photosensitivity than other available BRAF-MEK inhibitor combinations do (56). Considerable evidence supports that the median progression-free survival was 14.9 months with encorafenib plus binimetinib, compared with 7.3 months with vemurafenib (57). Therefore, it is an effective therapeutic option in patients with unresectable or metastatic melanoma, with a BRAF V600E or V600K mutation.

CONCLUSIONS

In the new era of targeted therapy, treatment options are increasingly based on the precise molecular and genetic profiling of tumor cells (58). Currently, the main challenge for further novel drug development in targeted therapy is the clarification of specific molecular mechanisms underlying the varied forms of tumors in clinic. It has been acknowledged that cancer is caused by a set of driver mutations. In this regard, it is of great significance to: (1) identify and validate key mutant genes and proteins in cancers as new targets; (2) identify patients most likely and unlikely to benefit from certain targeted therapies; (3) evaluate the mechanism of mutation-driven drug resistance. In past decades, several key mutations which influence drug sensitivity have been identified in various cancers. In order to deal with mutation-driven drug resistance, new methods and drugs have been discovered and approved for clinical use (47). Even so, detailed individualized treatment strategies targeting specific tumorigenesis and drug resistant mechanisms are still required. Advances in these areas would allow for more targeted and effective therapeutic options for more cancer patients.

AUTHOR CONTRIBUTIONS

ML, JS, JL, YZ, JW, LQ, and QW were responsible for the review of the literature. JJ, JY, XW, QZ, CC, and ML wrote the manuscript. XW and LQ drew the Tables. XW, TY, and ZX designed the study and contributed with the valuable discussion and revision of the manuscript.

FUNDING

This work was supported by the National Natural Science Foundation of China (Grant nos. 81503093, 81602166, and 81672444) and the Joint Funds of the Southwest Medical University and Luzhou (2016LZXNYD-T01, 2017LZXNYD-Z05, and 2017LZXNYD-J09). The funding from National Natural Science Foundation of China (Grant nos. 81503093) will cover open access fee.

REFERENCES

1. Scotti L, Mendonca Junior FJ, Ishiki HM, Ribeiro FF, Singla RK, Barbosa Filho JM, et al. Docking studies for multi-target drugs. *Curr Drug Targ.* (2017) 18:592–604. doi: 10.2174/138945011666615082511818
2. Tomasetti C, Li L, Vogelstein B. Stem cell divisions, somatic mutations, cancer etiology, and cancer prevention. *Science.* (2017) 355:1330–4. doi: 10.1126/science.aaf9011
3. Curtin JA, Fridlyand J, Kageshita T, Patel HN, Busam KJ, Kutzner H, et al. Distinct sets of genetic alterations in melanoma. *N Engl J Med.* (2005) 353:2135–47. doi: 10.1056/NEJMoa050092
4. Davies H, Bignell GR, Cox C, Stephens P, Edkins S, Clegg S, et al. Mutations of the BRAF gene in human cancer. *Nature.* (2002) 417:949–54. doi: 10.1038/nature00766
5. Hauschild A, Grob JJ, Demidov LV, Jouary T, Gutzmer R, Millward M, et al. Dabrafenib in BRAF-mutated metastatic melanoma: a multicentre, open-label, phase 3 randomised controlled trial. *Lancet.* (2012) 380:358–65. doi: 10.1016/s0140-6736(12)60868-x
6. Drilon A, Laetsch TW, Kummar S, DuBois SG, Lassen UN, Demetri GD, et al. Efficacy of larotrectinib in TRK fusion–positive cancers in adults and children. *N Engl J Med.* (2018) 378:731–9. doi: 10.1056/NEJMoa1714448
7. Shigematsu H, Lin L, Takahashi T, Nomura M, Suzuki M, Wistuba II, et al. Clinical and biological features associated with epidermal growth factor receptor gene mutations in lung cancers. *J Natl Cancer Inst.* (2005) 97:339–46. doi: 10.1093/jnci/dji055
8. Kobayashi S, Boggon TJ, Dayaram T, Janne PA, Kocher O, Meyerson M, et al. EGFR mutation and resistance of non-small-cell lung cancer to gefitinib. *N Engl J Med.* (2005) 352:786–92. doi: 10.1056/NEJMoa044238
9. Mok TS, Wu YL, Ahn MJ, Garassino MC, Kim HR, Ramalingam SS, et al. Osimertinib or platinum-pemetrexed in EGFR T790M-positive lung cancer. *N Engl J Med.* (2017) 376:629–40. doi: 10.1056/NEJMoa1612674
10. Callegari D, Ranaghan KE, Woods CJ, Minari R, Tiseo M, Mor M, et al. L718Q mutant EGFR escapes covalent inhibition by stabilizing a non-reactive conformation of the lung cancer drug osimertinib. *Chem Sci.* (2018) 9:2740–9. doi: 10.1039/c7sc04761d
11. Cappuzzo F, Bemis L, Varella-Garcia M. HER2 mutation and response to trastuzumab therapy in non-small-cell lung cancer. *N Engl J Med.* (2006) 354:2619–21. doi: 10.1056/NEJMc060020
12. De Greve J, Teugels E, Geers C, Decoster L, Galdermans D, De Mey J, et al. Clinical activity of afatinib (BIBW 2992) in patients with lung

adenocarcinoma with mutations in the kinase domain of HER2/neu. *Lung Cancer.* (2012) 76:123–7. doi: 10.1016/j.lungcan.2012.01.008

13. Hanker AB, Brewer MR, Sheehan JH, Koch JP, Sliwoski GR, Nagy R, et al. An acquired HER2(T798I) gatekeeper mutation induces resistance to neratinib in a patient with HER2 mutant-driven breast cancer. *Cancer Discov.* (2017) 7:575–85. doi: 10.1158/2159-8290.cd-16-1431
14. Rexer BN, Ghosh R, Narasanna A, Estrada MV, Chakrabarty A, Song Y, et al. Human breast cancer cells harboring a gatekeeper T798M mutation in HER2 overexpress EGFR ligands and are sensitive to dual inhibition of EGFR and HER2. *Clin Cancer Res.* (2013) 19:5390–401. doi: 10.1158/1078-0432.ccr-13-1038
15. Hyman DM, Piha-Paul SA, Won H, Rodon J, Saura C, Shapiro GI, et al. HER kinase inhibition in patients with HER2- and HER3-mutant cancers. *Nature.* (2018) 554:189–94. doi: 10.1038/nature25475
16. Katayama R, Lovly CM, Shaw AT. Therapeutic targeting of anaplastic lymphoma kinase in lung cancer: a paradigm for precision cancer medicine. *Clin Cancer Res.* (2015) 21:2227–35. doi: 10.1158/1078-0432.ccr-14-2791
17. Shaw AT, Kim DW, Mehra R, Tan DS, Felip E, Chow LQ, et al. Ceritinib in ALK-rearranged non-small-cell lung cancer. *N Engl J Med.* (2014) 370:1189–97. doi: 10.1056/NEJMoa1311107
18. Shaw AT, Friboulet L, Leshchiner I, Gainor JF, Bergqvist S, Brooun A, et al. Resensitization to crizotinib by the lorlatinib ALK resistance mutation L1198F. *N Engl J Med.* (2016) 374:54–61. doi: 10.1056/NEJMoa1508887
19. Choi YL, Soda M, Yamashita Y, Ueno T, Takashima J, Nakajima T, et al. EML4-ALK mutations in lung cancer that confer resistance to ALK inhibitors. *N Engl J Med.* (2010) 363:1734–9. doi: 10.1056/NEJMoa1007478
20. Sasaki T, Koivunen J, Ogino A, Yanagita M, Nikiforow S, Zheng W, et al. A novel ALK secondary mutation and EGFR signaling cause resistance to ALK kinase inhibitors. *Cancer Res.* (2011) 71:6051–60. doi: 10.1158/0008-5472.can-11-1340
21. Hamid O, Robert C, Daud A, Hodi FS, Hwu WJ, Kefford R, et al. Safety and tumor responses with lambrolizumab (anti-PD-1) in melanoma. *N Engl J Med.* (2013) 369:134–44. doi: 10.1056/NEJMoa1305133
22. Peters S, Kerr KM, Stahel R. PD-1 blockade in advanced NSCLC: a focus on pembrolizumab. *Cancer Treat Rev.* (2018) 62:39–49. doi: 10.1016/j.ctrv.2017.10.002
23. Zaretsky JM, Garcia-Diaz A, Shin DS, Escuin-Ordinas H, Hugo W, Hu-Lieskovan S, et al. Mutations associated with acquired resistance to PD-1 blockade in melanoma. *N Engl J Med.* (2016) 375:819–29. doi: 10.1056/NEJMoa1604958
24. Condorelli R, Spring L, O'Shaughnessy J, Lacroix L, Bailleux C, Scott V, et al. Polyclonal RB1 mutations and acquired resistance to CDK 4/6 inhibitors in patients with metastatic breast cancer. *Ann Oncol.* (2018) 29:640–5. doi: 10.1093/annonc/mdx784
25. Cancer Genome Atlas Network. (2012). Comprehensive molecular portraits of human breast tumours. *Nature.* 490, 61–70. doi: 10.1038/nature 11412
26. Herrera-Abreu MT, Palafox M, Asghar U, Rivas MA, Cutts RJ, Garcia-Murillas I, et al. Early adaptation and acquired resistance to CDK4/6 inhibition in estrogen receptor-positive breast cancer. *Cancer Res.* (2016) 76:2301–13. doi: 10.1158/0008-5472.can-15-0728
27. Renhowe PA. Inhibitors of growth factor receptor kinase-dependent signaling pathways in anticancer chemotherapy–clinical progress. *Curr Opin Drug Discov Devel.* (2002) 5:214. doi: 10.2174/09298670246 06957
28. Pao W, Miller V, Zakowski M, Doherty J, Politi K, Sarkaria I, et al. EGF receptor gene mutations are common in lung cancers from "never smokers" and are associated with sensitivity of tumors to gefitinib and erlotinib. *Proc Natl Acad Sci USA.* (2004) 101:13306–11. doi: 10.1073/pnas.04052 20101
29. Morin MJ. From oncogene to drug: development of small molecule tyrosine kinase inhibitors as anti-tumor and anti-angiogenic agents. *Oncogene.* (2000) 19:6574–83. doi: 10.1038/sj.onc.1204102
30. Inoue A, Kobayashi K, Usui K, Maemondo M, Okinaga S, Mikami I, et al. First-line gefitinib for patients with advanced non-small-cell lung cancer harboring epidermal growth factor receptor mutations without indication for chemotherapy. *J Clin Oncol.* (2009) 27:1394–400. doi: 10.1200/JCO.2008.18.7658
31. Maemondo M, Inoue A, Kobayashi K, Sugawara S, Oizumi S, Isobe H, et al. Gefitinib or chemotherapy for non-small-cell lung cancer with mutated EGFR. *N Engl J Med.* (2010) 362:2380–8. doi: 10.1056/NEJMoa0909530
32. Bell DW, Gore I, Okimoto RA, Godin-Heymann N, Sordella R, Mulloy R, et al. Inherited susceptibility to lung cancer may be associated with the T790M drug resistance mutation in EGFR. *Nat Genet.* (2005) 37:1315–6. doi: 10.1038/ng1671
33. Bose R, Kavuri SM, Searleman AC, Shen W, Shen D, Koboldt DC, et al. Activating HER2 mutations in HER2 gene amplification negative breast cancer. *Cancer Discov.* (2013) 3:224–37. doi: 10.1158/2159-8290.cd-12-0349
34. Xu X, De Angelis C, Burke KA, Nardone A, Hu H, Qin L, et al. HER2 Reactivation through acquisition of the HER2 L755S mutation as a mechanism of acquired resistance to HER2-targeted therapy in HER2(+) breast cancer. *Clin Cancer Res.* (2017) 23:5123–34. doi: 10.1158/1078-0432.ccr-16-2191
35. Dienstmann R, Tabernero J. Spectrum of gene mutations in colorectal cancer: implications for treatment. *Cancer J.* (2016) 22:149–55. doi: 10.1097/ppo.0000000000000191
36. Ross JS, Fakih M, Ali SM, Elvin JA, Schrock AB, Suh J, et al. Targeting HER2 in colorectal cancer: the landscape of amplification and short variant mutations in ERBB2 and ERBB3. *Cancer.* (2018) 124:1358–73. doi: 10.1002/cncr.31125
37. Ou SH. Crizotinib: a novel and first-in-class multitargeted tyrosine kinase inhibitor for the treatment of anaplastic lymphoma kinase rearranged non-small cell lung cancer and beyond. *Drug Des Devel Ther.* (2011) 5:471–85. doi: 10.2147/dddt.s19045
38. Kimura AGM. Molecularly targeted therapy: past, present and future. *Chemotherapy* 1:105. doi: 10.4172/2167-7700.1000105
39. Zhang S, Wang F, Keats J, Zhu X, Ning Y, Wardwell SD, et al. Crizotinib-resistant mutants of EML4-ALK identified through an accelerated mutagenesis screen. *Chem Biol Drug Des.* (2011) 78:999–1005. doi: 10.1111/j.1747-0285.2011.01239.x
40. Soda M, Choi YL, Enomoto M, Takada S, Yamashita Y, Ishikawa S, et al. Identification of the transforming EML4-ALK fusion gene in non-small-cell lung cancer. *Nature.* (2007) 448:561–6. doi: 10.1038/nature05945
41. Heuckmann JM, Holzel M, Sos ML, Heynck S, Balke-Want H, Koker M, et al. ALK mutations conferring differential resistance to structurally diverse ALK inhibitors. *Clin Cancer Res.* (2011) 17:7394–74. doi: 10.1158/1078-0432.ccr-11-1648
42. Zhang S, Anjum R, Squillace R, Nadworny S, Zhou T, Keats J, et al. The potent ALK inhibitor brigatinib (AP26113) overcomes mechanisms of resistance to first- and second-generation ALK inhibitors in preclinical models. *Clin Cancer Res.* (2016) 22:5527–38. doi: 10.1158/1078-0432.ccr-16-0569
43. Shaw AT, Felip E, Bauer TM, Besse B, Navarro A, Postel-Vinay S, et al. Lorlatinib in non-small-cell lung cancer with ALK or ROS1 rearrangement: an international, multicentre, open-label, single-arm first-in-man phase 1 trial. *Lancet Oncol.* (2017) 18:1590–9. doi: 10.1016/s1470-2045(17)30680-0
44. Uchibori K, Inase N, Araki M, Kamada M, Sato S, Okuno Y, et al. Brigatinib combined with anti-EGFR antibody overcomes osimertinib resistance in EGFR-mutated non-small-cell lung cancer. *Nat Commun.* (2017) 8:14768. doi: 10.1038/ncomms14768
45. Iranzo J, Martincorena I, Koonin EV. Cancer-mutation network and the number and specificity of driver mutations. *Proc Natl Acad Sci USA.* (2018) 115:E6010–9. doi: 10.1073/pnas.1803155115
46. Yue X, Zhao Y, Xu Y, Zheng M, Feng Z, Hu W. Mutant p53 in cancer: accumulation, gain-of-function, and therapy. *J Mol Biol.* (2017) 429:1595–606. doi: 10.1016/j.jmb.2017.03.030
47. Wang L, Wang H, Song D, Xu M, Liebmen M. New strategies for targeting drug combinations to overcome mutation-driven drug resistance. *Semin Cancer Biol.* (2017) 42:44–51. doi: 10.1016/j.semcancer.2016.11.002
48. Wu YL, Cheng Y, Zhou X, Lee KH, Nakagawa K, Niho S, et al. Dacomitinib versus gefitinib as first-line treatment for patients with EGFR-mutation-positive non-small-cell lung cancer (ARCHER 1050): a randomised, open-label, phase 3 trial. *Lancet Oncol.* (2017) 18:1454–66. doi: 10.1016/s1470-2045(17)30608-3
49. Engelman JA, Zejnullahu K, Gale CM, Lifshits E, Gonzales AJ, Shimamura T, et al. PF00299804, an irreversible pan-ERBB inhibitor, is effective in lung cancer models with EGFR and ERBB2 mutations that are resistant to gefitinib. *Cancer Res.* (2007) 67:11924–32. doi: 10.1158/0008-5472.can-07-1885

50. Chen G, McQuade JL, Panka DJ, Hudgens CW, Amin-Mansour A, Mu XJ, et al. Clinical, molecular, and immune analysis of dabrafenib-trametinib combination treatment for BRAF inhibitor-refractory metastatic melanoma: a phase 2 clinical trial. *JAMA Oncol.* (2016) 2:1056–64. doi: 10.1001/jamaoncol.2016.0509
51. Planchard D, Smit EF, Groen HJM, Mazieres J, Besse B, Helland A, et al. Dabrafenib plus trametinib in patients with previously untreated BRAF(V600E)-mutant metastatic non-small-cell lung cancer: an open-label, phase 2 trial. *Lancet Oncol.* (2017) 18:1307–16. doi: 10.1016/s1470-2045(17)30679-4
52. Gilmartin AG, Bleam MR, Groy A, Moss KG, Minthorn EA, Kulkarni SG, et al. GSK1120212 (JTP-74057) is an inhibitor of MEK activity and activation with favorable pharmacokinetic properties for sustained *in vivo* pathway inhibition. *Clin Cancer Res.* (2011) 17:989–1000. doi: 10.1158/1078-0432.ccr-10-2200
53. Puszkiel A, Noe G, Bellesoeur A, Kramkimel N, Paludetto MN, Thomas-Schoemann A, et al. Clinical pharmacokinetics and pharmacodynamics of dabrafenib. *Clin Pharmacokinet.* (2019) 58:451–67. doi: 10.1007/s40262-018-0703-0
54. Subbiah V, Kreitman RJ, Wainberg ZA, Cho JY, Schellens JHM, Soria JC, et al. Dabrafenib and trametinib treatment in patients with locally advanced or metastatic BRAF V600-mutant anaplastic thyroid cancer. *J Clin Oncol.* (2018) 36:7–13. doi: 10.1200/jco.2017.7 3.6785
55. Dummer R, Ascierto PA, Gogas HJ, Arance A, Mandala M, Liszkay G, et al. Overall survival in patients with BRAF-mutant melanoma receiving encorafenib plus binimetinib versus vemurafenib orencorafenib (COLUMBUS): a multicentre, open-label, randomised, phase 3 trial. *Lancet Oncol.* (2018b) 19:1315–27. doi: 10.1016/s1470-2045(18)30497-2
56. Sullivan RJ, Weber JS, Patel SP, Dummer R, Miller WH, Cosgrove D, et al. A phase Ib/II study of BRAF inhibitor (BRAFi) encorafenib (ENCO) plus MEK inhibitor (MEKi) binimetinib (BINI) in cutaneous melanoma patients naive to BRAFi treatment. *J Clin Oncol.* (2015) 33:9007–9007. doi: 10.1200/jco.2015.33.15_suppl.9007
57. Dummer R, Ascierto PA, Gogas HJ, Arance A, Mandala M, Liszkay G, et al. Encorafenib plus binimetinib versus vemurafenib or encorafenib in patients with BRAF-mutant melanoma (COLUMBUS): a multicentre, open-label, randomised phase 3 trial. *Lancet Oncol.* (2018) 19:603–15. doi: 10.1016/s1470-2045(18)30142-6
58. Huang M, Shen A, Ding J, Geng M. Molecularly targeted cancer therapy: some lessons from the past decade. *Trends Pharmacol Sci.* (2014) 35:41–50. doi: 10.1016/j.tips.2013.11.004

10

USP7: Novel Drug Target in Cancer Therapy

Zhiru Wang[1,2,3], Wenting Kang[1,2], Yinghua You[1,2], Jingru Pang[1,2], Hongmei Ren[1,2], Zhenhe Suo[3]*, Hongmin Liu[1,2]* and Yichao Zheng[1,2]**

[1] School of Pharmaceutical Sciences, Zhenghzou University, Zhengzhou, China, [2] Collaborative Innovation Centre of New Drug Research and Safety Evaluation, Henan Province, and Key Laboratory of Advanced Drug Preparation Technologies, Zhengzhou University, and Key Laboratory of Henan Province for Drug Quality and Evaluation, Ministry of Education of China, Zhengzhou, China, [3] Pathology, Institute of Clinical Medicine, Faculty of Medicine, University of Oslo, Oslo, Norway

***Correspondence:**
Zhiru Wang
simplearu@163.com
Zhenhe Suo
zhenhe.suo@medisin.uio.no
Hongmin Liu
liuhm@zzu.edu.cn
Yichao Zheng
yichaozheng@zzu.edu.cn

Ubiquitin specific protease 7 (USP7) is one of the deubiquitinating enzymes (DUB) that erases ubiquitin and protects substrate protein from degradation. Full activity of USP7 requires the C-terminal Ub-like domains fold back onto the catalytic domain, allowing the remodeling of the active site to a catalytically competent state by the C-terminal peptide. Until now, numerous proteins have been identified as substrates of USP7, which play a key role in cell cycle, DNA repair, chromatin remodeling, and epigenetic regulation. Aberrant activation or overexpression of USP7 may promote oncogenesis and viral disease, making it a target for therapeutic intervention. Currently, several synthetic small molecules have been identified as inhibitors of USP7, and applied in the treatment of diverse diseases. Hence, USP7 may be a promising therapeutic target for the treatment of cancer.

Keywords: deubiquitination, USP7, structure, immune, DNA damage

INTRODUCTION

Post-translational modification (PTM) is generally enzymatic modification of proteins following protein biosynthesis. Examples of PTM include methylation, acetylation, phosphorylation, glycosylation, ubiquitination, S-nitrosylation, and so on (Chatterjee and Thakur, 2018). As one of the most studied PTMs, ubiquitination involves in the intracellular proteolytic machinery and regulates numerous physical activities in the cell (Dybas et al., 2018). The process of the addition of ubiquitin to a substrate protein is named ubiquitination, which may contribute to the protein degradation. Ubiquitination of target protein can be catalyzed by a cascade reaction comprising the ubiquitin-activating enzymes (E1), the ubiquitin conjugation enzymes (E2) and the ubiquitin ligases (E3). First, ubiquitin is activated by E1 with the participation of ATP and transferred to E2 through a trans-thiolation reaction, and then conjugated to a lysine or α-amino group of the substrate protein in the presence of E3 (Cheon and Baek, 2006). Eventually, proteins labels with more than four ubiquitin molecules can be recognized and subjected to the 26S proteasome at which they are degraded, generating small polypeptides (**Figure 1**).

Deubiquitinating enzymes (DUBs) are responsible for the removal of ubiquitin and keeping the stability of the substrate by rescuing them from degradation (Nijman et al., 2005; Clague et al., 2013). Until now, approximately 100 DUBs have been identified and can be classified into five subclasses based on their Ub-protease domains: ubiquitin-specific proteases (USPs), ubiquitin C-terminal hydrolases (UCHs), ovarian tumor proteases (OTUs), Machado-Joseph disease proteases (MJDs) belonging to cysteine-dependent proteases, and JAB1/MPN/Mov34 (JAMMs) belonging to zinc metalloproteases (Zhou et al., 2018). With approximately 50 members, the USPs family is the largest one among all the DUB subfamilies. All these members include conserved domains, i.e., three primary functional domains of Cys, His and Asp/Asn boxes which are in charge of the reorganization of ubiquitin conjugated molecules.

Among the members of USP family, ubiquitin specific protease USP7, also known as herpes-associated ubiquitin-specific protease (HAUSP), is a unique deubiquitinating enzyme which was identified in 1997, and it characterized as a novel member of the ubiquitin-specific protease family to interact with herpes simplex virus type 1 immediate-early protein (Vmw110) of the herpes simplex virus type 1 (HSV-1) regulatory protein (Everett et al., 1997). Later, USP7 was found to interact with other viral proteins such as the Epstein-Barr nuclear antigen 1 (EBNA1) of Epstein-Barr virus (EBV) and the vIRF1 (viral interferon regulatory factor 1) protein of Kaposi's sarcoma associated herpesvirus (KSHV) (Holowaty et al., 2003), therefore indicating it as a general target of herpes viruses and giving it the name herpes-associated ubiquitin specific protease. Up to now, USP7 is the most widely studied deubiquitinating enzymes, and is considered as an oncogene by promoting tumor growth and negatively affecting the patient immune response to tumors (Everett, 2014; Lu et al., 2016).

STRUCTURE OF USP7

The full length USP7 includes 1102 amino acids. There are four domains: an N-terminal poly-glutamine stretch (poly Q), the tumor necrosis factor receptor- associated factors (TRAF) domain (amino acids 62–205), the catalytic domain (amino acids 208–560), and the C-terminal tandem ubiquitin-like (Ubl) domain (amino acids 560–1102) (Kim and Sixma, 2017) (**Figure 2A**).

As reported, the amino acids 62–205 of USP7 (**Figure 2B**) bind to EBNA1 (Holowaty et al., 2003), mouse double minute 2 homolog (MDM2) and p53 (Hu et al., 2006; Sheng et al., 2006) through a PA-x-x-S motif (Saridakis et al., 2005), and the TRAF (amino acids 62–205) domain contributes to the nuclear localization of the USP7 (Fernandez-Montalvan et al., 2007). Besides, the USP7 truncation (amino acids 208–1102) performed similar activity as the full length protein (Ma et al., 2010).

Hu et al. (2002) identified a 40 kDa fragment of USP7 as the catalytic domain (amino acids 208–560), which mediates ubiquitin binding and deubiquitination of the substrate. The structure of the catalytic core domain reveals novel three-domain architecture, including Fingers, Palm, and Thumb domains (**Figure 2C**). This catalytic core domain binds to ubiquitin aldehyde, which reveals a conformational change in the active site (Hu et al., 2002). With the aid of molecular dynamics simulations, it is found that the transition of USP7 from the inactive to the active can only be captured when H294 was neutralized with a deprotonated C223 and charged H464. In the inactive apo state, positively charged H294 stabilizes an electrostatic network with W285, E298, and Y224. However, neutral H294 in the active state cannot make charge interactions, so the electrostatic network is disrupted. That would results in the C223 unfavorable backbone angles improved by helical refolding, thus, the active site is formed (Ozen et al., 2018).

Ubl shares the ubiquitin β-grasp fold, however, it lacks the C-terminal Gly–Gly residues that are required for conjugation to a target and is located outside the boundaries of the catalytic core domain (Faesen et al., 2011). There are five Ubl domains that are detected in the C-terminal and are organized in a 2-1-2 manner as Ubl-12, Ubl-3, and Ubl-45 (**Figure 2D**) (Zhu et al., 2007). Among them, Ubl-45 is sufficient to reconstitute the USP7 activation *in vitro* and *in vivo*. In the C-terminal, the 19 residues of USP7 (amino acids 1084–1102) are conserved across species (Faesen et al., 2011). Rouge et al. (2016) revealed how the C terminal 19 amino acids of the USP7 contribute to the enhancement of USP7 activity by stabilizing the ubiquitin binding conformation of the catalytic domain. And the individual point mutations at residues I1100 or I1098 are able to abolish the deubiquitinase activity of USP7 (Rouge et al., 2016).

USP7: ONE PROTEIN, MULTIPLE ROLES

Many proteins have been identified as potential substrates and binding partners of USP7, such as viral proteins, transcription factors, and epigenetic modulators (**Figure 8**), and most of these substrates play important roles in viral replication, immune response, tumor suppression, epigenetic control, and DNA repair. Here, functions of USP7 on these substrate are as detailed below (**Table 1**).

Viral Proteins

EBNA1

EBNA1 of EBV is important for the replication, segregation, and transcriptional activation of latent EBV genomes, it has been implicated in host cell immortalization, and avoids proteasome processing and cell-surface presentation. The amino acids 395–450 of EBNA1 bind to the USP7 N-terminal domain with a dissociation constant of 0.9–2 μM. The Δ395–450 mutant that selectively disrupted the binding to USP7 was found to increase fourfold EBNA1 replication activity than wild-type, but performed no impact on EBNA1 turnover and cell-surface presentation (Holowaty et al., 2003). As p53 and EBNA1 share similar binding sites with USP7, EBNA1 peptide efficiently competes with p53 peptide for USP7 binding, which results the decreasing stability of p53, and protects cells from apoptosis (Saridakis et al., 2005).

ICP0

Infected cell protein 0 (ICP0) of HSV is a multifunctional protein containing 775 amino acids that acts as a promiscuous trans-activator linked to the degradation of several proteins. The ^{618}PRKCARKT^{625} of ICP0 binds to a negatively charged region on Ubl2, where the residues K620 and K624 of ICP0 form direct contacts with residues D762 and D764 in Ubl2 of USP7 (Pfoh et al., 2015). Overexpression of USP7 had no effect on the mRNA level of ICP0, but could accelerate the mRNA accumulation of thymidine kinase (TK) and gI, which are important for HSV infection of non-replicating cells. The mutations at residues 620

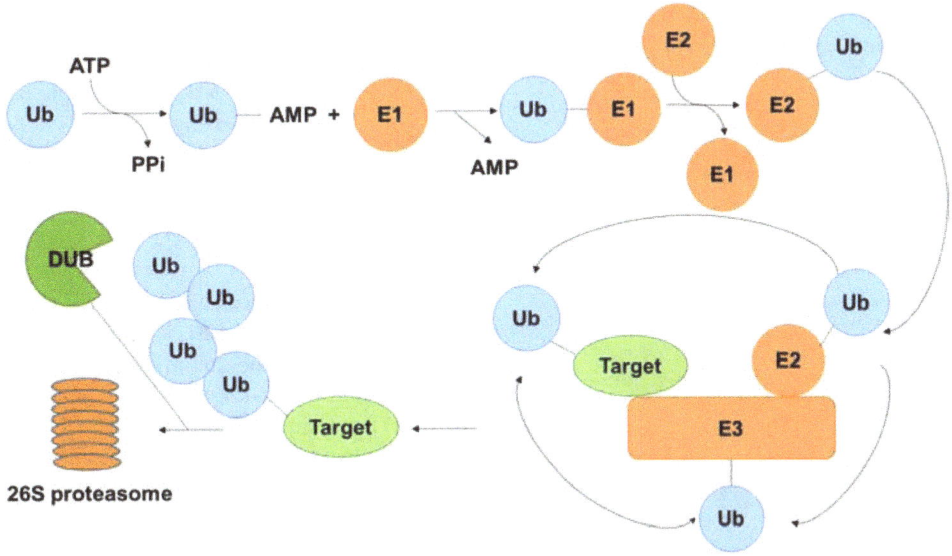

FIGURE 1 | Schematic of the ubiquitin-proteasome system. Ubiquitin is activated by E1 in the presence of ATP and transferred to E2 and then conjugated to a lysine or α-amino group of the substrate protein with the aid of E3. Polyubiquinated targets are recognized and degraded by the 26S proteasome, while the ubiquitin on the substrate can be erased by DUBs to protect it from degradation.

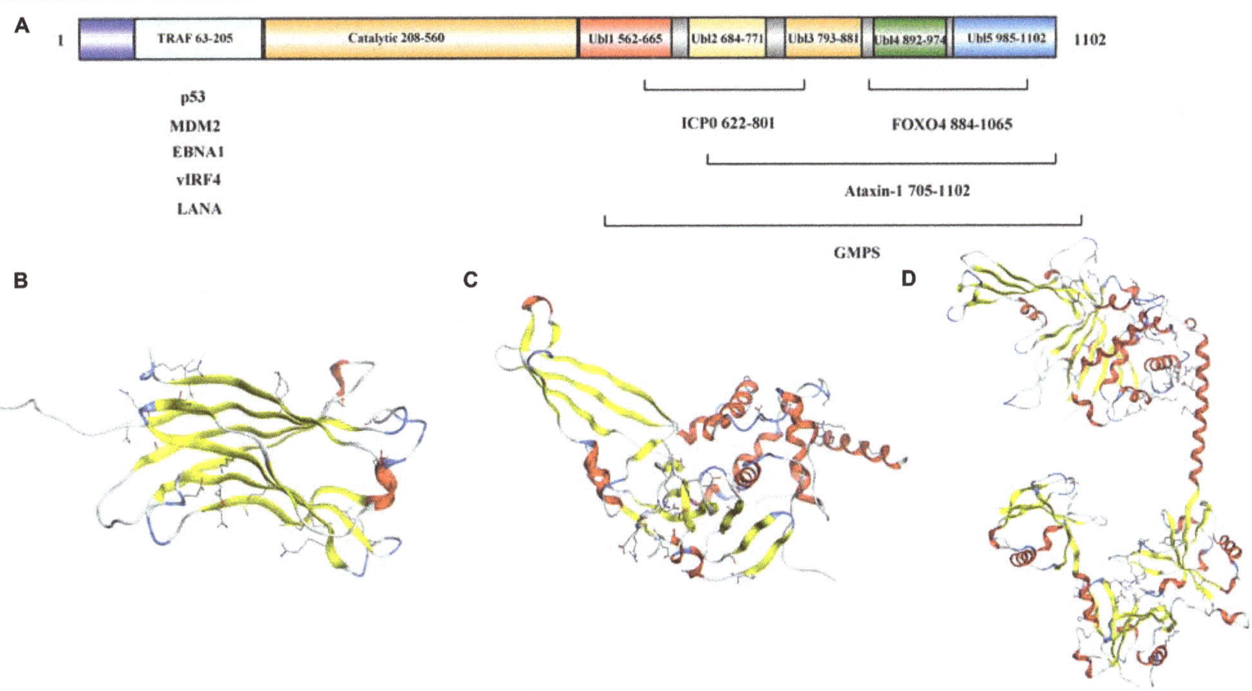

FIGURE 2 | Structure analysis of USP7. **(A)** USP7 primary sequence map. **(B)** Structure of the USP7 N-terminal domain (PDB 2F1W). **(C)** Structure of USP7 catalytic domain and five UBl-domains (PDB 1NB8). **(D)** Structure of the inactive state of USP7 catalytic domain (PDB 5FWI).

to 626 of ICP0 (named as R6702) can abolish the interaction between USP7 and ICP0, and the replication of R6702 in cells cannot be impaired (Kalamvoki et al., 2012). Hence, inhibition of USP7 and/or its interaction with ICP0 using small molecule inhibitors may decrease the virulence of HSV.

vIRFs

Among the vIRFs, vIRF1 could interact with the TRAF domain of USP7 via EGPS motif. The vIRF1 interaction with USP7 can decrease p53 levels by blocking the deubiquitination and stabilization of USP7 on p53. Thus the KSHV could have a

TABLE 1 | Proteins regulated by USP7.

USP7 substrates	Processes	Related cancer	References
EBNA1	Viral proteins		Holowaty et al., 2003
ICPO			Pfoh et al., 2015
vIRFs			Chavoshi et al., 2016; Xiang et al., 2018
LANA			Jager et al., 2012
E1B-55K			Ching et al., 2013
Tat			Ali et al., 2017
Foxp3	Immune response	Non-small cell lung cancer	van Loosdregt et al., 2013; Wang L. et al., 2016
TRIM27		Cervical carcinoma	Cai et al., 2018
NLRP3		Leukemia	Palazon-Riquelme et al., 2018
C-Myc and N-Myc	Oncoproteins	Neuroblastoma	Bhattacharya and Ghosh, 2015
p53	Tumor suppressor proteins	Ovarian cancers	Oliner et al., 1992; Li et al., 2002
DAXX		Breast cancer	Tang et al., 2006
PTEN		Chronic lymphocytic leukemia	Morotti et al., 2014
FOXOs family		Lung carcinoma	Huang et al., 2005
DNMT1	Epigenetics	Colon cancer	Du et al., 2010; Bronner, 2011
SUMO			Lecona et al., 2016
LSD1		Medulloblastoma	Yi et al., 2016
CHK1	DNA damage and repair		Alonso-de Vega et al., 2014
UVSSA			Sarasin, 2012; Zhang et al., 2012
ANXA1		Hela	Park et al., 2015
XPC			He et al., 2014
HLTF, Rad18			Qing et al., 2011
Polη			Qian et al., 2015
RNF168		Breast cancer	Malapelle et al., 2017
PHF8		Breast cancer	Wang Q. et al., 2016
MDC1		Cervical cancer	Su et al., 2018
Wnt/β-catenin signaling pathway	Several canonical signaling pathways	Colorectal cancer	Novellasdemunt et al., 2017
NF-κB signaling pathway		Multiple myeloma	Colleran et al., 2013
NOTCH signaling pathway		Lymphoblastic leukemia	Shan et al., 2018

lifelong infection when p53 is destabilized by USP7 coupled with vIRF1 (Chavoshi et al., 2016). Besides, vIRF3 is expressed in human herpes virus 8 (HHV-8) – infected primary effusion lymphoma (PEL) cells. The vIRF3 has two copies of EGPS, and both support the vIRF3 – USP7 interaction. This interaction plays important roles in PEL cell growth and viability and contributes to the suppression of productive virus replication (Xiang et al., 2018). For another vIRF family member, amino residues 210–216 of KSHV vIRF4 bind to the same surface groove of the USP7 TRAF domain as that can be recognized by MDM2 and p53. Moreover, the amino residues 202–208 of vIRF4 interact with the β-sheet in TRAF domain. The vIRF4-derived vif1 and vif2 peptides can restore p53 dependent apoptosis in wild-type p53 cancer cells by suppressing the USP7 activity. Thus the two peptides may be considered as potential backbones for peptide mimic small molecule inhibitors development for anti-cancer therapies (Lee et al., 2011).

LANA

The viral latency-associated nuclear antigen 1 (LANA) is expressed in all latency KSHV-infected cells and involves in viral latent replication and maintenance of the viral genome. The amino residues 971–986 of LANA interact with TRAF domain of USP7 with similar binding sites as EBNA1, while the △971–986 mutant shows an enhanced ability to replicate latent viral DNA. These results indicate that USP7 may influence accessibility of the viral DNA for latent replication or LANA-mediated viral persistence (Jager et al., 2012). Because of the role of USP7 in EBNA1 – dependent latent replication of EBV, USP7 may play the same role in the replication of latent viral DNA among gamma-1 and gamma-2 herpesviridae.

E1B-55K

Adenovirus E1B protein refers to one or two proteins transcribed from the E1B gene of the adenovirus: a 55 kDa protein and a 19 kDa protein. The N-terminal 79 amino acids of E1B-55K interact with the TRAF domain of USP7. Abrogation of USP7 decreases the protein level of E1B-55K and reduces progeny viral production. Therefore, the small inhibitors of USP7 may be used to treat adenovirus infections (Ching et al., 2013).

Tat

Human immunodeficiency virus (HIV) Tat is synthesized early after infection and mainly responsible for enhancing viral production. USP7 deubiquitinates and stabilizes Tat and enhances HIV-1 production. In turn, HIV-1 infection leads to the overexpression of USP7. These results show that the small inhibitors of USP7 can be used as a novel anti-HIV approach (Ali et al., 2017).

In sum, these results show that USP7 is recruited by these viruses to promote their survival in the host. So we speculate that USP7 may be an attractive target for controlling infection and other malignancies caused by these viruses.

Immune Response

Foxp3

Recent years, more and more reports have identified the importance of USP7 on keeping T regulatory cells (Treg) functions. As the major factor that restrains autoimmune responses, Treg cell expresses the forkhead transcription factor Foxp3, which is necessary for Treg cell development (Bettelli et al., 2005; Laurence et al., 2013). According to a report in 2016, five distinct lysine residues (K249, K251, K263, K267, and K393) in Foxp3 were identified to be ubiquitinated, and Foxp3 can be stabilized by USP7 mediated deubiquitination, resulting in the maintenance of Treg cell number and function (Wang L. et al., 2016). In fact, a study in 2013 showed that aberrant USP7 overexpression decreases Foxp3 polyubiquitination and protects it from proteasome degradation, resulting in Treg-cell-mediated suppression and tumor growth. On the contrary, USP7 knockdown decreases Foxp3 level and abrogates Treg cell-induced suppression of autoimmune responses *in vitro* and *in vivo* (van Loosdregt et al., 2013).

Later studies gave the mechanism how the level of Foxp3 is regulated. Foxp3 could be ubiquitinated and degraded by the E3 ubiquitin ligase stress inducible protein 1 homology and U-Box containing protein 1 (STUB1). In addition, Foxp3, Heat Shock Protein 70 (Hsp70) and STUB1 associate together as a complex, indicating that these proteins bind and promote Foxp3 ubiquitination (**Figure 3**) (van Loosdregt and Coffer, 2014). Moreover, it is found that mesenchymal stem cells (MSCs) - induced Treg cells express high level of USP7 and low level of STUB1. Besides, Foxp3 mRNA expression was positively associated with USP7 and negatively associated with STUB1 (Khosravi et al., 2018). So, it provides us an opportunity to find a new way to study the unique role of USP7 in Treg cells and makes USP7 as a target in immunology.

TRIM27

Among the binding partners of USP7, tripartite motif 27 (TRIM27) is an ubiquitin E3 ligase that negatively regulates antiviral signaling by promoting the ubiquitination and degradation of TRAF family member-associated NF-κ-B activator - binding kinase 1 (TBK1). USP7 interacts with TRIM27 and forms the USP7-TRIM27-TBK1 complex, and the interaction between USP7 and TRIM27 can be enhanced after Sendai virus (SeV) infection. When USP7 was overexpressed, TRIM27 can be protected from degradation, which contributed to the ubiquitination and degradation of TBK1, resulting in decreased type I interferons (IFNs) signaling (Cai et al., 2018). As IFNs are a series of signaling proteins which are produced and released by host cells to cope with the presence of pathogens, USP7 can enhance the effects of TRIM27 on TBK1-induced IFN - stimulated response element (ISRE) and IFN-β activation (Zaman et al., 2013). Therefore, USP7 may act as a significant host protein to bridge the viral proteins with the antiviral immune response. Therapeutic methods against the USP7-TRIM27 complex may overcome the immune escape mediated by various viruses.

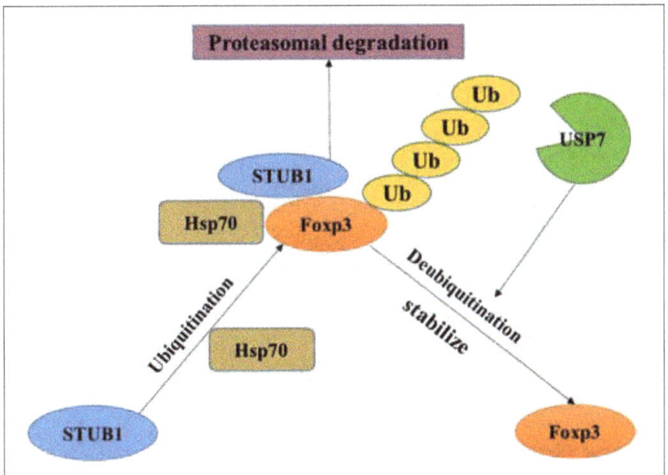

FIGURE 3 | Regulation of Foxp3 by USP7. Foxp3 is ubiquitinated by STUB1 and then produces a complex containing Foxp3, Hsp70 and STUB1, which leading to proteasome degradation of Foxp3. USP7 can remove the ubiquitin on Foxp3 and stabilize it.

NLRP3

USP7 may also impact on regulating NLR family pyrin domain containing 3 (NLRP3) inflammasome activation. NLRP3 is expressed primarily in macrophages as a component of the inflammasome to monitor products of damaged cells such as extracellular ATP and crystalline uric acid. The ubiquitination status of NLRP3 itself can be altered by USP7 and USP47. Furthermore, researchers discovered that the activity of USP7 and USP47 were augmented once the inflammasome was activated. In the meantime, they discovered that abrogation of both USP7 and USP47 resulted in reduction of inflammasome activation (Palazon-Riquelme et al., 2018).

To sum up, there is a remarkable connection between USP7 and immune-associated proteins, and so many studies have shown that the important roles of USP7 on regulating these proteins. It's worth thinking about USP7 inhibitors in combination with immunotherapy will be applied to cancer therapy so that the antitumor effect can be promoted. We hope to see their potential dual antitumor activity will be applied to clinical trials on day.

Oncoproteins

C-Myc and N-Myc

There are three members in Myc family: C-Myc, l-Myc, and N-Myc. Myc family is the most frequent amplified oncogene in human, which contributing to the formation of cancer. Among them, C-Myc and N-Myc are the substrates of USP7. USP7 overexpression can promote C-Myc stability by deubiquitination as well as transformation/transcription domain-associated protein (TRRAP), which is an adaptor protein known as a regulator of C-Myc. On the other hand, C-Myc mRNA can be accumulated by TRRAP indirectly (Bhattacharya and Ghosh, 2015).

N-Myc is another transcription factor that can be stabilized by USP7 via deubiquitination (Tavana et al., 2016). Hence, USP7 inhibitor p5091 was applied to decrease N-Myc expression in a dose dependent manner in neuroblastoma (Tavana et al., 2016). As a consequence, USP7 can be considered as a drug target to modulate C-Myc and N-Myc amount in order to block tumor development.

Tumor Suppressor Proteins

p53

p53 participates in cell cycle arrest, DNA repair, apoptosis, senescence and plays a key role in maintaining normal cell growth (Levine, 1997). USP7 plays a paradoxical role in regulating p53 functions through a variety of mechanisms. On one hand, p53 binds to TRAF domain and C-terminal (amino acids

880–1050) of USP7, and then USP7 ubiquitinates p53 directly and prevents it from degradation. On the other hand, TRAF domain and C-terminal (amino acids 801–1050) of USP7 can interact with MDM2 to increase its stability by erasing the ubiquitin on MDM2, an E3 ligase of p53 (Oliner et al., 1992), and protect it from proteasome degradation. Subsequently, MDM2 ubiquitinates p53 and causes its proteasome degradation, resulting in low expression of p53 in cancer cells (**Figure 4**) (Li et al., 2002, 2004). In addition, MDM2 can also inhibit the transcription of p53 (Wade et al., 2013). Therefore, inhibition of the interaction between MDM2 and p53 can stabilize p53 (Vassilev et al., 2004). It is noteworthy that, crystal structures analysis and binding studies suggest that the MDM2 peptide and p53 peptide bind to the same surface groove in USP7, but MDM2 performs more extensive interaction and stronger affinity (Hu et al., 2006). Taken together, the activation of USP7-MDM2-p53 interaction can promote the occurrence and development of tumors. The design of small molecules that disrupt or prevent the interaction may be an important target for cancer therapy by regulating p53 pathway.

DAXX

Death-domain-associated protein (DAXX) is a highly conserved and developmentally essential nuclear protein, which participates in many cellular processes (Lindsay et al., 2008). The N-terminal 160 amino acids and amino acids 347–570 of DAXX associate with USP7, which are far from the binding sites of MDM2 on DAXX. In unstressed cells, DAXX interacts with USP7 and MDM2, and mediates the stabilization of USP7 on MDM2, thus blocking p53 activation. In response to DNA damage, self-ubiquitination of MDM2 is accelerated when MDM2 is stripped from DAXX and USP7. That is to say, DAXX directs the ligase activity of MDM2 through regulating USP7 (Tang et al., 2006). Recent reports also show that USP7 and DAXX are critical in regulating the correct execution of mitosis by forming a tertiary complex as MDM2/DAXX/USP7 (Zhang et al., 2010). DAXX binding increases USP7 activity toward MDM2. Disassemble the MDM2-DAXX-USP7 complex can increase MDM2 self-ubiquitination and degradation, which leads to the stabilization and accumulation of p53 (Kumar et al., 2018).

PTEN

Phosphatase and tensin homolog (PTEN) is a tumor suppressor gene that displays dual specific phosphatase activity. PTEN inhibits the proliferation and migration of tumor cells (Blanco-Aparicio et al., 2007). It is reported that nuclear PTEN import is promoted by its mono-ubiquitination (Trotman et al., 2007). However, USP7 can remove the mono-ubiquitination of PTEN, triggering its nuclear exclusion and PTEN inactivation (Morotti et al., 2014). Likewise, USP7 inhibitor, P5091, regains PTEN nuclear pool and restores its tumor suppressive functions in chronic lymphocytic leukemia (CLL) (Carra et al., 2017). In addition, PTEN deletion leads to accumulation of activated AKT, and subsequent phosphorylation of MDM2 by AKT (Blanco-Aparicio et al., 2007), which results in the ubiquitination and degradation of p53 (Freeman et al., 2003). Therefore, PTEN deficiency causes p53-dependent cancer-promoting processes. This suggests how important it is to inhibit USP7 to ensure PTEN protein localization and activity.

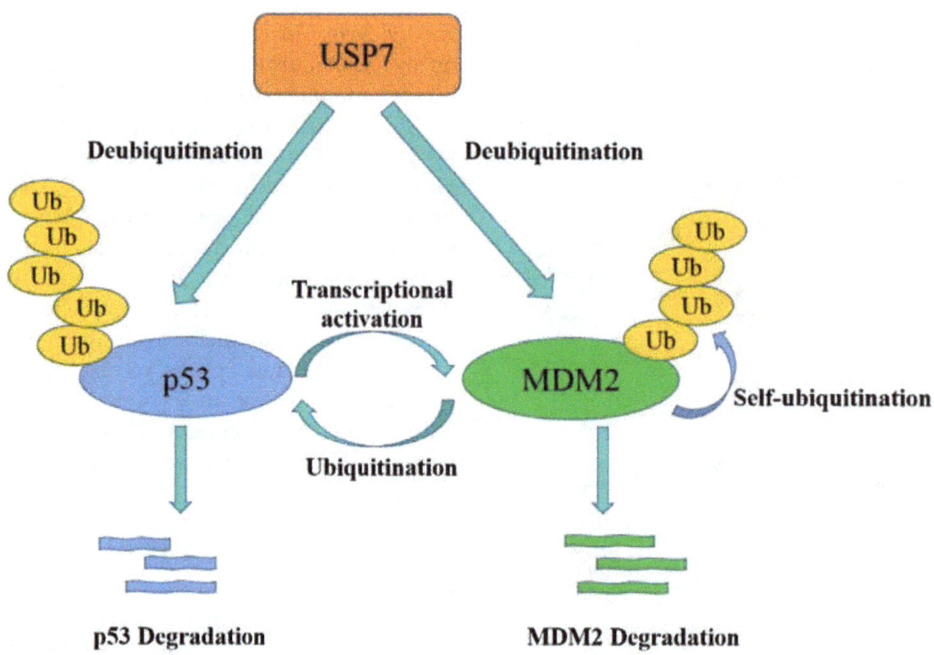

FIGURE 4 | USP7-p53-MDM2 axis interactions control the stability of p53 and MDM2. USP7 can stabilize p53 by deubiquitination, meanwhile, USP7 can also remove the ubiquitin of MDM2, which promotes to p53 degradation.

FOXOs Family

The Forkhead box O (FOXO) family members, including FOXO1, FOXO3, FOXO4 and FOXO6, are transcription factors that take part in regulating several cellular responses, including cell cycle progression and apoptosis and so on (van der Horst and Burgering, 2007). It is reported that USP7 can remove ubiquitin from FOXO1, which is written by Skp2 as an E3 ligase (Huang et al., 2005). Besides, mono-ubiquitination FOXO4 localizes in the nucleus and exhibits stronger transcriptional promotion activity (Brenkman et al., 2008). USP7 can suppress FOXO4 activity due to its deubiquitination and re-localization (van der Horst et al., 2006). In a word, USP7 affects tumor progression by interacting with FOXOs and affecting their activity and localization.

Epigenetics

DNMT1

DNMT1 (DNA methyltransferase 1) contributes to the maintenance of DNA methylation. As reported, USP7 can deubiquitinate and stabilize DNMT1 when its acetylation is erased by histone deacetylase 1 (HDAC1), which protects DNMT1 from proteasome degradation (Bronner, 2011). When the KG linker of DNMT1 is acetylated by Tip60, USP7 breaks away from DNMT1 and results in the degradation of DNMT1 mediated by proteasome system (**Figure 5**) (Du et al., 2010). Thus, HDAC and USP7 inhibitors can be applied in combination for cancer treatment (Cheng et al., 2015).

SUMO

Small ubiquitin related modifier (SUMO) is a ubiquitin-like molecule, which binds to its substrate by E3 SUMO ligase in a similar way as ubiquitination (Geoffroy and Hay, 2009). Like ubiquitin, proteins can be SUMOylated as mono-SUMOylation or poly-SUMOylation, but differently, poly-SUMOylation cannot lead to target degradation directly (Smits and Freire, 2016). Recent research shows that USP7 is associated with DNA synthesis (Smits and Freire, 2016). USP7 associates with an active DNA replication fork and inhibition of USP7 can reduce DNA replication. Moreover, Lecona et al. (2016) identified SUMO2 as a new USP7 substrate and demonstrated that USP7 can deubiquitinate SUMO2 *in vitro* and *in vivo*. However, the fate of SUMO2 after deubiquitination and its biological function are still unclear (Lecona et al., 2016).

LSD1

Histone lysine specific demethylase 1 (LSD1) is the first histone demethylase identified in 2004 and can remove methyl groups of histone H3K4, H3K9 (Shi et al., 2004). As reported, LSD1 can be ubiquitinated by E3 ligase JADE2 (Han et al., 2014). Since ubiquitination of LSD1 is considered as reversible process as ubiquitination and deubiquitination always exit in pair, LSD1 was identified to be deubiquitinated by USP7 and protected it from proteasome degradation (Yi et al., 2016). Besides, patients with high expression of USP7, REST, and LSD1 performed poorer outcomes in medulloblastoma (Callegari et al., 2018). And they found that p53 was a vital downstream transcription factor in the action of USP7 and LSD1.

DNA Damage and Repair

CHK1

USP7 can regulate CHK1 in three manners. The first one is the indirect regulation, USP7 deubiquitinated and prolonged the half-life of Claspin, which leaded to the sustaining phosphorylation of checkpoint kinase 1 (Chk1) in response to genotoxic stress (Faustrup et al., 2009). For the rest two manners, in DNA damage, USP7 deubiquitinates and stabilizes Chk1 via direct deubiquitination in the presence of zinc finger E-box binding homeobox 1 (ZEB1) (Zhang et al., 2014) or not (Alonso-de Vega et al., 2014), while ZEB1 binds to USP7 may result in promoting homologous recombinant-dependent DNA repair and resistant to radiation. In addition, USP7 can also directly regulate the stability of CDC25A, a Cdk-activating phosphatase as the substrate of CHK1, with the aid of brain and reproductive organ expressed protein (BRE). These results show that USP7 is an important modulator of Chk1.

CHFR

Checkpoint with Forkhead and Ring domains (CHFR), a RING family Ub-ligase, is a mitotic checkpoint that delays the transition to metaphase in response to mitotic stress. USP7 binds with CHFR *in vivo* and regulates its stability (**Figure 6**). These results indicate that USP7 may play a role in the cell cycle progression via the deubiquitination of CHFR (Oh et al., 2007).

UVSSA

Transcription-coupled nucleotide excision repair (TC-NER) removes DNA damage of actively transcribed genes. Defect in TC-NER is associated with cockayne syndrome (CS) and ultraviolet – sensitive syndrome (UVSS). Cockayne syndrome B (CSB/ERCC6) and UVSS protein are two important proteins in TC-NER. UVSSA binds with USP7 to stabilize CSB and restores the hypophosphorylated form of RNA polymerase II after UV irradiation (**Figure 6**) (Zhang et al., 2012). UVSSA and USP7 play roles in controlling the fate of stalled RNA polymerase II, the steady-state level of CSB, the efficiency of TC-NER and cell survival following DNA damage (Sarasin, 2012).

ANXA1

ANXA1 is a 37-kDa protein identified as the first member of the annexin superfamily. In response to DNA damage, ANXA1 is cleaved and generates the N-terminal fragment (Ac2-26) and the cleaved form of ANXA1. Both the full length of ANXA1 and Ac2-26 can be translocated to the cell membrane and induce apoptotic cell clearance through recruiting monocytes. The N-terminal of ANXA1 shares the USP7-binding motif sequences (AMVS and ALLS) and interacts with USP7. Hence, USP7 can deubiquitinate and stabilize ANXA1 (**Figure 6**). USP7 may participate in the DDR after UV-induced DNA damage in certain types via ANXA1 (Park et al., 2015).

XPC

Xeroderma pigmentosum complementation group C (XPC) is a critical damage recognition factor which binds to helix-distorting DNA lesions and initiates nucleotide excision repair (NER).

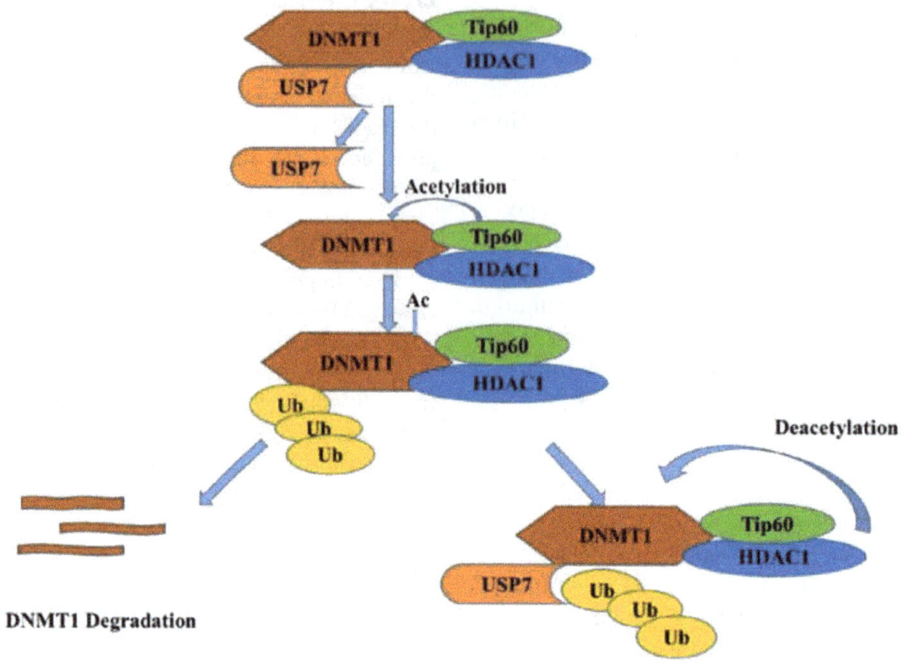

FIGURE 5 | USP7 and HDAC1 protect DNMT1 from degradation while Tip60 acetylates DNMT1 and promotes its degradation.

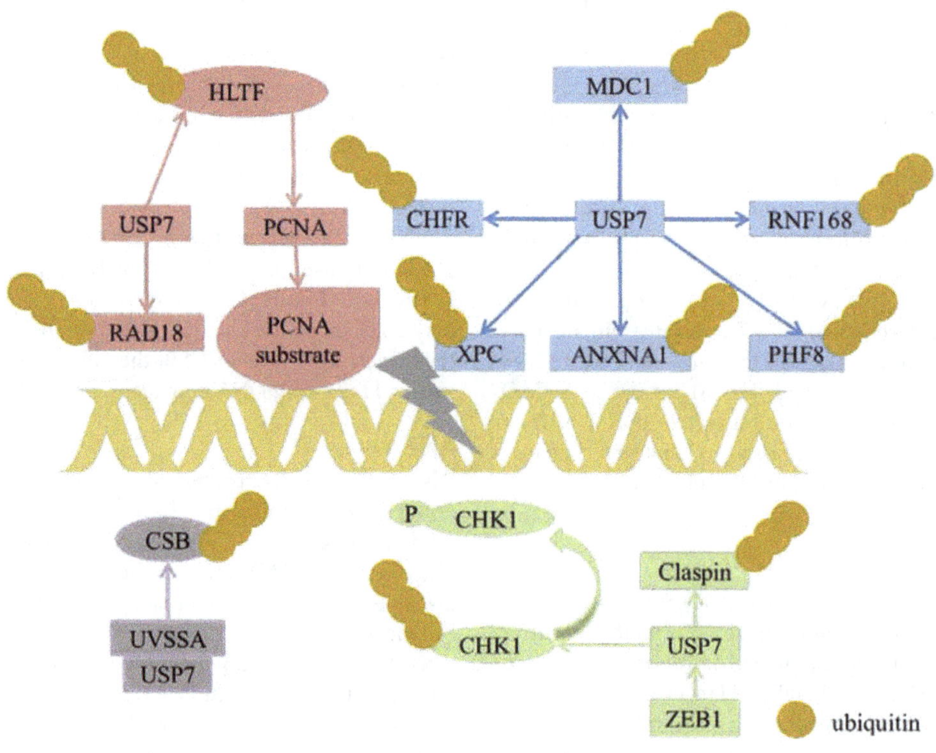

FIGURE 6 | USP7 interacts with a number of substrates in DNA damage response.

During the early stage of NER of UV light-induced DNA lesions, XPC is ubiquitinated. Ubl1 domain (amino acids 560–644) of USP7 can bind and erase the ubiquitination on XPC and prevents XPC from proteolysis (**Figure 6**). Taken together, USP7 plays a vital role in regulating NER through deubiqitinating XPC (He et al., 2014).

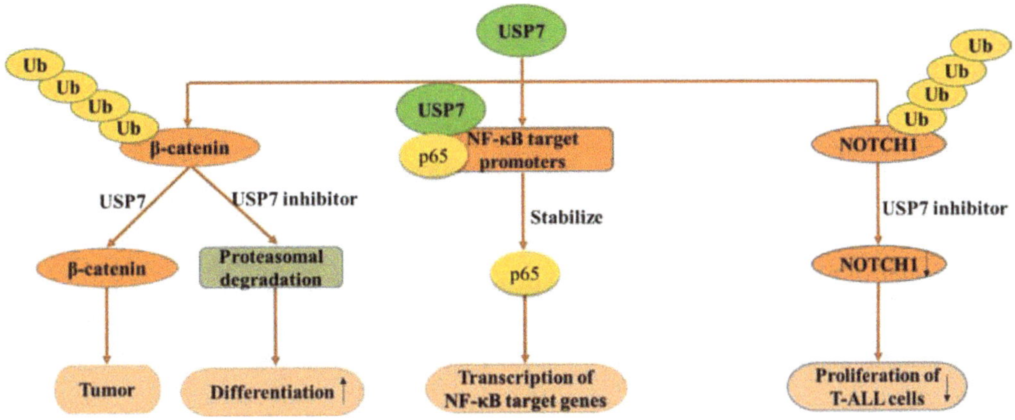

FIGURE 7 | USP7 functions in several canonical signaling pathways. USP7 functions in Wnt/β-catenin signaling pathway **(left)**, NF-κB signaling pathway **(middle)**, NOTCH signaling pathway **(right)**.

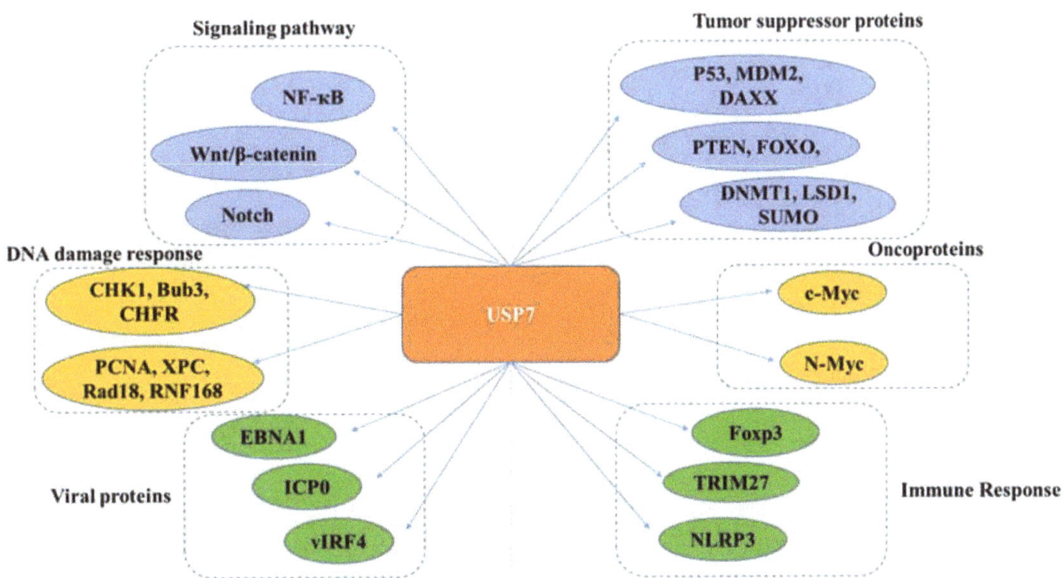

FIGURE 8 | Overview of USP7 functions.

HLTF, Rad18, and Polη

Helicase-like transcription factor (HLTF) is a double-stranded DNA translocase that can promote the polyubiquitination of proliferating cell nuclear antigen (PCNA), while Rad6–Rad18 monoubiquitinates PCNA, both of which make PCNA work as a molecular switch between various DNA damage bypass processes. On one hand, USP7 stabilizes HLTF after genotoxic stress, resulting in prolonging the half-life of HLTF, thus in turn increases polyubiquitination of PCNA (**Figure 6**) (Qing et al., 2011). Besides, USP7 and DNA polymerase eta (Polη), a key player in several DNA damage-tolerance pathways, interact with each other, and USP7 increases UV-induced PCNA ubiquitination through stabilizing Polη and in turn facilitates the recruitment of DNA translesion synthesis (TLS) polymerases to bypass DNA lesions. Therefore USP7 promotes monoUb-PCNA mediated stress-tolerance pathways via the stabilization of Polη. These results provide new mechanistic for USP7-related tumorigenesis and therapeutic strategy (Qian et al., 2015). On the other hand, the amino acids 110–251 of Rad18 interact with USP7 and contain two USP7-binding motifs. Loss of USP7 destabilizes Rad18 and compromises UV-induced PCNA monoubiquitylation and Polη recruitment to stalled replication forks (Zlatanou et al., 2016).

RNF168

During DDR, histone ubiquitination by RNF168 orchestrates the recruitment of downstream DDR factors, e.g., breast cancer type 1 susceptibility protein (BRCA1) and p53 binding protein

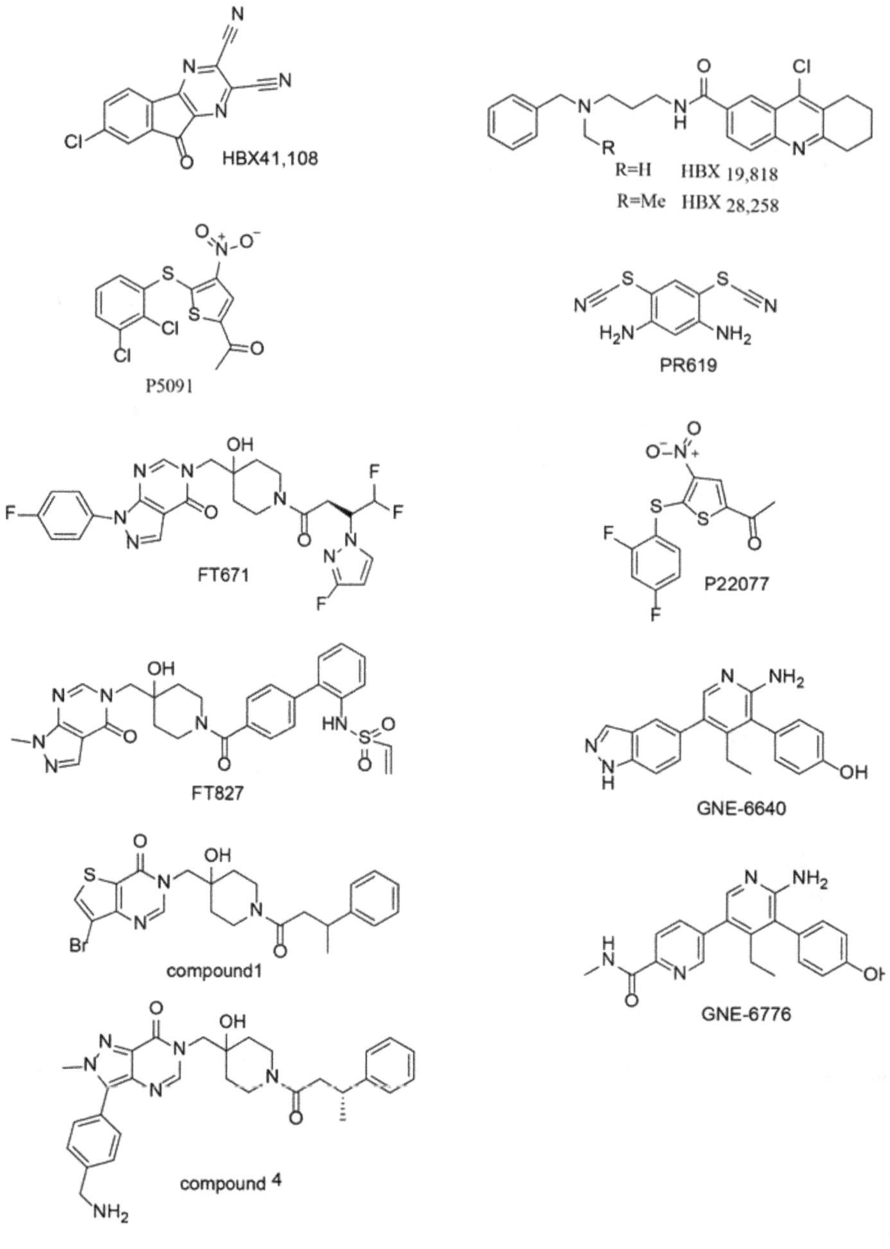

FIGURE 9 | Chemical structures of USP7 inhibitors.

1 (53BP1). The Ubl1 domain of USP7 binds to RNF168 (**Figure 6**). USP7 regulates H2A monoubiquitination and H2A/X polyubiquitination via its regulation on RNF168. In summary, USP7 plays a vital role in regulation of Ub-dependent signaling in DDR via monitoring RNF168 (Malapelle et al., 2017).

PHF8

Plant homeodomain finger-containing protein 8 (PHF8) consists of an N-terminal plant homeodomain and recognizes and binds tri-methyl histone 3 lysine 4 at transcription start sites. The C-terminal region of PHF8 binds with the TRAF domain of USP7, and USP7 promotes the stability of PHF8 via deubiquitinase activity and contributes to the maintenance of genome integrity, which is implemented in DDR (**Figure 6**). The USP7/PHF8 is involved in breast carcinogenesis, indicating these molecules may be as potential targets for breast cancer intervention (Wang Q. et al., 2016).

MDC1

DNA damage checkpoint protein 1 (MDC1) is important for the initiation and amplification of the DDR. USP7 deubiquitinates and stabilizes of MDC1, resulting in sustaining the DDR, while depletion of USP7 influences the engagement of MRE11-RAD50-NBS1(MRN)-MDC1 complex and the

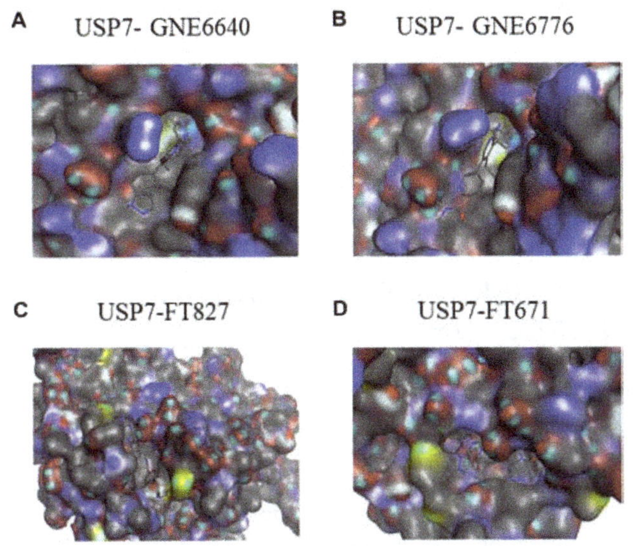

FIGURE 10 | Co-crystal structures of USP7 in complex with inhibitors. The electrostatic surface representation of the CD of USP7 is shown along with compounds **(A)** USP7-GNE6640 (PDB code 5UQV). **(B)** USP7-GNE6776 (PDB code 5UQX). **(C)** USP7-FT827 (PDB code 5NGF). **(D)** USP7-FT671 (PDB code 5NGE). The images were generated with molecular operating environment (MOE).

recruitment of the downstream factors 53BP1 and BRCA1 at DNA lesions. USP7 promotes cervical cancer cell survival and confrere cellular resistance to genotoxic insults via the stabilization of MDC1 (Su et al., 2018).

In a nutshell, USP7 plays a vital role in the DNA damage response (**Figure 6**), and it can be targeted for the treatment of malignancies with DDR defects. Besides, USP7 inhibitors can be combined with genotoxic agents as a novel therapeutic strategy for the treatment of cancer.

USP7 stabilizes HLTF to result in polyubiquitination of PCNA and induces monoubiquitination of PCNA through regulating Rad18. USP7 plays a role in DDR through regulating MDC1, CHFR, XPC, ANXNA1, RNF168, and PHF8. USP7 and UVSSA interact with each other to control steady state of CSB following DNA damage. USP7 can regulate stability of CDC25A via deubiquitination CDC25A directly and through regulating Claspin and CHK1 expression.

Several Canonical Signaling Pathways

Wnt/β-Catenin Signaling Pathway

Wnt signaling was initially found for its function in cancer and embryonic development and then was found responsible for tissue regeneration in adult bone marrow, skin and intestine. β-Catenin, a key element in Wnt signaling pathway, is regulated by diverse PTMs, including ubiquitination (Ma et al., 2014). According to a research in 2017, β-catenin can be deubiquitinated and stabilized by USP7 in adenomatous polyposis coli (APC) truncating mutated colorectal cancer (CRC) but not APC wide type CRC, which resulting in the activation of Wnt pathway (Novellasdemunt et al., 2017). Mechanism study suggested that APC β-catenin inhibitory domain (CID) protects β-catenin from USP7-mediated deubiquitination, while APC lacking CID exposes β-catenin to USP7 for deubiquitination. Hence, abrogation of USP7 in APC-mutated CRC suppresses Wnt activation by regaining β-catenin ubiquitination, which leads to the cell differentiation, and inhibits tumor growth (Novellasdemunt et al., 2017). With the aid of USP7 inhibitor P5091, Wnt pathway can be inactivated by improving ubiquitination and degradation of β-catenin, which provides evidence for the rationality for developing USP7 inhibitors as anti-CRC agent (**Figure 7A**) (An et al., 2017). In a nutshell, USP7 can be considered as a Wnt activator for tumor-specific therapeutic target for most CRCs.

NF-κB Signaling Pathway

Nuclear factor kappa B (NF-κB) signaling pathway is responsible for the transcription of a series of genes that controlling inflammation and immunity. As an essential regulator of Toll-like-receptor (TLR) and tumor necrosis factor receptor (TNFR)-inducible inflammatory gene expression, NF-κB is regulated by USP7 in a research in 2013. Different from other USP7 partners and substrates, NF-κB p65 and USP7 interact together after USP7 is recruited to NF-κB target promoters. Besides, the inhibition of USP7 lead to decreased TLR and TNFR-induced expression of Interleukin (IL-6), TNFα (NF-κB reporter) indicates that the deubiquitination of NF-κB by USP7 may have therapeutic potential (**Figure 7B**) (Colleran et al., 2013).

In 2018, some researchers found that knockout of USP7 dramatically increased the sensitivity of multiple myeloma (MM) cells to bortezomib (BTZ) which led to myeloma cell death and inhibited NF-κB activation by stabilizing IκBα. As expected, usage of USP7 inhibitors also inhibited the activation of NF-κB and the combination of USP7 inhibitor with BTZ triggered the synergistic antitumor activity in bortezomib-resistant MM cells. Taken together, this study provides a new application for USP7 inhibitors alone or in combination with BTZ to overcome BTZ resistance and improve the patient prognosis in MM (Yao et al., 2018).

In all, several reports have illustrated the mechanism that how USP7 and its related proteins regulate NF-κB signaling pathway. However, more deep studies should be conducted to make the mechanism more clearly and logically and there are still great challenges for researchers to face.

NOTCH Signaling Pathway

Notch signaling pathway is highly conserved and presents in most multicellular organisms. This intercellular signaling cascade is involved in cell differentiation, proliferation, and contributes to the fate of cells and occurs in multiple organisms and tissues, containing early T cell development in the thymus and peripheral T cell differentiation (Auderset et al., 2012; Bailis et al., 2013; Amsen et al., 2015). There are four notch receptors in mammals possessing NOTCH1-4 in which NOTCH1 can be stabilized through USP7-mediated deubiquitination. Previous studies have revealed that ubiquitination regulates the stability, activity, and localization of NOTCH1. However, the specific deubiquitinase that affects NOTCH1 protein stability was clarified recently.

Researchers reported that USP7 can deubiquitinate and stabilize NOTCH1 *in vivo* and *in vitro*, on the other hand, knockdown of USP7 increased the ubiquitination of NOTCH1. Used up of USP7 significantly restrained the proliferation of T-cell acute lymphoblastic leukemia (T-ALL) cells *in vitro* and *in vivo*, accompanied by downregulation of the NOTCH1 protein level, suggesting that targeting the USP7/NOTCH1 axis is a novel strategy to combat T-ALL and other NOTCH1-related malignancies (**Figure 7C**) (Shan et al., 2018). Almost at the same time, researchers found USP7 can bind several oncogenes by interacting and stabilizing NOTCH1 and JmjC Domain-Containing Protein 3 (JMJD3) in order to control leukemia growth. What's more, USP7 and NOTCH1 bind T-ALL superenhancers, and inhibition of USP7 leads to a decrease of the transcriptional levels of NOTCH1 targets and T-ALL cell growth *in vitro* and *in vivo*. Therefore, USP7 cooperating with NOTCH1 can improve the oncogenic transcriptional program in T-ALL (Jin et al., 2018).

The functions of USP7 on different signaling pathways indicate the brand new role of USP7 as a great target. To be sure, other classical signaling pathways which may be regulated by USP7 is yet to be found. It provides us a great challenge to find the new mechanisms between USP7 and other classical signaling pathways.

USP7 in Cancer

USP7 is highly expressed in a wide variety of cancers and affects the progression of cancer diseases. Moreover, USP7 assumes different roles in different tumors. In prostate cancer, high expression of USP7 is directly related to tumor invasion (Song et al., 2008). USP7 plays a key role in carcinogenesis via p53-dependent pathways in non-small cell lung carcinoma (NSCLCs) (Masuya et al., 2006). Studies have shown that changes of USP7 regulate colon carcinoma growth and apoptotic sensitivity *in vivo* (Becker et al., 2008). USP7 maintains DNA damage response and promotes cervical cancer, and is positively correlated with poor survival rate in patients with cervical cancer (Su et al., 2018). USP7 regulates human terminal erythroid differentiation by stabilizing GATA1, providing a certain treatment for leukemia (Liang et al., 2019). In short, USP7 plays an important role in a variety of pathologies and is a good target from a therapeutic point of view.

USP7 INHIBITORS

USP7 is a promising target not only for its roles in cellular pathways including regulators of viral proteins, immune response, oncogenes, and DNA damage but also because of its aberrant expression in various cancers. Due to lack of co-crystal structures between USP7 and small molecule inhibitors, there is no potent and selective USP7 inhibitor for a long time (Colland et al., 2009; Altun et al., 2011; Chauhan et al., 2012; Reverdy et al., 2012) (**Figure 9**). However, several groups reported the structures of USP7 in complex with small molecule inhibitors last year (Kategaya et al., 2017; Turnbull et al., 2017) (**Figure 10**) and these structures gives guidance to obtain structure-based small molecule inhibitors.

CONCLUSION AND FUTURE PERSPECTIVES

This review illustrates our current knowledge of USP7, including its source and characterization, structure, binding partners and substrates in various biological processes. Besides, how USP7 regulates various aspects of a cell under both normal and pathological states are elaborated in detail. As the processes of ubiquitination and deubiquitination are extremely dynamic and context-specific, a series of studies have linked USP7 to different cancers. The biology, particularly the immune oncology mechanisms, reveal that USP7 inhibitors would be useful drugs, thus it is vital to develop highly selective and specific inhibitors of USP7. The association of USP7 with several canonical signaling pathways still needs characterized in order to search new targets and regulatory mechanisms. Last but not least, USP7 may be a promising target for cancer therapy and it therefore merits further studies.

AUTHOR CONTRIBUTIONS

ZW discusses the structure of USP7, the viral protein targets of USP7, the DNA damage substrates of USP7 and conclusion. WK talks about the introduction, immune function of USP7, Wnt/β-catenin signaling pathway, and NF-κB signaling pathway. YY illustrates oncoproteins and tumor suppressor proteins. JP states about the epigenetics substrates of USP7. HR talks about the NOTCH signaling pathway. ZS and YZ provide expertise and feedback. HL provides funding.

FUNDING

This work was supported by National Natural Science Foundation of China (Project No. 81602961 for YZ; Project Nos. 81430085 and 81773562 for HL); Outstanding Young Talent Research Fund of Zhengzhou University (Project No. 1521331002 for YZ); National Key Research Program of Proteins (Project No. 2016YFA0501800 for HL; Project No. 2017YFD0501401 for YZ); and Key Research Program of Henan Province (Project No. 161100310100 for HL).

REFERENCES

1. Ali, A., Raja, R., Farooqui, S. R., Ahmad, S., and Banerjea, A. C. (2017). USP7 deubiquitinase controls HIV-1 production by stabilizing Tat protein. *Biochem. J.* 474, 1653–1668. doi: 10.1042/bcj20160304
2. Alonso-de Vega, I., Martin, Y., and Smits, V. A. (2014). USP7 controls Chk1 protein stability by direct deubiquitination. *Cell Cycle* 13, 3921–3926. doi: 10.4161/15384101.2014.973324
3. Altun, M., Kramer, H. B., Willems, L. I., McDermott, J. L., Leach, C. A., Goldenberg, S. J., et al. (2011). Activity-based chemical proteomics

accelerates inhibitor development for deubiquitylating enzymes. *Chem. Biol.* 18, 1401–1412. doi: 10.1016/j.chembiol.2011.08.018
4. Amsen, D., Helbig, C., and Backer, R. A. (2015). Notch in T Cell differentiation: all things considered. *Trends Immunol.* 36, 802–814. doi: 10.1016/j.it.2015.10.007
5. An, T., Gong, Y., Li, X., Kong, L., Ma, P., Gong, L., et al. (2017). USP7 inhibitor P5091 inhibits Wnt signaling and colorectal tumor growth. *Biochem. Pharmacol.* 131, 29–39. doi: 10.1016/j.bcp.2017.02.011
6. Auderset, F., Coutaz, M., and Tacchini-Cottier, F. (2012). The role of notch in the differentiation of CD4(+) T helper cells. *Curr. Top. Microbiol. Immunol.* 360, 115–134. doi: 10.1007/82_2012_227
7. Bailis, W., Yashiro-Ohtani, Y., Fang, T. C., Hatton, R. D., Weaver, C. T., Artis, D., et al. (2013). Notch simultaneously orchestrates multiple helper T cell programs independently of cytokine signals. *Immunity* 39, 148–159. doi: 10.1016/j.immuni.2013.07.006
8. Becker, K., Marchenko, N. D., Palacios, G., and Moll, U. M. (2008). A role of HAUSP in tumor suppression in a human colon carcinoma xenograft model. *Cell Cycle* 7, 1205–1213. doi: 10.4161/cc.7.9.5756
9. Bettelli, E., Dastrange, M., and Oukka, M. (2005). Foxp3 interacts with nuclear factor of activated T cells and NF-kappa B to repress cytokine gene expression and effector functions of T helper cells. *Proc. Natl. Acad. Sci. U.S.A.* 102, 5138–5143. doi: 10.1073/pnas.0501675102
10. Bhattacharya, S., and Ghosh, M. K. (2015). HAUSP regulates c-MYC expression via de-ubiquitination of TRRAP. *Cell Oncol.* 38, 265–277. doi: 10.1007/s13402-015-0228-6
11. Blanco-Aparicio, C., Renner, O., Leal, J. F., and Carnero, A. (2007). PTEN, more than the AKT pathway. *Carcinogenesis* 28, 1379–1386. doi: 10.1093/carcin/bgm052
12. Brenkman, A. B., de Keizer, P. L., van den Broek, N. J., Jochemsen, A. G., and Burgering, B. M. (2008). Mdm2 induces mono-ubiquitination of FOXO4. *PLoS One* 3:e2819. doi: 10.1371/journal.pone.0002819
13. Bronner, C. (2011). Control of DNMT1 abundance in epigenetic inheritance by acetylation, ubiquitylation, and the histone code. *Sci. Signal.* 4:pe3. doi: 10.1126/scisignal.2001764
14. Cai, J., Chen, H. Y., Peng, S. J., Meng, J. L., Wang, Y., Zhou, Y., et al. (2018). USP7- TRIM27 axis negatively modulates antiviral type I IFN signaling. *FASEB J.* 32, 5238–5249. doi: 10.1096/fj.201700473RR
15. Callegari, K., Maegawa, S., Bravo-Alegria, J., and Gopalakrishnan, V. (2018). Pharmacological inhibition of LSD1 activity blocks REST- dependent medulloblastoma cell migration. *Cell Commun. Signal.* 16:60. doi: 10.1186/s12964-018-0275-5
16. Carra, G., Panuzzo, C., Torti, D., Parvis, G., Crivellaro, S., Familiari, U., et al. (2017). Therapeutic inhibition of USP7-PTEN network in chronic lymphocytic leukemia: a strategy to overcome TP53 mutated/deleted clones. *Oncotarget* 8, 35508–35522. doi: 10.18632/oncotarget.16348
17. Chatterjee, B., and Thakur, S. S. (2018). Investigation of post-translational modifications in type 2 diabetes. *Clin. Proteomics* 15:32. doi: 10.1186/s12014-018-9208-y
18. Chauhan, D., Tian, Z., Nicholson, B., Kumar, K. G., Zhou, B., Carrasco, R., et al. (2012). A small molecule inhibitor of ubiquitin-specific protease-7 induces apoptosis in multiple myeloma cells and overcomes bortezomib resistance. *Cancer Cell* 22, 345–358. doi: 10.1016/j.ccr.2012.08.007
19. Chavoshi, S., Egorova, O., Lacdao, I. K., Farhadi, S., Sheng, Y., and Saridakis, V. (2016). Identification of kaposi sarcoma herpesvirus (KSHV) vIRF1 protein as a novel interaction partner of human deubiquitinase USP7. *J. Biol. Chem.* 291, 6281–6291. doi: 10.1074/jbc.M115.710632
20. Cheng, J., Yang, H., Fang, J., Ma, L., Gong, R., Wang, P., et al. (2015). Molecular mechanism for USP7-mediated DNMT1 stabilization by acetylation. *Nat. Commun.* 11:7023. doi: 10.1038/ncomms8023
21. Cheon, K. W., and Baek, K. H. (2006). HAUSP as a therapeutic target for hematopoietic tumors (review). *Int. J. Oncol.* 28, 1209–1215.
22. Ching, W., Koyuncu, E., Singh, S., Arbelo-Roman, C., Hartl, B., Kremmer, E., et al. (2013). A ubiquitin-specific protease possesses a decisive role for adenovirus replication and oncogene-mediated. *PLoS Pathog.* 9:e1003273. doi: 10.1371/journal.ppat.1003273
23. Clague, M. J., Barsukov, I., Coulson, J. M., Liu, H., Rigden, D. J., and Urbe, S. (2013). Deubiquitylases from genes to organism. *Physiol. Rev.* 93, 1289–1315. doi: 10.1152/physrev.00002.2013
24. Colland, F., Formstecher, E., Jacq, X., Reverdy, C., Planquette, C., Conrath, S., et al. (2009). Small-molecule inhibitor of USP7/HAUSP ubiquitin protease stabilizes and activates p53 in cells. *Mol. Cancer Ther.* 8, 2286–2295. doi: 10.1158/1535-7163.mct-09-0097
25. Colleran, A., Collins, P. E., O'Carroll, C., Ahmed, A., Mao, X., McManus, B., et al. (2013). Deubiquitination of NF-kappaB by ubiquitin-specific protease-7 promotes transcription. *Proc. Natl. Acad. Sci. U.S.A.* 110, 618–623. doi: 10.1073/pnas.1208446110
26. Du, Z., Song, J., Wang, Y., Zhao, Y., Guda, K., Yang, S., et al. (2010). DNMT1 stability is regulated by proteins coordinating deubiquitination and acetylation-driven ubiquitination. *Sci. Signal.* 3:ra80. doi: 10.1126/scisignal.2001462
27. Dybas, J. M., Herrmann, C., and Weitzman, M. D. (2018). Ubiquitination at the interface of tumor viruses and DNA damage responses. *Curr. Opin. Virol.* 32, 40–47. doi: 10.1016/j.coviro.2018.08.017
28. Everett, R. D. (2014). HSV-1 biology and life cycle. *Methods Mol. Biol.* 1444, 1–17. doi: 10.1007/978-1-4939-0428-0_1
29. Everett, R. D., Meredith, M., Orr, A., Cross, A., Kathoria, M., and Parkinson, J. (1997). A novel ubiquitin-specific protease is dynamically associated with the PML nuclear domain and binds to a herpesvirus regulatory protein. *EMBO J.* 16, 1519–1530. doi: 10.1093/emboj/16.7.1519
30. Faesen, A. C., Dirac, A. M., Shanmugham, A., Ovaa, H., Perrakis, A., and Sixma, T. K. (2011). Mechanism of USP7/HAUSP activation by its C-terminal ubiquitin-like domain and allosteric regulation by GMP-synthetase. *Mol. Cell* 44, 147–159. doi: 10.1016/j.molcel.2011.06.034
31. Faustrup, H., Bekker-Jensen, S., Bartek, J., Lukas, J., and Mailand, N. (2009). USP7 counteracts SCFbetaTrCP- but not APCCdh1-mediated proteolysis of Claspin. *J. Cell Biol.* 184, 13–19. doi: 10.1083/jcb.200807137
32. Fernandez-Montalvan, A., Bouwmeester, T., Joberty, G., Mader, R., Mahnke, M., Pierrat, B., et al. (2007). Biochemical characterization of USP7 reveals post-translational modification sites and structural requirements for substrate processing and subcellular localization. *FEBS J.* 274, 4256–4270. doi: 10.1111/j.1742-4658.2007.05952.x
33. Freeman, D. J., Li, A. G., Wei, G., Li, H. H., Kertesz, N., Lesche, R., et al. (2003). PTEN tumor suppressor regulates p53 protein levels and activity through phosphatase-dependent and -independent mechanisms. *Cancer Cell* 3, 117–130. doi: 10.1016/s1535-6108(03)00021-7
34. Geoffroy, M. C., and Hay, R. T. (2009). An additional role for SUMO in ubiquitin- mediated proteolysis. *Nat. Rev. Mol. Cell Biol.* 10, 564–568. doi: 10.1038/nrm2707
35. Han, X., Gui, B., Xiong, C., Zhao, L., Liang, J., Sun, L., et al. (2014). Destabilizing LSD1 by Jade-2 promotes neurogenesis: an antibraking system in neural development. *Mol. Cell* 55, 482–494. doi: 10.1016/j.molcel.2014.06.006
36. He, J., Zhu, Q., Wani, G., Sharma, N., Han, C., Qian, J., et al. (2014). Ubiquitin-specific protease 7 regulates nucleotide excision repair through deubiquitinating XPC protein and preventing XPC protein from undergoing ultraviolet light-induced and VCP/p97 protein-regulated proteolysis. *J. Biol. Chem.* 289, 27278–27289. doi: 10.1074/jbc.M114.589812
37. Holowaty, M. N., Zeghouf, M., Wu, H., Tellam, J., Athanasopoulos, V., Greenblatt, J., et al. (2003). Protein profiling with epstein-barr nuclear antigen-1 reveals an interaction with the herpesvirus-associated ubiquitin-specific protease HAUSP/USP7. *J. Biol. Chem.* 278, 29987–29994. doi: 10.1074/jbc.M303977200
38. Hu, M., Gu, L., Li, M., Jeffrey, P. D., Gu, W., and Shi, Y. (2006). Structural basis of competitive recognition of p53 and MDM2 by HAUSP/USP7: implications for the regulation of the p53-MDM2 pathway. *PLoS Biol.* 4:e27. doi: 10.1371/journal.pbio.0040027
39. Hu, M., Li, P., Li, M., Li, W., Yao, T., Wu, J. W., et al. (2002). Crystal structure of a UBP-family deubiquitinating enzyme in isolation and in complex with ubiquitin aldehyde. *Cell* 111, 1041–1054. doi: 10.1016/s0092-8674(02)01199-6
40. Huang, H., Regan, K. M., Wang, F., Wang, D., Smith, D. I., van Deursen, J. M., et al. (2005). Skp2 inhibits FOXO1 in tumor suppression through ubiquitin-mediated degradation. *Proc. Natl. Acad. Sci. U.S.A.* 102, 1649–1654. doi: 10.1073/pnas.0406789102
41. Jager, W., Santag, S., Weidner-Glunde, M., Gellermann, E., Kati, S., Pietrek, M., et al. (2012). The ubiquitin-specific protease USP7 modulates the replication of Kaposi's sarcoma-associated herpesvirus latent episomal DNA. *J. Virol.* 86, 6745–6757. doi: 10.1128/jvi.06840-11
42. Jin, Q., Martinez, C. A., Arcipowski, K. M., Zhu, Y., Gutierrez-Diaz, B. T., Wang, K. K., et al. (2018). USP7 cooperates with NOTCH1 to drive the

oncogenic transcriptional program in T cell leukemia. *Clin. Cancer Res.* 25, 222–239. doi: 10.1158/1078-0432.CCR-18-1740
43. Kalamvoki, M., Gu, H., and Roizman, B. (2012). Overexpression of the ubiquitin- specific protease 7 resulting from transfection or mutations in the ICP0 binding site accelerates rather than depresses herpes simplex virus 1 gene expression. *J. Virol.* 86, 12871–12878. doi: 10.1128/jvi.01981-12
44. Kategaya, L., Di Lello, P., Rouge, L., Pastor, R., Clark, K. R., Drummond, J., et al. (2017). USP7 small-molecule inhibitors interfere with ubiquitin binding. *Nature* 550, 534–538. doi: 10.1038/nature24006
45. Khosravi, M., Bidmeshkipour, A., Cohen, J. L., Moravej, A., Hojjat-Assari, S., Naserian, S., et al. (2018). Induction of CD4(+)CD25(+)FOXP3(+) regulatory T cells by mesenchymal stem cells is associated with modulation of ubiquitination factors and TSDR demethylation. *Stem Cell Res. Ther.* 9:273. doi: 10.1186/s13287-018-0991-1
46. Kim, R. Q., and Sixma, T. K. (2017). Regulation of USP7: a high incidence of E3 complexes. *J. Mol. Biol.* 429, 3395–3408. doi: 10.1016/j.jmb.2017.05.028
47. Kumar, S., Brown, A., and Tchounwou, P. B. (2018). Trisenox disrupts MDM2-DAXX-HAUSP complex and activates p53, cell cycle regulation and apoptosis in acute leukemia cells. *Oncotarget* 9, 33138–33148. doi: 10.18632/oncotarget.26025
48. Laurence, A., Belkaid, Y., and O'Shea, J. J. (2013). A degrading view of regulatory T cells. *Immunity* 39, 201–203. doi: 10.1016/j.immuni.2013.08.017
49. Lecona, E., Rodriguez-Acebes, S., Specks, J., Lopez-Contreras, A. J., Ruppen, I., Murga, M., et al. (2016). USP7 is a SUMO deubiquitinase essential for DNA replication. *Nat. Struct. Mol. Biol.* 23, 270–277. doi: 10.1038/nsmb. 3185
50. Lee, H. R., Choi, W. C., Lee, S., Hwang, J., Hwang, E., Guchhait, K., et al. (2011). Bilateral inhibition of HAUSP deubiquitinase by a viral interferon regulatory factor protein. *Nat. Struct. Mol. Biol.* 18, 1336–1344. doi: 10.1038/nsmb.2142
51. Levine, A. J. (1997). p53, the cellular gatekeeper for growth and division. *Cell* 88, 323–331. doi: 10.1016/s0092-8674(00)81871-1
52. Li, M., Brooks, C. L., Kon, N., and Gu, W. (2004). A dynamic role of HAUSP in the p53-Mdm2 pathway. *Mol. Cell* 13, 879–886. doi: 10.1016/s1097-2765(04)00157-1
53. Li, M., Chen, D., Shiloh, A., Luo, J., Nikolaev, A. Y., Qin, J., et al. (2002). Deubiquitination of p53 by HAUSP is an important pathway for p53 stabilization. *Nature* 416, 648–653. doi: 10.1038/nature737
54. Liang, L., Peng, Y., Zhang, J., Zhang, Y., Roy, M., Han, X., et al. (2019). Deubiquitylase USP7 regulates human terminal erythroid differentiation by stabilizing GATA1. *Haematologica*
55. Lindsay, C. R., Morozov, V. M., and Ishov, A. M. (2008). PML NBs (ND10) and Daxx: from nuclear structure to protein function. *Front. Biosci.* 13, 7132–7142. doi: 10.2741/3216
56. Lu, Y., Orr, A., and Everett, R. D. (2016). Stimulation of the replication of ICP0-null mutant herpes simplex virus 1 and pp71-deficient human cytomegalovirus by epstein-barr virus tegument protein BNRF1. *J. Virol.* 90, 9664–9673. doi: 10.1128/jvi.01224-16
57. Ma, J., Martin, J. D., Xue, Y., Lor, L. A., Kennedy-Wilson, K. M., Sinnamon, R. H., et al. (2010). C-terminal region of USP7/HAUSP is critical for deubiquitination activity and contains a second mdm2/p53 binding site. *Arch. Biochem. Biophys.* 503, 207–212. doi: 10.1016/j.abb.2010.08.020
58. Ma, P., Yang, X., Kong, Q., Li, C., Yang, S., Li, Y., et al. (2014). The ubiquitin ligase RNF220 enhances canonical Wnt signaling through USP7-mediated deubiquitination of beta-catenin. *Mol. Cell Biol.* 34, 4355–4366. doi: 10.1128/mcb.00731-14
59. Malapelle, U., Morra, F., Ilardi, G., Visconti, R., Merolla, F., Cerrato, A., et al. (2017). USP7 inhibitors, downregulating CCDC6, sensitize lung neuroendocrine cancer cells to PARP-inhibitor drugs. *Lung Cancer* 107, 41–49. doi: 10.1016/j.lungcan.2016.06.015
60. Masuya, D., Huang, C., Liu, D., Nakashima, T., Yokomise, H., Ueno, M., et al. (2006). The HAUSP gene plays an important role in non-small cell lung carcinogenesis through p53-dependent pathways. *J. Pathol.* 208, 724–732. doi: 10.1002/path.1931
61. Morotti, A., Panuzzo, C., Crivellaro, S., Pergolizzi, B., Familiari, U., Berger, A. H., et al. (2014). BCR-ABL disrupts PTEN nuclear-cytoplasmic shuttling through phosphorylation-dependent activation of HAUSP. *Leukemia* 28, 1326–1333. doi: 10.1038/leu.2013.370
62. Nijman, S. M., Luna-Vargas, M. P., Velds, A., Brummelkamp, T. R., Dirac, A. M., Sixma, T. K., et al. (2005). genomic and functional inventory of deubiquitinating enzymes. *Cell* 123, 773–786. doi: 10.1016/j.cell.2005.11.007
63. Novellasdemunt, L., Foglizzo, V., Cuadrado, L., Antas, P., Kucharska, A., Encheva, V., et al. (2017). USP7 Is a tumor-specific WNT activator for APC-mutated colorectal cancer by mediating beta-catenin deubiquitination. *Cell Rep.* 21, 612–627. doi: 10.1016/j.celrep.2017.09.072
64. Oh, Y. M., Yoo, S. J., and Seol, J. H. (2007). Deubiquitination of Chfr, a checkpoint protein, by USP7/HAUSP regulates its stability and activity. *Biochem. Biophys. Res. Commun.* 357, 615–619. doi: 10.1016/j.bbrc.2007.03.193
65. Oliner, J. D., Kinzler, K. W., Meltzer, P. S., George, D. L., and Vogelstein, B. (1992). Amplification of a gene encoding a p53-associated protein in human sarcomas. *Nature* 358, 80–83. doi: 10.1038/358080a0
66. Ozen, A., Rouge, L., Bashore, C., Hearn, B. R., Skelton, N. J., and Dueber, E. C. (2018). Selectively modulating conformational states of USP7 catalytic domain for activation. *Structure* 26, 72–84.e7. doi: 10.1016/j.str.2017.11.010
67. Palazon-Riquelme, P., Worboys, J. D., Green, J., Valera, A., Martin-Sanchez, F., Pellegrini, C., et al. (2018). USP7 and USP47 deubiquitinases regulate NLRP3 inflammasome activation. *EMBO Rep.* 19:e44766. doi: 10.15252/embr.201744766
68. Park, J. J., Lim, K. H., and Baek, K. H. (2015). Annexin-1 regulated by HAUSP is essential for UV-induced damage response. *Cell Death Dis.* 2015:e1654. doi: 10.1038/cddis.2015.32
69. Pfoh, R., Lacdao, I. K., Georges, A. A., Capar, A., Zheng, H., Frappier, L., et al. (2015). Crystal structure of USP7 ubiquitin-like domains with an ICP0 peptide reveals a novel mechanism used by viral and cellular proteins to target. *PLoS Pathog.* 11:e1004950. doi: 10.1371/journal.ppat.1004950
70. Qian, J., Pentz, K., Zhu, Q., Wang, Q., He, J., Srivastava, A. K., et al. (2015). USP7 modulates UV-induced PCNA monoubiquitination by regulating DNA polymerase eta stability. *Oncogene* 34, 4791–4796. doi: 10.1038/onc.2014.394
71. Qing, P., Han, L., Bin, L., Yan, L., and Ping, W. X. (2011). USP7 regulates the stability and function of HLTF through deubiquitination. *J. Cell Biochem.* 112, 3856–3862. doi: 10.1002/jcb.23317
72. Reverdy, C., Conrath, S., Lopez, R., Planquette, C., Atmanene, C., Collura, V., et al. (2012). Discovery of specific inhibitors of human USP7/HAUSP deubiquitinating enzyme. *Chem. Biol.* 19, 467–477. doi: 10.1016/j.chembiol.2012.02.007
73. Rouge, L., Bainbridge, T. W., Kwok, M., Tong, R., Di Lello, P., Wertz, I. E., et al. (2016). Molecular understanding of USP7 substrate recognition and C-terminal activation. *Structure* 24, 1335–1345. doi: 10.1016/j.str.2016.05.020
74. Sarasin, A. (2012). UVSSA and USP7: new players regulating transcription-coupled nucleotide excision repair in human cells. *Genome Med.* 4:44. doi: 10.1186/gm343
75. Saridakis, V., Sheng, Y., Sarkari, F., Holowaty, M. N., Shire, K., Nguyen, T., et al. (2005). Structure of the p53 binding domain of HAUSP/USP7 bound to Epstein-Barr nuclear antigen 1 implications for EBV-mediated immortalization. *ESE Mol. Cell* 18, 25–36. doi: 10.1016/j.molcel.2005.02.029
76. Shan, H., Li, X., Xiao, X., Dai, Y., Huang, J., Song, J., et al. (2018). USP7 deubiquitinates and stabilizes NOTCH1 in T-cell acute lymphoblastic leukemia. *Signal. Transduct. Target. Ther.* 3:29. doi: 10.1038/s41392-018-0028-3
77. Sheng, Y., Saridakis, V., Sarkari, F., Duan, S., Wu, T., Arrowsmith, C. H., et al. (2006). Molecular recognition of p53 and MDM2 by USP7/HAUSP. *Nat. Struct. Mol. Biol.* 13, 285–291. doi: 10.1038/nsmb1067
78. Shi, Y., Lan, F., Matson, C., Mulligan, P., Whetstine, J. R., Cole, P. A., et al. (2004). Histone demethylation mediated by the nuclear amine oxidase homolog LSD1. *Cell* 119, 941–953. doi: 10.1016/j.cell.2004.12.012
79. Smits, V. A., and Freire, R. (2016). USP7/HAUSP: a SUMO deubiquitinase at the heart of DNA replication. *Bioessays* 38, 863–868. doi: 10.1002/bies.201600096
Song, M. S., Salmena, L., Carracedo, A., Egia, A., Lo-Coco, F., Teruya-Feldstein, J., et al. (2008). The deubiquitinylation and localization of PTEN are regulated by a HAUSP-PML network. *Nature* 455, 813–817. doi: 10.1038/nature07290
80. Su, D., Ma, S., Shan, L., Wang, Y., Wang, Y., Cao, C., et al. (2018). Ubiquitin-specific protease 7 sustains DNA damage response and promotes cervical carcinogenesis. *J. Clin. Invest.* 128, 4280–4296. doi: 10.1172/jci120518
81. Tang, J., Qu, L. K., Zhang, J., Wang, W., Michaelson, J. S., Degenhardt, Y. Y., et al. (2006). Critical role for Daxx in regulating Mdm2. *Nat. Cell Biol.* 8, 855–862. doi: 10.1038/ncb1442
82. Tavana, O., Li, D., Dai, C., Lopez, G., Banerjee, D., Kon, N., et al. (2016). HAUSP deubiquitinates and stabilizes N-Myc in neuroblastoma. *Nat. Med.* 22, 1180–1186. doi: 10.1038/nm.4180
83. Trotman, L. C., Wang, X., Alimonti, A., Chen, Z., Teruya-Feldstein, J., Yang,

H., et al. (2007). Ubiquitination regulates PTEN nuclear import and tumor suppression. *Cell* 128, 141–156. doi: 10.1016/j.cell.2006.11.040

84. Turnbull, A. P., Ioannidis, S., Krajewski, W. W., Pinto-Fernandez, A., Heride, C., Martin, A. C. L., et al. (2017). Molecular basis of USP7 inhibition by selective small-molecule inhibitors. *Nature* 550, 481–486. doi: 10.1038/nature24451
85. van der Horst, A., and Burgering, B. M. (2007). Stressing the role of FoxO proteins in lifespan and disease. *Nat. Rev. Mol. Cell Biol.* 8, 440–450. doi: 10.1038/nrm2190
86. van der Horst, A., de Vries-Smits, A. M., Brenkman, A. B., van Triest, M. H., van den Broek, N., Colland, F., et al. (2006). FOXO4 transcriptional activity is regulated by monoubiquitination and USP7/HAUSP. *Nat. Cell Biol.* 8, 1064–1073. doi: 10.1038/ncb1469
87. van Loosdregt, J., and Coffer, P. J. (2014). Post-translational modification networks regulating FOXP3 function. *Trends Immunol.* 35, 368–378. doi: 10.1016/j.it. 2014.06.005
88. van Loosdregt, J., Fleskens, V., Fu, J., Brenkman, A. B., Bekker, C. P., Pals, C. E., et al. (2013). Stabilization of the transcription factor Foxp3 by the deubiquitinase USP7 increases Treg-cell-suppressive capacity. *Immunity* 39, 259–271. doi: 10.1016/j.immuni.2013.05.018
89. Vassilev, L. T., Vu, B. T., Graves, B., Carvajal, D., Podlaski, F., Filipovic, Z., et al. (2004). In vivo activation of the p53 pathway by small-molecule antagonists of MDM2. *Science* 303, 844–848. doi: 10.1126/science.1092472
90. Wade, M., Li, Y. C., and Wahl, G. M. (2013). MDM2, MDMX and p53 in oncogenesis and cancer therapy. *Nat. Rev. Cancer* 13, 83–96. doi: 10.1038/nrc3430
91. Wang, L., Kumar, S., Dahiya, S., Wang, F., Wu, J., Newick, K., et al. (2016). Ubiquitin-specific protease-7 inhibition impairs Tip60-dependent Foxp3+ T-regulatory Cell function and promotes antitumor immunity. *EBioMedicine* 13, 99–112. doi: 10.1016/j.ebiom.2016.10.018
92. Wang, Q., Ma, S., Song, N., Li, X., Liu, L., Yang, S., et al. (2016). Stabilization of histone demethylase PHF8 by USP7 promotes breast carcinogenesis. *J. Clin. Invest.* 126, 2205–2220. doi: 10.1172/jci85747
93. Xiang, Q., Ju, H., Li, Q., Mei, S. C., Chen, D., and Choi, Y. B. (2018). Human herpesvirus 8 interferon regulatory factors 1 and 3 mediate replication and latency activities via interactions with USP7 Deubiquitinase. *J. Virol.* 92:e2003-17. doi: 10.1128/jvi.02003-17
94. Yao, Y., Zhang, Y., Shi, M., Sun, Y., Chen, C., Niu, M., et al. (2018). Blockade of deubiquitinase USP7 overcomes bortezomib resistance by suppressing NF-kappaB signaling pathway in multiple myeloma. *J. Leukoc. Biol.* 104, 1105–1115. doi: 10.1002/JLB.2A1017-420RR
95. Yi, L., Cui, Y., Xu, Q., and Jiang, Y. (2016). Stabilization of LSD1 by deubiquitinating enzyme USP7 promotes glioblastoma cell tumorigenesis and metastasis through suppression of the p53 signaling pathway. *Oncol. Rep.* 36, 2935–2945. doi: 10.3892/or.2016.5099
96. Zaman, M. M., Nomura, T., Takagi, T., Okamura, T., Jin, W., Shinagawa, T., et al. (2013). Ubiquitination-deubiquitination by the TRIM27-USP7 complex regulates tumor necrosis factor alpha-induced apoptosis. *Mol. Cell Biol.* 33, 4971–4984. doi: 10.1128/mcb.00465-13
97. Zhang, P., Wei, Y., Wang, L., Debeb, B. G., Yuan, Y., Zhang, J., et al. (2014). ATM-mediated stabilization of ZEB1 promotes DNA damage response and radioresistance through CHK1. *Nat. Cell Biol.* 16, 864–875. doi: 10.1038/ncb3013
98. Zhang, X., Gu, L., Li, J., Shah, N., He, J., Yang, L., et al. (2010). Degradation of MDM2 by the interaction between berberine and DAXX leads to potent apoptosis in MDM2-overexpressing cancer cells. *Cancer Res.* 70, 9895–9904. doi: 10.1158/0008-5472.can-10-1546
99. Zhang, X., Horibata, K., Saijo, M., Ishigami, C., Ukai, A., Kanno, S., et al. (2012). Mutations in UVSSA cause UV-sensitive syndrome and destabilize ERCC6 in transcription-coupled DNA repair. *Nat. Genet.* 44, 593–597. doi: 10.1038/ng. 2228
100. Zhou, J., Wang, J., Chen, C., Yuan, H., Wen, X., and Sun, H. (2018). USP7: target validation and drug discovery for cancer therapy. *Med. Chem.* 14, 3–18. doi: 10.2174/1573406413666171020115539
101. Zhu, X., Menard, R., and Sulea, T. (2007). High incidence of ubiquitin-like domains in human ubiquitin-specific *proteases. Proteins* 69, 1–7. doi: 10.1002/prot.21546
102. Zlatanou, A., Sabbioneda, S., Miller, E. S., Greenwalt, A., Aggathanggelou, A., Maurice, M. M., et al. (2016). USP7 is essential for maintaining Rad18 stability and DNA damage tolerance. *Oncogene* 35, 965–976. doi: 10.1038/onc.2015.149

11

Epigenetic Enzyme Mutations: Role in Tumorigenesis and Molecular Inhibitors

Mei Han[†], Lina Jia[†], Wencai Lv, Lihui Wang[*] and Wei Cui[*]

Department of Pharmacology, Shenyang Pharmaceutical University, Shenyang, China

Correspondence:
Lihui Wang
lhwang@syphu.edu.cn
Wei Cui
cuiwei@syphu.edu.cn

[†] *These authors have contributed equally to this work*

Epigenetic modifications, such as DNA methylation and histone modification, result in heritable changes in gene expression without changing the DNA sequence. Epigenetic regulatory enzymes such as DNA methyltransferases, histone methyltransferases, and histone deacetylases are involved in epigenetic modification. Studies have shown that the dysregulation caused by changes in the amino acid sequence of these enzymes is closely correlated with tumor onset and progression. In addition, certain amino acid changes in the metabolic enzyme isocitrate dehydrogenase (IDH) are linked to altered epigenetic modifications in tumors. Some small molecule inhibitors targeting these aberrant enzymes have shown promising anti-cancer efficacy in preclinical and clinical trials. For example, the small molecule inhibitor ivosidenib, which targets IDH1 with a mutation at R132, has been approved by the FDA for the clinical treatment of acute myeloid leukemia. In this review, we summarize the recurrent "hotspot" mutations in these enzymes in various tumors and their role in tumorigenesis. We also describe candidate inhibitors of the mutant enzymes which show potential therapeutic value. In addition, we introduce some previously unreported mutation sites in these enzymes, which may be related to tumor development and provide opportunities for future study.

Keywords: DNMT, mutation, small molecule inhibitors, tumor, histone modification enzyme

INTRODUCTION

The term "epigenetics" describes inheritable changes of gene expression with no alteration of the DNA sequence (1). As the field of epigenetics has expanded, the connection between epigenetic changes and the occurrence and development of tumors has received more attention (2). The structure of chromatin is the basis for modulating gene expression: euchromatin has an open structure that is typically associated with active transcription, while heterochromatin is tightly compacted and usually associated with transcriptional repression. Epigenetic modification such as DNA methylation and histone modification are important for regulating chromatin structure and therefore gene expression. These modifications are catalyzed by epigenetic regulatory enzymes, including DNA methyltransferases, histone methyltransferases and histone deacetylases.

Recent studies have shown that the dysregulation (e.g., overexpression) of these enzymes plays a crucial role in tumorigenesis. Some small molecule inhibitors targeting these aberrantly expressed epigenetic regulatory enzymes have been approved by the FDA for the treatment of certain cancers. For example, the small molecule inhibitor 5-azacytidine, which targets the DNA methyltransferase DNMT3A, has been approved for clinical treatment of patients with acute lymphoblastic leukemia (AML) (3), and belinostat, which targets histone deacetylases (HDACs) in peripheral T-cell lymphoma (PTCL), was approved for use in 2014 (4). In addition, the inhibitor EPZ6438, which targets EZH2, a histone methyltransferase, has been approved for testing in the clinic (5).

In recent years, increasing evidence has shown that epigenetic regulatory enzymes are mutated in various types of cancer, and mutations of these enzymes are closely related to the malignant phenotype (6, 7). Hence, inhibitors that target these mutant enzymes have gradually entered preclinical and clinical research. In this review, we first summarize the epigenetic regulatory enzymes and their mutations in different types of tumors, and then we explain how the mutations are correlated with tumorigenesis. Finally, we present some small molecule inhibitors which target epigenetic regulatory enzymes, especially their mutated forms, and may have potential therapeutic value in the future.

DNMTS AND THEIR MUTATIONS IN CANCER

DNMTs in Cancer

DNA methylation, which is one of the major epigenetic regulatory mechanisms, plays a crucial role in many life processes (8). In eukaryotic cells, DNA methylation is a stable gene silencing modification that is copied during DNA replication (9). DNA methylation predominately occurs at cytosine residues in 5′-CpG-3′ dinucleotides, with S-adenosyl methionine (SAM) as the methyl donor (10). In mammals, DNA methylation is catalyzed by enzymes in the DNA methyltransferase (DNMT) family, mainly DNMT1, DNMT3A, and DNMT3B. DNMT1 maintains the methylation status of newly replicated (hemi-methylated) DNA, whereas DNMT3A and DNMT3B are responsible for *de novo* DNA methylation (11). The mechanism by which DNA methylation regulates gene expression involves blocking the binding of transcription factors to DNA and the recruitment of proteins containing a methylated CpG-binding domain to inhibit gene expression in tumor cells (12). The methylation profiles in different cells are not the same, and this has functional consequences. In normal cells, gene promoters containing CpG islands are usually unmethylated, which maintains the chromatin in an open structure, and hence enhances the transcription of the gene. However, in tumor cells, the CpG island-containing promoters of tumor suppressor genes are usually methylated, and thus the euchromatin is converted to compacted heterochromatin (13). These findings indicate that DNA methylation regulates tumorigenesis and progression by inhibiting the expression of tumor suppressor genes.

DNMT Mutations in Cancer

Recently, studies have shown that mutations of DNMT family, especially DNMT3A, are prominent features of many tumors and can lead to malignant transformation (14). DNMT3A is one of the most frequently mutated DNA methyltransferase in AML (6) and myelodysplastic syndromes (MDS) (15). Some reports have shown that mutations in DNMT3A are present in up to 20% of AML cases and are associated with poor prognosis (8, 16). Although a large number of mutations in the DNMT3A have been reported, ~50% of the changes are in the catalytic domain at position R882 (most commonly R882H) (8, 17, 18). **Table 1** shows DNMT3A mutations, including hotspots and non-reported mutation sites, in various tumors. In addition, mutations in DNMT1 have been described in colorectal (29), prostate and hematological malignancies (30). The gene encoding DNMT3B was reported to be mutated in immunodeficiency syndrome, but mutations have rarely been reported in tumors (31). In addition, except DNMTs' mutations in various cancers, DNA hydroxymethylase TET2, which catalyzes the conversion of 5-methyl-cytosine to 5-hydroxymethyl-cytosine, has been reported in recent years for its mutations in various diseases, especially AML and MDS (32). The above results indicated that the mutations in DNMT and its related enzyme are frequent, which suggesting the potential role of them in tumorigenesis.

Function of DNMT Mutations

Mutations in DNMTs are closely correlated with the biological characteristics of malignant tumors and they increase the ability of cancer cells to undergo proliferation, migration, colony formation, and self-renewal. Recently, the relationship between the DNMT3A R882C mutation and the migration of tumor cells has been investigated *in vitro* (33). The results showed that the OCI-AML3 cell line, which carries the R882C mutation, had a greater migration ability than cell lines carrying wild-type (WT) DNMT3A, and infiltrated into the meninges of mice after intravenous infusion. This indicates that the DNMT3A R882 mutation contributes to the enhanced migration of malignant cells. It was also shown that the DNMT3A R882H mutation increases the proliferative capacity of hematopoietic cells and actively promotes the growth of monocytes and macrophages (33). Mechanistically, DNMT3A R882 mutant proteins interact with polycomb repressive complex 1 (PRC1) to block the differentiation of hematopoietic stem cells and lymphocytes by down-regulating differentiation-associated genes (34). Furthermore, cells with DNMT3A R882 mutations have a higher colony forming capacity than WT cells (34). In addition, it was reported that DNMT3A R882 mutations may induce chemotherapy resistance in AML patients. Guryanova et al. reported that the DNMT3A R882H mutation increases the risk of AML patients being resistant to anthracycline therapy by dysregulating nucleosome remodeling (35). Some reports have shown that the DNMT3A R882 mutation was negatively correlated with the prognosis of AML patients. The 5-year overall survival of AML patients with DNMT3A mutations was significantly shorter than AML patients without such mutations (36, 37). Accordingly, Delhommeau et al. reported that TET2 mutations are early events in patients with some MDS and secondary AML and confirmed the important role of TET2 in maintaining the balance between hematopoietic cell survival, growth and differentiation (38). Studies have shown that leukemia-associated missense mutations impair the enzymatic activity of TET2 and lead to a decrease in the genomic level of 5-hydroxymethyl-cytosine, which disrupts normal hematopoiesis and may accelerate leukemia formation (32). All of the above

TABLE 1 | Epigenetic regulatory enzymes mutation sites and their function in different types of cancer.

Enzyme	Gain-of-function mutation	Function of mutation	Non-reported mutation	Cancer type (references)	Inhibitor
DNMT3A	R882(H/C/P);	Migration;	Y735F, V716F, R729(Q/H/W), R803S, R736H, K829R, P718L, C497Y, D781G, G646V, A741V, F909C, M801V;	**Leukemia (6, 8, 16)**	5-azacytidine;
	R882C	Proliferation;	R792H, G26V, S708C, G412W, A254P, E629D, G293W, V763F, R771Q, Y533C, Q485H, K680R, S878P, E725V, R209P, P59L,	Lung cancer	Dichlone;
		Colony formation;	R379L, M864I, R326P, P804S, V258M, W327G, C494S, S312F, D781H, G413S, S669C, A116S, F909S, R458Q, R55H, Y724C,		SYC-52221;
		Blocking differentiation	V563M, D857V, W795C, P89R, D618N, Y735C, V560L, G570W, M78I, D279V, E392D, M224V, Q248R, V895M, V401L,		EPZ004777;
			G685V, C559Y, E854Q, G49R, G890C, E323K, P709L, Y359C, E213D, G746V, P58L, R885S, V687F, P425T		EPZ5676; (pan-inhibitors)
EZH2	Y641(S/H/F/N), A687V, A677G, Y646H;	Migration;	E740K, R679H, G159R, N670K, S271F, W113C, K660R, K660E, D185H, T53M, D183E, M701V, Y447H, V702G, C642S, T144I,	**Lymphoma (19–21)**	EPZ005687;
		Proliferation;	E636D, R685H, D659A, F672L;		GSK126;
	Y641(S/H/N/F), Y646(S/H);	Tumor growth;	S533L, R342Q, R216(Q/W), P132S, P219S, G2(D/S), D316G, R34P, P746S, S229L, S405L, T4(I/P), D142V, A226V, S228F,	**Melanoma (22)**	EPZ-6438;
		Poor prognosis;	P426S, R355G, C530W, G704S, G459E, R81S, P417Q, R456S, P535H, R382M, P262H, P631H, L338F, S474F, E391K, P527L, N366S, K510R, V675M, D511N, A590V, H521Y, I651T;		CPI-1205; (pan-inhibitors)
	Y646H, A687V		K426Q, S652(C/F), P493A, I633M, T467P, S624C, K550T, I150V, E173Q, H129D, Q653E, K545T, L315V, Q648E, S647C;	Breast cancer	
			K510R, E374Q, Q548E, N310S, A340T, P262(L/T/I), R685G, E650Q, R308L, A715V, A622, R497Q, D233Y, R34L, E341K, R64M, D186N, K39E, H613Q, S647C, Q66R, R357L, E312K, Q94R, P481S, F667L, H502Q, R52I, G5R, S647F, R527W,S40C	Lung cancer	
IDH1	R132(C/S/G/H/L);	Proliferation;	G339E, G161R;	**Glioma (7, 23)**	Ivosidenib (specific targeting mutant IDH1 in R132);
	R132(C/H);	Migration;	V178I, G370D, S210N, R20Q;	**Lymphoma (24)**	
	R132(C/G/H);	Colony formation;	R119Q, E306D, T106M;	**Prostate cancer (25)**	
	R132(C/S/G/L);	Blocking differentiation;	N349S;	**Cholangiocarcinoma (26)**	FT-2120 (specific targeting mutant IDH1 in R132);
	R132(C/G/L);	Angiogenesis;	C297S, Q198P, N171T, M182V;	**Hepatic carcinoma (27)**	
	R132(C/H);	Inhibition of apoptosis	D160E, D79N, T327A, G263V, L88F, K217N, Y235C, R338T, K81N, K151N, A179D, I189V, E84Q;	Breast cancer	IDH-305 (specific targeting mutant IDH1);
	R132(C/L)		R49C, M290I, Q228R, E361K, E360K, S94P, A341V, G339W, G284V, A282V;	Melanoma	
			I102T, E28Q, R109K, D375Y, A179D, Y34C, I333V, V294L, I189F, A193S, D299E, G175V, G221(L/V/W), L359F, E262Q, K406E T302R, R119W, G310V, I380F, N961	Lung cancer	AGI-881 (pan-inhibitor)
DH2	R172(S/K/G/W/M);	Proliferation;	G383V, K251N;	**Glioma (7, 28)**	Enasidenib (specific targeting mutant IDH2);
	R172(K/G/M/S);	Migration;	H430Y, R140(Q/L/G), D225N, N156I;	**Lymphoma (24)**	
	R172K;	Colony formation;	I62V, I61V;	**Prostate cancer (25)**	
	R172(K/S);	Blocking differentiation;	S301L, N156S, R60G, F270S, I419T;	**Hepatic carcinoma (27)**	AGI-881(pan-inhibitor)
	R172K	Angiogenesis;	R122(C/S), I139F, G137E, G387W, E68K, M248I, P198T, G176N, A321V,	Melanoma	
			M221I, R362W;	Lung cancer	
			R188W, H273D, Q267E, S249G, Q322K, I62M; I240V, F192L, T146S, E345K;	Breast cancer	
HDAC2	–	–	Q354L, D175N, D231H, S118P, K466Q, N470I;	Leukemia	–
			M65V, G28R, A257T, P102A, R78(L/W), L42F, D456N, A120V, C101F, E109Q, A122S, D426Y	Lung cancer	

Publications reporting cancers with the indicated gain-of-function mutations are in bold. Non-reported mutations in the same proteins were identified from the cBioPortal website.

observations show that mutations in DNMT3A and TET2, to some extent, promote oncogenesis, and tumor progression.

HMTS AND THEIR MUTATIONS IN CANCER

HMTs in Cancer

Histone methylation is involved in the regulation of various biological processes such as gene expression, DNA repair, differentiation, replication and growth (39). Histone methyltransferases catalyze the transfer of the methyl group of SAM to histone arginine or lysine residues. A number of HMTs have been identified, including histone lysine methyltransferases (HKMTs) and histone arginine methyltransferases (HRMTs), which have specific substrates and residues. EZH2 belongs to the HKMT family and is frequently overexpressed in various cancerous tissue types such as breast, prostate and lung (19, 20, 40).

HMT Mutations in Cancer

EZH2 is a histone methyltransferase that catalyzes the trimethylation of arginine 27 in histone H3 (H3K27). Reports of EZH2 mutations in cancer have increased in recent years. Mutations in epigenetic regulatory enzymes are either gain-of-function or loss-of-function (3). EZH2 gain-of-function mutations were previously reported in lymphoma, and the probability of EZH2 mutation in melanoma was recently reported to be about 2%. Popov et al. found that 27% of follicular lymphoma cases had EZH2 mutations at 3 recurrent hotspots (Y646, A682, and A692) (24). Other gain-of-function hotspot mutations including Y641, A677, and A687 in the catalytic SET domain of EZH2 are prevalent, accounting for ~10–24% of non-Hodgkin's lymphoma (26). In addition to these hotspot mutations, we have summarized some non-reported mutation sites that have yet to be studied, as shown in **Table 1**.

Function of HMT Mutations

The dysregulation of H3K27 trimethylation (H3K27me3) is important in human tumorigenesis (25), and some reports have shown that mutant EZH2 increases the level of H3K27me3 in follicular lymphoma, germinal center B-cell type diffuse large B-cell lymphomas (21, 24, 41) and metastatic skin melanoma (42). The level of H3K27 monomethylation and dimethylation in cancer cells and tumor tissues with heterozygous EZH2 mutations at Y641 and A677 is decreased, while the level of H3K27 trimethylation is increased, resulting from the changed substrate preference of the mutant enzymes (22, 41). Barsotti et al. revealed that cells with a gain-of-function EZH2 mutation at Y641 displayed enhanced motility compared to control cells, forming highly dynamic collective migrating chains under 3D culture conditions (42). The Y641 EZH2 gain-of-function mutant cells also had a significant growth advantage in melanoma xenografts. Others have reported that mutations in EZH2 can promote lymphocyte proliferation and maintain the enhanced histone methyltransferase activity *in vivo*, subsequently increasing tumorigenicity (26). Somatic mutations in EZH2 have been shown in many reports to correlate with poor prognosis in patients with AML and myeloproliferative neoplasms (6, 43). Thus, mutations in EZH2 may contribute to the enhancement of the malignant phenotype.

HMT-RELATED ENZYMES AND THEIR MUTATIONS IN CANCER

HMT-Related Enzymes in Cancer

Isocitrate dehydrogenase (IDH) plays a key role in the Kreb's cycle, catalyzing the conversion of isocitrate into α-ketoglutarate (α-KG). The two major human IDH proteins, IDH1 and IDH2, are not HMTs, but their mutant forms indirectly contribute to effects on histone methylation by catalyzing the conversion of α-KG to 2-hydroxyglutarate (2-HG). Accumulation of 2-HG can inhibit the activity of a broad range of histone demethylases, inducing hypermethylation which is observed in certain cancers such as gliomas (44). In addition, high levels of 2-HG can inhibit α-KG-dependent prolyl hydroxylase, which is important for the degradation of hypoxia-inducible factor (HIF)-1α, a regulator of histone demethylases (7, 23, 28). Mutated forms of IDH therefore mimic the effects of HMTs.

HMT-Related Enzyme Mutations in Cancer

As mentioned above, specific mutants of IDH can catalyze the conversion of α-KG to 2-HG, and 2-HG inhibits not only histone demethylases but also TET DNA demethylases. This can cause increased methylation of both DNA and histones (3). Therefore, mutant IDH may be an oncoprotein and 2-HG may be an "oncometabolite" (7). In recent years, hotspot mutations in IDH1/2 have been reported in various tumors (**Table 1**). It has been reported that mutations of IDH1 and IDH2 occur in the vast majority of low-grade gliomas and secondary high-grade gliomas, and also in some cases of AML (27). In addition, IDH mutations have been found in solid tumors such as cholangiocarcinoma and prostate cancer (45, 46). The hotspot mutation of IDH1 is located at R132, while the hotspot mutation of IDH2 is located at R172, which is homologous to R132 in IDH1. We also found that other mutations of IDH1, including G339(E/W), R49C, R119(Q/W), and V294L, may be hotspot mutations in various tumors (**Table 1**). In addition to mutations in the enzyme of IDH family in the Kreb's cycle, two other metabolic enzymes involved in epigenetic regulation, SDH and FH, have also been reported in recent years to mutate in germline frequently. Ciccarone et al. concluded that SDH mutations in germline are responsible for the formation of hereditary paragangliomas and adrenal gland pheochromocytoma, whereas FH mutations are typical of hereditary leiomyomatosis and renal cell cancer (HLRCC) (47).

Function of HMT-Related Enzyme Mutations

Several groups have investigated the effect of IDH hotspot mutations, which mimic the activity of HMTs, in cancer. Cohen et al. elucidated that mutant IDH can trigger tumorigenesis. In detail, they found that somatic mutations in IDH1 at R132 or IDH2 at R172 led to increased risk of glioma, hemangiomas and chondrosarcoma, and they demonstrated that the mutated IDH contributed to the increased cell proliferation, colony formation, and inability to differentiate (7). In addition, Fu et al. showed that the IDH2 R172 mutation accelerated the migration and growth of C6 glioma cells by increasing the stability of HIF-1α (48). They also reported that IDH mutations promoted glioma cell metastasis and resistance to chemotherapy through up-regulation of the HIF-1α signaling pathway (49). IDH mutations also play an important role in blocking cell differentiation. Mutant IDH blocks hepatocyte differentiation by inhibiting the HNF-4α pathway (50). Other studies have shown that high levels of 2-HG caused by mutations in IDH can inhibit histone and DNA demethylases, resulting in hypermethylation of histones and DNA which eventually blocks cell differentiation (51, 52). Interestingly, there is no significant difference in the median overall survival rate of intrahepatic cholangiocarcinoma patients with mutant or WT IDH (53). In general, mutated IDH catalyzes the production of high levels of 2-HG, which has multiple effects including the inhibition of α-KG-dependent prolyl hydroxylase, which leads to the accumulation of HIF-1α in cells. This results in the induction of HIF-1α target genes that influence growth, migration, differentiation and angiogenesis as well as cell apoptosis (7), ultimately promoting tumor onset and progression (see **Figure 1**).

HDACS, HATS, AND THEIR MUTATIONS IN CANCER

Histone acetylation is an important epigenetic modification that mainly occurs in the N-terminal region of the histone tail. This modification weakens the binding between histones and DNA, which relaxes the chromatin and enhances gene expression (54). Histone acetyltransferases (HATs) mediate the acetylation in histones, whereas histone deacetylases (HDACs) catalyze the removal of acetyl groups from histones. The HATs are mainly divided into five major families, including GCN5/PCAF, MYST, TAFII250, CBP/p300, and SRC (55). The HDACs are divided into four classes. Class I HDACs include HDAC1, HDAC2, HDAC3, HDAC8; class II HDACs are further divided into two groups, class IIa (HDAC4, HDAC5, HDAC7, HDAC9) and class IIb (HDAC6, HDAC10); class III contains SIRT1-7; and class IV contains one enzyme, HDAC11 (56, 57). Class I, II, and IV HDACs are all Zn^{2+}-dependent enzymes, while class III HDACs do not show any sequence similarity to the other three classes and depend on NAD+ as a co-factor (56, 57). By reversing the histone acetylation status, HDACs mostly regulate the expression of tumor suppressor genes (4). The dysregulation of HATs and HDACs is correlated with the occurrence and development of various diseases, including cancer.

Mutations in genes encoding HDACs are associated with the progression of tumors, owing to the abnormal transcription of key genes that regulate important cellular functions such as cell proliferation, cell cycle regulation and apoptosis. Some studies have shown that HDACs are mutated in certain cancers. For example, somatic mutations of HDAC1 were detected in ~8% of dedifferentiated human liposarcomas, and the dysfunction of HDAC2 expression caused by a frame-shift mutation was investigated in human epithelial cancers and in colorectal cancer (58). **Table 1** summarizes some of the mutated sites in HDAC2, which may correlate with the development and progression of tumors. However, most of the mutations in HDACs have not been studied and require further investigation. In addition to the discovery that HDACs are mutated in a variety of cancers, there have been many reports in recent years that the HAT CREBBP somatic mutations are more frequent in lymphomas, lung cancer, urothelial carcinoma, and other human tumor types. Jiang et al. reported that somatic mutations in CREBBP occur in 6.4–22.3% of patients with DLBCL and 30.8–68% of follicular lymphoma. Their findings suggest that CREBBP mutation can promote lymphomagenesis *in vivo* (59). Similarly, the results of Jia et al. showed that *CREBBP* acts as a tumor suppressor gene, and its inactivating mutations can promote tumorigenesis of pre-neoplastic neuroendocrine cells and accelerate small cell lung cancer in the autochthonous mouse model (60). The above results suggested that the mutations in HATs and HDACs, although relative low in frequency, might also be involved into the carcinogenesis in various tumors.

INHIBITORS TARGETING MUTATIONS OF EPIGENETIC REGULATORY ENZYMES

Inhibitors Targeting DNMT Mutants

The DNMT inhibitors 5-azacytidine and decitabine (5-aza-2′-deoxycytidine) have already been approved by the FDA (3). These inhibitors are nucleoside analogs which are incorporated into DNA and then covalently trap DNMTs. The results of research by Xu et al. showed that 5-azacytidine might be a suitable drug for the treatment of AML with DNMT3A mutations (8). In a study comparing small molecule inhibitors of DNMT3A R882H, compound 9 (dichlone) displayed superior efficacy, indicating its potential for targeting mutant DNMT3A (61). Interestingly, a recent study showed that targeting DOT1L, a histone lysine methyltransferase without a SET domain, also has an obvious antitumor effect in DNMT3A mutant leukemia. Rau et al. found that the DOT1L inhibitors SYC-52221 and EPZ004777 decreased tumor cell proliferation and induced cell apoptosis, cycle arrest and terminal differentiation in DNMT3A mutant cell lines in a dose- and time-dependent manner (62). Furthermore, they reported that the DOT1L inhibitor EPZ5676 showed promising efficacy in a nude mouse xenograft model of AML with mutant DNMT3A (62). Since pharmacological inhibitors of DOT1L have been tested in clinical trials, DOT1L may be an indirect therapeutic target for the treatment of AML with DNMT3A mutations. These results suggesting a novel approach for treating patients with DNMT3A mutations.

For the TET2, although inhibitors targeting TET2 mutations have not yet been developed, the results of Bejar et al. indicated that cells in MDS patients with TET2-deficient are more sensitive to azacitidine treatment, and this suggests that patients with MDS carrying the TET2 mutation can improve their response to hypomethylating agents (63). However, the detailed mechanisms mediating this process need further study.

Inhibitors Targeting EZH2 Mutants

Recently, studies have shown that small molecule inhibitors can effectively target tumors driven by EZH2 mutations.

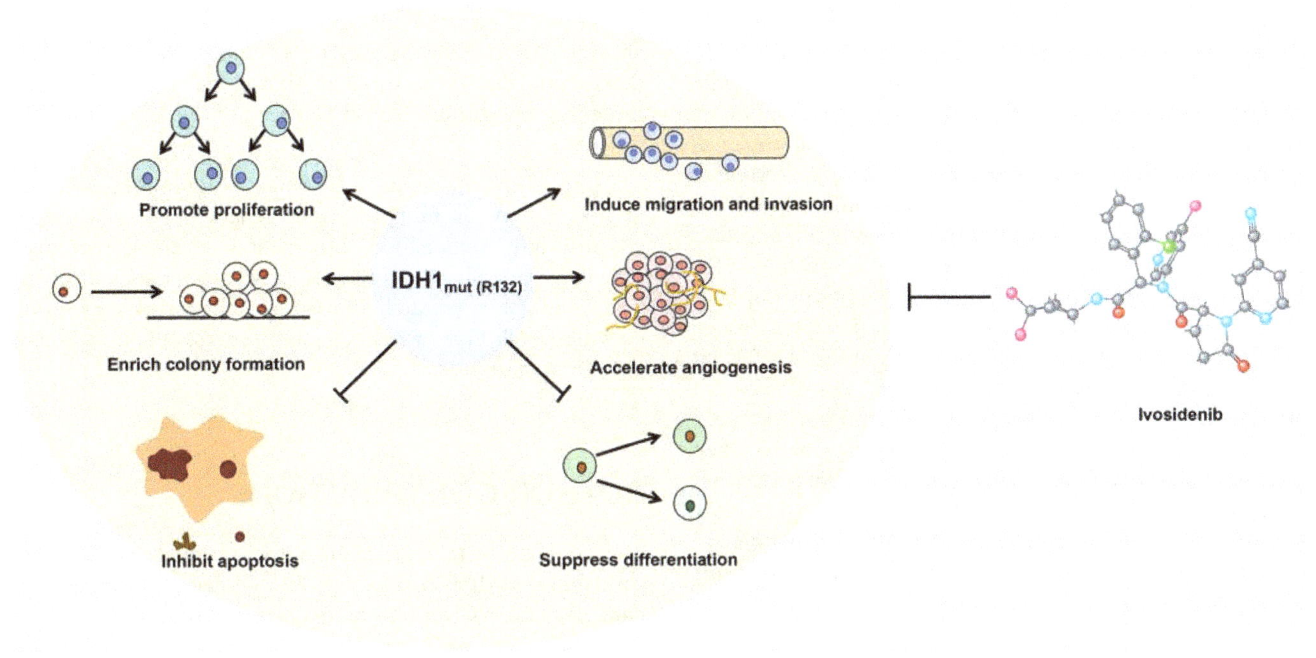

FIGURE 1 | The IDH1 R132 mutant is shown as an example to illustrate how a gain-of-function mutation in an epigenetic enzyme affects the growth and differentiation of cells. Ivosidenib, a specific inhibitor of the IDH1 R132 mutant, is shown at the right.

Knutson et al. have reported that the SAM-competitive EZH2 inhibitor EPZ005687, which is highly selective for EZH2 over other methyltransferases, significantly reduced the viability of lymphoma cell lines carrying the EZH2 Y641 and A677 mutations (64). McCabe et al. discovered that GSK126 is a SAM-competitive small molecule inhibitor of EZH2 methyltransferase activity that efficiently and selectively reduced H3K27me3 levels and reactivated the silenced target genes of polycomb repressive complex 2 (PRC2) (41). Their results also revealed that GSK126 effectively inhibited the proliferation of EZH2-mutant diffuse large B-cell lymphoma (DLBCL) cell lines and retarded the growth of EZH2-mutant DLBCL xenografts in mice (41). In addition, EPZ-6438, another selective inhibitor of EZH2, exerted potent antitumor activity against EZH2-mutant non-Hodgkin's lymphoma (65). Also, CPI-1205, an orally available selective inhibitor of EZH2, killed cells in both EZH2-WT and EZH2-mutant B-cell non-Hodgkin's lymphoma by altering PRC2 target gene expression in a dose- and time-dependent manner (5). All of the above inhibitors markedly reduced the high level of H3K27 trimethylation caused by EZH2 mutations, indicating that inhibition of EZH2 methyltransferase activity may be an effective way of treating EZH2 mutant lymphomas. EPZ005687 is currently in preclinical research, whereas GSK126, EPZ-6438 and CPI-1205 are under phase I/II investigation to assess their efficacy in patients with non-Hodgkin's lymphoma and certain solid tumors (5). In view of the high rate of EZH2 mutation in certain cancers, the application of these inhibitors in the clinic is expected to be successful in the future.

However, in addition to focusing on the effects of the EZH2 inhibitor itself on EZH2 mutant enzymes, we also need to consider the use of EZH2 inhibitors in synthetic lethality. Recently, targeting chromatin deficiency in cancer based on synthetic lethality has been used in cancer treatment. Synthetic lethality defines a relationship between two genes, where the loss of either gene is compatible with cell viability, but the loss of both genes causes cell death. Morel *et al.* summarized that the deficiency of SMARCB1, ARID1A, SMARCA4, and PBRM1, which constitute the chromatin remodeling complex SWI/SNF subunit, led to an EZH2 oncogenic dependence in tumor cells, and pharmacological EZH2 inhibitors such as tazemetostat induced dramatic tumor shrinkage in these subunits-deficient tumors (66). Therefore, synthetic lethality strategy may pave the way to potential epigenetic drugs targets.

Inhibitors Targeting IDH Mutants

Inhibitors targeting mutant IDH enzymes have also been widely investigated. In preclinical studies, it is reported that inhibitors targeting mutated forms of IDH1 and IDH2 can inhibit the growth of glioma cells and induce the differentiation of primary human IDH mutant AML cells *in vitro* (67). Encouragingly, clinical studies of inhibitors targeting mutated IDH have entered the phase I stage, and two inhibitors have been approved by the FDA for clinical use (68). For example, enasidenib (AG-221), a novel-specific small molecule inhibitor targeting mutant IDH2, was approved by the FDA in August 2017 for the treatment of relapsed AML (69). Another novel specific small molecule inhibitor, ivosidenib (AG-120), was approved by the FDA in July 2018 for clinical treatment of relapsed and refractory AML. Ivosidenib targets IDH1 with a mutation at the R132 site (see **Figure 1**) (70). Three other small molecule inhibitors, AGI-881,

IDH305, and FT-2102, are currently in phase I clinical trials. AGI-881 is a non-specific small molecule inhibitor which can target the mutant forms of both IDH1 and IDH2, whereas IDH-305 and FT-2102 target mutant IDH1 (68). These inhibitors prevent the reduction of α-KG to 2-HG by binding to the active site of the mutated IDH enzyme. High levels of 2-HG can inhibit DNA and histone demethylation, leading to hypermethylation. Borodovsky et al. have demonstrated that hypomethylating agents strongly induce differentiation, reduce colony formation ability, and suppress the growth of IDH mutant cells *in vivo* (71). Therefore, inhibitors targeting DNA and histone modifications may have potential therapeutic value. The DNA methyltransferase inhibitors decitabine (DAC) and 5-azacytidine have been approved by the FDA for clinical application and may have a therapeutic effect on tumors caused by IDH mutations (72). These findings also suggest that there is crosstalk among different epigenetic regulatory enzymes. In contrast to IDH mutation inhibitors, studies on inhibitors targeting SDH and FH mutations are currently lagging behind, which may lay the foundation for the development of new anti-tumor drugs.

CONCLUSION AND PERSPECTIVES

DNA methylation and histone modification are common epigenetic changes in eukaryotes, and the dysregulation of epigenetic regulatory enzymes is closely related to the onset and progression of various types of cancer. Mutations, especially gain-of-function mutations, may be responsible for some changes in epigenetic enzyme activity. Mutant epigenetic regulatory enzymes, and mutant forms of IDH that affect epigenetic changes, can enhance the ability of cancer cells to proliferate, migrate and form colonies. Therefore, these mutations are closely related to tumor onset and progression. Some inhibitors that specifically target the mutant forms of epigenetic regulatory enzymes and IDH have now entered clinical trials. The potential therapeutic effects of these inhibitors on tumors caused by mutations are summarized in **Figure 1**.

Many of the mechanisms by which mutations cause changes in the activity or function of epigenetic regulatory enzymes are not fully understood. Elucidation of these mechanisms may drive our understanding of the characteristics of different tumors. Further research into drugs that target these mutant enzymes will also accelerate the process of individualized treatment of tumors.

AUTHOR CONTRIBUTIONS

MH contributes to draft manuscript and analysis the data. LJ contributes to draft manuscript. WL contributes to analysis the data. LW and WC contribute to design and draft the manuscript.

FUNDING

This work was financially supported by the National Natural Science Foundation of China (No. 81673652, 81572947, 81773780, 81773216), the Natural Science Foundation of Liaoning Province (No. 20170540841, 20180550076), the Scientific Research Fund of Liaoning Provincial Education Department (No. 2017LFW01) and the Science Foundation of Shenyang Pharmaceutical University (No. DFJJ2018210).

REFERENCES

1. Egger G, Liang G, Aparicio A, Jones PA. Epigenetics in human disease and prospects for epigenetic therapy. *Nature.* (2004) 429:457–63. doi: 10.1038/nature02625
2. Lund AH, Lohuizen MV. Epigenetics and cancer. *Genes Dev.* (2004) 18:2315–35. doi: 10.1101/gad.1232504
3. Carlberg C, Molnár F. Cancer epigenomics. *Hum Epigenomics.* (2018) 159–74. doi: 10.1007/978-981-10-7614-5_10
4. Mottamal M, Zheng S, Huang T, Wang G. Histone deacetylase inhibitors in clinical studies as templates for new anticancer agents. *Molecules.* (2015) 20:3898–941. doi: 10.3390/molecules20033898
5. Gulati N, Béguelin W, Giulino-Roth L. Enhancer of zeste homolog 2 (EZH2) inhibitors. *Leuk Lymphoma.* (2018) 59:1574–85. doi: 10.1080/10428194.2018.1430795
6. Tatton-Brown K, Seal S, Ruark E, Harmer J, Ramsay E, Rahman N, et al. Mutations in the DNA methyltransferase gene DNMT3A cause an overgrowth syndrome with intellectual disability. *Nat Genet.* (2014) 46:385–8. doi: 10.1038/ng.2917
7. Cohen AL, Holmen SL, Colman H. IDH1 and IDH2 mutations in gliomas. *Curr Neurol Neurosci Rep.* (2013) 13:345. doi: 10.1007/s11910-013-0345-4
8. Xu J, Wang YY, Dai YJ, Zhang W, Zhang WN, Xiong SM, et al. DNMT3A Arg882 mutation drives chronic myelomonocytic leukemia through disturbing gene expression/DNA methylation in hematopoietic cells. *Proc Natl Acad Sci USA.* (2014) 111:2620–5. doi: 10.1073/pnas.1400150111
9. Ballestar E. The impact of chromatin in human cancer: linking DNA methylation to gene silencing. *Carcinogenesis.* (2002) 23:1103–9. doi: 10.1093/carcin/23.7.1103
10. Singal R, Ginder GD. DNA methylation. *Blood.* (1999) 93:4059–70. doi: 10.1016/S0887-7963(99)80035-2
11. Chen QW, Zhu XY, Li YY, Meng ZQ. Epigenetic regulation and cancer. *Oncol Rep.* (2014) 31:523–32. doi: 10.3892/or.2013.2913
12. Boyes J, Bird A. DNA methylation inhibits transcription indirectly via a methyl-CpG binding protein. *Cell.* (1991) 64:1123–34. doi: 10.1016/0092-8674(91)90267-3
13. Costello JF, Frühwald MC, Smiraglia DJ, Rush LJ, Robertson GP, Gao X, et al. Aberrant CpG-island methylation has non-random and tumour-type-specific patterns. *Nat Genet.* (2000) 24:132–8. doi: 10.1038/72785
14. Baylin SB, Jones PA. A decade of exploring the cancer epigenome — biological and translational implications. *Nat Rev Cancer.* (2011) 11:726–34. doi: 10.1038/nrc3130
15. Yamashita Y, Yuan J, Suetake I, Suzuki H, Ishikawa Y, Choi YL, et al. Array-based genomic resequencing of human leukemia. *Oncogene.* (2010) 29:3723–31. doi: 10.1038/onc.2010.117
16. Elsayed GM, Fahmi AEA, Shafik NF, Elshimy RAA, Abd Elhakeem HK, Attea SA. Study of DNA methyl transferase 3A mutation in acute myeloid leukemic patients. *Egypt J Med Hum Genet.* (2018) 19:315–9. doi: 10.1016/j.ejmhg.2018.05.005
17. Russler-Germain DA, Spencer DH, Young MA, Lamprecht TL, Miller CA, Fulton R, et al. The R882H DNMT3A mutation associated with AML

dominantly inhibits wild-type DNMT3A by blocking its ability to form active tetramers. *Cancer Cell.* (2014) 25:442–54. doi: 10.1016/j.ccr.2014.02.010
18. Pløen GG, Nederby L, Guldberg P, Hansen M, Ebbesen LH, Jensen UB, et al. Persistence of DNMT3A mutations at long-term remission in adult patients with AML. *Br J Haematol.* (2014) 167:478–86. doi: 10.1111/bjh.13062
19. Varambally S, Dhanasekaran SM, Zhou M, Barrette TR, Kumar-Sinha C, Sanda MG, et al. The polycomb group protein EZH2 is involved in progression of prostate cancer. *Nature.* (2002) 419:624–9. doi: 10.1038/nature01075
20. Behrens C, Solis LM, Lin H, Yuan P, Tang X, Kadara H, et al. EZH2 Protein Expression Associates with the early pathogenesis, tumor progression, and prognosis of non-small cell lung carcinoma. *Clin Cancer Res.* (2013) 19:6556–65. doi: 10.1158/1078-0432.ccr-12-3946
21. Zhou Z, Gao J, Popovic R, Wolniak K, Parimi V, Winter JN, et al. Strong expression of EZH2 and accumulation of trimethylated H3K27 in diffuse large B-cell lymphoma independent of cell of origin and EZH2 codon 641 mutation. *Leuk Lymphoma.* (2015) 56:2895–901. doi: 10.3109/10428194.2015.1006220
22. Sneeringer CJ, Scott MP, Kuntz KW, Knutson SK, Pollock RM, Richon VM, et al. Coordinated activities of wild-type plus mutant EZH2 drive tumor-associated hypertrimethylation of lysine 27 on histone H3 (H3K27) in human B-cell lymphomas. *Proc Natl Acad Sci USA.* (2010) 107:20980–5. doi: 10.1073/pnas.1012525107
23. Kickingereder P, Sahm F, Radbruch A, Wick W, Heiland S, Deimling A, et al. Wiestler, B. (2015). IDH mutation status is associated with a distinct hypoxia/angiogenesis transcriptome signature which is non-invasively predictable with rCBV imaging in human glioma. *Sci Rep.* 5:16238. doi: 10.1038/srep16238
24. Bodor C, Grossmann V, Popov N, Okosun J, O'Riain C, Tan K, et al. EZH2 mutations are frequent and represent an early event in follicular lymphoma. *Blood.* (2013) 122:3165–8. doi: 10.1182/blood-2013-04-496893
25. Souroullas GP, Jeck WR, Parker JS, Simon JM, Liu J-Y, Paulk J, et al. An oncogenic Ezh2 mutation induces tumors through global redistribution of histone 3 lysine 27 trimethylation. *Nat Med.* (2016) 22:632–40. doi: 10.1038/nm.4092
26. Majer CR, Jin L, Scott MP, Knutson SK, Kuntz KW, Keilhack H, et al. A687V EZH2 is a gain-of-function mutation found in lymphoma patients. *FEBS Lett.* (2012) 586:3448–51. doi: 10.1016/j.febslet.2012.07.066
27. Dang L, Jin S, Su SM. IDH mutations in glioma and acute myeloid leukemia. *Trends Mol Med.* (2010) 16:387–97. doi: 10.1016/j.molmed.2010.07.002
28. Pollard PJ, Loenarz C, Mole DR, McDonough MA, Gleadle JM, Schofield CJ, et al. Regulation of Jumonji-domain-containing histone demethylases by hypoxia-inducible factor (HIF)-1α. *Bioch J.* (2008) 416:387–94. doi: 10.1042/bj20081238
29. Kanai Y, Ushijima S, Nakanishi Y, Sakamoto M, Hirohashi S. Mutation of the DNA methyltransferase (DNMT) 1 gene in human colorectal cancers. *Cancer Lett.* (2003) 192:75–82. doi: 10.1016/s0304-3835(02)00689-4
30. Yang L, Rau R, Goodell MA. DNMT3A in haematological malignancies. *Nat Rev Cancer.* (2015) 15:152–65. doi: 10.1038/nrc3895
31. Hansen RS, Wijmenga C, Luo P, Stanek AM, Canfield TK, Weemaes CMR, et al. The DNMT3B DNA methyltransferase gene is mutated in the ICF immunodeficiency syndrome. *Proc Natl Acad Sci USA.* (1999) 96:14412–7. doi: 10.1073/pnas.96.25.14412
32. Ko M, Bandukwala HS, An J, Lamperti ED, Thompson EC, Hastie R, et al. Ten-Eleven-Translocation 2 (TET2) negatively regulates homeostasis and differentiation of hematopoietic stem cells in mice. *Proc Natl Acad Sci USA.* (2011) 108:14566–71. doi: 10.1073/pnas.1112317108
33. Xu J, Zhang W, Yan XJ, Lin XQ, Li W, Mi JQ, et al. DNMT3A mutation leads to leukemic extramedullary infiltration mediated by TWIST1. *J Hematol Oncol.* (2016) 9:106. doi: 10.1186/s13045-016-0337-3
34. Koya J, Kataoka K, Sato T, Bando M, Kato Y, Tsuruta-Kishino T, et al. DNMT3A R882 mutants interact with polycomb proteins to block haematopoietic stem and leukaemic cell differentiation. *Nat Commun.* (2016) 7:10924. doi: 10.1038/ncomms10924
35. Guryanova OA, Shank K, Spitzer B, Luciani L, Koche RP, Garrett-Bakelman FE, et al. DNMT3A mutations promote anthracycline resistance in acute myeloid leukemia via impaired nucleosome remodeling. *Nat Med.* (2016) 22:1488–95. doi: 10.1038/nm.4210
36. Ley TJ, Ding L, Walter MJ, McLellan MD, Lamprecht T, Larson DE, et al. DNMT3A mutations in acute myeloid leukemia. *New Engl J Med.* (2010) 363:2424–33. doi: 10.1056/nejmoa1005143
37. Ferreira HJ, Heyn H, Vizoso M, Moutinho C, Vidal E, Gomez A, et al. DNMT3A mutations mediate the epigenetic reactivation of the leukemogenic factor MEIS1 in acute myeloid leukemia. *Oncogene.* (2015) 35:3079–82. doi: 10.1038/onc.2015.359
38. Delhommeau F, Dupont S, Valle VD, James C, Trannoy S, Massé A, et al. Mutation inTET2in Myeloid Cancers. *New Engl J Med.* (2009) 360:2289–301. doi: 10.1056/nejmoa0810069
39. Wei S, Li C, Yin Z, Wen J, Meng H, Xue L, et al. Histone methylation in DNA repair and clinical practice: new findings during the past 5-years. *J Cancer.* (2018) 9:2072–81. doi: 10.7150/jca.23427
40. Simon JA, Lange CA. Roles of the EZH2 histone methyltransferase in cancer epigenetics. *Mutat Res Fund Mol Mech Mutag.* (2008) 647:21–9. doi: 10.1016/j.mrfmmm.2008.07.010
41. McCabe MT, Ott HM, Ganji G, Korenchuk S, Thompson C, Van Aller GS, et al. EZH2 inhibition as a therapeutic strategy for lymphoma with EZH2-activating mutations. *Nature.* (2012) 492:108–12. doi: 10.1038/nature11606
42. Barsotti AM, Ryskin M, Zhong W, Zhang W-G, Giannakou A, Loreth C, et al. Epigenetic reprogramming by tumor-derived EZH2 gain-of-function mutations promotes aggressive 3D cell morphologies and enhances melanoma tumor growth. *Oncotarget.* (2015) 6:2928–38. doi: 10.18632/oncotarget.2758
43. Vannucchi AM, Lasho TL, Guglielmelli P, Biamonte F, Pardanani A, Pereira A, et al. Mutations and prognosis in primary myelofibrosis. *Leukemia.* (2013) 27:1861–9. doi: 10.1038/leu.2013.119
44. Saldanha SN, Tollefsbol TO. Epigenetic approaches to cancer therapy. *Epigenet Hum Dis.* (2018) 219–47. doi: 10.1016/b978-0-12-812215-0.00007-8
45. Kipp BR, Voss JS, Kerr SE, Barr Fritcher EG, Graham RP, Zhang L, et al. Isocitrate dehydrogenase 1 and 2 mutations in cholangiocarcinoma. *Hum Pathol.* (2012) 43:1552–8. doi: 10.1016/j.humpath.2011.12.007
46. Ghiam AF, Cairns RA, Thoms J, Dal Pra A, Ahmed O, Meng A, et al. IDH mutation status in prostate cancer. *Oncogene.* (2011) 31:3826. doi: 10.1038/onc.2011.546
47. Ciccarone F, Vegliante R, Di Leo L, Ciriolo MR. The TCA cycle as a bridge between oncometabolism and DNA transactions in cancer. *Sem Cancer Biol.* (2017) 47:50–6. doi: 10.1016/j.semcancer.2017.06.008
48. Fu Y, Zheng Y, Li K, Huang R, Zheng S, An N, et al. Mutations in isocitrate dehydrogenase 2 accelerate glioma cell migration via matrix metalloproteinase-2 and 9. *Biotechnol Lett.* (2011) 34:441–6. doi: 10.1007/s10529-011-0800-8
49. Fu Y, Zheng S, Zheng Y, Huang R, An N, Liang A, et al. Glioma derived isocitrate dehydrogenase-2 mutations induced up-regulation of HIF-1α and β-catenin signaling: Possible impact on glioma cell metastasis and chemo-resistance. *Int J Biochem Cell Biol.* (2012) 44:770–5. doi: 10.1016/j.biocel.2012.01.017
50. Saha SK, Parachoniak CA, Ghanta KS, Fitamant J, Ross KN, Najem MS, et al. Mutant IDH inhibits HNF-4α to block hepatocyte differentiation and promote biliary cancer. *Nature.* (2014) 513:110–4. doi: 10.1038/nature13441
51. Figueroa ME, Abdel-Wahab O, Lu C, Ward PS, Patel J, Shih A, et al. Leukemic IDH1 and IDH2 Mutations result in a hypermethylation phenotype, disrupt TET2 function, and impair hematopoietic differentiation. *Cancer Cell.* (2010) 18:553–67. doi: 10.1016/j.ccr.2010.11.015
52. Lu C, Ward PS, Kapoor GS, Rohle D, Turcan S, Abdel-Wahab O, et al. IDH mutation impairs histone demethylation and results in a block to cell differentiation. *Nature.* (2012) 483:474–8. doi: 10.1038/nature10860
53. Goyal L, Govindan A, Sheth RA, Nardi V, Blaszkowsky LS, Faris JE, et al. Prognosis and clinicopathologic features of patients with advanced stage Isocitrate Dehydrogenase (IDH) Mutant and IDH wild-type intrahepatic cholangiocarcinoma. *Oncologist.* (2015) 20:1019–27. doi: 10.1634/theoncologist.2015-0210
54. Kelly AD, Issa JPJ. The promise of epigenetic therapy: reprogramming the cancer epigenome. *Curr Opin Genet Dev.* (2017) 42:68–77. doi: 10.1016/j.gde.2017.03.015

55. Marmorstein R, Roth SY. Histone acetyltransferases: function, structure, and catalysis. *Curr Opin Genet Dev.* (2001) 11:155–61. doi: 10.1016/s0959-437x(00)00173-8
56. Yanginlar C, Logie C. HDAC11 is a regulator of diverse immune functions. *Biochim Biophys Acta Gene Regul Mech.* (2018) 1861:54–9. doi: 10.1016/j.bbagrm.2017.12.002
57. Wang L, Beier UH, Akimova T, Dahiya S, Han R, Samanta A, et al. Histone/protein deacetylase inhibitor therapy for enhancement of Foxp3+ T-regulatory cell function posttransplantation. *Am J Transpl.* (2018) 18:1596–603. doi: 10.1111/ajt.14749
58. Ropero S, Esteller M. The role of histone deacetylases (HDACs) in human cancer. *Mol Oncol.* (2007) 1:19–25. doi: 10.1016/j.molonc.2007.01.001
59. Jiang Y, Ortega-Molina A, Geng H, Ying H-Y, Hatzi K, Parsa S, et al. CREBBP inactivation promotes the development of HDAC3-dependent lymphomas. *Cancer Disc.* (2016) 7:38–53. doi: 10.1158/2159-8290.cd-16-0975
60. Jia D, Augert A, Kim DW, Eastwood E, Wu N, Ibrahim AH, et al. Crebbp loss drives small cell lung cancer and increases sensitivity to HDAC inhibition. *Cancer Disc.* (2018) 8:1422–37. doi: 10.1158/2159-8290.cd-18-0385
61. Emperle M, Rajavelu A, Kunert S, Arimondo PB, Reinhardt R, Jurkowska RZ, et al. The DNMT3A R882H mutant displays altered flanking sequence preferences. *Nucleic Acids Res.* (2018) 46:3130–9. doi: 10.1093/nar/gky168
62. Rau RE, Rodriguez BA, Luo M, Jeong M, Rosen A, Rogers JH, et al. DOT1L as a therapeutic target for the treatment of DNMT3A-mutant acute myeloid leukemia. *Blood.* (2016) 128:971–81. doi: 10.1182/blood-2015-11-684225
63. Bejar R, Lord A, Stevenson K, Bar-Natan M, Perez-Ladaga A, Zaneveld J, et al. TET2 mutations predict response to hypomethylating agents in myelodysplastic syndrome patients. *Blood.* (2014) 124:2705–12. doi: 10.1182/blood-2014-06-582809
64. Knutson SK, Wigle TJ, Warholic NM, Sneeringer CJ, Allain CJ, Klaus CR, et al. A selective inhibitor of EZH2 blocks H3K27 methylation and kills mutant lymphoma cells. *Nat Chem Biol.* (2012) 8:890–6. doi: 10.1038/nchembio.1084
65. Knutson SK, Kawano S, Minoshima Y, Warholic NM, Huang K-C, Xiao Y, et al. Selective inhibition of EZH2 by EPZ-6438 leads to potent antitumor activity in EZH2-mutant non-hodgkin lymphoma. *Mol Cancer Ther.* (2014) 13:842–54. doi: 10.1158/1535-7163.mct-13-0773
66. Morel D, Almouzni G, Soria JC, Postel-Vinay S. Targeting chromatin defects in selected solid tumors based on oncogene addiction, synthetic lethality and epigenetic antagonism. *Ann Oncol.* (2016) 28:254–69. doi: 10.1093/annonc/mdw552
67. Dang L, Yen K, Attar EC. IDH mutations in cancer and progress toward development of targeted therapeutics. *Ann Oncol.* (2016) 27:599–608. doi: 10.1093/annonc/mdw013
68. Montalban-Bravo G, DiNardo CD. The role of IDH mutations in acute myeloid leukemia. *Future Oncol.* (2018) 14:979–93. doi: 10.2217/fon-2017-0523
69. Kim ES. Enasidenib: first global approval. *Drugs.* (2017) 77:1705–11. doi: 10.1007/s40265-017-0813-2
70. Popovici-Muller J, Lemieux RM, Artin E, Saunders JO, Salituro FG, Travins J, et al. Discovery of AG-120 (Ivosidenib): a first-in-class mutant IDH1 inhibitor for the treatment of IDH1 mutant cancers. *ACS Med Chem Lett.* (2018) 9:300–5. doi: 10.1021/acsmedchemlett.7b00421
71. Borodovsky A, Salmasi V, Turcan S. 5-azacytidine reduces methylation, promotes differentiation and induces tumor regression in a patient-derived IDH1 mutant glioma xenograft. *Oncotarget.* (2013) 4:1737–47. doi: 10.18632/oncotarget.1408
72. Roy DM, Walsh LA, Chan TA. Driver mutations of cancer epigenomes. *Protein Cell.* (2014) 5:265–96. doi: 10.1007/s13238-014-0031-6

12

Glucose-Regulated Protein 78 Signaling Regulates Hypoxia-Induced Epithelial–Mesenchymal Transition in A549 Cells

*Ling-Ling Sun, Chang-Ming Chen, Jue Zhang, Jing Wang, Cai-Zhi Yang and Li-Zhu Lin**

Integrative Cancer Centre, the First Affiliated Hospital of Guangzhou University of Chinese Medicine, Guangzhou, China

Correspondence:
Li-Zhu Lin
lizhulin26@yahoo.com

Objective: Metastasis and therapeutic resistance are the major determinants of lung cancer progression and high mortality. Epithelial–mesenchymal transition (EMT) plays a key role in the metastasis and therapeutic resistance. Highly expressed glucose-regulated protein 78 (GRP78) is a poor prognostic factor in lung cancer and possibly correlated with EMT. This study aims to examine whether the up-regulation of GRP78 is involved in EMT in lung adenocarcinoma and explore the underlying downstream molecular pathways.

Study Design: EMT was assessed by analysis of cell morphology and expression of EMT protein markers in A549 cells under normoxia, hypoxia and silencing GRP78 conditions. The expression levels of Smad2/3, Src, and MAPK (p38, ERK, and JNK) proteins were examined by Western blot analysis under hypoxia and treatments with phosphorylation inhibitors.

Results: Under hypoxic conditions, the EMT morphology significantly changed and the GRP78 expression was significantly up-regulated in A549 cells compared with those in normoxia control. The expression and phosphorylation levels of smad2/3, Src, p38, ERK, and JNK were also upregulated. When GRP78 was silenced, EMT was inhibited, and the levels of phospho-smad2/3, phospho-Src, phospho-p38, phospho-ERK, and phospho-JNK were suppressed. When the activation of Smad2/3, Src, p38, ERK, and JNK was inhibited, EMT was also inhibited. The inhibition effect on EMT by these phosphorylation inhibitors was found to be weaker than that of GRP78 knockdown.

Conclusions: Hypoxia-induced EMT in A549 cells is regulated by GRP78 signaling pathways. GRP78 promotes EMT by activating Smad2/3 and Src/MAPK pathways. Hence, GRP78 might be a potential target for treatment of lung adenocarcinoma.

Keywords: lung cancer, lung adenocarcinoma, epithelial mesenchymal transition, hypoxia, glucose-regulated protein 78, GRP78

INTRODUCTION

Lung cancer is the leading cause of cancer death worldwide; according to the estimated data from GLOBOCAN in 2012, one of five cancer deaths is due to lung cancer (1.59 million deaths, 19.4% of the total cancer deaths) (1). Despite significant progress in the development of new therapies for lung cancer, metastasis and therapeutic resistance remain the major determinants of lung cancer progression and high mortality (2).

Mounting evidence demonstrated that epithelial–mesenchymal transition (EMT) is involved in the metastasis and therapeutic resistance of lung cancer. EMT refers to the biological process by which epithelial cells are transformed into mesenchymal phenotypes through specific procedures. EMT inhibits the expression of E-cadherin and cytokeratin in epithelial cells, upregulates the expression of N-cadherin and vimentin in mesenchymal cells and promotes the ability of cells to secrete matrix metalloproteinase and fibronectin. EMT can be induced by various factors, such as TGF-beta, which increases the expression of key nuclear transcription factors including Twist, Snail and ZEB (3) and causes phenotypic changes by activating intrinsic cellular signal molecules including Src, MAPK, Smad2/3, and other signals (4–6).

Hypoxia is a common hallmark of several human malignancies and an independent and unfavorable prognostic factor associated with the occurrence of EMT (7–9). Previous studies found that cAMP-dependent protein kinase, hypoxia factor Hif-1alpha(HIF1a) and unfolded protein response can potentiate EMT; moreover, treatment with insulin-like growth factor 1 receptor inhibitor reverses hypoxia-induced EMT (8–11), However, the mechanisms of hypoxia-induced EMT remain unknown. Understanding the biology of hypoxia-induced EMT and their implications in therapeutic relapse may provide new crucial approaches for development of improved therapeutic strategies.

The 78-kDa glucose-regulated protein (GRP78), also known as BiP and HSPA5, is highly expressed in many types of cancers, including lung, hepatocellular cancer, and breast cancer (12–15). It could inhibit apoptosis of cancer cells, and induce chemoresistance of cancer (16–18). What's more, it is closely related to EMT. Zhang et al. (19) reported that high expressed GRP78 induced EMT in hepatocellular carcinoma cell lines. Lizardo et al. (20) that up-regulation of GRP78 in metastatic cancer cells is necessary for lung metastasis in some highly metastatic cell line models, such as osteosarcomas and murine mammary adenocarcinoma. Zhang et al. (21) demonstrated that overexpressing GRP78 facilitated the expression and secretion of TGF-beta1, which further activated EMT. However, Chang et al. (22) stated that overexpressing GRP78 inhibited the metastasis of colon cancer through EMT biomarkers. Thus far, the relationship between GRP78 expression and EMT remains controversial. Whether GRP78 expression has causality link with EMT in lung cancer also remains unknown. Hence, the present study aims to examine the role of up-regulation of GRP78 in EMT in lung adenocarcinoma and explore the downstream molecular pathways involved.

METHODS

Cell Culture and Conditioning

Human lung adenocarcinoma A549 cells were purchased from the Cell Bank of the Chinese Academy of Sciences (Shanghai, China) and cultured in RPMI-1640 medium (Gibco, USA) supplied with 10% FBS (Gibco, USA) and 100 U/ml penicillin/streptomycin in 5% CO_2 incubator at 37°C. The medium was changed every 3 days. The cells were treated with normal O_2 as control.

A549 cells were cultured with 2% O_2 for hypoxia condition. The concentration of protein inhibitors for treatment of A549 cells were as follows: 550 nM SB505124 (phospho-Smad2/3 inhibitor), 25 nM KX2-391 (phospho-Src inhibitor), 100 nM JNK-IN-8 (phospho-JNK inhibitor), 2.5 μM SB203580 (phospho-p38 inhibitor), and 1.5 μM FR180204 (phospho-ERK). All of the inhibitors were purchased from Celleck Chemicals (USA).

Assessment of Cell Morphology

Morphological changes were examined using phase-contrast microscopy (Olympus, Japan).

Real-Time Quantitative Fluorescent PCR

Experiments were performed following the methods in our previous study. The cells were collected to extract total RNA using Trizol method. The cDNA was synthesized with Prime Script TMRT Master Mix (RR036A; Takara, Japan) through reverse transcription and used as template to amplify target genes with real-time quantitative fluorescent PCR with SYBR® Premix Ex TaqII (RR820A; Takara, Japan). The specific primers (Invitrogen, USA) of each transcription factor (Snail1, Snail2, Twist, ZEB1 and ZEB2) were also based on such study (23). The reaction condition was 95°C for 30 s, followed by 95°C for 5 s and 60°C for 30 s with 40 cycles. The amplified productions were quantitatively analyzed with 2-ΔΔCt method. All tests were repeated three times.

Western Blot Analysis

Experiments were performed following the methods in our previous study. The specific program and concentration of each antibody were also based on such study (23). Briefly, the protein was extracted with PIRA buffer and centrifuged at 12,000 g for 15 min at 4°C. Fifty microgram total proteins were separated with 10%SDS-PAGE. After electrophoresis, proteins were blotted to polyvinylidene fluoride (PVDF) membranes and then blocked with 5% skim milk powder with 0.1% Tween-20. The blots were then probed at 4°C overnight with the relevant primary antibodies respectively, and incubated in 4°C for overnight. The membranes were rinsed with TBST for 3 times, 10 min each time. Then secondary goat anti-rabbit or anti-mouse IgG-HRP antibodies were added for incubation in room temperature for 2 h. The membranes were rinsed with TBST for 3 times, and 10 min per time. Then the membranes were developed with ECL (Beijing Kangwei Biotech, China) and taken photos to analyze the relative expression of proteins with GAPDH as internal referral. All tests were repeated three times.

Immunofluorescence Staining

Cells were cultured on six-well chamber slides for immunofluorescent staining. The cells were fixed in 4% paraformaldehyde for 30 min at room temperature. After washing with PBS three times for 10 min each time, the cells were permeabilised with 0.1% Triton X-100 in PBS for 15 min. After three washes with PBS, the cells were blocked with 5%

BSA for 30 min at room temperature. The cells were incubated with the indicated GRP78 antibody (1:250) overnight at 4°C, washed three times with PBS and incubated with fluorescent secondary antibodies. Nuclear staining was performed in the dark with DAPI at room temperature. Phase contrast and fluorescent microscopy was performed using an NikonTi-U Inverted Fluorescence Microscope (Nikon, Japan).

Plasmid Transfection and Identification

GRP78 short hairpin RNA(GRP78shRNA) eukaryotic expression plasmid was designed and synthesized by Invitrogen, USA. Transfection and identification were conducted according to the protocol of Lipofectamine 3000. using previously published methods (24). Briefly, 7.5 μl Lipofectamine 3000 Reagent was diluted with 125 μl Opti-MEM media, then blended with a diluted plasmid DNA which diluted by 10 μl P3000 Reagent and 125 μl Opti-MEM media. After incubating for 5 min, the overall mixture was added into the culture cells and cultured for 72 h. The cells carrying green fluorescence are plasmids transfected successfully in inverted microscope. 20 μg/ml blasticidin was used to screen the cells and the maintenance concentration of blasticidin is 10 μg/ml. Blank shRNA was used as a control. The mRNA and protein expression levels of GRP78 decreased by 70 and 85.33%, respectively, suggesting successful transfection.

Statistical Analysis

Data were expressed as mean ± SD. Comparison between two groups was performed with *t*-test for independent samples. Comparison among multiple groups was performed with one-way ANOVA following LSD (equal variances) or Dunnett's *t*-test (unequal variances). $P<0.05$ was set as the significance level. All analyses were performed using SPSS 22.0 software.

RESULTS

Activation of EMT by Hypoxia in A549 Cells

A549 cells cultured under hypoxia condition for 72 h showed morphological changes, from oblate fusiform-shaped epithelial cells to elongated spindle-shaped mesenchymal cells (**Figure 1A**). The expression levels of EMT-related genes including Snail1, Snail2, Twist, ZEB1, and ZEB2 were increased by approximately three times under hypoxic condition compared with that in the control group. The Western blot analysis showed that the protein expression of E-cadherin (biomarker of epithelial phenotype) under hypoxia found to be approximately three times less than that in the control group. The expression levels of vimentin and fibronectin (biomarker of mesenchymal phenotype) were increased by 1.48 and 1.22 times, respectively, under hypoxia condition compared with that in the control group ($P < 0.05$ compared with Normoxia, **Figures 1B,C**).

Expression of GRP78 Under Normoxia and Hypoxia Conditions

The expression and location of the GRP78 protein in A549 cells under hypoxia and normoxia conditions were determined by immunofluorescence staining. Under normoxia condition, GRP78 (green fluorescence) showed weak staining intensity and was mainly distributed in the cytoplasm (**Figure 1A**). By contrast, under hypoxia, A549 cells showed an elongated spindle-shaped mesenchymal phenotype, and GRP78 showed strong staining intensity and was mainly distributed in the cytoplasm and cell membrane (**Figure 1A**). The Western blot analysis showed that the expression of GRP78 in A549 cells under hypoxia was found to be 1.36 times more than that under normoxia (**Figure 1B**).

Effect of GRP78 Knockdown on the Expression of EMT Markers

The expression of GRP78 in GRP78 knockdown A549 cells under hypoxia was reduced by 70% compared with that under hypoxia. In A549 cells transfected with GRP78 shRNA under hypoxia, the expression levels of vimentin and fibronectin significantly decreased by 52 and 60%, respectively. Meanwhile, the mRNA expression levels of transcription factors (Snail1, Snail2, Twist, ZEB1, and ZEB2) were significantly inhibited under hypoxia condition and decreased by approximately 70% compared with that in the normoxia group (**Figures 1B,C**). The significant change in the expression of EMT biomarkers and its transcription factor mRNAs after GRP78 knockdown indicated that GRP78 might play an important role in hypoxia-induced EMT.

Expression of Smad2/3, Src, p38, ERK and JNK in A549 Cells Under Hypoxia Condition

The expression levels of phosphorylated Smad2/3, p38, and JNK in A549 cells significantly increased by approximately 2.4 times under hypoxia condition compared with those under normoxia condition, whereas the levels of the phosphorylated Src and ERK increased by approximately 1.8 times (all $p < 0.05$, **Figure 2A**). Hence, these signaling pathways were activated under hypoxia condition.

The inhibitors of Smad2/3, Src, p38, ERK, and JNK were used to treat A549 cells under hypoxia condition to further verify the relationship between these signaling molecules with hypoxia-induced EMT. The expression levels of EMT protein markers and transcription factor mRNAs were also examined. The changes in EMT protein markers and transcription factor mRNAs in A549 cells were approximately similar to that in the group treated with Smad2/3 and Src inhibitors. The levels of vimentin, fibronectin and mRNAs decreased by approximately 50%, whereas that of E-cadherin increased by 2-fold compared with those in the cells under hypoxia. The change in the three other groups was found to be smaller than that in the group treated with Smad2/3 and Src inhibitors. The levels of vimentin, fibronectin and mRNAs were reduced by approximately 30%. Hence, EMT is inhibited in A549 cells when the activation of Smad2/3, Src, p38, ERK, and JNK proteins is inhibited under hypoxia (**Figure 2B**).

The changes in the expression of EMT protein markers were compared in A549 cells transfected by GRP78shRNA or treated by different protein inhibitors under hypoxia condition. The changes in the mRNA expression of EMT markers and signaling molecules were the most evident in GRP78 knockdown cells ($P < 0.05$ compared with the other groups, **Figures 3A,B**). Similar results were obtained on the protein expression of signaling molecules (Smad2/3, Src, p38, ERK, and JNK). After GRP78

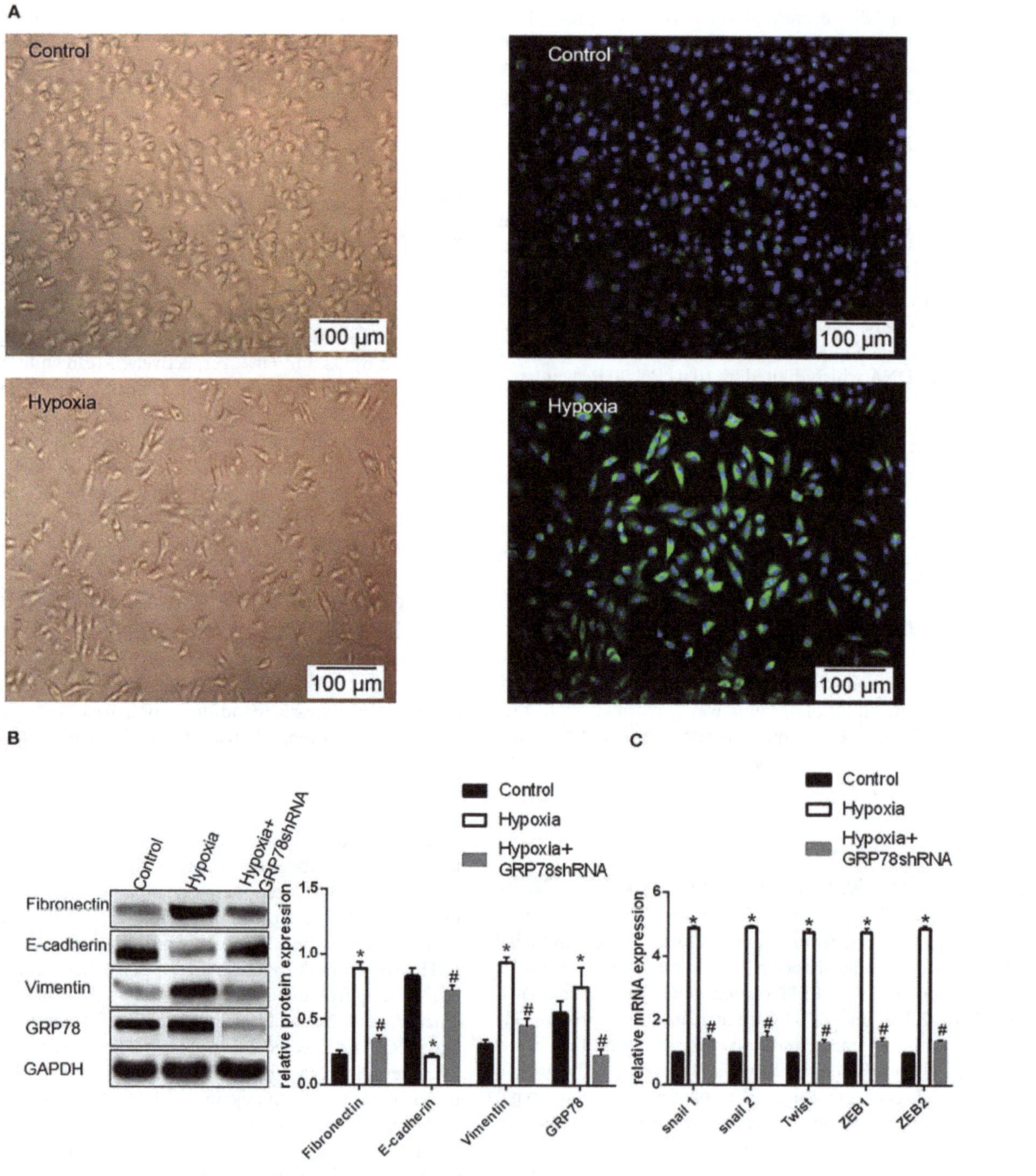

FIGURE 1 | Up-regulation of GRP78 plays an important role in hypoxia-induced EMT in A549 cells. **(A)** A549 cells acquire spindle-shaped mesenchymal morphology after 72 h of 2% O_2 hypoxia (left, 100×). GRP78 (green fluorescence) is highly expressed in A549 cells with spindle-shaped mesenchymal morphology (right, 100×). **(B)** EMT-related markers (E-cadherin, Vimentin and Fibronectin) and GRP78 were examined by Western blot analysis (left). GAPDH was used as internal control. The protein relative value (GAPDH) is plotted in the right panel (mean ± SD in three separate experiments). *$P < 0.05$, compared with A549 cells under the condition of normal oxygen, the expression of E-cadherin decreases, while those of Vimentin and Fibronectin increase in A549 cells under hypoxia (2% O_2 72 h). The expression of GRP78 also increases in A549 cells under hypoxia. #$P < 0.05$, compared with the A549 cells under the condition of hypoxia; the expression of E-cadherin increases, and those of Vimentin and Fibronectin decrease in GRP78 knockdown A549 cells under hypoxia. **(C)** EMT-related genes including Snail1, Snail2, Twist, ZEB1, and ZEB2 were examined by real-time quantitative PCR; mRNA expression relative value (control group) is plotted (mean ± SD in three separate experiments). *$P < 0.05$, compared with A549 cells in the control group, the mRNA expression levels of EMT-related genes including Snail1, Snail2, Twist, ZEB1, and ZEB2 increase under hypoxic condition (2% O_2 72 h); #$P < 0.05$, compared with A549 cells under the condition of hypoxia, the mRNA expression levels of EMT-related genes decrease in GRP78 knockdown A549 cells under hypoxia.

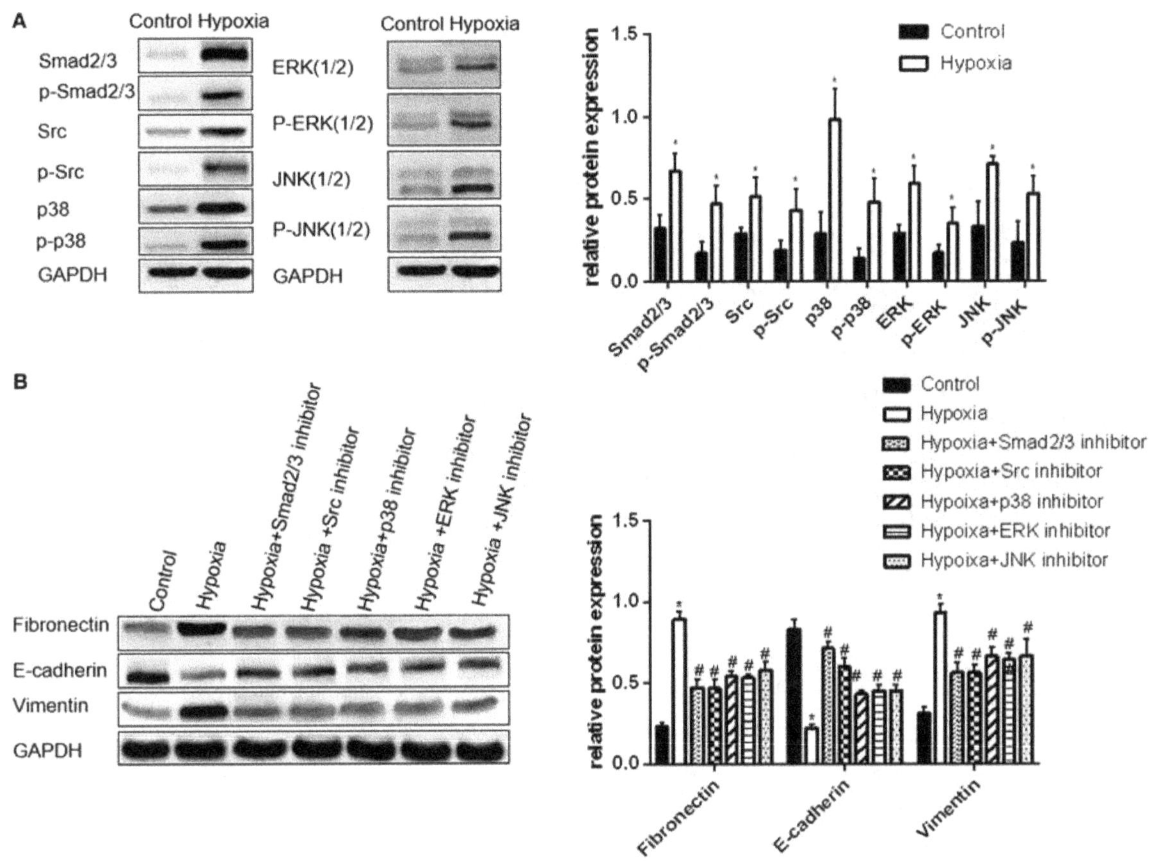

FIGURE 2 | Activation of Smad2/3, Src, p38, ERK, and JNK is important in hypoxia-induced EMT in A549 cells. **(A)** Smad2/3, Src, p38, ERK, JNK, and their phosphorylated forms were examined by Western blot analysis (left). GAPDH was used as internal control. The protein relative value (GAPDH) is plotted in the right panel (mean ± SD in three separate experiments). *$P < 0.05$, compared with A549 cells in the normal oxygen environments, the Smad2/3, Src, and MAPK proteins of A549 cells are highly regulated and activated in hypoxia environments. **(B)** EMT markers were examined by Western blot analysis (left). GAPDH was used as internal control. The protein relative value (GAPDH) is plotted in the right panel (mean ± SD in three separate experiments). *$P < 0.05$, compared with A549 cells in the normal oxygen environments, the EMT process of A549 cells under hypoxia is activated; #$P < 0.05$, compared with A549 cells in the hypoxia environments, the EMT process of A549 cells under hypoxia is inhibited separately by Smad2/3, Src, p38, ERK, and JNK inhibitors. The expression levels of Fibronectin and Vimentin decrease, and that of E-cadherin increases.

silencing, the expression of Smad2/3, Src, p38, ERK, and JNK and their phosphorylated proteins in hypoxia cells was significantly inhibited compared with that in the vehicle control under hypoxia ($P < 0.05$, **Figures 3C, 4A**).

Different effects were observed on the expression of the signaling molecules after inhibition of a particular pathway. After Smad2/3 inhibition, the expression of the four other signaling molecules did not significantly change ($P > 0.05$, **Figures 4A,B**). After inhibition of Src, JNK, ERK, and p38 pathways, the expression of Smad2/3 was not significantly changed ($P>0.05$, **Figures 4A,C**). After inhibiting Src, the activation of p38, ERK, and JNK (MAPK pathway) was also inhibited ($P < 0.05$, **Figures 4A,D**).

DISCUSSION

This study shows that GRP78 highly expressed under hypoxia condition is likely to play an essential role in hypoxia-induced EMT in A549 cells. This main finding is supported by the following observations: (1) the expression of GRP78 was significantly elevated under hypoxia condition and closely associated with the changes in the EMT markers; (2) GRP78 silencing significantly inhibited hypoxia-induced EMT markers; and (3) GRP78 silencing inhibited the expression of several signaling molecules, especially Smad2/3. This work is the first to demonstrate that GRP78 has a causal relationship with hypoxia-induced EMT in lung adenocarcinoma. Hence, targeted inhibition on GRP78 might could hamper EMT, which could further inhibit metastasis and overcome therapeutic resistance.

GRP78 was highly expressed in lung cancer cells under hypoxia condition; this finding is consistent with those reported by Song and Pi (25, 26). Chronic hypoxia induced GRP78 in human cancer cells possibly through the protein kinase C-epsilon/ERK/AP-1 signaling cascade (25).

A causal relationship between high GRP78 expression and EMT was confirmed by the GRP78 knock-down experiment. A very strong correlation was found between changes in the expression of GRP78 and EMT markers. Previous studies

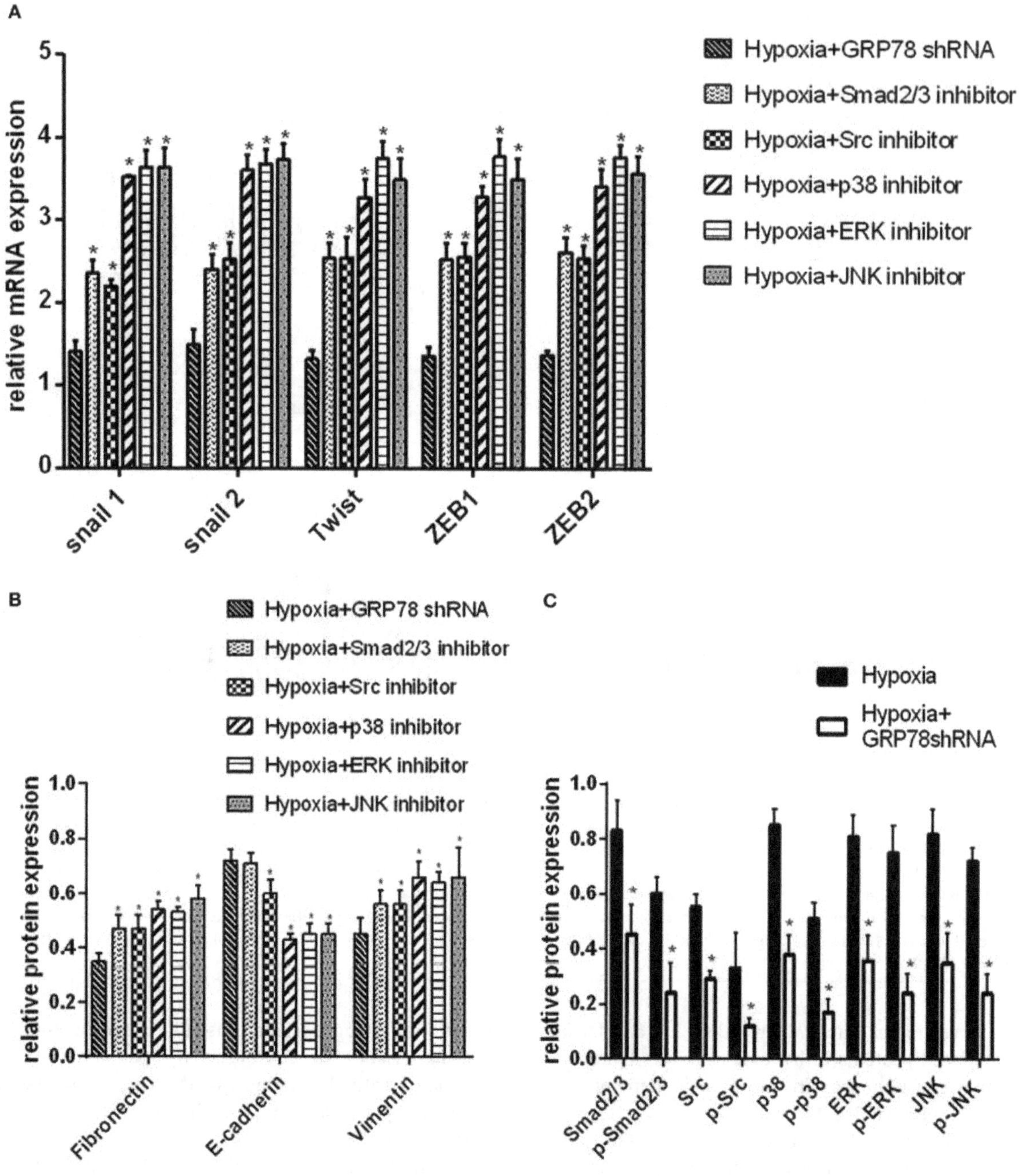

FIGURE 3 | GRP78 is the upper reaches of the Smad2/3, Src and MAPK pathways in hypoxia-induced EMT in A549 cells. **(A)** The mRNA relative value (control group) of EMT transcription factors is plotted (mean ± SD in three separate experiments). $^{*}P < 0.05$, compared with EMT transcription factors in A549 cells under hypoxia condition separately inhibited by Smad2/3, Src, p38, ERK, and JNK inhibitors, the expression is higher than that in GRP78 knockdown A549 cells under hypoxia. **(B)** The protein relative value (GAPDH) of EMT markers was examined by Western blot analysis and plotted (mean ± SD in three separate experiments). $^{*}P < 0.05$, compared with EMT markers of A549 cells under hypoxia condition separately inhibited by Smad2/3, Src, p38, ERK, and JNK inhibitors, the expression is higher than that in GRP78 knockdown A549 cells in the hypoxia. **(A,B)** indicate that the inhibition effect of GRP78 silencing is more powerful than those of the five other inhibitors. **(C)** The protein relative values (GAPDH) of Smad2/3, Src, p38, ERK, JNK, and their phosphorylated forms were examined by Western blot analysis and plotted (mean ± SD in three separate experiments). $^{*}P < 0.05$, compared with A549 cells under hypoxia, the expression levels of Smad2/3, Src, p38, ERK, JNK, and their activation forms decrease compared with those in GRP78 knockdown A549 cells under hypoxia. After GRP78 silencing, the expression and activation of these proteins are inhibited significantly.

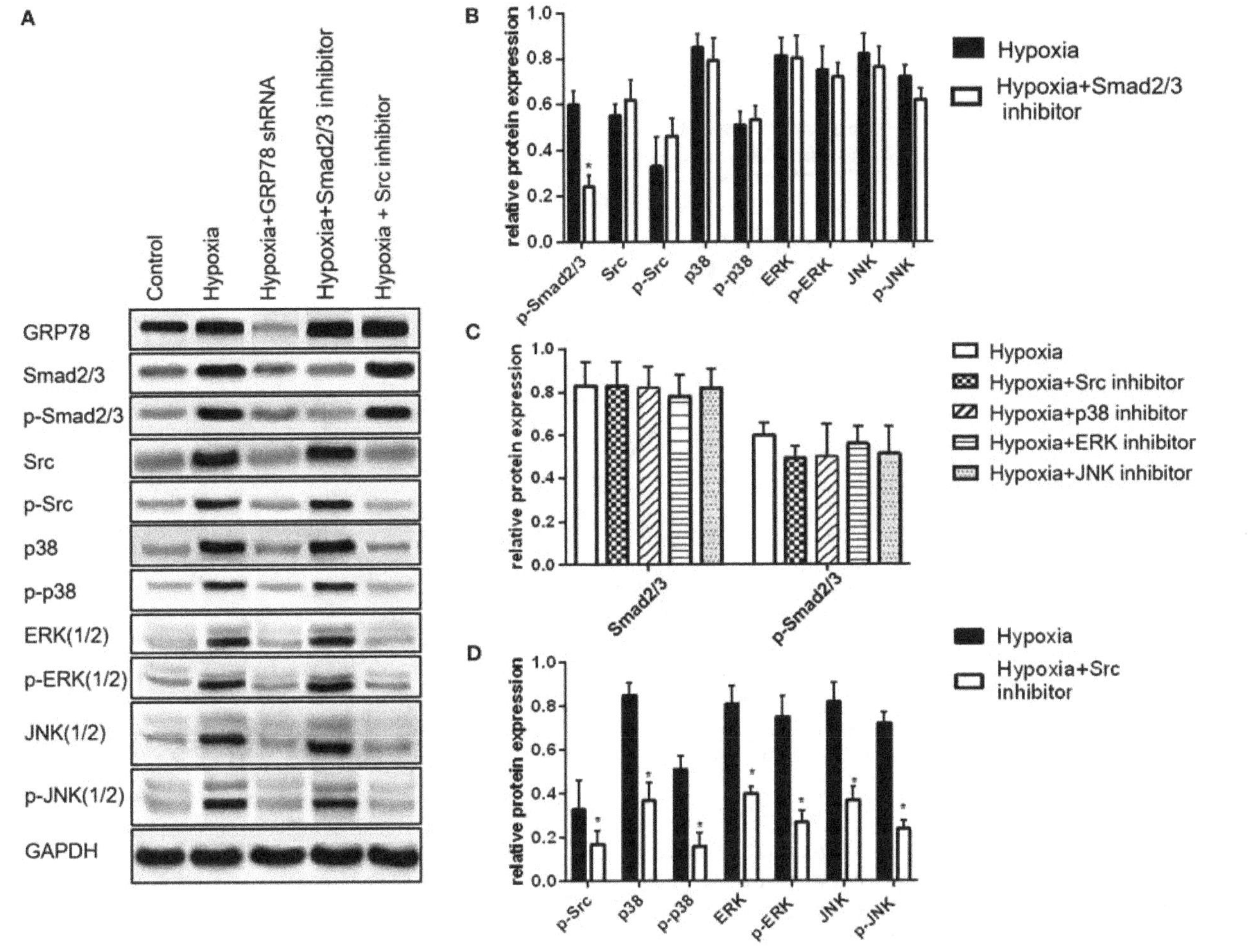

FIGURE 4 | Smad2/3 and Src/MAPK are two dependent signaling pathways in hypoxia-induced EMT in A549 cells. **(A)** Smad2/3, Src, p38, ERK, JNK, and their phosphorylated forms were examined by Western blot analysis. **(B)** Compared with the expression levels of Src, JNK, p38, ERK, and their activation forms in A549 cells under hypoxia, their expression levels do not change after inhibiting the activation of Smad2/3. **(C)** Compared with the expression levels of Smad2/3 and p-Smad2/3 in A549 cells under hypoxia, their expression does not change after inhibiting the activation of Src, JNK, ERK and p38. **(D)** *$P < 0.05$, compared with the expression levels of p38, ERK, JNK (three forms of MAPK) and their activated forms in A549 cells under hypoxia, their expression levels decrease after inhibiting the activation of Src. MAPK is the downstream pathway of Src.

suggested that other methods for silencing GRP78 could inhibit EMT. For example, neutralization of endogenous GRP78 on the cell surface with the anti-GRP78 antibody inhibited the ability of adhesion and invasion of hepatocellular carcinoma cell lines Mahlavu and SMMC7721 (19). The mitigation of GRP78 up-regulation by using short hairpin RNA or treatment with the small molecule IT-139 inhibited metastatic growth in the lung microenvironment in four highly metastatic cell line models (three human osteosarcomas and one murine mammary adenocarcinoma) (20). However, no rational interpretation is available regarding the inconsistency on the relationship between GRP78 expression and EMT in colorectal cancer.

The mechanism of GRP78 downstream signaling for EMT promotion has been demonstrated. Cell surface GRP78 can accelerate breast cancer cell proliferation and migration by activating STAT3 (27). We found two key molecular pathways (Smad2/3 and Src/MAPK) of GRP78 that may play an important role in hypoxia-induced EMT by using multiple protein inhibitors. These findings were consistent with those of previous works. Li et al. reported that overexpressing or knocking down GRP78 induced the corresponding activation or inhibition of the Smad2/3 pathway in colon cancer cells (28). Zhao et al. reported that GRP78 interacted directly with Src, thereby promoting the phosphorylation of Src in hepatocellular cancer cells (29). Tanjore et al. also suggested that the combination of the Smad2/3 inhibitor (SB431542) and the Src kinase inhibitor (PP2) blocked the EMT of alveolar epithelial cells induced by ER stress inducer tunicamycin, which also induced high GRP78 expression (30). In the present study, the activation of the Smad2/3 and Src/MAPK pathways follows the same trend with the up-regulation of GRP78; moreover, knockdown of GRP78 inhibited the activation of Smad2/3 and Src, suggesting a causal link between GRP78

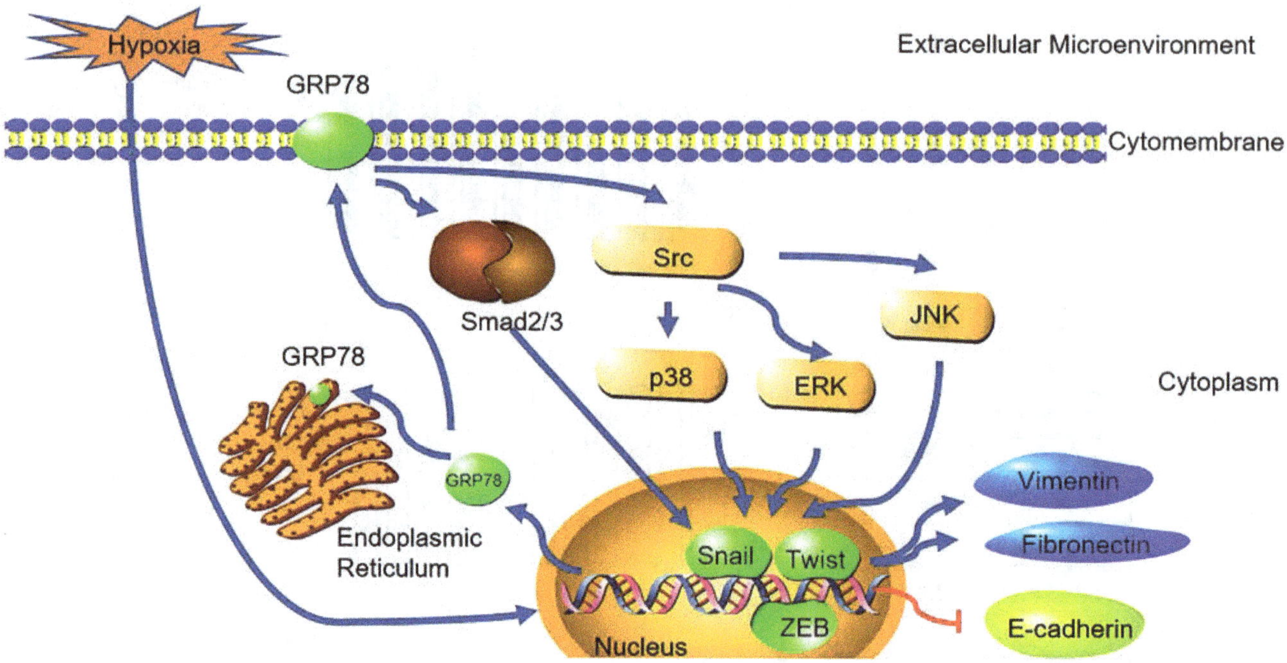

FIGURE 5 | GRP78 mediates hypoxia-induced EMT through smad2/3 and SRC/MAPK signaling. Hypoxia induced the high expression of GRP78. High expressed GRP78 activated the smad2/3 and Src/MAPK pathway. The pathway activated the expression of EMT transcription factor (snail, Twist and ZEB) and collaborated with them to induce the expression of Fibronectin, Vimentin and inhibit the expression of E-cadherin.

and activation of the two pathways in lung cancer. Smad2/3 inhibition did not interact with the inhibition of Src, p38, ERK, and JNK. By contrast, inhibiting the activation of Src was accompanied by the inhibition of p38, ERK, and JNK. Hence, the Smad2/3 and Src/MAPK pathways are two independent downstream signaling pathways of GRP78 during hypoxia-induced EMT in A549 cells. However, we did not perform the knockdown experiment of Smad2/3 and Src, and the co-immunoprecipitation experiment; as such, we cannot provide additional evidence for such link. And the control shRNA was not applied in the present study, which might limiting its evidence.

Other pitfall of the present study is that we have not explored the relationship between GRP78 and HIF1a, which is a key regulator on hypoxia induced EMT. But there are some evidences in other cell lines, that the expression of GRP78 is regulated by HIF1a (31). What's more, all the results in the study are limited to one cell line, limiting its evidence.

In summary, this study demonstrated the possible causal link between GRP78 and hypoxia-induced EMT in A549 cells (**Figure 5**). Together with its roles in anti-apoptosis and chemoresistance, it indicates that GRP78 might be a potential target for treatment of lung adenocarcinoma. Further, studies are needed to elucidate the exact mechanisms involved in the GRP78-EMT pathway in hypoxia and their relevant clinical significance.

AUTHOR CONTRIBUTIONS

L-ZL and L-LS: designed the experiments. L-LS, C-MC, and JW: performed the experiments. JZ and C-ZY: analyzed the data. L-LS and C-ZY: prepared the figures. L-LS and JZ: wrote the main manuscript. All authors reviewed the manuscript.

FUNDING

This study was supported by grant from the National Natural Science Foundation of China (NSFC) (Nos. 81403227 to L-LS and 81573870 to L-ZL).

ACKNOWLEDGMENTS

We would like to thank the colleagues from First Affiliated Hospital of Guangzhou University of Chinese Medicine, China. We would also like to thank the support from Prof. Chunguang Li, Prof. Xiaoshu Zhu, Prof. Alan Bensussan from the Western Sydney University, Australia and Prof. Kevin Chang from New South Wales Association of Chinese Medicine, Australia.

REFERENCES

1. Ferlay J, Soerjomataram I, Dikshit R, Eser S, Mathers C, Rebelo M, et al. Cancer incidence and mortality worldwide: sources, methods and major patterns in GLOBOCAN 2012. *Int J Cancer.* (2015) 136:E359–86. doi: 10.1002/ijc.29210
2. Zhao Y, Adjei AA. New strategies to develop new medications for lung cancer and metastasis. *Cancer Metastasis Rev.* (2015) 34:265–75. doi: 10.1007/s10555-015-9553-5
3. Skovierova H, Okajcekova T, Strnadel J, Vidomanova E, Halasova E. Molecular regulation of epithelial-to-mesenchymal transition in tumorigenesis (Review). *Int J Mol Med.* (2018) 41:1187–200. doi: 10.3892/ijmm.2017.3320
4. Xu J, Lamouille S, Derynck R. TGF-beta-induced epithelial to mesenchymal transition. *Cell Res.* (2009) 19:156–72. doi: 10.1038/cr.2009.5
5. Patel A, Sabbineni H, Clarke A, Somanath PR. Novel roles of Src in cancer cell epithelial-to-mesenchymal transition, vascular permeability, microinvasion and metastasis. *Life Sci.* (2016) 157:52–61. doi: 10.1016/j.lfs.2016.05.036
6. Zhao L, Li X, Song N, Li A, Hou K, Qu X, et al. Src promotes EGF-induced epithelial-to-mesenchymal transition and migration in gastric cancer cells by upregulating ZEB1 and ZEB2 through AKT. *Cell Biol Int.* (2018) 42:294–302. doi: 10.1002/cbin.10894
7. Ruan J, Zhang L, Yan L, Liu Y, Yue Z, Chen L, et al. Inhibition of hypoxia-induced epithelial mesenchymal transition by luteolin in non-small cell lung cancer cells. *Mol Med Rep.* (2012) 6:232–8. doi: 10.3892/mmr.2012.884
8. Shaikh D, Zhou Q, Chen T, Ibe JC, Raj JU, Zhou G. cAMP-dependent protein kinase is essential for hypoxia-mediated epithelial-mesenchymal transition, migration, and invasion in lung cancer cells. *Cell Signal.* (2012) 24:2396–406. doi: 10.1016/j.cellsig.2012.08.007
9. Nurwidya F, Takahashi F, Kobayashi I, Murakami A, Kato M, Minakata K, et al. Treatment with insulin-like growth factor 1 receptor inhibitor reverses hypoxia-induced epithelial-mesenchymal transition in non-small cell lung cancer. *Biochem Biophys Res Commun.* (2014) 455:332–8. doi: 10.1016/j.bbrc.2014.11.014
10. Barriga EH, Maxwell PH, Reyes AE, Mayor R. The hypoxia factor Hif-1alpha controls neural crest chemotaxis and epithelial to mesenchymal transition. *J Cell Biol.* (2013) 201:759–76. doi: 10.1083/jcb.201212100
11. Shen X, Xue Y, Si Y, Wang Q, Wang Z, Yuan J, et al. The unfolded protein response potentiates epithelial-to-mesenchymal transition (EMT) of gastric cancer cells under severe hypoxic conditions. *Med Oncol.* (2015) 32:447. doi: 10.1007/s12032-014-0447-0
12. Su R, Li Z, Li H, Song H, Bao C, Wei J, et al. Grp78 promotes the invasion of hepatocellular carcinoma. *BMC Cancer.* (2010) 10:20. doi: 10.1186/1471-2407-10-20
13. Sun Q, Hua J, Wang Q, Xu W, Zhang J, Zhang J, et al. Expressions of GRP78 and Bax associate with differentiation, metastasis, and apoptosis in non-small cell lung cancer. *Mol Biol Rep.* (2012) 39:6753–61. doi: 10.1007/s11033-012-1500-8
14. Chang YW, Chen HA, Tseng CF, Hong CC, Ma JT, Hung MC, et al. De-acetylation and degradation of HSPA5 is critical for E1A metastasis suppression in breast cancer cells. *Oncotarget.* (2014) 5:10558–70. doi: 10.18632/oncotarget.2510
15. Chen HA, Chang YW, Tseng CF, Chiu CF, Hong CC, Wang W, et al. E1A-mediated inhibition of HSPA5 suppresses cell migration and invasion in triple-negative breast cancer. *Ann Surg Oncol.* (2015) 22:889–98. doi: 10.1245/s10434-014-4061-3
16. Roller C, Maddalo D. The molecular chaperone GRP78/BiP in the development of chemoresistance: mechanism and possible treatment. *Front Pharmacol.* (2013) 4:10. doi: 10.3389/fphar.2013.00010
17. Xie J, Tao ZH, Zhao J, Li T, Wu ZH, Zhang JF, et al. Glucose regulated protein 78 (GRP78) inhibits apoptosis and attentinutes chemosensitivity of gemcitabine in breast cancer cell via AKT/mitochondrial apoptotic pathway. *Biochem Biophys Res Commun.* (2016) 474:612–9. doi: 10.1016/j.bbrc.2016.03.002
18. Gifford JB, Hill R. GRP78 Influences Chemoresistance and Prognosis in Cancer. *Curr Drug Targets.* (2018) 19:701–8. doi: 10.2174/1389450118666170615100918
19. Zhang XX, Li HD, Zhao S, Zhao L, Song HJ, Wang G, et al. The cell surface GRP78 facilitates the invasion of hepatocellular carcinoma cells. *Biomed Res Int.* (2013) 2013:917296. doi: 10.1155/2013/917296
20. Lizardo MM, Morrow JJ, Miller TE, Hong ES, Ren L, Mendoza A, et al. Upregulation of glucose-regulated protein 78 in metastatic cancer cells is necessary for lung metastasis progression. *Neoplasia.* (2016) 18:699–710. doi: 10.1016/j.neo.2016.09.001
21. Zhang L, Li Z, Fan Y, Li H, Li Z, Li Y. Overexpressed GRP78 affects EMT and cell-matrix adhesion via autocrine TGF-beta/Smad2/3 signaling. *Int J Biochem Cell Biol.* (2015) 64:202–11. doi: 10.1016/j.biocel.2015.04.012
22. Chang YJ, Chen WY, Huang CY, Liu HH, Wei PL. Glucose-regulated protein 78 (GRP78) regulates colon cancer metastasis through EMT biomarkers and the NRF-2/HO-1 pathway. *Tumour Biol.* (2015) 36:1859–69. doi: 10.1007/s13277-014-2788-x
23. Chen CM, Sun LL, Fang RM, Lin LZ. YiQi ChuTan recipe inhibits epithelial mesenchymal transition of A549 cells under hypoxia. *Cell Mol Biol (Noisy-le-grand).* (2016) 62:10–5. doi: 10.14715/cmb/2016.62.1.3
24. Chen C, Sun L, Lin L. Construction of eukaryotic expression vector for glucose regulated protein 78-shRNA and establishment of stably transfected A549 cell line. *Chi J Biologic.* (2016) 29:348–53. doi: 10.13200/j.cnki.cjb.001289
25. Song MS, Park YK, Lee JH, Park K. Induction of glucose-regulated protein 78 by chronic hypoxia in human gastric tumor cells through a protein kinase C-epsilon/ERK/AP-1 signaling cascade. *Cancer Res.*(2001) 61:8322–30. Available online at: http://cancerres.aacrjournals.org/content/61/22/8322
26. Pi L, Li X, Song Q, Shen Y, Lu X, Di B. Knockdown of glucose-regulated protein 78 abrogates chemoresistance of hypopharyngeal carcinoma cells to cisplatin induced by unfolded protein in response to severe hypoxia. *Oncol Lett.* (2014) 7:685–92. doi: 10.3892/ol.2013.1753
27. Yao X, Liu H, Zhang X, Zhang L, Li X, Wang C, et al. Cell surface GRP78 accelerated breast cancer cell proliferation and migration by activating STAT3. *PLoS ONE.* (2015) 10:e0125634. doi: 10.1371/journal.pone.0125634
28. Li Z, Zhang L, Zhao Y, Li H, Xiao H, Fu R, et al. Cell-surface GRP78 facilitates colorectal cancer cell migration and invasion. *Int J Biochem Cell Biol.* (2013) 45:987–94. doi: 10.1016/j.biocel.2013.02.002
29. Zhao S, Li H, Wang Q, Su C, Wang G, Song H, et al. The role of c-Src in the invasion and metastasis of hepatocellular carcinoma cells induced by association of cell surface GRP78 with activated alpha2M. *BMC Cancer.* (2015) 15:389. doi: 10.1186/s12885-015-1401-z
30. Tanjore H, Cheng DS, Degryse AL, Zoz DF, Abdolrasulnia R, Lawson WE, et al. Alveolar epithelial cells undergo epithelial-to-mesenchymal transition in response to endoplasmic reticulum stress. *J Biol Chem.* (2015) 290:3277. doi: 10.1074/jbc.A110.181164
31. Lee JH, Yoon YM, Lee SH. Hypoxic preconditioning promotes the bioactivities of mesenchymal stem cells via the HIF-1alpha-GRP78-Akt Axis. *Int J Mol Sci.* (2017) 18:E1320. doi: 10.3390/ijms18061320

13

Midostaurin Reverses ABCB1-Mediated Multidrug Resistance, an *in vitro* Study

Ning Ji[1,2], *Yuqi Yang*[2], *Chao-Yun Cai*[2], *Jing-Quan Wang*[2], *Zi-Ning Lei*[2], *Zhuo-Xun Wu*[2], *Qingbin Cui*[2], *Dong-Hua Yang*[2], *Zhe-Sheng Chen*[2*] *and Dexin Kong*[1,3*]

[1] *Tianjin Key Laboratory on Technologies Enabling Development of Clinical Therapeutics and Diagnostics, School of Pharmacy, Tianjin Medical University, Tianjin, China,* [2] *Department of Pharmaceutical Sciences, College of Pharmacy and Health Sciences, St. John's University, Queens, NY, United States,* [3] *Research Center, School of Medicine, Tianjin Tianshi College, Tianyuan University, Tianjin, China*

Correspondence:
Zhe-Sheng Chen
chenz@stjohns.edu
Dexin Kong
kongdexin@tmu.edu.cn

Overexpression of ABC transporters in cancer cells is an underlying mechanism of multidrug resistance (MDR), leading to insensitive response to chemotherapeutic strategies. Thus, MDR is often results in treatment failure in the clinic. In this study, we found midostaurin, a Food and Drug Administration (FDA)-approved anti-leukemia drug, can antagonize ATP-binding cassette subfamily B member 1 (ABCB1)-mediated MDR. Our results indicated that midostaurin has the capacity to antagonize ABCB1-mediated MDR, while no significant reversal effect was found on ATP-binding cassette subfamily G member 2 (ABCG2)-mediated MDR. Our subsequent resistance mechanism studies showed that midostaurin directly inhibited the efflux function of the ABCB1 transporter without alteration of the expression level or the subcellular localization of ABCB1 transporter. In addition, midostaurin inhibited the ATPase activity of ABCB1 transporter in a dose-dependent manner. Moreover, our *in silico* docking study predicted that midostaurin could interact with the substrate-binding sites of ABCB1 transporter. This novel finding could provide a promising treatment strategy that co-administrating midostaurin with anticancer drugs in the clinic could overcome MDR and improve the efficiency of cancer treatment.

Keywords: midostaurin, multidrug resistance, ATP-binding cassette (ABC) transporter, ABC, chemotherapy

INTRODUCTION

Multidrug resistance (MDR) in cancer, a phenomenon leading to synchronous resistance of cancer cells to structurally unrelated antineoplastic drugs, is one of the most critical factors responsible for the failure of chemotherapeutics and the poor survival rate of patients (1). Several mechanisms are involved in cancer MDR, including reduced apoptosis, advanced DNA damage repair mechanisms, or altered drug metabolism. However, the most prominent factor is ABC transporter-mediated efflux of antineoplastic drugs (3, 51).

The transport system superfamily of ABC transporters plays critical roles in physiological and pharmacological processes (2). The human ABC protein family has been divided into seven subfamilies (ABCA to ABCG). The ABC transporter family has 49 ABC proteins and 48 of them have identified functions (3, 4). As one of the main contributors, ABCB1 (P-gp/MDR1) is widely expressed not only in the placenta, but in the blood-brain barrier (BBB), intestines, livers and kidneys, in order to protect the body from xenobiotics (5, 6). The ABCB1 transporter also mediates the transport of a wide range of physiological substrates like lipids, porphyrins, and sterols (7). Furthermore, a broad range of chemotherapeutic drugs are substrates of the ABCB1 transporter, such as taxanes and anthracyclines. ABCB1 transporter significantly increases the efflux of such anticancer drugs, a major reason leading to ABCB1-mediated MDR (8). It has been documented that ABCB1 is strongly related to the chemotherapy prognosis and the progression of malignancy (9). Thus, it is critical to elude MDR by either decreasing the expression level of ABCB1 proteins or inhibiting the efflux function of ABCB1 through specific and potent inhibitors.

Midostaurin, a multi-kinase inhibitor that was originally developed as a protein kinase C (PKC) inhibitor for treatment of patients with solid malignancy (10), has already been approved by the FDA for treatment of acute myelocytic leukemia (AML) with Fms-like tyrosine kinase 3 (FLT3)-mutant subtype (11). It has recently been reported that the combination of midostaurin with standard chemotherapy can significantly prolong overall and event-free survival in patients who suffer from AML with a FLT3 mutation (12). Here, we report the reversal effects of midostaurin on ABCB1-mediated MDR when co-administrated with conventional antineoplastic drugs.

MATERIALS AND METHODS

Chemicals

Midostaurin was obtained from Thermo Fisher Scientific Inc. (Rockford, IL). Bovine serum albumin (BSA), fetal bovine serum (FBS), Dulbecco's modified Eagle's Medium (DMEM), penicillin/streptomycin and 0.25% trypsin were products from Corning Incorporated (Corning, NY). The monoclonal antibody for GAPDH (catalog number MA5-15738, lot number SA247966, clone GA1R), Alexa Fluor 488 conjugated goat anti-mouse IgG secondary antibody, were purchased from Thermo Fisher Scientific Inc. (Rockford, IL). Paclitaxel, doxorubicin, colchicine, cisplatin, mitoxantrone, verapamil, the monoclonal antibodies for ABCB1 (catalog number P7965, lot number 067M4761V, clone F4), dimethylsulfoxide (DMSO), 3-(4,5-dimethylthiazol-yl)-2,5-diphenyltetrazolium bromide (MTT), Triton X-100, 4',6-diamidino-2-phenylindole (DAPI), and paraformaldehyde, were obtained from Sigma-Aldrich (St. Louis, MO). HRP-conjugated rabbit anti-mouse IgG secondary antibody (catalog number 7076S, Lot number 32) were obtained from Cell Signaling Technology Inc. (Danvers, MA). Ko143 was a product from Enzo Life Sciences (Farmingdale, NY). [^{3}H]-paclitaxel (15 Ci/mmol) was purchased from Moravek Biochemicals, Inc. (Brea, CA). All other chemicals were purchased from Sigma Chemical Co (St. Louis, MO).

Cell Lines and Cell Culture

The ABCB1-overexpressing KB-C2 cell line was created by gradually adding colchicine to parental human epidermoid carcinoma KB-3-1 cells, and was kindly provided by Dr. Shin-ichi Akiyama (Kagoshima University, Kagoshima, Japan). The KB-C2 line was cultured in medium containing 2 μg/mL colchicine (13) to maintain its drugresistant characteristics. The SW620/Ad300 cells were cultured in medium with 300 ng/mL doxorubicin (14). KB-3-1, KB-C2, SW620, and SW620/Ad300 cells were used for ABCB1 reversal study. The human non-small cell lung cancer (NSCLC) NCI-H460 cell line and its subline of ABCG2-overexpressing NCI-H460/MX20 cells were used for ABCG2 reversal study. The NCI-H460/MX20 cells were selected by using a high dose of mitoxantrone and maintained in medium with 20 ng/mL mitoxantrone (15). HEK293/pcDNA3.1 and HEK293/ABCB1 were established by transfecting the human embryonic kidney HEK293 cells with empty and ABCB1 expressing vector, respectively (16). SW620 and SW620/Ad300 cells, NCI-H460 and NCI-H460/MX20 cells, were kindly provided by Drs. Susan Bates and Robert Robey (NCI, NIH, Bethesda, MD). HEK293/ABCB1 were kindly provided by Dr. Suresh V. Ambudkar (NCI, NIH, Bethesda, MD). All aforementioned cell lines were maintained in DMEM medium containing 10% fetal bovine serum and 1% penicillin/streptomycin at 37°C in a humidified atmosphere containing 5% CO_2. All cells were grown as an adherent monolayer and drug-resistant cells were grown in drug-free culture media for more than 20 days before assay.

MTT Cytotoxicity Assay

Cell viability was determined by MTT assay as we previously described (17). Each type of cell was harvested and resuspended before being seeded onto a 96-well plate at a final quantity of 5×10^3 cells per well in 160 μL of medium, and was then incubated overnight. Midostaurin and positive control drugs were added 2 h prior to incubation with or without anticancer drugs. After 72 h of further incubation, MTT solution (4 mg/mL) was added to each well and the cells were incubated for an additional 4 h at 37°C. Subsequently, the supernatant was discarded and 100 μL of DMSO was added to each well in order to dissolve the formazan crystals. An accuSkanTM GO UV/Vis Microplate Spectrophotometer from Fisher Sci. (Fair Lawn, NJ) was used to determine the absorbance at 570 nm. The concentration for 50% inhibition of cell viability (IC_{50}) of the anticancer drug was calculated as previously described (18). For positive control drugs, verapamil (3 μM) and Ko143 (3 μM) were used as reference inhibitors to reverse ABCB1- and ABCG2-mediated MDR, respectively. Cisplatin, which is not a substrate of ABCB1 or ABCG2, was used as a negative control chemotherapeutic drug.

Western Blotting and Immunofluorescence Analysis

Western blotting analysis was performed as previously described (19). Briefly, cells were lysed after incubated with or without midostaurin (500 nM) for varying amounts of time (0, 24, 48, and 72 h). The concentration of protein was determined by BCA Protein Assay Kit from Pierce (Rockford, IL). Equal amounts (20 μg) of proteins were subjected to 10% sodium dodecyl sulfate polyacrylamide gel electrophoresis (SDS-PAGE) and transferred to PVDF membranes from Millipore (Billerica, MA). The presence of ABCB1 was determined using monoclonal antibody F4 (dilution 1:500). GAPDH was used as a loading control. The resulting protein bands were analyzed using Image J software. The immunofluorescence assay was performed as previously described (17). Briefly, after being cultured overnight in 24-well plates, cells (2×10^4/well) were treated with midostaurin for 72 h at 500 nM concentration. Then, cells were fixed in 4% paraformaldehyde for 10 min and permeabilized by 0.1% Triton X-100 for 10 min before being blocked with 6% BSA for 1 h at 37°C. The presence of ABCB1 was determined using monoclonal antibody F4 (dilution 1:100) for incubation at 4°C overnight. Cells were washed with iced PBS after each incubation time. Alexa Fluor 488 (Ex = 499 nm, Em = 519 nm) conjugated secondary antibody (1:1,000) was used after washing with iced PBS. DAPI (Ex = 345 nm, Em = 455 nm) was used to counterstain the nuclei. The cells were washed with ice-cold PBS before being imaged. Immunofluorescence images were collected using an EVOS FL Auto fluorescence microscope from Life Technologies Corporation (Gaithersburg, MD).

Doxorubicin Accumulation and Fluorescence Microscopic Analysis

Cells were grown in 6-well plates and washed twice with phosphate-buffered saline (PBS) before the pre-treatment of 500 nM of midostaurin. After 1 h of midostaurin pretreatment, 10 μM of doxorubicin was then added to each well for further incubation (1 h). Immunofluorescence images were collected using an EVOS FL Auto fluorescence microscope from Life Technologies Corporation (Gaithersburg, MD). Excitation and emission wavelengths of doxorubicin were 475 and 585 nm, respectively.

[^{3}H]-Paclitaxel Accumulation and Efflux Assay

We conducted [^{3}H]-paclitaxel accumulation assay using KB-3-1 and its drug-resistant subline KB-C2 cells. As previously described (20), 5×10^5 cells/well were cultured in 24-well plates overnight before the assay, and midostaurin was added 2 h prior to the addition of [^{3}H]-paclitaxel. After incubating with [^{3}H]-paclitaxel with or without midostaurin for 2 h at 37°C, cells were washed twice with iced PBS, and lysed with 0.25% trypsin before being placed in 5 mL scintillation fluid, and radioactivity was measured in the Packard TRI-CARB 1900CA liquid scintillation analyzer from Packard Instrument (Downers Grove, IL).For the efflux assay, KB-3-1 and KB-C2 cells (20) were incubated with midostaurin for 2 h followed by incubation with [^{3}H]-paclitaxel, with or without midostaurin for 2 h at 37°C. The cells were washed with iced PBS twice and then lysed at various time points (0, 30, 60, and 120 min) with trypsin. Subsequently, cells were placed in 5 mL of scintillation fluid and radioactivity was measured in the Packard TRI-CARB 1900CA liquid scintillation analyzer from Packard Instrument (Downers Grove, IL).

ATPase Assay

The ABCB1-associated ATPase activities were measured using PREDEASY ATPase Kits from TEBU-BIO nv (Boechout, Belgium) with modified protocols. Briefly, cell membranes that overexpressed ABCB1 were thawed and diluted before use. Sodium orthovanadate (Na_3VO_4) was used as an ATPase inhibitor. Various concentrations of midostaurin were incubated with membranes for 5 min. The ATPase reactions were initiated by adding 5 mM Mg^{2+}-ATP. Luminescence signals of P_i were initiated and measured after incubation at 37°C for 40 min with brief mixing. The changes of relative light units were determined by comparing Na_3VO_4-treated samples with midostaurin-treated groups.

Molecular Modeling of Human ABCB1 Homology Model

In silico docking analysis was conducted using software Maestro 11.5 (Schr'odinger, LLC, New York, NY, 2018) (21). Human ABCB1 homology model was established by Dr. Aller based on refined mouse ABCB1 (PDB ID: 4M1M) (22). Afterwards, the docking grid at the drug-binding pocket was generated (23). The ligand was essentially prepared to perform glide XP docking with the default protocols.

Statistical Analysis

All data are expressed as the mean ± SD and were analyzed using one-way ANOVA. All experiments were repeated at least three times. Differences were considered significant when $P < 0.05$.

RESULTS

Midostaurin Significantly Antagonized ABCB1-Mediated MDR in ABCB1-Overexpressing Cancer Cells

Firstly, to avoid cytostatic-induced reversal phenomenon, we conducted MTT assays to evaluate the cytostatic effects of midostaurin in the ABCB1-overexpressing cells and corresponding parental cells that we would use. Hence, we could choose concentrations that would not significantly influence cell viability. We conducted further experiments with 200 and 500 nM doses of midostaurin (**Figure 1**).

As shown in **Figure 2**, midostaurin significantly sensitized ABCB1-overexpressing cancer cells KB-C2 (**Figures 2A–C**) and SW620/Ad300 (**Figures 2E–G**) to ABCB1 substrates (doxorubicin, paclitaxel, and colchicine), compared with their control resistance cells, and this sensitization occurred in a dose-dependent manner. At 200 or 500 nM, midostaurin could not alter the IC_{50} values of the above chemotherapeutic drugs to parental KB-3-1 (**Figures 2A–C**) and SW620 (**Figures 2E–G**) cells. In addition, when combined with cisplatin, a platinum drug which is known to not be a substrate of ABCB1, midostaurin showed no significant difference in its cytotoxic effect in neither the resistant cell lines nor the parental cell lines (**Figures 2D,H**). In this study, verapamil, a potent ABCB1 inhibitor, was used as a positive control drug (24).

Midostaurin Significantly Antagonized ABCB1-Mediated MDR in ABCB1-Gene-Transfected Cells

We next evaluated the reversal effect of midostaurin on ABCB1-gene-transfected cells. As shown in **Figure 3**, midostaurin could significantly lower the IC_{50} values of ABCB1 substrate-drugs

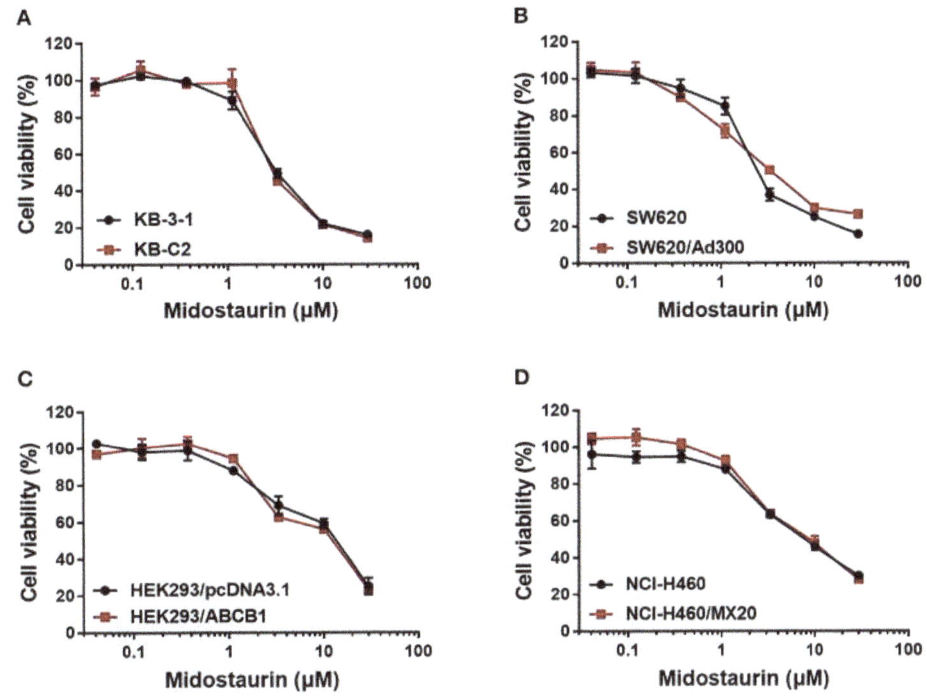

FIGURE 1 | Dose-viability curves of cells used in this study incubated with midostaurin for 72 h. Dose-viability curves for **(A)** KB-3-1 and KB-C2, **(B)** SW620 and SW620/Ad300, **(C)** HEK293/pcDNA3.1 and HEK293/ABCB1, and **(D)** NCI-H460 and NCI-H460/MX20.

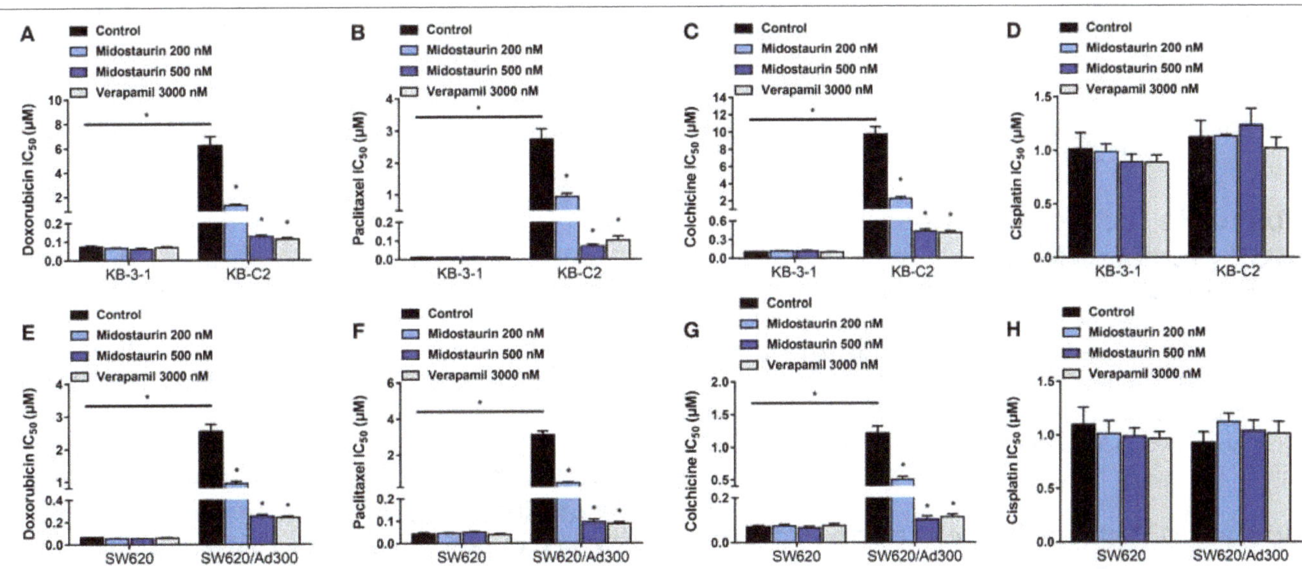

FIGURE 2 | The reversal effect of midostaurin on ABCB1-mediated MDR in ABCB1-overexpression cancer cells. IC_{50} values of **(A)** doxorubicin, **(B)** paclitaxel, **(C)** colchicine, and **(D)** cisplatin in parental KB-3-1 and drug-selected ABCB1-overexpression resistant KB-C2 cells with or without treatment of midostaurin. IC_{50} of **(E)** doxorubicin, **(F)** paclitaxel, **(G)** colchicine, and **(H)** cisplatin in parental SW620 and drug-selected ABCB1-overexpression resistant SW620/Ad300 cells with or without treatment of midostaurin. Data are expressed as mean ± SD, representative of at least three independent experiments. *$p < 0.05$, compared with control group.

(doxorubicin, paclitaxel, and colchicine) to HEK293/ABCB1 cells at 200 and 500 nM in a concentration-dependent manner (**Figures 3A–C**). More importantly, midostaurin did not significantly alter the efficacy of these ABCB1-substrate chemotherapeutic drugs in parental HEK293/pcDNA3.1 cells (**Figures 3A–C**). Furthermore, at 200 or 500 nM,

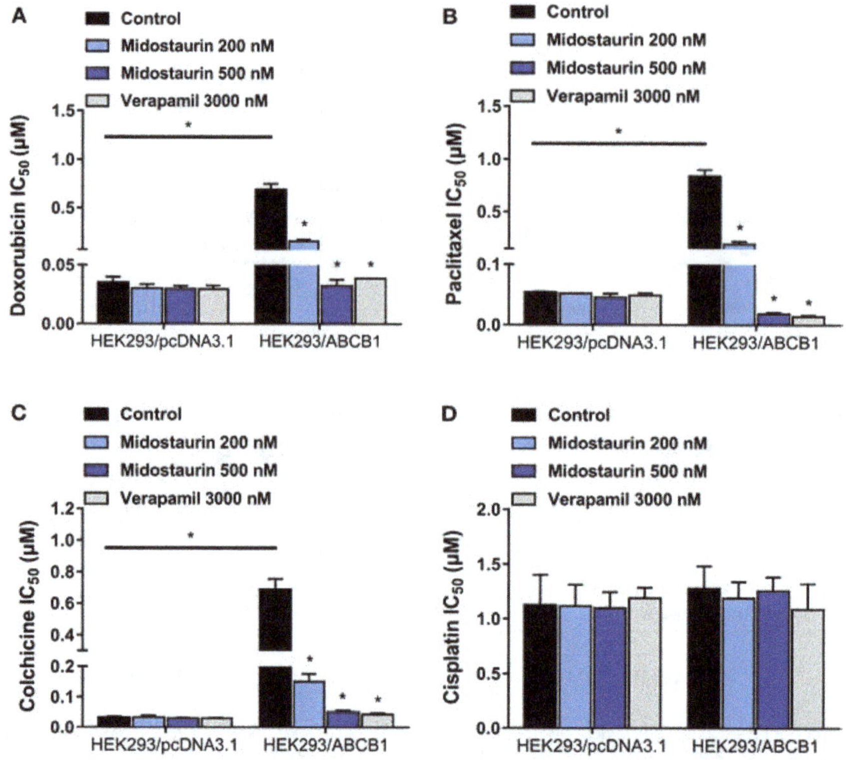

FIGURE 3 | The reversal effect of midostaurin on ABCB1-mediated MDR in ABCB1-gene-transfected cells. IC_{50} values of **(A)** doxorubicin, **(B)** paclitaxel, **(C)** colchicine, and **(D)** cisplatin in parental HEK293/pcDNA3.1 and transfected ABCB1-overexpression HEK293/ABCB1 cells with or without treatment of midostaurin. Data are expressed as mean ± SD, representative of at least three independent experiments. $^{*}p < 0.05$, compared with control group.

midostaurin did not significantly change the IC_{50} values of cisplatin (**Figure 3D**).

Midostaurin Did Not Reverse ABCG2-Mediated MDR

As shown in **Figure 4**, midostautrin (200 and 500 nM) could not significantly lower the IC_{50} value of mitoxantrone, a known substrate of ABCG2-mediated MDR, to drug-selected NCI-H460/MX20 cells. In this study, we chose Ko143 as a positive control drug because it is a potent ABCG2 inhibitor (21). Cisplatin was used as a negative substrate drug as previously described (25).

Midostaurin Did Not Influence the Protein Expression Level or Subcellular Localization of ABCB1 Transporters

The next step was to figure out the mechanism of action of midostaurin. Theoretically, there are varied mechanisms involved in the reversal of ABCB1-mediated MDR. For examples, the reversal effect could be due to down-regulation of ABCB1 protein expression level and/or the change of ABCB1 transporter subcellular localization. To evaluate the effect of midostaurin on the protein level of ABCB1 transporter, we conducted Western blotting and immunofluorescence assays to detect whether midostaurin could impact the ABCB1 protein expression and/or subcellular localization. As shown in **Figure 5A**, after incubation for 24, 48, and 72 h, respectively, midostaurin did not significantly change the expression level of ABCB1 protein (170 kDa) in ABCB1-overexpressing KB-C2 cells. Furthermore, midostaurin did not change the localization of ABCB1 at the subcellular level after incubating for up to 72 h in ABCB1-overexpressing KB-C2 cells (**Figure 5B**). These results suggested that midostaurin influenced neither the expression level nor the subcellular localization of ABCB1 protein even at high concentrations.

Midostaurin Significantly Increased the Intracellular Drug Accumulation in ABCB1-Overexpressing Cancer Cells

The above results indicated that midostaurin could reverse ABCB1-mediated MDR without altering the protein expression level or subcellular localization in ABCB1-overexpressing cancer cells. We then conducted our drug accumulation assay to further understand the mechanism of the reversal effect of midostaurin. Firstly, we conducted our doxorubicin accumulation assay with 500 nM of midostaurin. As shown in **Figure 6A**, midostaurin significantly enhanced the accumulation level of doxorubicin in ABCB1-overexpressing KB-C2 cells. We also conducted our $[^3H]$-paclitaxel accumulation assay to get a digitized result. The intracellular level of $[^3H]$-paclitaxel was measured in

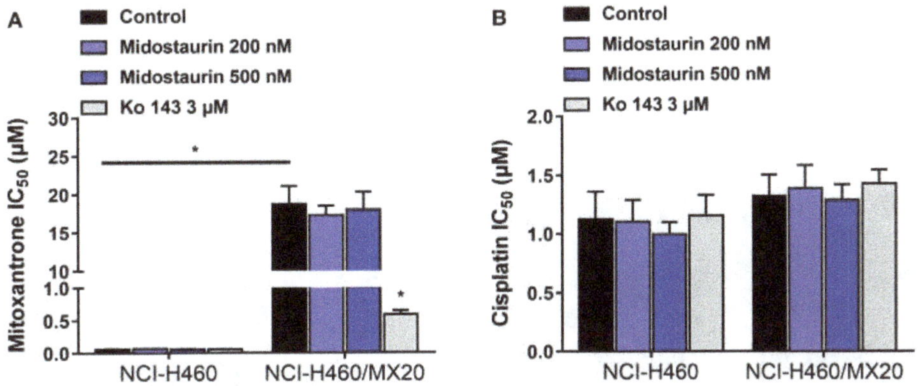

FIGURE 4 | The reversal effect of midostaurin on ABCG2-mediated MDR in ABCG2-overexpression cancer cells. **(A)** IC_{50} values of mitoxantrone in parental NCI-H460 cells and resistant NCI-H460/MX20 cells. **(B)** IC_{50} values of cisplatin in parental NCI-H460 cells and resistant NCI-H460/MX20 cells. *$p < 0.05$, compared with control group.

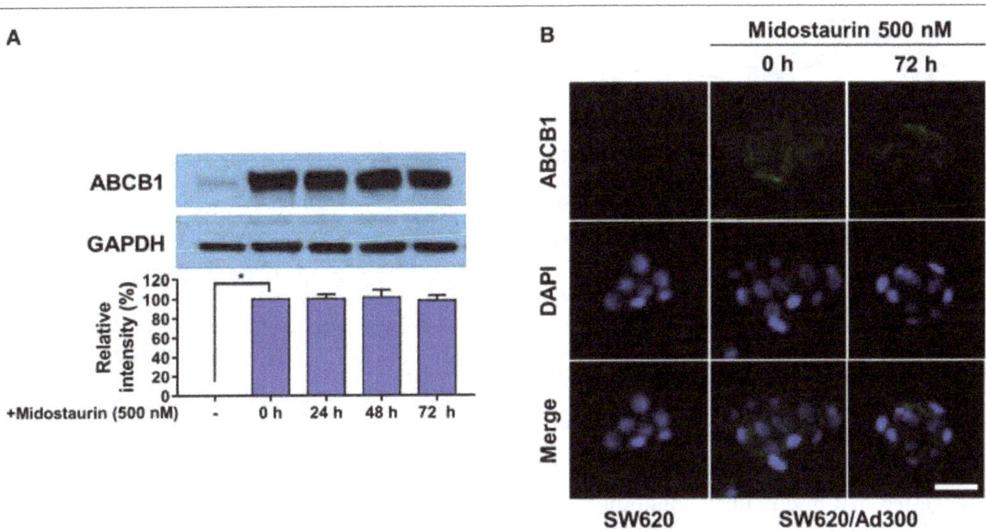

FIGURE 5 | Midostaurin did not alter the protein expression and subcellular localization of ABCB1 transporter. **(A)** Detection and relative intensity of ABCB1 expression in KB-C2 cells incubated with 500 nM of midostaurin for 0, 24, 48, and 72 h. **(B)** Sub-cellular localization of ABCB1 expression in SW620/Ad300 cells incubated with 500 nM of midostaurin for 72 h. Scale bar, 100 μm. *$p < 0.05$, compared with control group.

cells overexpressing ABCB1 transporter in the presence or absence of midostaurin. As shown in **Figure 6B**, midostaurin significantly increased the intracellular levels of [^{3}H]-paclitaxel in ABCB1-overexpressing KB-C2 cells in a dose-dependent manner. However, in parental KB-3-1 cells, no significant change in [^{3}H]-paclitaxel was found. In this study, verapamil was used as a positive control reversal reagent.

Midostaurin Significantly Inhibited the Efflux Function of ABCB1 Transporter in ABCB1-Overexpressing Cancer Cells

The efflux of antineoplastic drugs through ABCB1 transporter is involved in ABCB1-mediated MDR. We conducted an efflux assay at different time points (0, 30, 60, and 120 min) to determine whether midostaurin could inhibit the efflux function of ABCB1 transporter. As shown in **Figures 6C,D**, midostaurin significantly decreased the efflux level of [^{3}H]-paclitaxel in ABCB1-overexpressing KB-C2 cells in a dose-dependent manner, but this change was not shown in parental KB-3-1 cells. These results suggested that midostaurin could significantly increase the accumulation of anticancer drugs by inhibiting the efflux function mediated by ABCB1.

Midostaurin Significantly Inhibited the ATPase Activity of ABCB1 Transporter

The hydrolysis of ATP is the energy source of substrate-efflux mediated by ABCB1. Hence, we conducted the ABCB1-mediated ATP hydrolysis in the presence or absence of midostaurin at 0–40 μM serial concentrations. As shown in **Figure 7A**, midostaurin significantly inhibited the ATPase activity of ABCB1 transporters in a dose-dependent manner. The concentration of midostaurin required to obtain 50% of maximal inhibition

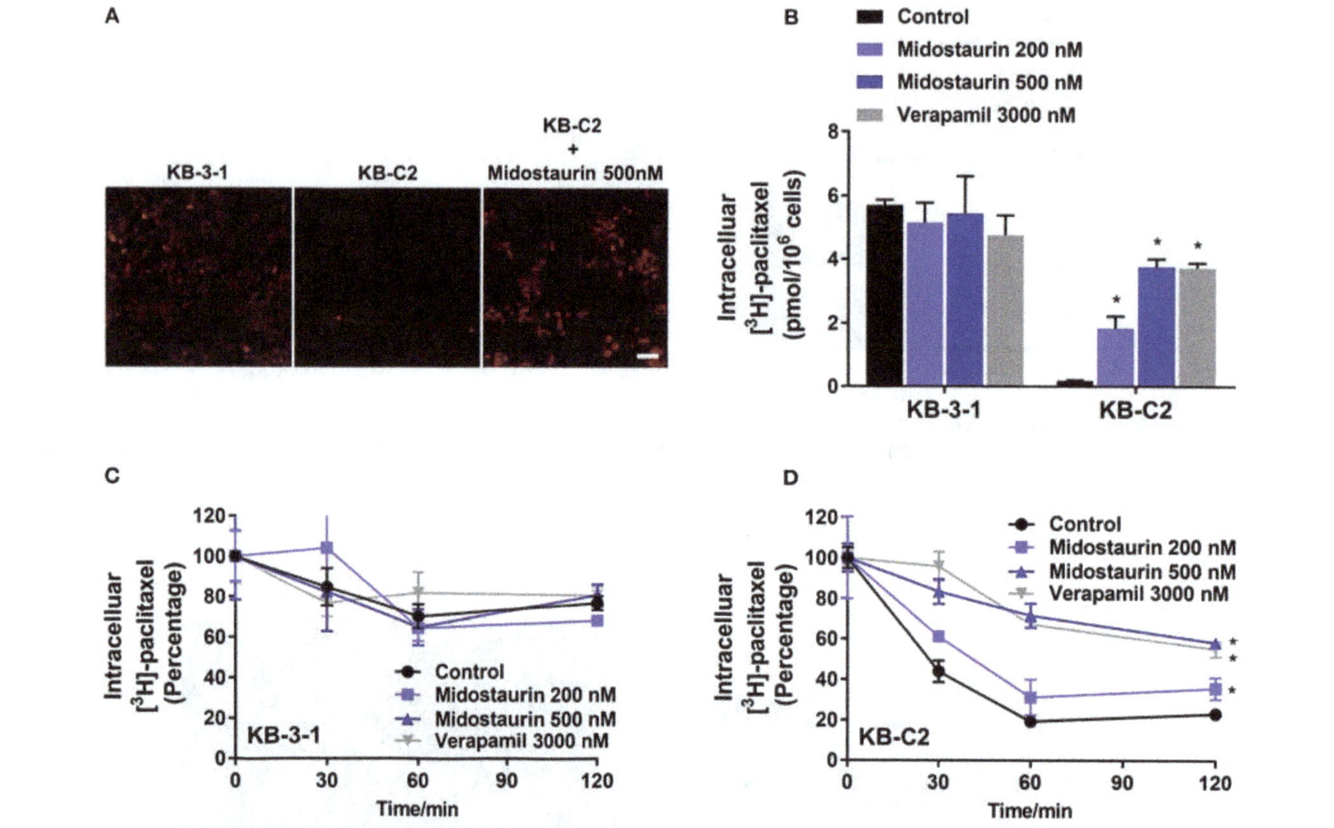

FIGURE 6 | The effect of midostaurin on accumulation and efflux activity in cancer cells overexpression ABCB1 transporter. Scale bar, 50 μm. **(A)** The effect of midostaurin on accumulation of doxorubicin. **(B)** The effect of midostaurin on accumulation of [^{3}H]-paclitaxel in KB-3-1 and KB-C2 cells. **(C,D)** The effects of midostaurin on efflux of [^{3}H]-paclitaxel in KB-3-1 and KB-C2 cells. $^*p < 0.05$, compared with control group.

(IC_{50}) was 3.1 μM with the maximum of inhibition being 0.4-fold. These results suggested that midostaurin could inhibit the ATPase activity in ABCB1 transporters by interacting with the drug-binding pocket of these transporters. Therefore, one of the reversal mechanisms of midostraurin includes a reduced energy source for ABCB1 efflux function through inhibition of ATPase activity.

Docking Analysis of the Binding of Midostaurin With ABCB1 Homology Model

The best-scored docked positions of midostaurin with ABCB1 transporter are shown in **Figure 7**. The phenol ring of the methylbenzamide moiety in midostaurin has π-π interactions with the residues Phe336 and Phe983 of human ABCB1 (**Figure 7C**). In addition, midostaurin has hydrophobic interactions with residues of ABCB1 including Met69, Leu339, Ile340, Phe343, Phe728, Met986, and Ala987 (**Figure 7D**), which stabilize midostaurin in the substrate-binding pocket of ABCB1.

DISCUSSION

Growing evidence has shown that the failure of clinical treatment resulting from drug resistance to chemotherapeutic drugs in a series of cancer cell lines is tightly correlated with the overexpression of ABC transporters. It has been widely reported that cancer cells overexpressing ABCB1 transporter is a key factor that could imply poor prognosis as well as low survival rate in cancer patients (26–30). Moreover, genetic polymorphisms in ABC transporters, especially in ABCB1 and ABCG2 transporters, could significantly increase the high risk of death in patients who suffer from colorectal malignancy or non-small cell lung cancer (NSCLC) (31, 32). In recent decades, many small-molecule target drugs have been reported to have the capacity to reverse ABC transporter-mediated MDR, via inhibiting the function, downregulating the protein expressing level, and/or changing the subcellular localization of ABC transporters. Previously, we have reported that selonsertib, ulixertinib, and VS-4718 can significantly antagonize ABC transporter-mediated MDR (21, 23, 33). Unfortunately, there was no successful clinical case study on the therapeutic strategies to develop ABC transporters inhibitors as reversal reagents to reverse drug resistance. Nonetheless, growing evidence has shown that the overexpression of ABC transporters is mainly involved in MDR in cancer, and it is also critical in regulating oral bioavailability of anticancer drugs and reagents. A series of first-line chemotherapeutic drugs, including doxorubicin, paclitaxel and mitoxantrone are substrates of ABC transporters, meaning

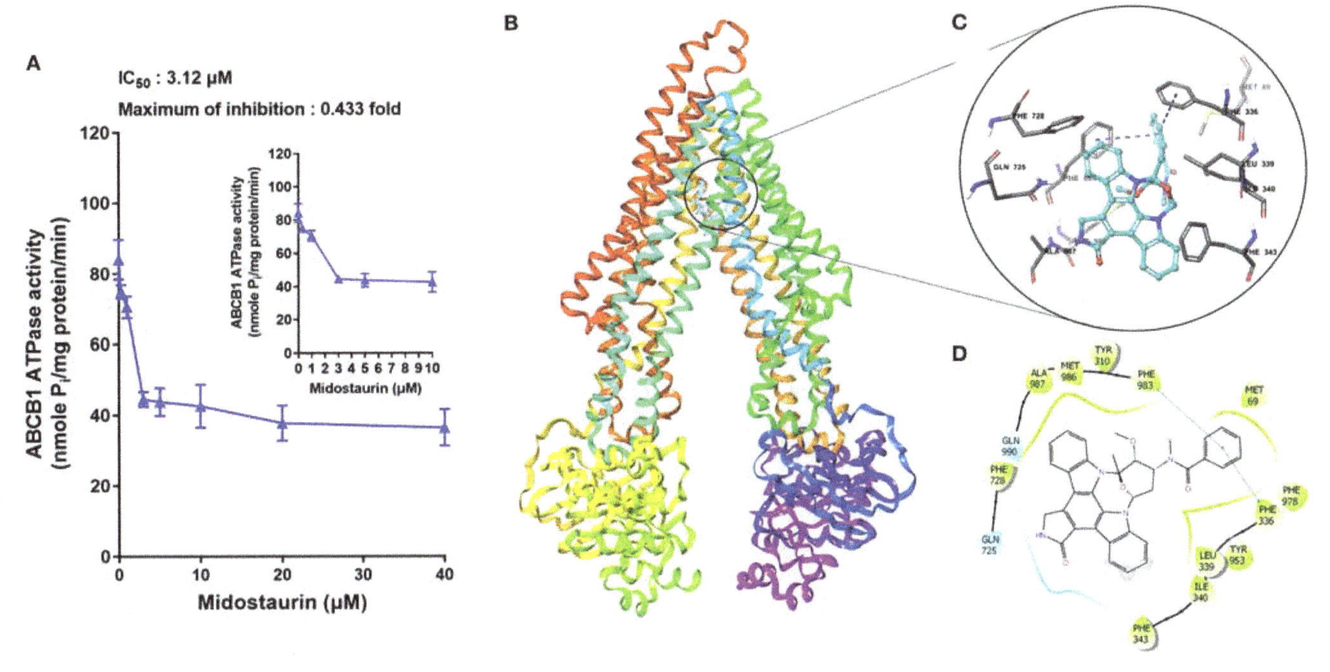

FIGURE 7 | The effects of midostaurin on the ATPase activity of ABCB1 and the molecular modeling study of midostaurin with human homology ABCB1. **(A)** Effect of midostaurin on the ATPase activity of ABCB1. The inset graphs illustrate the effect of 0–10 μM midostaurin on the ATPase activity of ABCB1. Data are mean, representative of three independent experiments. **(B)** Overall view of midostainrin-ABCB1 complex. **(C)** Docked position of midostaurin within the drug-binding site of human ABCB1 homology model by Glide docking. Midostaurin is shown as ball and stick mode with the atoms colored: carbon-cyan, hydrogen-white, nitrogen-blue, oxygen-red. Important residues are shown as sticks with gray color. π-π stacking interactions are indicated with blue dotted short line. **(D)** The two-dimensional ligand-receptor interaction diagram of midostaurin and human ABCB1. The amino acids within 3 Å are shown as colored bubbles, cyan indicates polar residues, and green indicates hydrophobic residues. The green short line shows π-π stacking interaction.

that these anti-cancer drugs will be pumped out from the cancer cells and finally lead to the failure of clinical carcinoma treatment (1–4, 34). Therefore, we confirm that screening small molecules to obtain the inhibitors of ABC transporters is still a potential and effective treatment strategy to circumvent MDR in cancer.

In this *in vitro* study, we evaluated the effect of midostaurin on ABCB1-mediated MDR. We mainly found that midostaurin, at non-toxic concentrations (200 and 500 nM), can significantly overcome ABCB1-mediated MDR in a series of cancer cell lines in a concentration-dependent manner. Firstly, to avoid potential reversal effects caused by the cytostatic effect of midostaurin, we performed our MTT assays to evaluate the anti-proliferative effect of midostaurin in the cells we would use in this study. Based on the results, we conducted further reversal studies using 200 and 500 nM of midostaurin. Our reversal study indicated that midostaurin could significantly reverse ABCB1-mediated MDR in KB-C2 and SW620/Ad300 cells, which were selected by treatment with colchicine or doxorubicin, respectively. Moreover, midostaurin could not alter the efficacy of certain chemotherapy substrate-drugs in their corresponding parental KB-3-1 or SW620 cells. In addition, midostaurin could not antagonize ABCG2-mediated MDR in ABCG2-overexpressing cancer cells NCI-H460/MX20. Based on these results, we hypothesized that the reversal effect of midostaurin was specific to interactions with the ABCB1 transporter. It is notable that we then verified this hypothesis by a reversal study in gene-transfected cells. We found that midostaurin could also lower the IC_{50} values of doxorubicin, paclitaxel, and colchicine in HEK293/ABCB1 cells compared with parental cells in a dose-dependent manner, but not those in parental HEK293/pcDNA3.1 cell line. Furthermore, midostaurin did not sensitize either parental HEK293/pcDNA3.1 cell line or HEK293/ABCB1 cells to cisplatin, a drug that does not use ABCB1 as a substrate. These results suggest that midostaurin exclusively reversed ABCB1-mediated MDR.

The reversal of MDR mediated by ABC transporters may be involved in the down-regulating and/or change of subcellular localization of certain ABC transporters. However, as shown in our Western blotting and immunofluorescence assays, no significant down-regulation of ABCB1 protein was found, and all ABCB1 protein was located on the membrane of KB-C2 cells after incubating with midostaurin for up to 72 h. In other words, these results signified that the mechanisms of midostaurin on the reversal of ABCB1 mediated-MDR were not due to the down-regulating of the protein level or change of subcellular localization of ABCB1 transporters. Nevertheless, as midostaurin is a multi-kinase inhibitor, we could not fully eliminate the possibility that part of the reversal effect of midostaurin could be associated with its effect to other proteins and/or potential cross-talk with other signals, which may impact the efflux function of ABCB1 transporter, and this needs to be studied further in the future. Further study should also evaluate the potential effect of midostaurin on the protein expression level of ABCB1 with increased concentration or prolonged incubation time. Moreover, a process named post-translational modifications (PTM) plays an important role in proteins, especially transporters' function (35). It has been reported that ABCB1 could be phosphorylated at S661, S667, S671, and S683 to modulate its cell surface trafficking (36), and Pim-1 kinase could prevent ABCB1 from degradation, enabling glycosylation and cell surface expression (36). These clues indicate that it is necessary to further determine the effects of midostaurin on PTM of ABCB1 using higher concentration and/or longer incubation time.

Subsequently, drug accumulation and efflux assays were conducted, so that we could deeply understand the mechanisms of midostaurin on ABC transporter-mediated MDR attenuation. Our results indicated that midostaurin could significantly increase the intracellular concentration of ABCB1 substrate-drugs (doxorubicin and [^{3}H]-paclitaxel) in ABCB1-overexpression KB-C2 cells. Midostaurin could also significantly prevent [^{3}H]-paclitaxel from being pumped out of KB-C2 cells in a concentration-dependent manner. However, there is no significant change in doxorubicin or [^{3}H]-paclitaxel in accumulation or efflux in parental KB-3-1 cells. These novel findings were congruent with our observed reversal effects of midostaurin. Our mechanism study also indicated that midostaurin could increase the accumulation of certain substrate-drugs (doxorubicin and [^{3}H]-paclitaxel) in ABCB1-overexpression cancer cells by targeting the function of ABCB1 transporter.

ABC transporters, including ABCB1, obtain energy via ATP hydrolysis, and this can be modulated by the presence of certain substrates or inhibitors (37, 38). In our ATPase assay, we found that midostaurin could significantly inhibit the ATPase activity of ABCB1 in a dose-dependent manner, and the maximal inhibition level was 0.4-fold. Nevertheless, the accurate binding site of midostaurin with ABCB1 transporter remained unclear. In the *in silico* modeling study, we predicted that midostaurin could interact with the drug-binding pocket in the transmembrane domain (TMD) of ABCB1 transporter.

Midostaurin is an anticancer drug approved by FDA for treatment of AML with FLT3-mutant subtype (11). Over the years, the effect of midostaurin on multidrug resistance mediated by ABCB1 has been investigated independently in great detail. At the very beginning, midostaurin, also known as PKC412 and CGP41215, was developed as a PKC inhibitor, and prior work has documented the effectiveness of midostaurin in reversing MDR. Utz et al. (39) and Fabbro et al. (40) have reported that midostaurin could sensitize CCRF-VCR1000 cells and KB-8551 cells to adriamycin and vinblastine, without altering the ABCB1 mRNA expressing level. As a derivative of staurosporine, midostaurin was also identified to have the capacity to increase doxorubicin accumulation in doxorubicin-resistant cell line A2780/Adr. Meanwhile, midostaurin also acted as a reversal reagent in P-gp mediated leukemia resistance (41, 42). Budworth et al. (43) have explored the reversal effects of midostaurin on P-gp mediated breast cancer MCF7/Adr cell line resistance and Beltran et al. (44) have confirmed that such an effect of midostaurin was related to alterions in the phosphorylation of P-gp. In the study conducted by Courage et al. (45), midostaurin-resistant A549/CGP human lung cancer cell line was identified that overexpressed P-gp, indicated that P-gp may play a key role in midostaurin-mediated MDR. Another research showed that midostaurin could not affect the development of RD cells resistance (RD is a cell line that is resistant to vincristine, and has a mutant P53 but does not have detectable P-gp). This finding, combined with the above evidence, suggests that midostaurin may influence P-gp-mediated MDR (46). Moreover, midostaurin was also documented to alter P-gp efflux function and induce cell death in FLT3 ITD/P-g-positive samples (47). Ganeshaguru et al. (48) studied the effect of midostaurin on malignant cells from B-CLL (B-cell chronic lymphocytic leukemia) patients, and the results showed that nearly 1/3 of B-CLL cells that were originally resistant to chlorambucil and fludarabine were sensitive to midostaurin. P-gp-mediated efflux activity of nearly half of B-CCL cells were observed to be modulated by midostaurin. This novel finding further supported the conclusion that midostaurin could reverse ABCB1-mediated MDR. However, due to technical restrictions in protein structure identification and the incomplete functional research on ABC transporters, few studies systematically explained the exact mechanisms of midostaurin on ABCB1-mediated MDR. In this study, we conducted a series of experiments to verify the reversal effects of midostaurin on ABCB1-mediated MDR in cell lines which were not involved in other studies. Furthermore, we used human ABCB1 homology model to conduct our *in silico* docking study, through which we determined the specific residues that midostaurin would bind to, indicated the potential combining mode of midostaurin with ABCB1 transporter. On the other hand, with the development of pharmacological and molecular biology, various resistant cell lines with definite mechanisms were established and identified. It is necessary to verify the reversal effect and to determine the mechanisms of midostaurin on MDR by utilizing different resistant cell lines. More recently, the results from Hsiao et al. (49) showed that midostaurin could sensitize ABCB1-overexpression KB-V-1, NCI-ADR-RES, and NIH3T3-G185 cells to paclitaxel, colchicine, and vincristine. They also found that midostaurin could enhance colchicine-induced apoptosis effect in KB-V-1 cells, without altering the expression level of ABCB1 transporter. This finding coincides with the results we found when we co-administrated midostaurin with ABCB1-substrate chemotherapeutic drugs. In conclusion, our study demonstrates that midostaurin could overcome ABCB1-mediated MDR by directly inhibiting the efflux function of ABCB1 transporter; as a result, midostaurin can increase the accumulation of antineoplastic drugs. This novel study also suggests that co-administration of midostaurin with certain substrate-chemotherapeutic drugs of ABCB1 may benefit cancer clinical treatment by circumventing MDR. However, we should not overstate the function of midostautin on MDR before further *in vivo* study and even clinical evaluation is completed as three generations of ABCB1 inhibitors have all failed to be applicable in clinic (50). Admittedly, it remains to be determined whether midostaurin could contribute to improving chemotherapeutic outcome in clinic. More recently, a global study of the efficacy and safety of midostaurin plus chemotherapy in newly diagnosed patients with FLT3 mutation negative (FLT3-MN) acute myeloid leukemia (AML) is recruiting (NCT03512197), and a phase II clinical evaluation is recruiting for midostaurin associated with standard chemotherapy in patients with core-binding factor leukemia (AML FLT3) (NCT03686345). These clinical trials may provide more potent evidence on combined utilization of midostaurin with conventional chemotherapeutic drugs, which would make midostaurin a sensitizing drug, not just a "reversal reagent."

AUTHOR CONTRIBUTIONS

DK and ZC conceived the general idea. NJ, YY, CC, JW, ZL, ZW, and QC performed experiments. NJ, ZC, DY, and DK analyzed the results. NJ, YY, CC, ZL, ZW, and QC wrote the first draft. DK and ZC revised the manuscript.

FUNDING

This work was supported by National Natural Science Foundation of China (81673464), Grant for Major Project of Tianjin for New Drug Development (17ZXXYSY00050), St. John's University Research Seed Grant (No. 579-1110-7002), and the Postgraduate Innovation Fund of 13th Five-Year comprehensive investment, Tianjin Medical University (YJSCX201712).

ACKNOWLEDGMENTS

We would like to thank Dr. Stephen Aller (The University of Alabama at Birmingham, Birmingham) for kindly providing the human ABCB1 homology model. We thank Tanaji T. Talele (St. John's University, New York, NY) for providing the computing resources for the docking analysis. We thank Drs. Susan E. Bates and Robert W. Robey (NCI, NIH, Bethesda, MD) for providing the cell lines. We thank Dr. Yanglu (Princeton University, NJ) for language editing. The first author thanks China Scholarship Council for reimbursing daily expenditures in America.

REFERENCES

1. Szakacs G, Paterson JK, Ludwig JA, Booth-Genthe C, Gottesman MM. Targeting multidrug resistance in cancer. *Nat Rev Drug Discov.* (2006) 5:219–34. doi: 10.1038/nrd1984
2. Dassa E, Bouige P. The ABC of ABCS: a phylogenetic and functional classification of ABC systems in living organisms. *Res Microbiol.* (2001) 152:211–29. doi: 10.1016/S0923-2508(01)01194-9
3. Eckford PD, Sharom FJ. ABC efflux pump-based resistance to chemotherapy drugs. *Chem Rev.* (2009) 109:2989–3011. doi: 10.1021/cr9000226
4. Stavrovskaya AA, Stromskaya TP. Transport proteins of the ABC family and multidrug resistance of tumor cells. *Biochemistry.* (2008) 73:592–604. doi: 10.1134/S0006297908050118
5. Linton KJ. Structure and function of ABC transporters. *Physiology.* (2007) 22:122–30. doi: 10.1152/physiol.00046.2006
6. Linton KJ, Higgins CF. Structure and function of ABC transporters: the ATP switch provides flexible control. *Pflugers Arch.* (2007) 453:555–67. doi: 10.1007/s00424-006-0126-x
7. Wu CP, Ambudkar VS. The pharmacological impact of ATP-binding cassette drug transporters on vemurafenib-based therapy. *Acta Pharm Sin B.* (2014) 4:105–11. doi: 10.1016/j.apsb.2013.12.001
8. Sauna ZE, Smith MM, Muller M, Kerr KM, Ambudkar SV. The mechanism of action of multidrug-resistance-linked P-glycoprotein. *J Bioenerg Biomembr.* (2001) 33:481–91. doi: 10.1023/A:1012875105006
9. Ali MA, Elsalakawy WA. ABCB1 haplotypes but not individual SNPs predict for optimal response/failure in Egyptian patients with chronic-phase chronic myeloid leukemia receiving imatinib mesylate. *Med Oncol.* (2014) 31:279. doi: 10.1007/s12032-014-0279-y
10. Propper DJ, McDonald AC, Man A, Thavasu P, Balkwill F, Braybrooke JP, et al. Phase I and pharmacokinetic study of PKC412, an inhibitor of protein kinase C. *J Clin Oncol.* (2001) 19:1485–92. doi: 10.1200/JCO.2001.19.5.1485
11. Rasko JEJ, Hughes TP. First approved kinase inhibitor for AML. *Cell.* (2017) 171:981. doi: 10.1016/j.cell.2017.11.007
12. Stone RM, Mandrekar SJ, Sanford BL, Laumann K, Geyer S, Bloomfield CD, et al. Midostaurin plus chemotherapy for acute myeloid leukemia with a FLT3 mutation. *N Engl J Med.* (2017) 377:454–64. doi: 10.1056/NEJMoa1614359
13. Akiyama S, Fojo A, Hanover JA, Pastan I, Gottesman MM. Isolation and genetic characterization of human KB cell lines resistant to multiple drugs. *Somat Cell Mol Genet.* (1985) 11:117–26. doi: 10.1007/BF01534700
14. Bates SE, Lee JS, Dickstein B, Spolyar M, Fojo AT. Differential modulation of P-glycoprotein transport by protein kinase inhibition. *Biochemistry.* (1993) 32:9156–64. doi: 10.1021/bi00086a022
15. Robey RW, Honjo Y, van de Laar A, Miyake K, Regis JT, Litman T, et al. A functional assay for detection of the mitoxantrone resistance protein, MXR (ABCG2). *Biochim Biophys Acta.* (2001) 1512:171–82. doi: 10.1016/S0005-2736(01)00308-X
16. Fung KL, Pan J, Ohnuma S, Lund PE, Pixley JN, Kimchi-Sarfaty C, et al. MDR1 synonymous polymorphisms alter transporter specificity and protein stability in a stable epithelial monolayer. *Cancer Res.* (2014) 74:598–608. doi: 10.1158/0008-5472.CAN-13-2064
17. Zhang XY, Zhang YK, Wang YJ, Gupta P, Zeng L, Xu M, et al. Osimertinib (AZD9291), a mutant-selective EGFR inhibitor, reverses ABCB1-mediated drug resistance in cancer cells. *Molecules.* (2016) 21:E1236. doi: 10.3390/molecules21091236
18. Zhang YK, Zhang H, Zhang GN, Wang YJ, Kathawala RJ, Si R, et al. Semi-synthetic ocotillol analogues as selective ABCB1-mediated drug resistance reversal agents. *Oncotarget.* (2015) 6:24277–90. doi: 10.18632/oncotarget.4493
19. Shi Z, Peng XX, Kim IW, Shukla S, Si QS, Robey RW, et al. Erlotinib (Tarceva, OSI-774) antagonizes ATP-binding cassette subfamily B member 1 and ATP-binding cassette subfamily G member 2-mediated drug resistance. *Cancer Res.* (2007) 67:11012–20. doi: 10.1158/0008-5472.CAN-07-2686
20. Sun YL, Kathawala RJ, Singh S, Zheng K, Talele TT, Jiang WQ, et al. Zafirlukast antagonizes ATP-binding cassette subfamily G member 2-mediated multidrug resistance. *Anticancer Drugs.* (2012) 23:865–73. doi: 10.1097/CAD.0b013e328354a196
21. Ji N, Yang Y, Lei ZN, Cai CY, Wang JQ, Gupta P, et al. Ulixertinib (BVD-523) antagonizes ABCB1- and ABCG2-mediated chemotherapeutic drug resistance. *Biochem Pharmacol.* (2018b) 158:274–85. doi: 10.1016/j.bcp.2018.10.028
22. Li J, Jaimes KF, Aller SG. Refined structures of mouse P-glycoprotein. *Protein Sci.* (2014) 23:34–46. doi: 10.1002/pro.2387

23. Ji N, Yang Y, Cai CY, Lei ZN, Wang JQ, Gupta P, et al. VS-4718 antagonizes multidrug resistance in ABCB1- and ABCG2-overexpression cancer cells by inhibiting the efflux function of ABC transporters. *Front Pharmacol.* (2018a) 9:1236. doi: 10.3389/fphar.2018.01236
24. Zhang H, Patel A, Wang YJ, Zhang YK, Kathawala RJ, Qiu LH, et al. The BTK inhibitor ibrutinib (PCI-32765) overcomes paclitaxel resistance in ABCB1- and ABCC10-overexpression cells and tumors. *Mol Cancer Ther.* (2017a) 16:1021–30. doi: 10.1158/1535-7163.MCT-16-0511
25. Zhang YK, Zhang XY, Zhang GN, Wang YJ, Xu H, Zhang D, et al. Selective reversal of BCRP-mediated MDR by VEGFR-2 inhibitor ZM323881. *Biochem Pharmacol.* (2017b) 132:29–37. doi: 10.1016/j.bcp.2017.02.019
26. Marsh S, Somlo G, Li X, Frankel P, King CR, Shannon WD, et al. Pharmacogenetic analysis of paclitaxel transport and metabolism genes in breast cancer. *Pharmacogenomics J.* (2007) 7:362–5. doi: 10.1038/sj.tpj.6500434
27. Campa D, Muller P, Edler L, Knoefel L, Barale R, Heussel CP, et al. A comprehensive study of polymorphisms in ABCB1, ABCC2 and ABCG2 and lung cancer chemotherapy response and prognosis. *Int J Cancer.* (2012) 131:2920–8. doi: 10.1002/ijc.27567
28. Hlavata I, Mohelnikova-Duchonova B, Vaclavikova R, Liska V, Pitule P, Novak P, et al. The role of ABC transporters in progression and clinical outcome of colorectal cancer. *Mutagenesis.* (2012) 27:187–96. doi: 10.1093/mutage/ger075
29. Litviakov NV, Cherdyntseva NV, Tsyganov MM, Denisov EV, Garbukov EY, Merzliakova MK, et al. Changing the expression vector of multidrug resistance genes is related to neoadjuvant chemotherapy response. *Cancer Chemother Pharmacol.* (2013) 71:153–63. doi: 10.1007/s00280-012-1992-x
30. Bartholomae S, Gruhn B, Debatin KM, Zimmermann M, Creutzig U, Reinhardt D, et al. Coexpression of multiple ABC-transporters is strongly associated with treatment response in childhood acute myeloid leukemia. *Pediatr Blood Cancer.* (2016) 63:242–7. doi: 10.1002/pbc.25785
31. Wu H, Kang H, Liu Y, Xiao Q, Zhang Y, Sun M, et al. Association of ABCB1 genetic polymorphisms with susceptibility to colorectal cancer and therapeutic prognosis. *Pharmacogenomics.* (2013) 14:897–911. doi: 10.2217/pgs.13.78
32. Wang F, Huang Z, Zheng K, Zhao H, Hu W. Two SNPs of ATP-binding cassette B1 gene on the risk and prognosis of colorectal cancer. *Int J Clin Exp Pathol.* (2015) 8:3083–9.
33. Ji N, Yang Y, Cai CY, Lei ZN, Wang JQ, Gupta P, et al. Selonsertib (GS-4997), an ASK1 inhibitor, antagonizes multidrug resistance in ABCB1- and ABCG2-overexpression cancer cells. *Cancer Lett.* (2019) 440–441:82–93. doi: 10.1016/j.canlet.2018.10.007
34. Kartal-Yandim M, Adan-Gokbulut A, Baran Y. Molecular mechanisms of drug resistance and its reversal in cancer. *Crit Rev Biotechnol.* (2016) 36:716–26. doi: 10.3109/07388551.2015.1015957
35. Czuba LC, Hillgren KM, Swaan PW. Post-translational modifications of transporters. *Pharmacol Ther.* (2018) 192:88–99. doi: 10.1016/j.pharmthera.2018.06.013
36. Germann UA, Chambers TC, Ambudkar SV, Licht T, Cardarelli CO, Pastan I, et al. Characterization of phosphorylation-defective mutants of human P-glycoprotein expressed in mammalian cells. *J Biol Chem.* (1996) 271:1708–16. doi: 10.1074/jbc.271.3.1708
37. Gottesman MM, Ambudkar SV. Overview: ABC transporters and human disease. *J Bioenerg Biomembr.* (2001) 33:453–8. doi: 10.1023/A:1012866803188
38. Wilkens S. Structure and mechanism of ABC transporters. *F1000Prime Rep.* (2015) 7:14. doi: 10.12703/P7-14
39. Utz I, Hofer S, Regenass U, Hilbe W, Thaler J, Grunicke H, et al. The protein kinase C inhibitor CGP 41251, a staurosporine derivative with antitumor activity, reverses multidrug resistance. *Int J Cancer.* (1994) 57:104–10. doi: 10.1002/ijc.2910570119
40. Fabbro D, Buchdunger E, Wood J, Mestan J, Hofmann F, Ferrari S, et al. Inhibitors of protein kinases: CGP 41251, a protein kinase inhibitor with potential as an anticancer agent. *Pharmacol Ther.* (1999) 82:293–301. doi: 10.1016/S0163-7258(99)00005-4
41. Sedlak J, Hunakova L, Duraj J, Chorvath B, Novotny L. Effects of protein kinase C inhibitor, staurosporine derivative CGP 41 251, on cell cycle, DNA synthesis and drug uptake in neoplastic cell lines. *Anticancer Drugs.* (1995) 6:70–6. doi: 10.1097/00001813-199502000-00008
42. Sedlak J, Hunakova L, Sulikova M, Chorvath B. Protein kinase inhibitor-induced alterations of drug uptake, cell cycle and surface antigen expression in human multidrug-resistant (Pgp and MRP) promyelocytic leukemia HL-60 cells. *Leuk Res.* (1997) 21:449–58. doi: 10.1016/S0145-2126(96)00088-4
43. Budworth J, Davies R, Malkhandi J, Gant TW, Ferry DR, Gescher A. Comparison of staurosporine and four analogues: their effects on growth, rhodamine 123 retention and binding to P-glycoprotein in multidrug-resistant MCF-7/Adr cells. *Br J Cancer.* (1996) 73:1063–8. doi: 10.1038/bjc.1996.205
44. Beltran PJ, Fan D, Fidler IJ, O'Brian CA. Chemosensitization of cancer cells by the staurosporine derivative CGP 41251 in association with decreased P-glycoprotein phosphorylation. *Biochem Pharmacol.* (1997) 53:245–7. doi: 10.1016/S0006-2952(96)00718-6
45. Courage C, Bradder SM, Jones T, Schultze-Mosgau MH, Gescher A. Characterisation of novel human lung carcinoma cell lines selected for resistance to anti-neoplastic analogues of staurosporine. *Int J Cancer.* (1997) 73:763–8.
46. Cocker HA, Tiffin N, Pritchard-Jones K, Pinkerton CR, Kelland LR. *In vitro* prevention of the emergence of multidrug resistance in a pediatric rhabdomyosarcoma cell line. *Clin Cancer Res.* (2001) 7:3193–8.
47. Hunter HM, Pallis M, Seedhouse CH, Grundy M, Gray C, Russell NH. The expression of P-glycoprotein in AML cells with FLT3 internal tandem duplications is associated with reduced apoptosis in response to FLT3 inhibitors. *Br J Haematol.* (2004) 127:26–33. doi: 10.1111/j.1365-2141.2004.05145.x
48. Ganeshaguru K, Wickremasinghe RG, Jones DT, Gordon M, Hart SM, Virchis AE, et al. Actions of the selective protein kinase C inhibitor PKC412 on B-chronic lymphocytic leukemia cells *in vitro*. *Haematologica.* (2002) 87:167–76.
49. Hsiao SH, Lusvarghi S, Huang YH, Ambudkar SV, Hsu SC, Wu CP. The FLT3 inhibitor midostaurin selectively resensitizes ABCB1-overexpression multidrug-resistant cancer cells to conventional chemotherapeutic agents. *Cancer Lett.* (2019) 445:34–44. doi: 10.1016/j.canlet.2019.01.001
50. Palmeira A, Sousa E, Vasconcelos MH, Pinto MM. Three decades of P-gp inhibitors: skimming through several generations and scaffolds. *Curr Med Chem.* (2012) 19:1946–2025. doi: 10.2174/0929867128001 67392
51. Gottesman MM, Fojo T, Bates SE. Multidrug resistance in cancer: role of ATP-dependent transporters. *Nat Rev Cancer.* (2002) 2:48–58. doi: 10.1038 nrc706

14

Molecular Targeted Therapy in the Treatment of Chordoma

Tong Meng [1,2,3†], Jiali Jin [4†], Cong Jiang [5], Runzhi Huang [1], Huabin Yin [2,3], Dianwen Song [2,3*] and Liming Cheng [1,6*]*

[1] Division of Spine, Department of Orthopedics, Tongji Hospital Affiliated to Tongji University School of Medicine, Shanghai, China, [2] Shanghai Bone Tumor Institution, Shanghai, China, [3] Department of Orthopedics, Shanghai General Hospital, School of Medicine, Shanghai Jiaotong University, Shanghai, China, [4] Department of Central Laboratory, Shanghai Tenth People's Hospital of Tongji University, School of Medicine, School of Life Sciences and Technology, Tongji University, Shanghai, China, [5] Beth Israel Deaconess Medical Center, BIDMC Cancer Center, Harvard Medical School, Cancer Research Institute, Boston, MA, United States, [6] Key Laboratory of Spine and Spinal Cord Injury Repair and Regeneration, Ministry of Education, Tongji University, Shanghai, China

***Correspondence:**
Huabin Yin
yinhuabin@aliyun.com
Dianwen Song
osongdianwen@126.com
Liming Cheng
limingcheng@tongji.edu.cn

† These authors have contributed equally to this work and share first authorship

Objectives: Chordoma is a rare bone malignancy that affects the spine and skull base. Treatment dilemma leads to a high rate of local relapse and distant metastases. Molecular targeted therapy (MTT) is an option for advanced chordoma, but its therapeutic efficacy and safety have not been investigated systematically. Therefore, a systematic review was conducted on studies reporting MTT regimens for chordoma.

Methods: Clinical trials, case series and case reports on chordoma MTT were identified using MEDLINE, Cochrane library and EMBASE, and systematically reviewed. Data on clinical outcomes, such as median overall survival, progression-free survival, response rate and adverse events (AEs) were extracted and analyzed.

Results: Thirty-three eligible studies were selected for the systematic review, which indicated that imatinib and erlotinib were the most frequently used molecular targeted inhibitors (MTIs) for chordoma. For PDGFR-positive and/or EGFR-positive chordoma, clinical benefits were achieved with acceptable AEs. Monotherapy is preferred as the first-line of treatment, and combined drug therapy as the second-line treatment. In addition, the brachyury vaccine has shown promising results.

Conclusions: The selection of MTIs for patients with advanced or relapsed chordoma should be based on gene mutation screening and immunohistochemistry (IHC). Monotherapy of TKIs is recommended as the first-line management, and combination therapy (two TKIs or TKI plus mTOR inhibitor) may be the choice for drug-resistant chordoma. Brachyury vaccine is a promising therapeutic strategy and requires more clinical trials to evaluate its safety and efficacy.

Keywords: molecular targeted therapy, bone tumor, chordoma, systematic review, imatinib, erlotinib

INTRODUCTION

Chordoma is a relatively rare malignant bone tumor with an incidence of 0.08 per 100,000 (1). It accounts for 1–4% of all bone malignancies, and ∼20% of primary spine tumors (2). Although it can occur at any segment of the spine, the predominant site of chordoma are fused segments like clivus and sacrococcyx (3). It is an indolent malignancy that progresses slowly, but exhibits strong local aggressiveness and often grows into huge masses that compress vital nerves and blood vessels (4). In addition, since chordoma is usually unresponsive to the conventional radiotherapy and cytotoxic chemotherapy, surgery is the primary therapeutic option (1, 5). Large case series including our previous one have shown that a total resection of the tumor, with the goal of negative microscopic margins, is crucial for long-term positive outcomes (6). However, the complex anatomy of the spine and the relatively large tumor volume make a clean resection technically challenging, leading to a high rate of local relapse and distant metastases (7). Regarding to this advanced setting, conventional therapeutic methods were shown to be not highly effective (1). Therefore, novel therapeutic strategies are needed to prolong patients' survival and improve the quality of life.

Pathologically, chordoma arises from residual notochord cells within the vertebral body (8), as verified on the basis of genetic and immuno-phenotypic biomarkers (9). New insights into the molecular mechanism underlying chordoma have also identified novel therapeutic targets (5). Molecular targeted therapy (MTT) in chordoma includes (1) imatinib and dasatinib against platelet-derived growth factor receptors (PDGFR) and stem cell factor receptor (KIT) (10, 11); (2) erlotinib, lapatinib, gefitinib, and cetuximab against epidermal growth factor receptor (EGFR) and erbB-2/human epidermal growth factor receptor 2 (HER2/neu) (12, 13); (3) sorafenib, pazopanib, and sunitinib that target angiogenic factors like vascular endothelial growth factor receptor (VEGFR) (14–16); and (4) temsirolimus and sirolimus that target the phosphoinositide 3-kinase (PI3K)/AKT/mammalian target of rapamycin (mTOR) pathway (17).

The indications for MTTs in chordoma patients are largely based on a few prospective clinical trials, small retrospective studies, and even case reports (10–17). However, the efficacy and safety of MTT regimens in chordoma patients, as well as the underlying molecular mechanisms, lack systematic investigation. Therefore, we conducted a systematic review on MTT regimens in chordoma patients to determine the clinical outcomes and underlying molecular mechanisms.

MATERIALS AND METHODS

Search Strategy

For this systematic review, we used standard procedures from PRISMA guidelines (18). A comprehensive, systematic search was performed using MEDLINE (via PubMed), Cochrane Library and EMBASE. To find appropriate studies in MEDLINE, we used a combination of terms related to the MeSH terms "Chordoma/drug therapy" OR the free-text searching "Chordoma" AND ("targeted therapy OR inhibitor OR inhibit OR inhibition"). This search was further modified as appropriate for Cochrane Library and EMBASE. Initial search was performed on January 17, 2018 and repeated on July 1, 2018.

Eligibility Criteria

Studies were deemed eligible for the assessment of MTTs in patients with chordoma, irrespective of previous and subsequent other treatment. Only English language publications were included. For clinical trials, case series and case reports published exclusively in abstract or news form, only those containing new data were analyzed. For literature reviews, new personal unpublished data is also included. Reference lists of selected studies and previous reviews associated with similar topics were screened manually. New clinical trials for chordoma were found from Chordoma Foundation, ClinicalTrials.gov, EU Clinical Trials Register and WHO International Clinical Trials Registry Platform. Although gray literature (such as unpublished reports, conference abstracts and dissertations) might provide some negative results and decrease the publication bias, we did not access them, because they were usually not peer reviewed and might be later published in peer-reviewed journals.

Data Extraction and Synthesis

After removal of duplicates, titles and abstracts of all identified publications were systematically screened by two independent reviewers (MT and YHB). Discrepancies between reviewers were resolved by discussion. When eligibility criteria seemed to be met, the two reviewers (MT and YHB) independently assessed retrieved full texts and extracted information. If disagreements were still remained, the third reviewer (SDW) helped to reach an agreement. We contacted with the Chordoma Foundation in order to get helpful information. Additionally, we corresponded with researchers clarify study eligibility if the published study was unclear, although responses were poor. Extracted data were study characteristics (study design, first author, year of publication), patient characteristics (total number, history of treatment) and tumor characteristics (gene mutation and immunohistochemistry), MTT information (type of agents, dosage, course of treatment and adverse events), evaluation criteria (Choi's criteria, the response evaluation criteria in solid tumor (RECIST), clinical and radiological or metabolic response), and survival (duration of follow-up, progression-free survival and overall survival).

RESULTS

Search Results

The flow-chart for the selection and exclusion of relevant publications is shown in **Figure 1**. We identified 293 studies in the initial screening, and after removing duplicates and papers based on their titles and abstracts, selected 64 publications for full-text assessment. Twenty-seven studies met our inclusion criteria, and six more were included—three from manually searching the reference list of the selected articles, two from repeated search and one with the help of the Chordoma

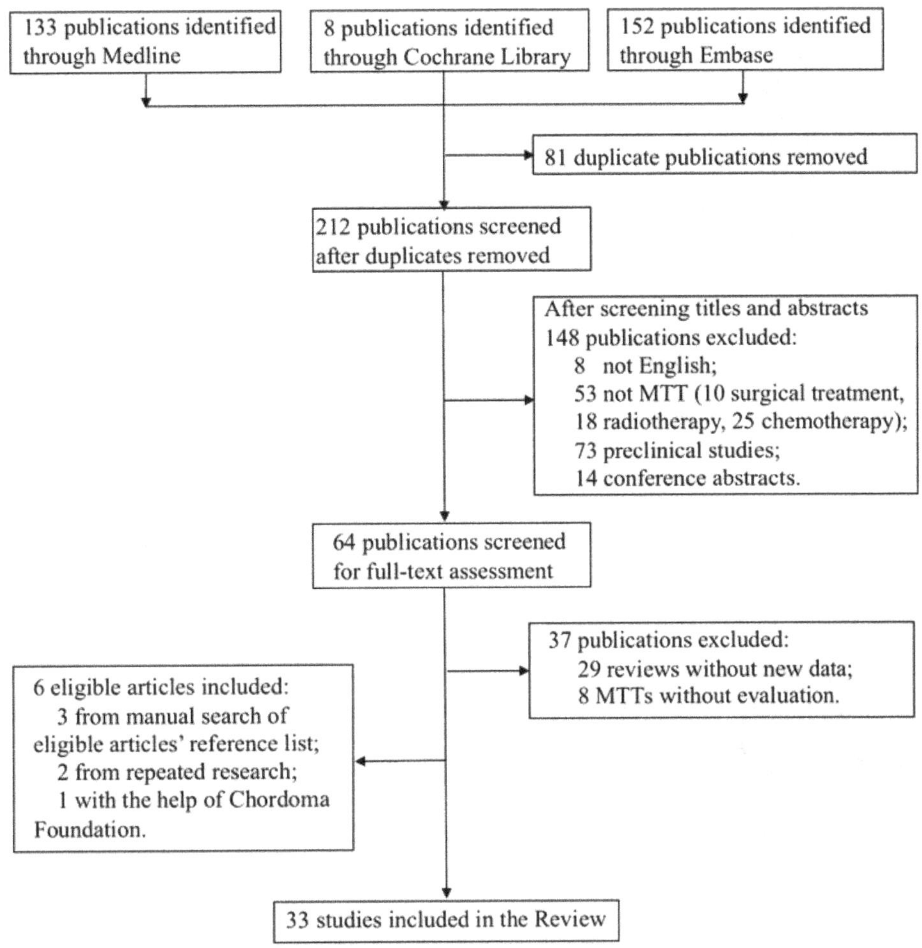

FIGURE 1 | PRISMA flow diagram of the study selection process.

Foundation. Finally, 33 studies were included in this systematic review.

Study Characteristics

Among 33 studies, nine studies were clinical trials (10–12, 14, 15, 19–22), with eight retrospective case series (16, 17, 23–28), and 16 case reports (13, 29–43). Imatinib was assessed in 18 studies with a total of 221 patients (10, 16, 17, 19, 23–28, 32, 34–36, 38, 39, 41, 42), erlotinib in 10 studies with 16 patients (13, 17, 22, 33, 35, 38, 40–42), cetuximab in five studies (seven patients) (13, 30, 31, 33, 41), sorafenib in four studies (65 patients) (15, 17, 21, 37), pazopanib in four studies with seven patients (16, 28, 41, 43) and sunitinib in three studies with 11 patients (14, 17, 28). Sirolimus, thalidomide, bevacizumab, gefitinib, linsitinib, and everolimus were accessed in two studies each (13, 22, 25, 28–31, 33, 34, 40–42), whereas dasatinib (32 patients) (11), lapatinib (18 patients) (12), rapamycin (one patients) (34), temosirolimus (one patients) (17) and yeast-brachyury (GI-6301) vaccine (11 patients) (20) were only analyzed in one study each (**Figures 2** and **3**). Monotherapy of MTTs was reported in 24 studies (10–12, 14–17, 20, 21, 23, 24, 26–28, 32, 34–39, 41, 43, 44) with combination therapy in 13 studies (13, 19, 22, 25, 28–31, 33, 39–42).

RECIST evaluation criteria was used in 19 studies (10–15, 17, 19, 20, 22, 25–28, 32, 40, 42, 43, 45) and Choi's criteria is applied in three studies (11, 12, 25). Twenty-one studies were evaluated by clinical/radiological or metabolic responses (16, 23–27, 29–43). Adverse events (AEs) were reported in 25 studies, including hematological anomalies like anemia, thrombocytopenia, as well as non-hematological AEs like fatigue, fever, anorexia, QTc prolongation, abnormal liver function, nausea, and vomiting (10–15, 19, 22, 23, 26–38, 40, 43, 45).

Efficacy and Safety of MTT Regimens in Chordoma Patients

PDGFR Inhibitors (Table 1)

Imatinib mesylate (IM), a specific tyrosine kinase inhibitor (TKI) targeting PDGFR and KIT (10, 46), was the most frequently-used MTT in chordoma patients. Eighteen studies investigated the therapeutic efficacy of IM on 221 patients (10, 16, 17, 19, 23–28, 32, 34–36, 38, 39, 41, 42), including three clinical trials (10, 19,

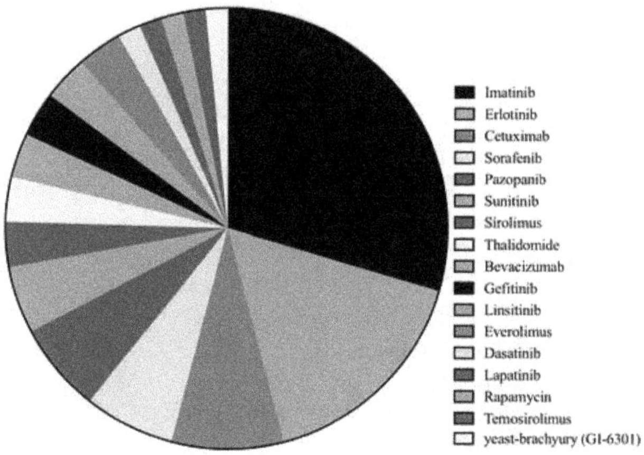

FIGURE 2 | Of the included studies, the proportion of studies reporting each molecular targeted inhibitor.

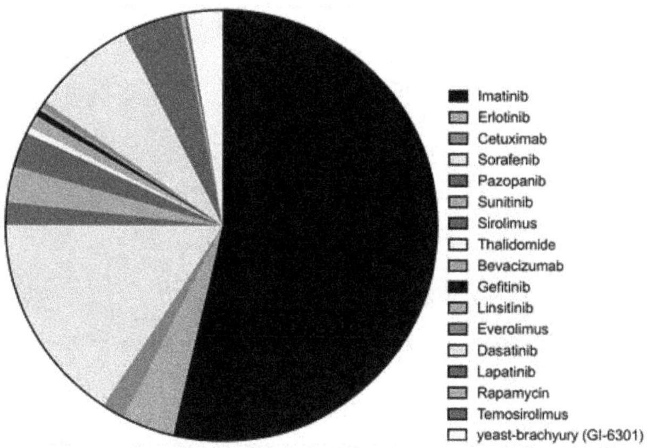

FIGURE 3 | Of the included chordoma patients, the proportion of patients received each molecular targeted inhibitor.

28), seven retrospective case series (16, 17, 23–27), and eight case reports (32, 34–36, 38, 39, 41, 42). Fourteen studies (204 patients) analyzed the efficacy of imatinib as monotherapy (10, 16, 17, 23, 24, 26–28, 32, 34–36, 39, 41), of which four studies (181 patients) used RECIST and 3 were focused on PDGFRβ-expressing chordoma. In these four studies, four patients achieved partial response (PR) (2.2%), 133 cases sustained stable disease (SD) (73.5%) and 44 cases experienced progressive disease (PD) (24.3%) (10, 17, 26, 27, 32). Clinical/radiological or metabolic responses were evaluated in 13 studies (85 patients), with 33 patients achieving PR (38.8%), 23 patients sustaining SD (27.1%) and 29 patients experiencing PD (34.1%) (16, 23, 24, 26–28, 32, 34–36, 38, 39, 41). Five of the above studies (73 patients) focused on PDGFRβ-expressing chordoma, with 45.2% PR, 31.5% SD, and 23.3% PD cases (23, 24, 26, 27, 36), and eight studies included 12 patients that experienced PD within a short period of time.

Progression-free survival (PFS) and overall survival (OS) are important indices of clinical outcome, and they were reported in two large case-studies (10, 27). Stacchiotti et al. conducted a phase II trial in 56 patients with chordoma, and the median PFS and OS were 9 and 35 months, respectively (10). A retrospective study on 46 chordoma patients reported a median PFS of 9.9 months (27).

AEs were reported in eight studies (10, 23, 27, 32, 34, 36), with skin rash being the most common, followed by oedema, chronic anemia, fatigue and fluid retention (10, 26). Subacute intraventricular hemorrhage was seen in one case of clivus chordoma treated with imatinib (36).

Dasatinib, an inhibitor of PDGFR and Src, was evaluated in a phase II study (NCT00464620) (11) on 32 patients. The median PFS and 6 months PFS rate were 6.3 months and 54%, respectively. The 2- and 5-years OS rate were 43 and 18%, respectively. Six patients had an objective response (OR) according to Choi criteria and one for RECIST. Fatigue, fever, anorexia, nausea, and vomiting occurred in more than 5% of the patients.

EGFR Inhibitors (Table 2)

Erlotinib was the most commonly used anti-EGFR agent and was analyzed in 10 studies (16 patients) for the treatment of chordoma (13, 17, 22, 32, 33, 35, 38, 40–42), including one clinical trials (22), one retrospective case study (17) and eight case reports (13, 17, 22, 32, 33, 35, 38, 40–42). Monotherapy with erlotinib was used in five studies (nine patients) (17, 32, 35, 38, 42), three (seven patients) of which were evaluated by RECIST (17, 32, 42), reporting PR in two patients and SD in five patients. Three case reports were evaluated by clinical/radiological or metabolic responses (32, 35, 38). All achieved PR and significant tumor bulk reduction was seen in two patients (70 and 46%, respectively). Skin rashes were commonly seen in the erlotinib-treated patients.

Lapatinib monotherapy was evaluated in a phase II clinical trial on 18 patients with EGFR-positive chordoma (12). Six patients achieved PR and seven sustained SD, with the median PFS of 6 months according to the Choi criteria. In contrast, all patients had SD by RECIST criteria with the median PFS of 8 months. Most patients experienced G $\geq$ 2 AEs.

Combined therapy with EGFR inhibitors was used in seven studies (eight patients) (13, 22, 30, 31, 33, 40, 41). Erlotinib was also the most common agents used in the combined MTT regimens (five studies, seven patients) (13, 22, 33, 40, 41).

Linsitinib, an inhibitor of IGF-1R/insulin receptor (INSR), was evaluated in a phase I study in combination with erlotinib (NCT00739453) (22). One patient with chordoma achieved PR for 18 months according to RECIST, with a PFS of 5 years. AEs included QTc prolongation, abnormal liver function, hyperglycemia and anorexia (22, 40).

The anti-EGFR monoclonal antibody (mAb) cetuximab was applied in combination with erlotinib in one patient with EGFR-positive chordoma, and he had a SD for 6 months (41). However, four patients with EGFR-negative chordoma experienced PD after receiving the same regimen. The treatment failure prompted a switch to bevacizumab, an anti-VEGF mAb (13, 33). Following this change, two patients achieved PR and another two presented SD. Treatment-related fatigue was observed in one patient (13, 33). Combined regimen of cetuximab and gefitinib was also effective in two cases of EGFR-positive chordoma (30, 31), where

TABLE 1 | Molecular targeted therapy of chordomas with PDGFR inhibitors (imatinib, dasatinib).

References	Study design	Levels of evidence	Sample size	Conditions	IHC positive	Drug (dosage)	Median treatment time (months)	AEs	Outcomes			Median follow-up (months)	Median PFS (months)	Median OS (months)
									Choi's criteria	RECIS	TRMR			
Stacchiotti et al. (10)	Phase II	IV	56	Advanced chordoma	PDGFRB/ PDGFB	Imatinib (800 mg/day)	9.1	Grade 3 toxicity: 72%	—	PR: 2%; SD: 70%; PD: 28%	—	26.4	9.2	35
Casali et al. (23)	Case series	IV	6	Advanced chordoma	PDGFRB	Imatinib (800 mg/day)	—	Toxicity: 33.3%	—	—	PR: 66.6%; SD: 16.7%; PD: 16.7%	—	—	—
Hindiet al. (27)	Case series	IV	46	Advanced chordoma	PDGFB/ PDGFRB	Imatinib (800 mg/day)	—	Toxicity: 87.5%	—	PR: 0; SD: 74%; PD: 26%	PR: 40%; SD: 28%; PD: 32%	24.5	9.9	30
Geoerger et al. (24)	Case series	IV	3	Chordoma	PDGFB/ PDGFRB/KIT	Imatinib (800 mg/day)	—	—	—	—	PR: 67%; SD: 33%	—	—	—
Ferraresi et al. (26)	Case series	IV	17	Advanced chordoma	PDGFRB	Imatinib (800 mg/day)	—	—	—	SD	PR: 54%; SD + PD: 46%	—	—	—
Launay et al. (35)	Case report	V	1	Advanced chordoma	EGFR	Imatinib (600 mg/day)	—	None	—	—	PD	—	—	—
Singhal et al. (32)	Case report	V	1	Recurrent chordoma	EMA/ cytokeratins	Imatinib (600 mg/day)	—	Grade 2 skin rash	—	—	PD	—	—	—
Trapani et al. (42)	Case report	V	1	Recurrent chordoma	PDGFRB, EGFR, pS6	Imatinib (400 mg/day) + everolimus	—	—	—	PD	—	—	—	—
Stacchiotti et al. (25)	Case series	IV	10	Advanced chordoma	mTOR effectors (AKT, S6) PDGFR	Imatinib (400 mg/day) + sirolimus (2 mg/day)	9	Grade 3 toxicity 30%	PR: 78%; SD: 11%; PD: 11%	PR: 11%; SD: 78%; PD: 11%	PR: 78%	—	—	—
Lebellec et al. (17)	Case series	IV	62	Advanced chordoma	—	Imatinib	—	—	—	PR: 5%; SD: 69%; PD: 26%	—	—	—	—
Adenis et al. (19)	Phase I	IV	7	Chordoma	—	MC (50 mg two times daily) + imatinib (400 mg/day)	—	Anemia, Nausea, vomiting, Fatigue	—	Long-lasting SD, PD at last	—	—	10.2	—
Lipplaa et al. (28)	Case series	IV	2	Metastatic chordoma	VEGFR	Imatinib	9		—	—	PD	—	—	—
Lipplaa et al. (28)	Case series	IV	1	Metastatic chordoma	VEGFR	Imatinib + sirolimus	—	Grade 2 fatigue, intermittent diarrhea	—	—	PD	—	—	—
Mercier et al. (36)	Case report	V	1	Recurrent chordoma	PDGFRB	Imatinib (400–800 mg/day)	2.25	Intracranial hemorrhage	—	—	PD	—	—	—

(Continued)

TABLE 1 | Continued

References	Study design	Levels of evidence	Sample size	Conditions	IHC positive	Drug (dosage)	Median treatment time (months)	AEs	Outcomes			Median follow-up (months)	Median PFS (months)	Median OS (months)
									Choi's criteria	RECIS	TRMR			
Chay et al. (34)	Case report	V	1	Recurrent chordoma	—	Imatinib	1.25	Persistent vomiting	—	—	PD	—	—	—
Houessinon et al. (38)	Case report	V	1	Recurrent chordoma	—	Imatinib (400–800 mg/day)	5	—	—	—	PD	—	—	—
Rohatgi et al. (39)	Case report	V	2	Metastatic chordoma	—	Imatinib (800 mg/day)	—	—	—	—	PR	—	60	—
Migliorini et al. (41)	Case report	V	2	Recurrent chordoma	Brachyury, EGFR, p53	Imatinib	—	—	—	—	PD	—	—	—
Jagersberg et al. (16)	Case series	V	2	Recurrent chordoma	—	Imatinib	—	—	—	—	PD	—	9	—
Schuetze et al. (11)	Phase II	IV	32	Incurable chordoma by conventional treatments	Src family of kinases, PDGFR, KIT, ephrin	Dasatinib (50–100 mg twice daily)	4	Grade 3 toxicity: 39.7%; Grade 4 toxicity: 6.9%	OR: 18.75%	OR: 3.125%	—	—	6.3	—

IHC, immunohistochemistry; AEs, adverse events; RMR, radiological or metabolic response; PR, partial response; SD, stable disease; PD, progressive disease; TVR, tumor volume regression; MC, metronomic cyclophosphamide.

one achieved a PR for 9 months and the other had a 44% reduction in tumor bulk. Pronounced AEs, such as rash, acne, diarrhea, and skin defects, were reported in both cases (30, 31).

VEGFR Inhibitors (Table 3)

Sorafenib, a TKI against VEGFR and PDGFR, was assessed in four studies (15, 17, 21, 37). A phase II trial was conducted on 27 patients with chordomas (NCT00874874) (15), and OR was observed in one patient as per RECIST. The 12 months PFS and OS rates were 73.0 and 86.5%, respectively. In a study on 11 patients treated with sorafenib, PR was obtained in one patient, with SD in nine patients and PD in one patient according to RECIST (17). Another study assessing sorafenib reported a PFS of 12 months (37). However, sorafenib was limited by severe AEs like thrombocytopenia and diarrhea, and the rates of grade 3 and 4 toxicity were 77.8 and 14.8%, respectively.

Sunitinib, a multi-targeting TKI against VEGFR and PDGFR, was assessed in three studies (14, 17, 28). A phase II trial on sunitinib was conducted on nine patients (14), four of which achieved SD according to RECIST, concurrent to a qualitative decrease in tumor density, along with a median PFS of 12 months (14). Two patients treated with sunitinib had at least SD according to RECIST (17, 28), and one achieved a PR after a 27 months SD (28). The major toxicities were of grade 1 or 2 (14).

Pazopanib, another VEGFR inhibitor, was analyzed in seven patients (16, 28, 41, 43), of which four sustained SD with the median PFS of 15 months and the remaining three experienced PD. Thalidomide, an inhibitor of VEGF, was used as a second-line treatment for chordoma after failure of imatinib, rapamycin and other chemotherapy (29, 34). While one patient achieved a 50% tumor reduction, another experienced a PD (29, 34). In addition, severe toxicities of grade 3 and 4 were reported in both cases.

Other Molecular Targeted Inhibitors (MTIs) (Table 4)

Monotherapy with the mTOR inhibitors rapamycin and everolimus were ineffective in chordoma patients (34, 41). The combined MTT regimen of everolimus and imatinib resulted in sustained SD in one patient, with a PFS of 16 months (42). In addition, IM plus sirolimus was used in 10 patients with IM-refractory chordoma and activated mTOR (25). Nine patients were assessed, of which one achieved PR, seven sustained SD and one experienced PD according to RECIST. According to Choi criteria, seven patients achieved PR, and one sustained SD and one experienced PD. The same MTT regimen was also used against IM- and sunitinib-refractory chordoma but was not effective due to short of the mTOR expression (28). A phase I trial evaluated the effect of IM plus metronomic cyclophosphamide (MC)-based chemotherapy on 7 IM- and sunitinib-refractory chordoma patients (19). The median PFS was 10.2 months, and the 12 months PFS and OS rates were 42.9 and 85.7%, respectively according to RECIST. No dose-limiting toxicity and drug pharmacokinetic interactions were observed.

Brachyury Vaccine (Table 4)

A phase I dose-escalation trial using a recombinant *Saccharomyces cerevisiae* (yeast) vaccine encoding brachyury (GI-6301) was conducted on 11 patients (20), and 10 evaluable

TABLE 2 | Molecular targeted therapy of chordomas with EGFR inhibitors (erlotinib, linsitinib, cetuximab, lapatinib, gefitinib).

References	Study design	Levels of evidence	Sample size	Conditions	IHC positive	Drug (dosage)	Median treatment time (months)	AEs	Outcomes			Median follow-up (months)	Median PFS (months)	Median OS (months)
									Choi's criteria	RECIST	RMR			
Launay et al. (35)	Case report	V	1	Advanced chordoma	EGFR	Erlotinib (150 mg/day)	40	None	–	–	TVR (70%)	40	12	40
Singhal et al. (32)	Case report	V	1	Recurrent chordoma	EMA, cytokeratins	Erlotinib (150 mg/day)	18	Grade 2 skin rash	–	PR	TVR (46%)	18	11	18
Trapani et al. (42)	Case report	V	1	Recurrent chordoma	PDGFR-β, EGFR, pS6	Erlotinib (150 mg/day)	–	–	–	PD (4 months), SD (16 months)	–	–	–	–
Asklund et al. (13)	Case report	V	3	Recurrent chordoma	–	Erlotinib (100–150 mg/day) + cetuximab;	–	Infection	–	–	–	–	–	–
Asklund et al. (13)	Case report	V	3	Recurrent chordoma	–	Erlotinib 100–150 mg/day + bevacizumab 10 mg/kg*week	–	Infection	–	PR: 33%, SD: 67%	–	–	–	–
Aleksic et al. (40)	Case report	V	1	Recurrent chordoma	brachyury, EGFR, IGF-1R	Erlotinib (100 mg/day) + linsitinib (50 mg/day)	61	Toxicity ≤ grade 2	–	PR	TVR	69	60	69
Lebellec et al. (17)	Case series	IV	5	Advanced chordoma	–	Erlotinib	–	–	–	PR: 20%, SD: 80%	–	–	4	–
Macaulay et al. (22)	Phase I	V	1	Advanced chordoma	–	Erlotinib + linsitinib	–	–	–	–	–	–	–	–
Migliorini et al. (41)	Case report	V	1	Recurrent and metastatic chordoma	Brachyury, EGFR, p53	Erlotinib + cetuximab	–	–	–	–	SD	–	–	–
Asklund et al. (33)	Case report	V	1	Advanced chordoma	–	Erlotinib + cetuximab	–	–	–	–	PD	–	–	–
Asklund et al. (33)	Case report	V	1	Advanced chordoma	–	Erlotinib + bevacizumab	–	–	–	–	TVR	–	–	–
Houessinon et al. (38)	Case report	V	1	Recurrent chordoma	–	Erlotinib (150 mg/day)	28	A moderate rash and diarrhea	–	–	PR	–	28	–
Stacchiotti et al. (12)	Phase II	V	18	Advanced chordoma	EGFR and HER2/neu	Lapatinib (1,500 mg/day)	–	G ≥ 2 toxicity	PR: 33%, SD: 39%, PD: 28%	PR: 40%, SD: 50%, PD: 10%	–	10.5	6 (Choi); 8 (RECIST)	25

(Continued)

TABLE 2 | Continued

References	Study design	Levels of evidence	Sample size	Conditions	IHC positive	Drug (dosage)	Median treatment time (months)	AEs	Outcomes			Median follow-up (months)	Median PFS (months)	Median OS (months)
									Choi's criteria	RECIST	RMR			
Lindén et al. (31)	Case report	V	1	Recurrent and metastatic chordoma	–	Cetuximab 500 mg/week + gefitinib 250 mg/day	4	Facial acne	–	–	TVR (44%)	4	4	4
Hof et al. (30)	Case report	V	1	Recurrent and metastatic chordoma	EGFR	Cetuximab 500 mg/week + gefitinib 250 mg/day	12	Facial acne, diarrhea and skin defects	–	–	TVR	12	12	12

IHC, immunohistochemistry; AEs, adverse events; RMR, radiological or metabolic response; PR, partial response; SD, stable disease; PD, progressive disease; TVR, tumor volume regression.

patients showed a median PFS of 8.3 months. One patient achieved PR, with eight sustaining SD and one experiencing PD at 3 months according to RECIST. Seven patients had no evidence of PD, giving a clinical benefit rate of 70% at 5 months. The most common AEs were injection site reactions.

Ongoing and planned clinical trials on chordoma MTT are listed in **Table 5**.

DISCUSSION

Novel therapeutic strategies against chordoma are urgently needed to prolong the overall survival and relieve symptoms. Elucidation of the underlying molecular mechanisms of chordoma have helped identify numerous potential therapeutic targets (47, 48), and several anti-chordoma agents are currently being tested in animal models and clinical trials. This systematic review is focused on the pharmacological management of chordoma patients and the clinical outcomes. Furthermore, the molecular mechanisms of MTT action have also been assessed.

Molecular Targets

Chordoma is a genetically heterogeneous tumor with frequent imbalances of large chromosomal regions. Somatic duplications of the notochordal transcription factor brachyury (47, 48), chromosomal copy loss of phosphatase and tensin homolog (PTEN) (49), tuberous sclerosis complex (TSC) (50), cyclin-dependent kinase inhibitor 2A and 2B (CDKN2A and CDKN2B) (51), SMARCB1 (49), and PIK3CA (9) mutations are key aspects of chordoma pathogenesis, and therefore potential targets.

RTKs are the key players in the development and progression of chordoma, and their mutated forms can activate signaling cascades resulting in dysregulation of many essential proteins. Therefore, mutational analyses and IHC can greatly assist oncologists to determine the optimal inhibitors (52–56). It needs to be emphasized that mutations in the molecular targets are clinically more relevant than their immunoreactivity, since target overexpression is not always driven by the activation of the corresponding signaling pathway. For example, high levels of EGFR in the chordoma cell line JHC7 was not accompanied by activated EGFR signaling (57).

Indications and Evaluation Criteria for MTTs

MTTs are not the first treatment options for chordoma, and only recommended for advanced or recurrent chordoma that are unresponsive to either surgical resection or radiotherapy.

The outcomes of MTTs is often difficult to evaluate in chordoma. Choi's criteria is based on changes in tumor size and density following contrast administration in CT or MRI (58). A radiological PR is defined as ≥10% decrease in tumor size or ≥15% decrease in tumor density/contrast enhancement in CT/MRI. RECIST defines PR as ≥20% decrease in tumor growth, which occurs later than that required for Choi criteria. Therefore, RECIST is not fully adequate to evaluate the clinical response in chordoma (59). Clinical/radiological and metabolic responses include symptom relief, anti-tumor effects (such as liquefaction) and changes in tumor density in the CT scan,

TABLE 3 | Molecular targeted therapy with VEGF and VEGFR inhibitors (sorafenib, sunitinib, thalidomide, pazopanib).

References	Study design	Levels of evidence	Sample size	Conditions	IHC positive	Drug (dosage)	Median treatment time (months)	AEs	Outcomes			Median follow-up (months)	Median PFS (months)	Median OS (months)
									Choi's criteria	RECIS	TRMR			
Bompas et al. (15)	Phase II	IV	27	Locally advanced and metastatic chordoma	—	Sorafenib (800 mg/day)	8.7	Grade 3 (77.8%); grade 4 (14.8%)	—	OR: 4%; PR: 4%; SD + PD: 92%	—	—	PFS rates: 6 m (85.3%), 9 m (73.0%), 12 m (73.0%)	OS rates: 6 m (100%), 9 m (86.5%), 12 m (86.5%)
Lebellec et al. (21)	Phase II	IV	26	Advanced chordoma	—	Sorafenib	—	—	—	—	—	—	—	—
Lebellec et al. (17)	Case series	IV	11	Advanced chordoma	—	Sorafenib	—	—	—	PR: 9%; SD: 82%; PD: 9%	—	—	—	—
Svoboda et al. (37)	Case report	IV	1	Recurrent and metastatic chordoma	—	Sorafenib (200 mg/day)	—	Thrombocytopenia; diarrhea		—	SD	—	12	—
George et al. (14)	Phase II	IV	9	Advanced chordoma	VEGFR, PDGFRB	Sunitinib (37.5 mg/day)	—	Grade 1 or 2 (fatigue, diarrhea, hypertension)	—	SD: 44%; PD: 56%	—	—	—	—
Lipplaa et al. (28)	Case series	IV	1	Metastatic chordoma	VEGFR	Sunitinib (37.5–50 mg/day)	—	Grade 2 nausea, fatigue	—	PR	TVR	—	27	—
Lebellec et al. (17)	Case series	IV	1	Advanced chordoma	—	Sunitinib	—	—	—	—	—	—	—	—
Schonegger et al. (29)	Case report	V	1	Recurrent and metastatic chordoma	—	Thalidomide	12	—	—	—	PD	—	—	—
Chay et al. (34)	Case report	V	1	Recurrent chordoma	—	Thalidomide (100–300 mg/day)	23+	—	—	—	TVR (more than 50%)	—	21	—
Lipplaa et al. (28)	Case series	IV	4	Unresectable or metastatic chordoma	VEGFR	Pazopanib (600–800 mg/day)	—	Grade 2 diarrhea, fatigue	—	SD: 50%; PD: 50%	—	—	8.5	—
Ribeiro et al. (43)	Case report	V	1	Recurrent chordoma	Cytokeratins, EMA and vimentin	Pazopanib (800 mg/day)	—	Grade 3 neutropenia	—	SD	TVR (23.1%)	—	15	—
Migliorini et al. (41)	Case report	V	1	Recurrent chordoma	Brachyury, EGFR, p53	Pazopanib	6	—	—	—	PD	—	—	—
Jagersberg et al. (16)	Case series	IV	1	Recurrent chordoma	—	Pazopanib	—	—	—	—	PR	—	24	—

IHC, immunohistochemistry; AEs, adverse events; RMR, radiological or metabolic response; OR, objective response; PR, partial response; SD, stable disease; PD, progressive disease; TVR, tumor volume regression.

TABLE 4 | Molecular targeted therapy of chordomas with other inhibitors (rapamycin, temsirolimus, yeast brachyury vaccine).

References	Study design	Levels of evidence	Sample size	Conditions	IHC positive	Drug (dosage)	Median treatment time (months)	AEs	Outcomes			Median follow-up (months)	Median PFS (months)	Median OS (months)
									Choi's criteria	RECIS	TRMR			
Chay et al. (34)	Case report	V	1	Recurrent chordoma	–	Rapamycin	2	–	–	–	PD	–	–	–
Migliorini et al. (41)	Case report	V	1	Recurrent and metastatic chordoma	Brachyury, EGFR, p53	Everolimus	–	–	–	–	PD	–	–	–
Lebellec et al. (17)	Case series	IV	1	Advanced chordoma	–	Temsirolimus	–	–	–	–	SD	–	–	–
Migliorini et al. (41)	Case report	V	1	Recurrent chordoma	Brachyury	Pembrolizumab	6	–	–	–	TVR	–	6	–
Heery et al. (20)	Phase I	IV	11	Advanced chordoma	–	Yeast-brachyury (GI-6301) vaccine (40-80 YU)	–	–	–	PR: 10%; SD: 80%; PD: 10%	–	–	8.3	–

IHC, immunohistochemistry; AEs, adverse events; RMR, radiological or metabolic response; PR, partial response; SD, stable disease; PD, progressive disease; TVR, tumor volume regression.

reduction in contrast enhancement in MR, and maximum standardized uptake (SUVmax) in PET (23). However, typical tumor tissue characteristics like component and scirrhosity may also affect tumor-related symptoms, even in the absence of any changes in tumor size, resulting in incorrect readings.

MTTs for Chordoma

Imatinib was the first effective agent tested against chordoma, and is currently the most commonly used MTIs (23). Most patients with PDGFRβ-positive chordoma benefited from imatinib treatment and avoided rapid PD, likely due to tumor necrosis and intra-tumoral subacute bleeding that manifest as liquefaction (36). A dosage of 800 mg/day is recommended, except in cases of high toxicity. The major AEs associated with imatinib include oedema, chronic anemia, fatigue and even subacute intraventricular hemorrhage (36).

Several trials have also reported the ineffectiveness of imatinib in chordoma (19, 28, 32, 35, 38, 42). In such cases, EGFR inhibitor is the second line of treatment, since PDGFRβ activation can also stimulate EGFR, given an EGFR gene copy number gain (CNG) or strong intra-tumoral EGFR staining is detected. Around 40% of chordoma patients show CNG of the chromosome band 7p12, where EGFR is located. Erlotinib has shown a good clinical effect EGFR-positive chordoma, and could serve as the second choice for imatinib-refractory chordoma (32, 35). The combination of gefitinib and cetuximab, two other inhibitors of EGFR, showed improved clinical benefits and decreased AEs (30, 31).

HER2/neu is involved in EGFR dimer formation, and the possibility of heterodimerization increases the sensitivity of EGFR-positive chordoma to 54% (60). Lapatinib, a bi-specific inhibitor blocking both EGFR and HER2/neu, achieved 33.3% PR and 38.9% SD as per Choi criteria and 100% SD according to RECIST in EGFR-positive chordoma (12). Afatinib, another bi-specific inhibitor of EGFR and HER2/neu, was the only agent which showed cytotoxic effects across multiple chordoma cell lines in a drug sensitivity assessment (57). On this basis, a new clinical trial on the effects of afatinib is currently enrolling patients (NCT03083678).

IGF signaling is also important in chordoma tumorigenesis, since IGF-1 and IGF-1R have been detected in 92 and 76% of chordoma tissues (61), and are absent in benign notochordal cell tumor and fetal notochord (52). Linsitinib, an IGF-1R inhibitor, was assessed in two studies (22, 40), and effectively controlled chordoma progression in combination with erlotinib (22, 40).

VEGF levels are significantly higher in chordoma tissues and associated with angiogenesis (62). Five VEGFR or VEGF inhibitors (sorafenib, sunitinib, pazopanib, thalidomide, bevacizumab) were evaluated in this systematic review. Although occasional severe AEs were observed occasionally, sorafenib, sunitinib, and pazopanib monotherapy resulted in substantial clinical effects. Although thalidomide was effective against drug-resistant chordomas, severe toxicities limit its clinical application. Bevacizumab can be used as a supplement for erlotinib in drug-resistant chordomas, and their combination showed good clinical effect and high tolerance. A new phase II trial evaluating the efficacy and safety of regorafenib, a

TABLE 5 | Clinical trials programs of chordomas in progress.

Official title	Trial registration number	Type	Medical condition:	Interventions	Mechanism	Sites	Status
Nilotinib with radiation for high risk chordoma	NCT01407198	Phase I	Histologically confirmed chordoma	Nilotinib (daily 200–400 mg BID) Radiation therapy	A Bcr-Abl kinase inhibitor	USA	Active, not recruiting
Study of Imatinib, a platelet-derived growth factor receptor inhibitor, and LBH589, a histone deacetylase inhibitor, in the treatment of newly diagnosed and recurrent chordoma	NCT01175109	Phase I	Histologically confirmed chordoma	Imatinib + LBH589	Imatinib: a PDGFR inhibitor LBH589: a HDAC inhibitor	USA	Unknown
CDK4/6 inhibition in locally advanced/metastatic chordoma	NCT03110744 EUDRACT 2016-004660-19	Phase II	Locally advanced or metastatic chordoma refractory to tyrosine kinase inhibitors	Palbociclib	A CDK4/6 inhibitor	Germany	Recruiting
Afatinib in locally advanced and metastatic chordoma	NCT03083678	Phase II	Locally advanced or metastatic, pathologically proven, EGFR expressing chordoma	Afatinib (40 mg/day)	A Her2 and EGFR kinases inhibitor	Italy, Netherlands, UK	Not yet recruiting
Phase I safety study of stereotactic radiosurgery with concurrent and adjuvant PD-1 antibody nivolumab in subjects with recurrent or advanced chordoma	NCT02989636	Phase I	Histologically confirmed chordoma	Nivolumab Stereotactic Radiosurgery	Nivolumab: a PD-1 Antibody	USA	Recruiting
A randomized, double-blind, phase 2 trial of GI-6301 (Yeast-Brachyury Vaccine) vs. placebo in combination with standard of care definitive radiotherapy in locally advanced, unresectable, chordoma	NCT02383498	Phase II	Histologically confirmed chordoma	GI-6301 Vaccine (Yeast-Brachyury) GI-6301 Placebo Radiotherapy	A heat-killed, recombinant yeast-based vaccine engineered to express the transcription factor, Brachyury	USA	Recruiting
Phase II trial of the immune checkpoint inhibitor nivolumab in patients with select rare CNS cancers	NCT03173950	Phase II	Primary brain sarcoma including chordoma	Nivolumab	A PD-1 Antibody	USA	Recruiting
A phase II trial of dasatinib in advanced sarcomas	NCT00464620	Phase II	Unresectable, recurrent, or metastatic soft tissue or bone sarcoma including chordoma	Dasatinib (70 mg, twice daily)	An inhibitor of Src family of kinases, PDGFR, KIT, ephrin	USA	Active, not recruiting
DART: dual anti-CTLA-4 and anti-PD-1 blockade in rare tumors	NCT02834013	Phase II	Rare tumors including chordoma	Ipilimumab Nivolumab	Ipilimumab: a CTLA-4 inhibitor Nivolumab: a PD-1 inhibitor	USA	Recruiting
A phase II, multicenter study of the EZH2 inhibitor tazemetostat in adult subjects with INI1-negative tumors or relapsed/refractory synovial sarcoma	NCT02601950 EUDRACT 2015-002469-41	Phase II	Poorly differentiated chordoma (or other chordoma with sponsor approval)	Tazemetostat (800 mg BID)	An EZH2 Inhibitor	USA, Australia, Belgium, Canada, France, Germany, Italy, Taiwan, UK	Recruiting
A phase 1 study of the EZH2 inhibitor tazemetostat in pediatric subjects with relapsed or refractory INI1-negative tumors or synovial sarcoma	NCT02601937 EUDRACT 2015-002468-18	Phase I	INI1-negative tumors including chordoma	Tazemetostat	An EZH2 Inhibitor	USA, Australia, Canada, Denmark, France, Germany, Italy, Netherlands, UK	Active, not recruiting

(Continued)

TABLE 5 | Continued

Official title	Trial registration number	Type	Medical condition:	Interventions	Mechanism	Sites	Status
A phase II multi-arm study to test the efficacy of immunotherapeutic agents in multiple sarcoma subtypes	NCT02815995	Phase II	Advanced and/or metastatic sarcoma including chordoma	Durvalumab Tremelimumab	Durvalumab: a PD-L1 inhibitor; Tremelimumab: a CTLA-4 inhibitor	USA	Recruiting
A randomized phase II study of Durvalumab (MEDI4736) and Tremelimumab compared to doxorubicin in patients with advanced or metastatic soft tissue sarcoma.	EUDRACT 2016-004750-15	Phase II	Advanced or metastatic soft tissue sarcoma including chordoma	Durvalumab Tremelimumab	Durvalumab: a PD-L1 inhibitor; Tremelimumab: a CTLA-4 inhibitor	Germany	Ongoing
A phase I, open-label, multiple-ascending dose trial to investigate the safety, tolerability, pharmacokinetics, biological and clinical activity of MSB0011359C in subjects with metastatic or locally advanced solid tumors and expansion to selected indications	NCT02517398	Phase I	Solid tumors including chordoma	MSB0011359C (M7824)	A PD-L1 inhibitor	USA	Recruiting
An open-label phase 1 trial to evaluate the safety and tolerability of a Modified Vaccinia Ankara (MVA) priming followed by fowlpox booster vaccines modified to express brachyury and T-cell costimulatory molecules (MVA-BN-Brachyury/FPV-Brachyury)	NCT03349983	Phase I	Metastatic or unresectable locally advanced malignant solid tumors including chordoma	MVA-BN-Brachyury FPV-Brachyury	A brachyury vaccine	USA	Recruiting
An open phase I clinical study assessing safety and tolerability of MVX-ONCO-1 in patients with solid tumor who are not/not any longer amenable to standard therapy	NCT02193503	Phase I	—	MVX-ONCO-1	An autologous tumor vaccine	Switzerland	Recruiting
Secured access to pembrolizumab for adult patients with selected rare cancer types	NCT03012620 EUDRACT 2016-002260-14	Phase II	Unresectable, recurrent, or metastatic soft tissue or bone sarcoma including chordoma	Pembrolizumab	A PD-L1 inhibitor	France	Recruiting
A randomized phase II, placebo-controlled, multicenter study evaluating efficacy and safety of regorafenib in patients with metastatic bone sarcomas	NCT02389244	Phase II	Advanced metastatic cancer in progression including chordoma	Regorafenib Placebo	A multi-kinase inhibitor; angiogenesis inhibitor	France	Recruiting
Phase 2 study on imatinib in combination with RAD001 in advanced chordoma	EUDRACT 2010-021755-34	Phase II	PDGFRB and mTOR (or S6 or 4BP1) positive advanced chordoma	Imatinib Everolimus	Imatinib: a PDGFRB inhibitor Everolimus: a mTOR inhibitor	Italy	Ongoing
A phase 2, single arm, European multi-center trial evaluating the efficacy of afatinib as first-line or later-line treatment in advanced chordoma.	EUDRACT 2016-002766-31	Phase II	Metastatic or unresectable chordoma	Afatinib	A Her2 and EGFR kinases inhibitor	Netherlands	Ongoing
Phase II study of lapatinib in EGFR/HER2NEU positive advanced chordoma	EUDRACT 2009-014456-29	Phase II	Advanced EGFR/Her2Neu positive chordoma	Lapatinib	EGFR/Her2Neu inhibitor	Germany	Ongoing

PDGFR, platelet-derived growth factor receptor; HDAC, histone deacetylase; Her2, human epidermal growth factor receptor 2; EGFR, epidermal growth factor receptor; PD-1, programmed cell death protein 1; CTLA4, cytotoxic T lymphocyte antigen 4.

multi-kinase inhibitor of VEGFR, is ongoing in France for metastatic bone sarcoma (NCT02389244).

Chordomas with indication of anti-RTK agents may also relapse or progress early. In TKI-resistant chordomas, p-AKT is a relative reliable indicator and its persistent expression following tyrphostin treatment resulted in relapse and progression (54). AKT is activated by mTOR, its downstream molecules (RPS6 and eIF4E), and Stat3. The combination of the antagonists of upstream RTKs and downstream mTOR/PI3K/MAPK/Stat not only synergistically reduced chordoma growth by avoiding the negative feedback loop (63) and PI3K-dependent feedback loop (64), but also significantly decreased the cytotoxicity of either agent (65). For example, monotherapy of rapamycin or everolimus was ineffective against tumor progression (34, 41), while combining imatinib with everolimus or sirolimus induced good clinical effects in 3 studies (12 patients) (25, 28, 42). Therefore, the combined therapy can be considered for drug-resistant chordoma.

Mutations in the downstream effectors of RTKs, like PTEN and PIK3CA, also impair TKI response (66, 67). PTEN deficient chordoma cell lines exhibit increased proliferation, reduced apoptosis and enhanced migration in chordoma cell lines (68). Reintroduction of PTEN in tumor cells increased their therapeutic sensitivity to PDGFR inhibitors, and the combination of histone deacetylase (HDAC) and PDGFR inhibitors effectively reduced the growth and invasion of chordoma cells, irrespective of PTEN status (69). On this basis, a new phase I trial of Imatinib and LBH589 (a HDAC inhibitor) is ongoing in chordoma patients (NCT01175109).

Chordomas frequently show deletions in the SMARCB1 locus (49). SMARCB1 directly antagonizes the histone methyltransferase EZH2 and regulates the cell-cycle by activating CDKN2A (45). A phase I trial on the EZH2 inhibitor tazemetostat, confirmed complete or partial responses were observed in two children with chordoma according to RECIST (NCT02601937) (45). Therefore, another phase II clinical trial on tazemetostat is ongoing in patients with SMARCB1/INI1 deleted chordoma (NCT02601950).

The loss of chromosome 9 or 9p region, which contains CDKN2A, has been reported in some chordoma patients (51). The inactivation of CDKN2A universally activates the CDK4/6 and Rb pathways (70), which are highly expressed in the chordoma tissues (71). The CDK4/6 inhibitors palbociclib and LY2835219 inhibited chordoma cell growth and proliferation *in vitro* efficiently (72, 73). A phase II clinical trial on palbociclib is currently enrolling patients with chordoma (NCT031 10744).

Somatic duplications of the notochordal transcription factor brachyury was demonstrated in chordoma, and enhanced tumor growth by activating YAP (9, 47, 48). Preclinical studies have shown that a recombinant *Saccharomyces cerevisiae* (yeast) vaccine encoding brachyury (GI-6301) activates human T cells *in vitro*. A phase II GI-6301 dose-escalation trial showed a 70% clinical benefit rate in chordoma patients (20). A phase II clinical trial on the combination of GI-6301 and radiotherapy is currently enrolling chordoma patients in the United States (NCT02383498). Additionally, a phase I trial of a Modified Vaccinia Ankara (MVA)-brachyury and a fowlpox (FPV)-brachyury vaccines is currently ongoing in patients with solid tumors, including chordoma (NCT03349983).

Limitations

In order to decrease the selection bias, this systematic review screened all published studies enrolling chordoma patients treated with MTT, including clinical trials, case series and even case reports, and provides the most detailed information. However, there were some limitations that need to be addressed. We included case reports on account of the rarity of chordoma and the paucity of available studies. However, a case report might overemphasize the final results due to lack of strong results. In addition, we only included English language publications which can also increase the selection bias. Furthermore, the baseline conditions of the patients and the evaluation criteria were not consistent across studies which is another factor contributing to selection bias. Therefore, large prospective randomized clinical trials are warranted to help clinicians determine the optimum treatment modality for chordoma patients.

CONCLUSIONS

The selection of MTIs for patients with advanced or relapsed chordoma should be based on gene mutation screening and immunohistochemistry (IHC). Monotherapy of TKIs is recommended as the first-line treatment. Combined therapy (two TKIs or TKI plus mTOR inhibitor) may be the choice for drug-resistant chordoma. Brachyury vaccine is a promising therapeutic strategy and requires more clinical trials to evaluate its safety and efficacy.

AUTHOR CONTRIBUTIONS

TM did the literature search, data and data analysis, and led the writing of the review. HY, JJ, and RH contributed to the design, data collection, and analysis. HY, DS, and LC contributed their experience of clinical practice in chordoma to ensure the relevance of findings. JJ and CJ contributed their experience in the discussion of the molecular mechanism underlying chordoma and drug interaction.

FUNDING

This work was supported in part by the National Natural Science Foundation of China [grant numbers 81702659, 81772856] and National Key R&D Program of China [grant numbers 2016YFA0100800].

ACKNOWLEDGMENTS

We acknowledge the contributions of Josh Sommer of the Chordoma Foundation, who assisted with the revision of concept and the final manuscript.

REFERENCES

1. Walcott BP, Nahed BV, Mohyeldin A, Coumans JV, Kahle KT, Ferreira MJ. Chordoma: current concepts, management, and future directions. *Lancet Oncol.* (2012) 13:e69–76. doi: 10.1016/S1470-2045(11)70337-0
2. Mcmaster ML, Goldstein AM, Bromley CM, Ishibe N, Parry DM. Chordoma: incidence and survival patterns in the United States, 1973–1995. *Cancer Causes Control.* (2001) 12:1–11. doi: 10.1023/A:1008947301735
3. Chugh R, Tawbi H, Lucas DR, Biermann JS, Schuetze SM, Baker LH. Chordoma: the nonsarcoma primary bone tumor. *Oncologist* (2007) 12:1344–50. doi: 10.1634/theoncologist.12-11-1344
4. Casali PG, Stacchiotti S, Sangalli C, Olmi P, Gronchi A. Chordoma. *Curr Opin Oncol.* (2007) 19:367–70. doi: 10.1097/CCO.0b013e3281214448
5. Stacchiotti S, Sommer J. Building a global consensus approach to chordoma: a position paper from the medical and patient community. *Lancet Oncol.* (2015) 16:e71–83. doi: 10.1016/S1470-2045(14)71190-8
6. Meng T, Yin H, Li B, Li Z, Xu W, Zhou W, et al. Clinical features and prognostic factors of patients with chordoma in the spine: a retrospective analysis of 153 patients in a single center. *Neuro Oncol.* (2015) 17:725–32. doi: 10.1093/neuonc/nou331
7. Stacchiotti S, Casali PG, Lo Vullo S, Mariani L, Palassini E, Mercuri M, et al. Chordoma of the mobile spine and sacrum: a retrospective analysis of a series of patients surgically treated at two referral centers. *Ann Surg Oncol.* (2010) 17:211–9. doi: 10.1245/s10434-009-0740-x
8. Arain A, Hornicek FJ, Schwab JH, Chebib I, Damron TA. Chordoma arising from benign multifocal notochordal tumors. *Skeletal Radiol.* (2017) 46:1745–52. doi: 10.1007/s00256-017-2727-1
9. Tarpey PS, Behjati S, Young MD, Martincorena I, Alexandrov LB, Farndon SJ, et al. The driver landscape of sporadic chordoma. *Nat Commun.* (2017) 8:890. doi: 10.1038/s41467-017-01026-0
10. Stacchiotti S, Longhi A, Ferraresi V, Grignani G, Comandone A, Stupp R, et al. Phase II study of imatinib in advanced chordoma. *J Clin Oncol.* (2012) 30:914–20. doi: 10.1200/JCO.2011.35.3656
11. Schuetze SM, Bolejack V, Choy E, Ganjoo KN, Staddon AP, Chow WA, et al. Phase 2 study of dasatinib in patients with alveolar soft part sarcoma, chondrosarcoma, chordoma, epithelioid sarcoma, or solitary fibrous tumor. *Cancer* (2017) 123:90–7. doi: 10.1002/cncr.30379
12. Stacchiotti S, Tamborini E, Lo Vullo S, Bozzi F, Messina A, Morosi C, et al. Phase II study on lapatinib in advanced EGFR-positive chordoma. *Ann Oncol.* (2013) 24:1931–6. doi: 10.1093/annonc/mdt117
13. Asklund T, Sandstrom M, Shahidi S, Riklund K, Henriksson R. Durable stabilization of three chordoma cases by bevacizumab and erlotinib. *Acta Oncol.* (2014) 53:980–4. doi: 10.3109/0284186X.2013.878472
14. George S, Merriam P, Maki RG, Van Den Abbeele AD, Yap JT, Akhurst T, et al. Multicenter phase II trial of sunitinib in the treatment of nongastrointestinal stromal tumor sarcomas. *J Clin Oncol.* (2009) 27:3154–60. doi: 10.1200/JCO.2008.20.9890
15. Bompas E, Le Cesne A, Tresch-Bruneel E, Lebellec L, Laurence V, Collard O, et al. Sorafenib in patients with locally advanced and metastatic chordomas: a phase II trial of the French Sarcoma Group (GSF/GETO). *Ann Oncol.* (2015) 26:2168–73. doi: 10.1093/annonc/mdv300
16. Jagersberg M, El Rahal A, Dammann P, Merkler D, Weber DC, Schaller K. Clival chordoma: a single-centre outcome analysis. *Acta Neurochir (Wien).* (2017) 159:1815–23. doi: 10.1007/s00701-017-3163-7
17. Lebellec L, Chauffert B, Blay JY, Le Cesne A, Chevreau C, Bompas E, et al. Advanced chordoma treated by first-line molecular targeted therapies: outcomes and prognostic factors. A retrospective study of the French Sarcoma Group (GSF/GETO) and the Association des Neuro-Oncologues d'Expression Francaise (ANOCEF). *Eur J Cancer* (2017) 79:119–28. doi: 10.1016/j.ejca.2017.03.037
18. Liberati A, Altman DG, Tetzlaff J, Mulrow C, Gotzsche PC, Ioannidis JP, et al. The PRISMA statement for reporting systematic reviews and meta-analyses of studies that evaluate healthcare interventions: explanation and elaboration. *BMJ* (2009) 339:b2700. doi: 10.1136/bmj.b2700
19. Adenis A, Ray-Coquard I, Italiano A, Chauzit E, Bui-Nguyen B, Blay JY, et al. A dose-escalating phase I of imatinib mesylate with fixed dose of metronomic cyclophosphamide in targeted solid tumours. *Br J Cancer* (2013) 109:2574–8. doi: 10.1038/bjc.2013.648
20. Heery CR, Singh BH, Rauckhorst M, Marte JL, Donahue RN, Grenga I, et al. Phase I trial of a yeast-based therapeutic cancer vaccine (GI-6301) targeting the transcription factor brachyury. *Cancer Immunol Res.* (2015) 3:1248–56. doi: 10.1158/2326-6066.CIR-15-0119
21. Lebellec L, Bertucci F, Tresch-Bruneel E, Bompas E, Toiron Y, Camoin L, et al. Circulating vascular endothelial growth factor (VEGF) as predictive factor of progression-free survival in patients with advanced chordoma receiving sorafenib: an analysis from a phase II trial of the french sarcoma group (GSF/GETO). *Oncotarget* (2016) 7:73984–94. doi: 10.18632/oncotarget.12172
22. Macaulay VM, Middleton MR, Eckhardt SG, Rudin CM, Juergens RA, Gedrich R, et al. Phase I dose-escalation study of linsitinib (OSI-906) and erlotinib in patients with advanced solid tumors. *Clin Cancer Res.* (2016) 22:2897–907. doi: 10.1158/1078-0432.CCR-15-2218
23. Casali PG, Messina A, Stacchiotti S, Tamborini E, Crippa F, Gronchi A, et al. Imatinib mesylate in chordoma. *Cancer* (2004) 101:2086–97. doi: 10.1002/cncr.20618
24. Geoerger B, Morland B, Ndiaye A, Doz F, Kalifa G, Geoffray A, et al. Target-driven exploratory study of imatinib mesylate in children with solid malignancies by the Innovative Therapies for Children with Cancer (ITCC) European Consortium. *Eur J Cancer* (2009) 45:2342–51. doi: 10.1016/j.ejca.2009.03.007
25. Stacchiotti S, Marrari A, Tamborini E, Palassini E, Virdis E, Messina A, et al. Response to imatinib plus sirolimus in advanced chordoma. *Ann Oncol.* (2009) 20:1886–94. doi: 10.1093/annonc/mdp210
26. Ferraresi V, Nuzzo C, Zoccali C, Marandino F, Vidiri A, Salducca N, et al. Chordoma: clinical characteristics, management and prognosis of a case series of 25 patients. *BMC Cancer* (2010) 10:22. doi: 10.1186/1471-2407-10-22
27. Hindi N, Casali PG, Morosi C, Messina A, Palassini E, Pilotti S, et al. Imatinib in advanced chordoma: a retrospective case series analysis. *Eur J Cancer* (2015) 51:2609–14. doi: 10.1016/j.ejca.2015.07.038
28. Lipplaa A, Dijkstra S, Gelderblom H. Efficacy of pazopanib and sunitinib in advanced axial chordoma: a single reference centre case series. *Clin Sarcoma Res.* (2016) 6:19. doi: 10.1186/s13569-016-0059-x
29. Schonegger K, Gelpi E, Prayer D, Dieckmann K, Matula C, Hassler M, et al. Recurrent and metastatic clivus chordoma: systemic palliative therapy retards disease progression. *Anticancer Drugs* (2005) 16:1139–43. doi: 10.1097/00001813-200511000-00015
30. Hof H, Welzel T, Debus J. Effectiveness of cetuximab/gefitinib in the therapy of a sacral chordoma. *Onkologie* (2006) 29:572–4. doi: 10.1159/000096283
31. Linden O, Stenberg L, Kjellen E. Regression of cervical spinal cord compression in a patient with chordoma following treatment with cetuximab and gefitinib. *Acta Oncol.* (2009) 48:158–9. doi: 10.1080/02841860802266672
32. Singhal N, Kotasek D, Parnis FX. Response to erlotinib in a patient with treatment refractory chordoma. *Anticancer Drugs* (2009) 20:953–5. doi: 10.1097/CAD.0b013e328330c7f0
33. Asklund T, Danfors T, Henriksson R. PET response and tumor stabilization under erlotinib and bevacizumab treatment of an intracranial lesion non-invasively diagnosed as likely chordoma. *Clin Neuropathol.* (2011) 30:242–6. doi: 10.5414/NP300371
34. Chay WY, Teo M, Sittampalam K, Toh HC. Effective use of thalidomide in the treatment of recurrent metastatic chordoma. *J Clin Oncol.* (2011) 29:e477–80. doi: 10.1200/JCO.2010.34.2139
35. Launay SG, Chetaille B, Medina F, Perrot D, Nazarian S, Guiramand J, et al. Efficacy of epidermal growth factor receptor targeting in advanced chordoma: case report and literature review. *BMC Cancer* (2011) 11:423. doi: 10.1186/1471-2407-11-423

36. Mercier F, Guiot MC, Bojanowski MW. Treatment of chordoma with imatinib complicated by intracranial hemorrhage: a case showing dissociation between biological effect and therapeutic outcome. *J Neurooncol.* (2012) 107:435–7. doi: 10.1007/s11060-011-0767-2
37. Svoboda RM, Mackay D, Welsch MJ, Anderson BE. Multiple cutaneous metastatic chordomas from the sacrum. *J Am Acad Dermatol.* (2012) 66:e246–7. doi: 10.1016/j.jaad.2011.07.037
38. Houessinon A, Boone M, Constans JM, Toussaint P, Chauffert B. Sustained response of a clivus chordoma to erlotinib after imatinib failure. *Case Rep Oncol.* (2015) 8:25–9. doi: 10.1159/000371843
39. Rohatgi S, Ramaiya NH, Jagannathan JP, Howard SA, Shinagare AB, Krajewski KM. Metastatic chordoma: report of the two cases and review of the literature. *Eurasian J Med.* (2015) 47:151–4. doi: 10.5152/eurasianjmed.2015.52
40. Aleksic T, Browning L, Woodward M, Phillips R, Page S, Henderson S, et al. Durable response of spinal chordoma to combined inhibition of IGF-1R and EGFR. *Front Oncol.* (2016) 6:98. doi: 10.3389/fonc.2016.00098
41. Migliorini D, Mach N, Aguiar D, Vernet R, Landis BN, Becker M, et al. First report of clinical responses to immunotherapy in 3 relapsing cases of chordoma after failure of standard therapies. *Oncoimmunology* (2017) 6:e1338235. doi: 10.1080/2162402X.2017.1338235
42. Trapani D, Conforti F, De Pas T. EGFR Inhibition in a pretreated sacral chordoma: a role for erlotinib? Case Report and a Brief Review of Literature. *Transl Med UniSa* (2017) 16:30–3.
43. Ribeiro M, De Sousa MC, Hanna SA, Maldaun MVC, Kurimori CO, De Lima L, et al. Tumor reduction with pazopanib in a patient with recurrent lumbar chordoma. *Case Rep Oncol Med.* (2018) 2018:4290131. doi: 10.1155/2018/4290131
44. Mcpherson CM, Suki D, Mccutcheon IE, Gokaslan ZL, Rhines LD, Mendel E. Metastatic disease from spinal chordoma: a 10-year experience. *J Neurosurg Spine* (2006) 5:277–80. doi: 10.3171/spi.2006.5.4.277
45. Chi S, Fouladi M, Shukla N, Bourdeaut F, Margol A, Makin G, et al. Phase 1 study of the EZH2 inhibitor, tazemetostat, in children with relapsed or refractory INI1-negative tumors including rhabdoid tumors, epithelioid sarcoma, chordoma, and synovial sarcoma. *Mol Cancer Ther.* (2018) 17:1. doi: 10.1158/1535-7163
46. Tamborini E, Miselli F, Negri T, Lagonigro MS, Staurengo S, Dagrada GP, et al. Molecular and biochemical analyses of platelet-derived growth factor receptor (PDGFR) B, PDGFRA, and KIT receptors in chordomas. *Clin Cancer Res.* (2006) 12:6920–8. doi: 10.1158/1078-0432.CCR-06-1584
47. Presneau N, Shalaby A, Ye H, Pillay N, Halai D, Idowu B, et al. Role of the transcription factor T (brachyury) in the pathogenesis of sporadic chordoma: a genetic and functional-based study. *J Pathol.* (2011) 223:327–35. doi: 10.1002/path.2816
48. Shah SR, David JM, Tippens ND, Mohyeldin A, Martinez-Gutierrez JC, Ganaha S, et al. Brachyury-YAP regulatory axis drives stemness and growth in cancer. *Cell Rep.* (2017) 21:495–507. doi: 10.1016/j.celrep.2017.09.057
49. Choy E, Macconaill LE, Cote GM, Le LP, Shen JK, Nielsen GP, et al. Genotyping cancer-associated genes in chordoma identifies mutations in oncogenes and areas of chromosomal loss involving CDKN2A, PTEN, and SMARCB1. *PLoS ONE* (2014) 9:e101283. doi: 10.1371/journal.pone.0101283
50. Lee-Jones L, Aligianis I, Davies PA, Puga A, Farndon PA, Stemmer-Rachamimov A, et al. Sacrococcygeal chordomas in patients with tuberous sclerosis complex show somatic loss of TSC1 or TSC2. *Genes Chromosomes Cancer* (2004) 41:80–5. doi: 10.1002/gcc.20052
51. Hallor KH, Staaf J, Jonsson G, Heidenblad M, Vult Von Steyern F, Bauer HC, et al. Frequent deletion of the CDKN2A locus in chordoma: analysis of chromosomal imbalances using array comparative genomic hybridisation. *Br J Cancer* (2008) 98:434–42. doi: 10.1038/sj.bjc.6604130
52. Sommer J, Itani DM, Homlar KC, Keedy VL, Halpern JL, Holt GE, et al. Methylthioadenosine phosphorylase and activated insulin-like growth factor-1 receptor/insulin receptor: potential therapeutic targets in chordoma. *J Pathol.* (2010) 220:608–17. doi: 10.1002/path.2679
53. Tamborini E, Virdis E, Negri T, Orsenigo M, Brich S, Conca E, et al. Analysis of receptor tyrosine kinases (RTKs) and downstream pathways in chordomas. *Neuro Oncol.* (2010) 12:776–89. doi: 10.1093/neuonc/noq003
54. De Castro CV, Guimaraes G, Aguiar S Jr, Lopes A, Baiocchi G, Da Cunha IW, et al. Tyrosine kinase receptor expression in chordomas: phosphorylated AKT correlates inversely with outcome. *Hum Pathol.* (2013) 44:1747–55. doi: 10.1016/j.humpath.2012.11.024
55. Akhavan-Sigari R, Gaab MR, Rohde V, Abili M, Ostertag H. Prognostic significance of immunohistochemical expression of VEGFR2 and iNOS in spinal chordoma. *Eur Spine J.* (2014) 23:2416–22. doi: 10.1007/s00586-014-3417-5
56. Hu Y, Mintz A, Shah SR, Quinones-Hinojosa A, Hsu W. The FGFR/MEK/ERK/brachyury pathway is critical for chordoma cell growth and survival. *Carcinogenesis* (2014) 35:1491–9. doi: 10.1093/carcin/bgu014
57. Magnaghi P, Salom B, Cozzi L, Amboldi N, Ballinari D, Tamborini E, et al. Afatinib is a new therapeutic approach in chordoma with a unique ability to target EGFR and brachyury. *Mol Cancer Ther.* (2018) 17:603–13. doi: 10.1158/1535-7163.MCT-17-0324
58. Choi H, Charnsangavej C, Faria SC, Macapinlac HA, Burgess MA, Patel SR, et al. Correlation of computed tomography and positron emission tomography in patients with metastatic gastrointestinal stromal tumor treated at a single institution with imatinib mesylate: proposal of new computed tomography response criteria. *J Clin Oncol.* (2007) 25:1753–9. doi: 10.1200/JCO.2006.07.3049
59. Eisenhauer EA, Therasse P, Bogaerts J, Schwartz LH, Sargent D, Ford R, et al. New response evaluation criteria in solid tumours: revised RECIST guideline (version 1.1). *Eur J Cancer* (2009) 45:228–47. doi: 10.1016/j.ejca.2008.10.026
60. Stommel JM, Kimmelman AC, Ying H, Nabioullin R, Ponugoti AH, Wiedemeyer R, et al. Coactivation of receptor tyrosine kinases affects the response of tumor cells to targeted therapies. *Science* (2007) 318:287–90. doi: 10.1126/science.1142946
61. Scheipl S, Froehlich EV, Leithner A, Beham A, Quehenberger F, Mokry M, et al. Does insulin-like growth factor 1 receptor (IGF-1R) targeting provide new treatment options for chordomas? A retrospective clinical and immunohistochemical study. *Histopathology* (2012) 60:999–1003. doi: 10.1111/j.1365-2559.2012.04186.x
62. Akhavan-Sigari R, Gaab MR, Rohde V, Brandis A, Tezval H, Abili M, et al. Expression of vascular endothelial growth factor receptor 2 (VEGFR-2), inducible nitric oxide synthase (iNOS), and Ki-M1P in skull base chordoma: a series of 145 tumors. *Neurosurg Rev.* (2014) 37:79–88. doi: 10.1007/s10143-013-0495-5
63. Roux PP, Shahbazian D, Vu H, Holz MK, Cohen MS, Taunton J, et al. RAS/ERK signaling promotes site-specific ribosomal protein S6 phosphorylation via RSK and stimulates cap-dependent translation. *J Biol Chem.* (2007) 282:14056–64. doi: 10.1074/jbc.M700906200
64. Carracedo A, Ma L, Teruya-Feldstein J, Rojo F, Salmena L, Alimonti A, et al. Inhibition of mTORC1 leads to MAPK pathway activation through a PI3K-dependent feedback loop in human cancer. *J Clin Invest.* (2008) 118:3065–74. doi: 10.1172/JCI34739
65. Yang C, Schwab JH, Schoenfeld AJ, Hornicek FJ, Wood KB, Nielsen GP, et al. A novel target for treatment of chordoma: signal transducers and activators of transcription 3. *Mol Cancer Ther.* (2009) 8:2597–605. doi: 10.1158/1535-7163.MCT-09-0504
66. Ohashi K, Maruvka YE, Michor F, Pao W. Epidermal growth factor receptor tyrosine kinase inhibitor-resistant disease. *J Clin Oncol.* (2013) 31:1070–80. doi: 10.1200/JCO.2012.43.3912
67. Chen K, Mo J, Zhou M, Wang G, Wu G, Chen H, et al. Expression of PTEN and mTOR in sacral chordoma and association with poor prognosis. *Med Oncol.* (2014) 31:886. doi: 10.1007/s12032-014-0886-7
68. Han S, Polizzano C, Nielsen GP, Hornicek FJ, Rosenberg AE, Ramesh V. Aberrant hyperactivation of akt and Mammalian target of rapamycin complex 1 signaling in sporadic chordomas. *Clin Cancer Res.* (2009) 15:1940–6. doi: 10.1158/1078-0432.CCR-08-2364
69. Lee DH, Zhang Y, Kassam AB, Park MJ, Gardner P, Prevedello D, et al. Combined PDGFR and HDAC inhibition overcomes PTEN disruption in chordoma. *PLoS ONE* (2015) 10:e0134426. doi: 10.1371/journal.pone.0134426
70. Wang L, Zehir A, Nafa K, Zhou N, Berger MF, Casanova J, et al. Genomic aberrations frequently alter chromatin regulatory genes in chordoma. *Genes Chromosomes Cancer* (2016) 55:591–600. doi: 10.1002/gcc.22362

71. Bosotti R, Magnaghi P, Di Bella S, Cozzi L, Cusi C, Bozzi F, et al. Establishment and genomic characterization of the new chordoma cell line Chor-IN-1. *Sci Rep.* (2017) 7:9226. doi: 10.1038/s41598-017-10044-3
72. Liu T, Shen JK, Choy E, Zhang Y, Mankin HJ, Hornicek FJ, et al. CDK4 Expression in chordoma: a potential therapeutic target running title: CDK4 expression in chordoma. *J Orthop Res.* (2018) 36:1581–9. doi: 10.1002/jor.23819
73. Levy J. *Chordoma Foundation In Vivo Drug Screening Program.* Chordoma Foundation (2018). Available online at: https://figshare.com/projects/Chordoma_Foundation_In_Vivo_Drug_Screening_Program/25948 (accessed January 25, 2018).

15

Bevacizumab Combined with Oxaliplatin/ Capecitabine in Patient with Refractory and Recurrent Mucinous Adenocarcinoma of the Appendix

Wenzhi Liu[1†], Lili Liu[2†], Ruoyu Wang[1†], Guanyu Gong[1,3], Xinjia Ding[4], Bin Yang[3,5], Yun Bao[1], Zhiqiang Wang[1], Bo Zhang[4], Dewei Zhao[1], Fei Wu[1] and Yan Ding[1,5*]*

[1] The Institute for Translational Medicine, The Affiliated Zhongshan Hospital of Dalian University, Dalian, China, [2] Department of Oncology, The Second Affiliated Hospital of Dalian Medical University, Dalian, China, [3] Genomic Future Inc., Lexington, MA, United States, [4] Department of Neurosurgery, The Second Affiliated Hospital of Dalian Medical University, Dalian, China, [5] Department of Pediatrics, Children's Hospital of Boston, Harvard Medical School, Boston, MA, United States

***Correspondence:**
Fei Wu
wufei0348@126.com
Yan Ding
yan.ding@childrens.harvard.edu

† These authors have contributed equally to this work

Primary appendiceal adenocarcinoma with peritoneal pseudomyxoma (PPM) has a high recurrence rate and refractory to medical interventions such as repetitive debulking surgery and systemic chemotherapy. Genome-based targeted therapy for such cases has not been well-documented. Here we present a 63-years-old women, who was diagnosed with recurrent mucinous adenocarcinoma of the appendix with local invasions and peritoneal carcinomatosis, was refractory to systemic chemotherapy after surgery. We used a regime developed using whole exome sequencing. Somatic mutations in the genes encoding VEGFR2, FGFR1, FGFR2, FGFR3, and KRAS were identified in the patient's tumor tissue. The patient was then treated with bevacizumab plus oxaliplatin. After 4 months of treatment, pelvic CT showed dramatic reduction of pseudomyoma and a decline of CA199 level from 5436.7 to 1121.4 U/ml. Continual treatment with bevacizumab-capecitabine remained effective and the patient's CA199 level further decreased to 401.26 U/ml according to the follow-up examination on Aug 15th, 2018. Results from this study show the evidence of gene mutations involving VEGF signal activation in the recurrence of appendiceal adenocarcinoma. Our results also suggest the association of these mutations with the effectiveness of anti-VEGF treatment using bevacizumab. Therefore, the screening of gene mutations involved in VEGF signaling and targeted therapy with anti-VEGF drugs may provide a new option to manage refractory/recurrent advanced-stage appendiceal adenocarcinoma.

Keywords: appendiceal adenocarcinoma, peritoneal carcinomatosis, next generation sequencing, bevacizumab, targeted therapy

BACKGROUND

Primary adenocarcinoma of the appendix is a rare malignancy and accounts for 0.4% of gastrointestinal tumors, according to a report of national cancer institute (NCI) (1). Mucinous adenocarcinoma is the most common histological subtype (37%), followed by colonic and carcinoid subtypes (2). The clinical presentations of appendiceal cancer are vague until advanced stage. As a result, early diagnosis of appendiceal cancer is often difficult. Common complications of late stage disease include rupture and acute appendicitis (accounting for ~1% appendectomy cases) (3), local invasion and peritoneal carcinomatosis (PC)/peritoneal pseudomyxoma (PPM) (4, 5). The advanced stage has a poor overall survival rate with median survival time of 5.2–12.6 months (5). Currently there is no standard medical care for the disseminated late-stage appendiceal cancer with PC/PPM. It has been generally recommended to perform cytoreductive surgery (CRS) combined with perioperative hyperthermic intraperitoneal chemotherapy (HIPEC) or postoperative intraperitoneal chemotherapy (EPIC) with mitomycin C, cisplatin, 5-FU, or a combination (5, 6). Unfortunately, most appendiceal cancer patients with PC/PPM experience recurrent and refractory to treatment, and fail to repetitive surgery and systemic chemotherapy (6).

Targeted therapy has been successfully used to treat many types of cancers including colorectal cancer. However, to the best of our knowledge, genome-based targeted therapy for the appendiceal cancer has never been reported. In the present case, a patient was diagnosed with mucinous adenocarcinoma of the appendix with peritoneal carcinomatosis and multiple local invasions. The patient received routine treatments by CRS-HEPIC-EPIC but relapsed after 1 year. Then the patient's condition deteriorated continuously and experienced recurrent and refractory to the treatment. Using whole exome sequencing and targeted medicine, optimal therapeutical efficacy was achieved with a gradual remission and remains progression-free until now.

CASE PRESENTATION

A 63-years-old Chinese female presented with asymptomatic palpable abdominal mass, increased carbohydrate antigen 19-9 (CA-199) level and pelvic mass on CT scan. An opening surgery observed an appendiceal mass involving the entire layer of the appendix, rupture, invasion of bilateral ovaries, wide-spreading nodular implantations with pseudomyxoma in peritoneal cavity, greater omentum, small intestine mesentery and hepatic and splenic regions. Debulking surgery with peritoneal nodule ablation and mucus reduction was performed in Beijing 301 Hospital. Postoperative pathology confirmed mucinous adenocarcinoma of the appendix T4NxM1, stage IV with peritoneal carcinomatosis (**Figure 1**). After surgery, the patient received one time standard perioperative hyperthermic intraperitoneal chemotherapy (HIPEC) with mitomycin C. Because of the excessive peritoneal carcinomatosis, the patient was given three cycles of postoperative intraperitoneal chemotherapy (EPIC) with 5-FU plus mitomycin C. The patient remained symptom free for 1 year until she developed progressive abdominal distension, loss of appetite and worsening nourishment. The patient failed to response to further systemic chemotherapy, and a large number of PPM (**Figures 2A,B**). Then a second surgery was performed, intestinal obstruction by mucous cavities was observed, and a colostomy was given. Shortly after operation, cetuximab, a monoclonal antibody binding to and inhibiting EGFR, was given to the patient for 20 days (yet without gene testing) at a local hospital, but failed to show any improvement. By then the patient had tried all available approved options and became refractory to the treatments.

TABLE 1 | Mutated genes identified in the present case of mucinous adenocarcinoma.

AKT1	ATM	CSFIR	ERBB2	FGFR1	FGFR2	FGFR3	FLT3
GNA11	JAK3	KDR	KIT	KRAS	NOTCH1	PIK3CA	PET
SMARCB1	SMO	STK11	TP53				

At the time when the patient visited us, she was severely wasted, with progressive abdominal distension and elevated CA-199 level at 5436.7 U/ml. Considering her weak constitution and failure of previous interventions, alternative treatment strategies, especially a rationally designed targeted therapy, emerged to be the last-ditch option to the patient. Targeted therapy is usually based on a patient's genomic profile by genetic testing. In order to find the accurate target, we decided to use the paraffin-embedded surgical tumor tissue from the patient, and detect gene mutations using the TruSeq Rapid Capture Exome Kit for whole exome sequencing (WES) on the Illumina NextSeq500 sequencing platform. The WES data was then analyzed using OncoDecoder^{TM} (Genomic Future, Inc. USA). Several key gene mutations were identified including a missense mutation p.Gln472His (exon 11) in KDR/VEGFR-2, a missense mutation p.Arg281Gln (exon 8) in FGFR1, a missense mutation p.Lys296Arg (exon 7) in FGFR2, a missense mutation p.Thr654Ser (exon 14) in FGFR3 and a missense mutation p.Gly12Asp (exon 2) in KRAS. Additional 38 gene mutations including TP53, ERBB2, KIT, GNA11, and JAK3 were also detected (**Table 1**).

Although no NCCN-guided targeted therapy regime for appendiceal mucinous adenocarcinoma is documented as of to-date, there are two approved drugs for colorectal cancer may be considered as potential candidates: bevacizumab and cetuximab. Bevacizumab is a monoclonal antibody blocking the VEGF ligand, and bevacizumab in combination with standard chemotherapy has been approved by FDA as first line treatment for metastatic colorectal cancer (7, 8). We predicted that bevacizumab may be a suitable targeted drug candidate for our case based on the following three reasons: Firstly, the gene testing results showed several mutations involving KDR/VEGFR-2, FGFR1, FGFR2, and FGFR3. Although these mutations are currently classified as variation of uncertain significance (VUS), hyperactive VEGF pathway is a common event in colorectal cancer and contributes to tumor metastatic activity (9). A recent study from the MD Anderson cancer center showed improved average overall survival and progression-free survival by providing anti-VEGF treatment to patients diagnosed with unresectable appendiceal epithelial neoplasm (yet no gene

Abbreviations: CT, computed tomography; PC, peritoneal carcinomatosis; PPM, peritoneal pseudomyxoma; CRS, cytoreductive surgery; HIPEC, hyperthermic intraperitoneal chemotherapy; EPIC, intraperitoneal chemotherapy; VEGFR, Vascular endothelial growth factor receptor; FGFR, Fibroblast growth factor receptor.

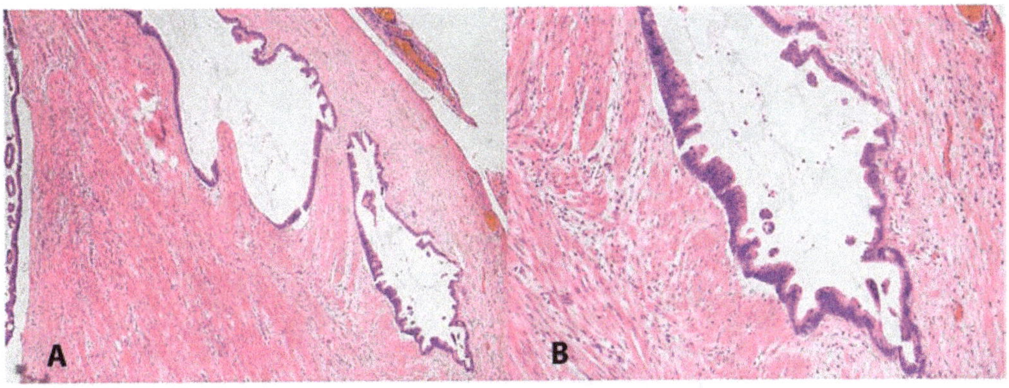

FIGURE 1 | Low (**A**, 40X) and high (**B**, 100X) magnification pictures of appendiceal mucinous adenocarcinoma. H&E stained.

testing was performed) (10). This finding suggests that VEGF hyperactivity could be a common event in appendiceal cancer, and bevacizumab could be a promising targeted drug. Next, it has been known that the efficacy of certain EGFR monoclonal antibody drugs, including cetuximab and panitumumab, could be affected by KRAS mutation (6). Indeed, in the present case, we identified KRAS p.Gly12Asp missense mutation, which could cause inefficient response to cetuximab (11). However, the efficacy of bevacizumab for colorectal cancer treatment has been testified to be independent from KRAS mutation (8). Thirdly, there was no contraindication of bevacizumab usage to the patient. The common risk factors include low WBC count, high blood pressure, impaired heart function and poor renal function.

Under our advice, the patient received treatment of bevacizumab (7.5 mg/Kg, in total 450 mg, IV-GTT) plus oxaliplatin (130 mg/m^2, in total 200 mg IV-GTT) on day 1 every 3 weeks for 6 cycles since August, 2016. Follow-up examination after treatment showed significant improvement of the patient's condition, and CT scan imaging results showed dramatic reduction of her peritoneal mucus (as shown in **Figures 2C,D**). In addition, the patient's CA-199 level decreased from 5,436.7 U/ml (before treatment) to 1121.4 U/ml (after treatment). Afterwards, the patient received continuous maintenance treatment using bevacizumab (7.5 mg/Kg, in total 450 mg, IV-GTT on day 1 each 3 weeks) plus capecitabine (1,500 mg, oral, twice a day) for days 1 to 14 until now. The patient has been followed up routinely to evaluate the treatment efficacy and to monitor the adverse effects. The main adverse effects were numbness in the hands and feet, dry nose and epistaxis, dry throat, fatigue, loss of appetite. The patient has been progression-free as of recent follow-up on September 26th, 2018 with the most recent CA-199 being 401.26 U/ml on August 15th, 2018.

DISCUSSION

Primary adenocarcinoma of the appendix is a rare neoplasm with an incidence of 1.2 cases per 100,000 people each year (12). The prognosis of appendiceal adenocarcinoma varies depending on the histology types, including colonic-type adenocarcinoma, typical carcinoid, mucinous adenocarcinoma, and singlet ring cell adenocarcinoma (3). The mucinous adenocarcinoma is similar to the ovarian adenocarcinoma, and peritoneal dissemination is a frequent metastatic route (12). Like most colorectal cancers, the appendiceal adenocarcinoma presents with non-specific symptoms and is difficult to be diagnosed preoperatively (4, 5). As a result, it is often found at an advanced stage in which the disease has already spread within abdomen (5). Appendiceal adenocarcinoma-derived peritoneal carcinomatosis (PC) or peritoneal pseudomyxoma (PPM) is a very poor prognostic factor with average life expectancy between half and 1 year (5). In the present case, the patient presented with asymptomatic abdominal mass, local invasions to greater omentum and fallopian tubes and peritoneal carcinomatosis with multiple pseudomyxoma cavities at the initial visit.

The management of mucinous appendiceal adenocarcinoma varies depending on the stages and does not have standard guideline. Right hemicolectomy remains the treatment of choice for the early stage local or regional appendiceal adenocarcinoma (5, 6). CRS-HIPEC or EPIC is usually recommended for the appendiceal or colonic-type carcinoma with confined peritoneal metastasis (5). However, there is no standardized protocol for HIPEC or EPIC (5), and it only achieved complete response in some patients (5, 6). In our case, the patient received CRS-HIPEC-EPIC regime but relapse of peritoneal carcinomatosis occurred 1 year later. Systemic 5-fluorouracil-based chemotherapy was barely beneficial.

Recently, genome-based precision medicine has made great progress to treat a variety of cancers, including colorectal cancer (13). Targeted drugs feature high efficiency and low toxicity. To the best of our knowledge, genome-based targeted therapy for metastatic appendiceal adenocarcinoma has not yet been reported. In order to seek for appropriate targeted therapy for the patient with recurrent and refractory appendiceal cancer, we performed whole exome sequencing with the patient surgical pathology tissue at our genetic testing lab. Several

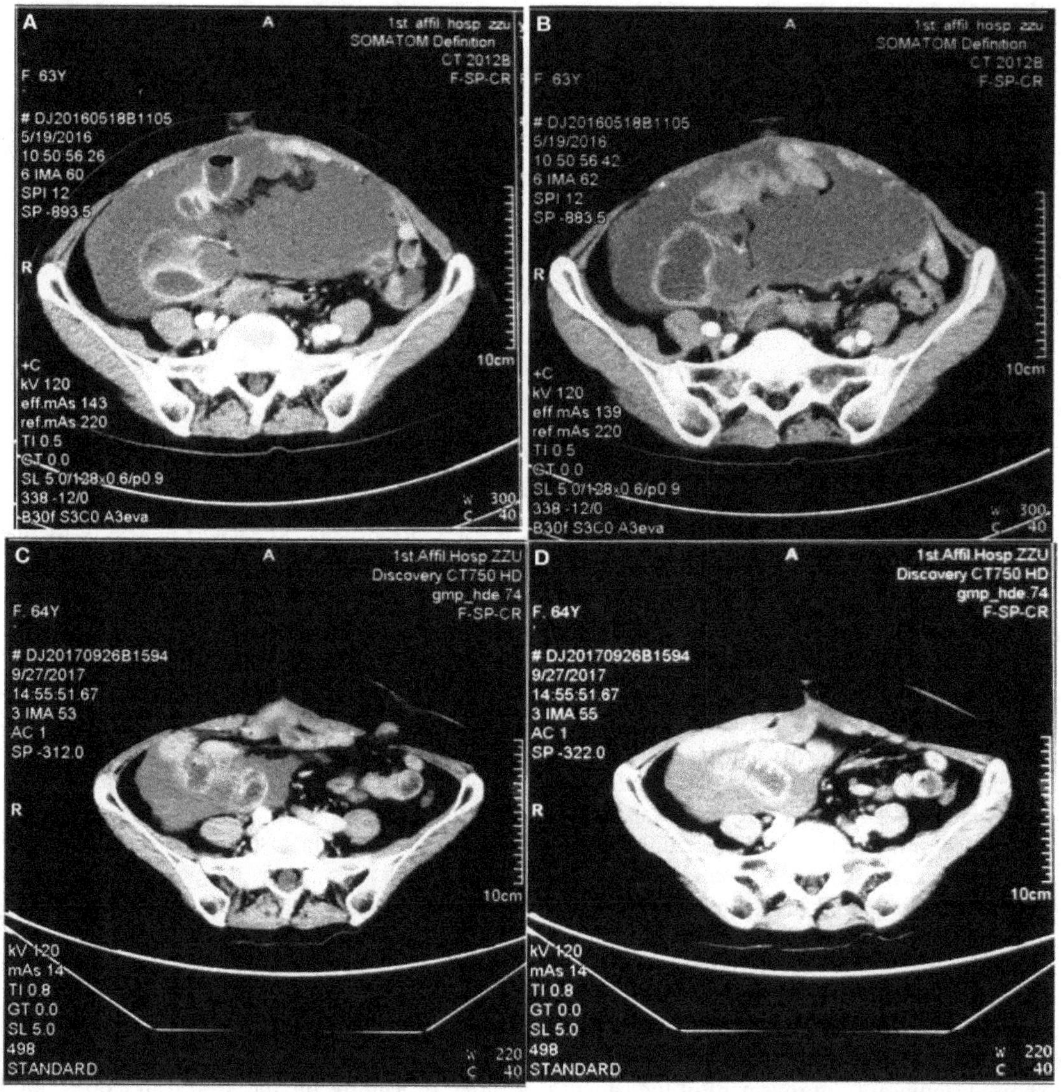

FIGURE 2 | Pelvic CT images before **(A,B)** vs. after **(C,D)** targeted therapy. **(A,B)** Prior to targeted therapy, images showed intraperitoneal multiple nodules, and a large number of peritoneal cavities filled up with mucus. **(C,D)** After targeted therapy using bevacizumab and oxaliplatin, image on the same sections showed significantly reduced peritoneal nodules and mucous cavities, suggesting stabilization of disease progression and partial response.

candidate target gene mutations involved in the angiogenesis pathway including KDR/VEGFR-2 and FGFR1, FGFR2, FGFR3 were identified. Both VEGF and FGF pathways function as angiogenetic mediators to promote metastasis of many neoplasms (9). Based on the gene mutation profile, the patient received the bevacizumab-oxaliplatin regime and then the bevacizumab-capecitabine as maintenance treatment. The results showed great effectiveness of the treatment and the patient remains progression-free and continuous decrease of CA-199 level as of to-date. The use of bevacizumab for metastatic appendiceal cancer treatment has been reported in a recent study (10). However, the treatment achieved therapeutical benefits in some patients but not the others, owing to the fact that no gene testing was performed before treatment (10). Therefore, our case report is the first study demonstrating evidence-based therapy for metastatic mucinous appendiceal adenocarcinoma. Indeed, we argue that certain level of cost-effective gene testing may be necessary prior to administration of targeted drugs in order to avoid the abuse of targeted medicines. A good example could be found in our case that the blind usage of anti-EGFR drug cetuximab without prior detection of KRAS mutation from the patient pathology tissue failed to achieve any treatment benefit.

In conclusion, accurate detection of gene mutation can help clinicians to make the optimal choice of individualized targeted drugs, and improve the prognosis and life quality of patients. The present report is one case and limited and waits for more cases to be filled in to expand our knowledge about the genome mutations and personalized medicine of appendiceal cancer.

ETHICS STATEMENT

The patient of this case report agreed and provided written informed consent in accordance with the Declaration of Helsinki. Written informed consent was obtained from the patient for the purpose of publication of the present case report and any relevant images.

AUTHOR CONTRIBUTIONS

All authors listed have made a substantial, direct and intellectual contribution to the work, and approved it for publication.

REFERENCES

1. Hesketh KT. The management of primary adenocarcinoma of the vermiform appendix. *Gut* (1963) 4:158. doi: 10.1136/gut.4.2.158
2. Turaga KK, Pappas SG, Gamblin T. Importance of histologic subtype in the staging of appendiceal tumors. *Ann Surg Oncol.* (2012) 19:1379–85. doi: 10.1245/s10434-012-2238-1
3. Connor SJ, Hanna GB, Frizelle FA. Appendiceal tumors: retrospective clinicopathologic analysis of appendiceal tumors from 7,970 appendectomies. *Dis Colon Rectum* (1998) 41:75–80. doi: 10.1007/BF022 36899
4. Ruoff C, Hanna L, Zhi W, Shahzad G, Gotlieb V, Salf MW. Cancers of the appendix: review of the literatures. *ISRN Oncol.* (2011) 2011:728579. doi: 10.5402/2011/728579
5. Winder T, Lenz HJ. Mucinous adenocarcinomas with intra-abdominal dissemination: a review of current therapy. *Oncologist* (2010) 15:836–44. doi: 10.1634/theoncologist.2010-0052
6. Pietrantonio F, Maggi C, Fanetti G, Iacovelli R, Di Bartolomeo M, Ricchini F, et al. FOLFOX-4 chemotherapy for patients with unresectable or relapsed peritoneal pseudomyxoma. *Oncologist* (2014) 19:845–50. doi: 10.1634/theoncologist.2014-0106
7. Saltz LB, Clarke S, Díaz-Rubio E, Scheithauer W, Figer A, Wong R, et al. Bevacizumab in combination with oxaliplatin-based chemotherapy as first-line therapy in metastatic colorectal cancer: a randomized phase III study. *J Clin Oncol.* (2008) 26:2013–9. doi: 10.1200/JCO.2007.14.9930.
8. Bencsikova B, Bortlicek Z, Halamkova J, Ostrizkova L, Kiss I, Melichar B, et al. Efficacy of bevacizumab and chemotherapy in the first-line treatment of metastatic colorectal cancer: broadening KRAS-focused clinical view. *BMC Gastroenterol.* (2015) 15:37. doi: 10.1186/s12876-015-0266-6
9. Ellis LM, Takahashi Y, Liu W, Shaheen RM. Vascular endothelial growth factor in human colon cancer: biology and therapeutic implications. *Oncologist.* (2000) 5 (Suppl. 1):11–5. doi: 10.1634/theoncologist.5-suppl_1-11
10. Choe JH, Overman MJ, Fournier KF, Royal RE, Ohinata A, Rafeeq S, et al. Improved survival with anti-VEGF therapy in the treatment of unresectable appendiceal epithelial neoplasms. *Ann Surg Oncol.* (2015) 22:2578–84. doi: 10.1245/s10434-014-4335-9
11. Karapetis CS, Khambata-Ford S, Jonker DJ, O'Callaghan CJ, Tu D, Tebbutt NC, et al. K-ras mutations and benefit from cetuximab in advanced colorectal cancer. *N Engl J Med.* (2008) 359:1757–65. doi: 10.1056/NEJMoa0804385
12. Arellano ML, Gonzalez-Dominguez Y, Molina-Ortiz F, Garceau MAH, Cantero R, Rodriguez-Montes JA. Primary adenocarcinoma of the appendix: experience at La Paz University Hospital of Madrid (1967-2014). *Int J Surg Open* (2016) 4:23–6. doi: 10.1016/j.ijso.2016.06.003
13. Linnekamp JF, Wang X, Medema JP, Vermeulen L. Colorectal cancer heterogeneity and targeted therapy: a case for molecular disease subtypes. *Cancer Res.* (2015) 75:245–9. doi: 10.1158/0008-5472.CAN-14-2240

16

An Insight into the Molecular Mechanism of Berberine Towards Multiple Cancer Types Through Systems Pharmacology

Pengfei Guo[1,2†], Chuipu Cai[1,3†], Xiaoqin Wu[4], Xiude Fan[4], Wei Huang[1], Jingwei Zhou[1], Qihui Wu[1], Yujie Huang[1], Wei Zhao[1], Fengxue Zhang[3], Qi Wang[1,5], Yongbin Zhang[2] and Jiansong Fang[1,4,5*]*

[1] Science and Technology Innovation Center, Guangzhou University of Chinese Medicine, Guangzhou, China, [2] Laboratory of Experimental Animal, Guangzhou University of Chinese Medicine, Guangzhou, China, [3] School of Basic Medical Sciences, Guangzhou University of Chinese Medicine, Guangzhou, China, [4] Lerner Research Institute, Cleveland Clinic, Cleveland, OH, United States, [5] Institute of Clinical Pharmacology, Guangzhou University of Chinese Medicine, Guangzhou, China

***Correspondence:**
Jiansong Fang
fangjs@gzucm.edu.cn;
fangj3@ccf.org
Yongbin Zhang
zyb-73@163.com

†These authors have contributed equally to this work.

Over the past several decades, natural products with poly-pharmacological profiles have demonstrated promise as novel therapeutics for various complex diseases, including cancer. Berberine (PubChem CID: 2353), a soliloquies quaternary alkaloid, has been validated to exert powerful effects in many cancers. However, the underlying molecular mechanism is not yet fully elucidated. In this study, we summarized the molecular effects of berberine against multiple cancers based on current available literatures. Furthermore, a systems pharmacology infrastructure was developed to discover new cancer indications of berberine and explore their molecular mechanisms. Specifically, we incorporated 289 high-quality protein targets of berberine by integrating experimental drug–target interactions (DTIs) extracted from literatures and computationally predicted DTIs inferred by network-based inference approach. Statistical network models were developed for identification of new cancer indications of berberine through integration of DTIs and curated cancer significantly mutated genes (SMGs). High accuracy was yielded for our statistical models. We further discussed three typical cancer indications (hepatocarcinoma, lung adenocarcinoma, and bladder carcinoma) of berberine with new mechanisms of actions (MOAs) based on our systems pharmacology framework. In summary, this study systematically provides a powerful strategy to identify potential anti-cancer effects of berberine with novel mechanisms from a systems pharmacology perspective.

Keywords: berberine, cancer, systems pharmacology, drug–target interactions, significantly mutated genes

INTRODUCTION

Natural products with diverse chemical scaffolds have been recognized as an invaluable source of candidates in drug discovery and development for multiple complex diseases, including cancer. Berberine, a plant-derived compound isolated from medicinal plants such as Coptis chinensis and Hydrastis canadensis, had a long history of medicinal application in traditional Chinese medicine

(Ayati et al., 2017). As one of the main alkaloids, berberine has been reported to exert potentially beneficial effects on many cancer types, including breast cancer (Kim et al., 2008), bladder cancer (Yan et al., 2011), and hepatocarcinoma (Liu et al., 2011; Zhu et al., 2016). For example, berberine had shown significant inhibitory effect on hepatocellular carcinoma cells and could reduce the volume and weight of tumors in an H22 transplanted tumor model in mice (Li et al., 2015).

Based on collection of hundreds of berberine-related pharmacological literatures, we systematically summarized eight key mechanisms of anti-cancer effects of berberine, including cell death, cell invasion and metastasis, cell cycle arrest, cell growth, transcription factors, inflammatory factors, angiogenic, chemo-sensitivity, and radio-sensitivity (**Figure 1** and **Supplementary Table S1**). Specifically, apoptosis (programmed cell death) plays a vital role in tumor cell development, differentiation, and proliferation (Ola et al., 2011). Recent study has revealed that berberine could induce apoptosis of human osteosarcoma U2OS cells through inhibiting the PI3K/Akt signaling pathway activation (Chen, 2016). In addition, anti-angiogenesis is a promising strategy for prevention and treatment of multicancer in preclinical or clinical studies in terms of many natural products (Khalid et al., 2016; Kotoku et al., 2016). Previous *in vitro* and *in vivo* experiments have validated that berberine exerted anti-angiogenic effect through inhibiting various proinflammatory and pro-angiogenic factors, including vascular endothelial growth factor (VEGF), interleukin-6 (IL-6), interleukin-2 (IL-2), and metalloproteinase inhibitor (TIMP) (Hamsa and Kuttan, 2012).

Collectively, berberine with polypharmacology has demonstrated its broad anti-cancer properties through targeting various oncogenic pathways and targets. Therefore, systematic exploration of the drug targets of berberine is of great significance for understanding its anti-cancer mechanisms of action (MOAs) and for further excavating its novel cancer indications.

Systems pharmacology-based approaches, as an emerging interdiscipline that combines experimental assays and computational tools, have provided an alternative to understand the therapeutic mechanisms of complex diseases (Fang et al., 2018). Recent studies have demonstrated advanced discovery of new indications for natural products based on systems pharmacology approaches (Fang et al., 2017b; Fang et al., 2019). For example, novel molecular mechanisms of several effective natural products (e.g., resveratrol, quercetin, caffeic acid, and wogonoside) for multiple complex diseases including multi-cancer types and age-related disorders have been identified and validated by various literatures and *in vitro* and *in vivo* experiments (Fang et al., 2017a; Huang et al., 2019). Collectively, systems pharmacology-based approaches have been proved as an effective tool for exploring the poly-pharmacological actions of natural products towards various complex diseases.

In this study, we proposed a systems pharmacology infrastructure to identify new cancer indications of berberine and explore their molecular mechanisms (**Figure 2**). Specifically, we constructed a global DTI network of berberine by integrating both experimentally reported DTIs obtained from literatures and DTIs computationally predicted by our previous predictive network models (Fang et al., 2017c). Besides, a high-quality

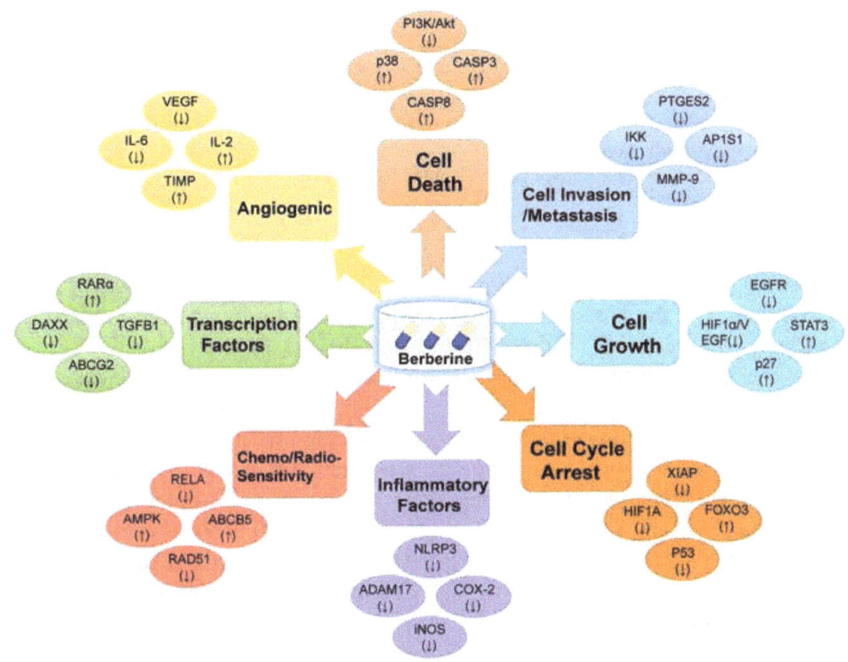

FIGURE 1 | Diagram illustrating the eight potential anti-cancer effects of berberine. Berberine exerts anti-cancer activities *via* targeting various cancer key protein targets, related to cell death, cell invasion and metastasis, cell cycle arrest, cell growth, transcription factors, inflammatory factors, angiogenic, chemo-sensitivity, and radio-sensitivity.

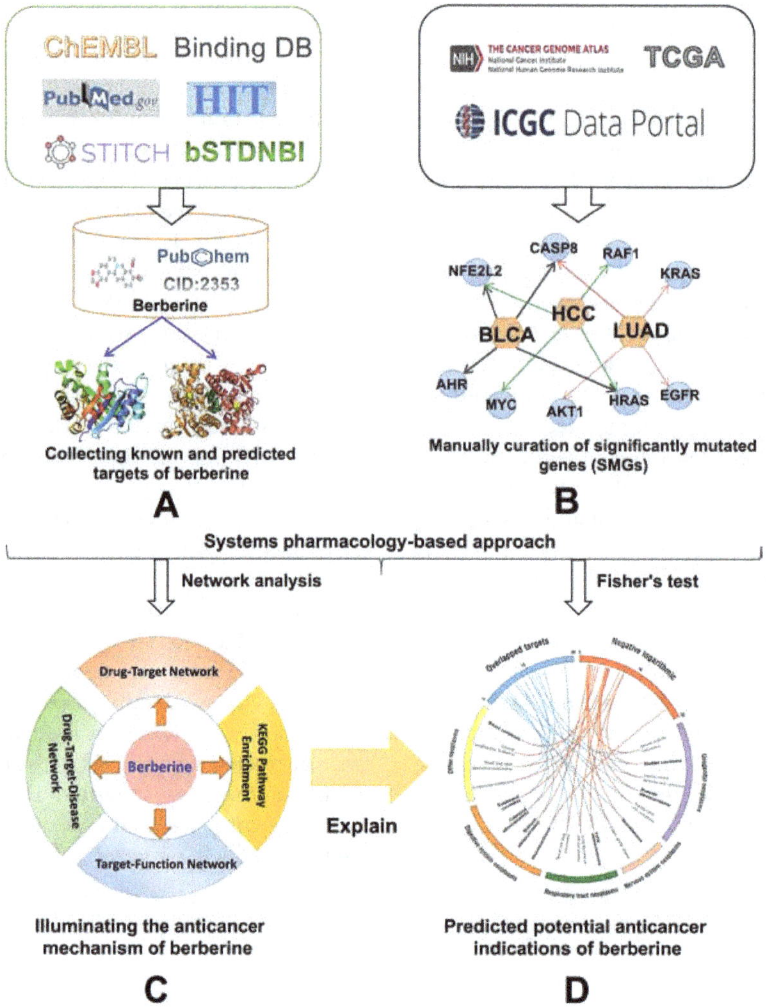

FIGURE 2 | Workflow of a systems pharmacology infrastructure for the identification of cancer indications and exploration of molecular mechanisms of berberine. **(A)** Construction of drug–target network for berberine, **(B)** manual curation of cancer significantly mutated genes (SMGs) for multiple cancer types, **(C)** performing network analyses to explore the anti-cancer mechanism of berberine, and **(D)** statistical network models for prioritizing novel anti-cancer indication of berberine through integrating computationally predicted and known drug targets into the curated cancer SMGs.

collection of significantly mutated genes (SMGs) for multiple cancer types was manually collected. On the basis of curated cancer SMGs and DTIs, we built statistical network models with high accuracy to prioritize new cancer indications of berberine and showcased its potential mechanisms. Overall, this study provides a useful systems pharmacology framework to interpret the multi-scale MOAs of berberine in multiple cancer type management, which may give some enlightenment for further treatment of cancer-associated diseases.

MATERIALS AND METHODS

Collection of Known Targets for Berberine

Known targets of berberine were collected by extracting data from four data sources, including HIT (Ye et al., 2011), STITCH (Kuhn et al., 2014), BindingDB (accessed June 2016) (Gilson et al., 2016), and ChEMBL (Bento et al., 2014). For STITCH, we only kept the targets with experimental evidence score higher than 0.7. We totally obtained 66 known targets *via* integrating the four available databases. Besides, we further gathered 238 extra targets of berberine by manually retrieving large-scale pharmacological literatures from PubMed (https://www.ncbi.nlm.nih.gov) with "berberine [title] and cancer" as search terms (**Supplementary Table S2**). After duplicated targets and DTIs were eliminated from non-*Homo sapiens*, 275 high-quality known DTIs were selected for further study (**Supplementary Table S3**).

Network-Based Target Prediction for Berberine

In a previous study, we have developed statistical network models to predict targets of natural products through a balanced substructure–drug–target network-based inference (bSDTNBI) approach (Fang et al., 2018). The bSDTNBI method utilizes resource-diffusion processes to prioritize potential targets for natural products through integrating known DTI network, drug–substructure linkages, and new input drug–substructure linkages (Wu et al., 2017). For a new input chemical, each of its substructures equally spreads resources to its neighbor nodes layer by layer, and targets obtaining final resources could be regarded as the potential targets of the new chemical. Four parameters ($\alpha = \beta = 0.1$, $\gamma = -0.5$, and $k = 2$) of bSDTNBI were adopted based on a previous study (Wu et al., 2016). Among them, parameter α was introduced to balance the initial resource allocation of different node types, while β was used to adjust weighted values of different edge types. The third parameter γ was imported to balance the influence of hub nodes in resource-diffusion processes, and the fourth parameter κ denotes the number of resource-diffusion processes. We calculated four substructure items for each compound based on four types of molecular fingerprints from PaDEL-Descriptor (version 2.18) (Yap, 2011), including Substructure (FP4), Klekota-Roth (KR), MACCS, and PubChem. Among the four network models generated with different types of fingerprints, bSDTNBI_KR performed best with the highest values of precision ($P = 0.049$), recall ($R = 0.752$), precision enhancement (Ep = 27.02), recall enhancement (eR = 27.24), and the area under the receiver operating characteristic curve (AUC = 0.959). Finally, the best model built based on KR molecular fingerprint was selected to predict the new targets of berberine. The top 20 predicted candidates were used for further study (**Supplementary Table S3**).

Significantly Mutated Genes (SMG) for Multiple Cancer Types

We collected 804 SMGs for 28 cancer types/subtypes from a previous study (Cheng et al., 2016), including glioblastoma multiforme (GBM), serous ovarian adenocarcinoma (SOC), stomach adenocarcinoma (STAD), colorectal adenocarcinoma (CRAC), breast carcinoma (BRCA), uterine corpus endometrioid (UCEC), medulloblastoma (MBL), acute myeloid leukemia (AML), cutaneous melanoma (CM), lung squamous cell (SQCC), thyroid carcinoma (THCA), lung adenocarcinoma (LUAD), kidney clear cell (CCSK), head and neck squamous (HNSCC), small cell lung (SCLC), lower grade glioma (LGG), bladder carcinoma (BLCA), esophageal carcinoma (EC), prostate adenocarcinoma (PRAD), hepatocarcinoma (HCC), neuroblastoma (NBL), chronic lymphocytic leukemia (CLL), pancreas adenocarcinoma (PAC), multiple myeloma (MM), acute lymphocytic leukemia (ALL), non-small cell lung (NSCLC), diffuse large B-cell lymphoma (DLBCL), and pilocytic astrocytoma (PA). Considering a lack of statistical power if the number of SMG for specific cancer types is lower than 20, we further excluded ALL, NSCLC, DLBCL, and PA. All SMGs are annotated using gene Entrez ID, chromosome location, and the official gene symbols from the National Center for Biotechnology Information (NCBI) database (Zhe and Huang, 2002). Finally, 24 cancer types/subtypes covering 804 SMGs were selected for further study (**Supplementary Table S4**).

Prioritizing Cancer Indications of Berberine

In this study, an integrated statistical network model was generated to prioritize cancer indication of berberine based on drug–target network and cancer SMGs (Cheng et al., 2016; Jiang et al., 2018). We assumed that berberine would exert high potential for the treatment of a specific cancer type if its targets tend to be SMGs of this cancer. For each cancer type/subtype, Fisher's exact test was utilized to calculate the statistical significance of the enrichment of SMGs for each cancer type in target profiles of berberine. The *P*-values were corrected by Benjamini–Hochberg method (Benjamini and Yekutieli, 2001). We set a cutoff adjusted *P*-value threshold (q) < 0.05 to define significantly predicted drug–cancer pairs.

Network Construction

To further explore the multi-scale MOAs of berberine in treating multiple cancer types, three types of networks were constructed by Cytoscape 3.2.1 software (Shannon et al., 2003): 1) drug-target (D-T) network, which presents the relationship between berberine and its targets; 2) target-function (T-F) network, which illustrates the relationship between cancer-related biological processes and SMGs; and 3) drug-target-disease (D-T-D) network, which reflects a global view of the molecular mechanism of berberine against multiple cancer types. After network analysis, the SMGs were further mapped to DAVID database (https://david.ncifcrf.gov/summary.jsp) for extracting the canonical pathways that were highly associated with these targets (Dennis et al., 2003). Finally, circos plot was used to visualize the predicted cancer indications.

RESULTS AND DISCUSSION

Construction of the Drug–Target (D-T) Network for Berberine

The constructed drug–target interaction network (**Figure 3**) of berberine contains 289 interactions, including 275 known targets and 20 predicted targets (**Supplementary Table S3**). *In vitro* and *in vivo* assays in previous studies have validated that five out of the 20 predicted targets could be mediated by berberine, indicating high accuracy of our target prediction approach. These five predicted targets are caspase-3 (CASP3) (Okubo et al., 2017), cellular tumor antigen p53 (TP53) (Qing et al., 2014), caspase-9 (CASP9) (Zhao et al., 2017), nuclear factor NF-kappa-B p105 subunit (NFKB1) (Yu et al., 2014), and mitogen-activated protein kinase 1 (MAPK1) (Song et al., 2015).

We further mapped the 289 protein targets of berberine into the curated cancer SMGs, resulting in 51 cancer-related targets encoded by SMGs (**Supplementary Table S3**). Accumulating evidences indicate that berberine may exert anti-cancer effects through regulating these targets. For instance, signal transducer and activator of transcription 3 (STAT3) are important in

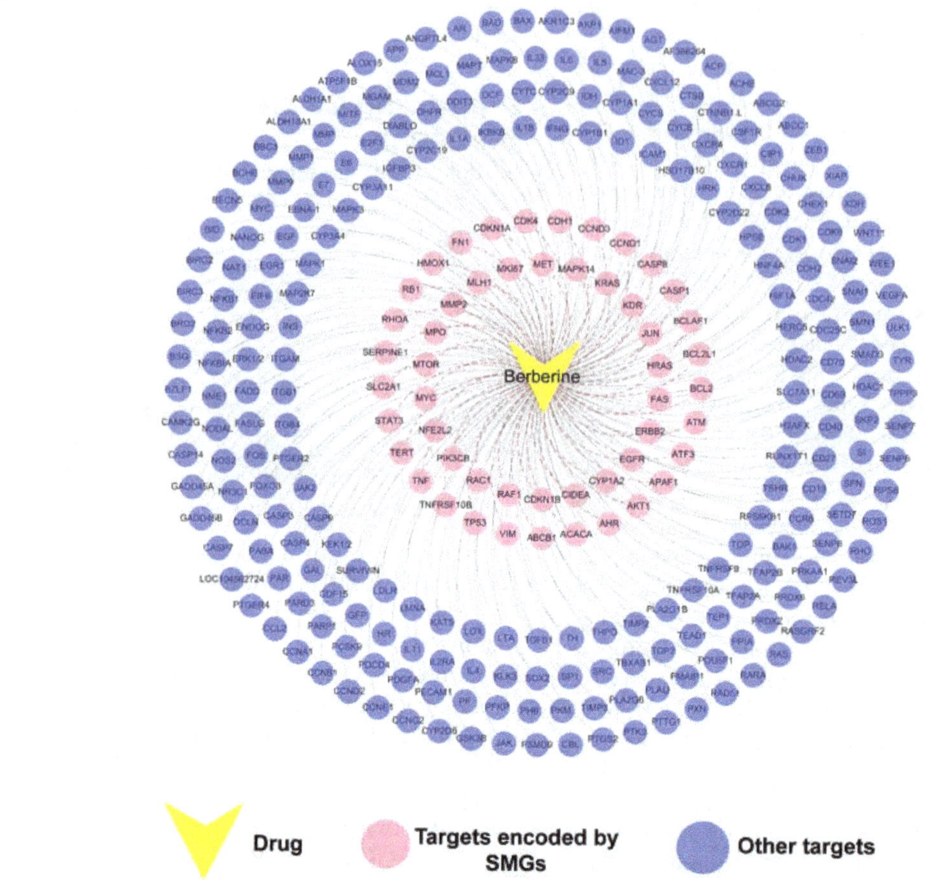

FIGURE 3 | Drug–target (D-T) network of berberine composed of known and predicted targets. The predicted targets were obtained by a balanced substructure–drug–target network-based inference (bSDTNBI) approach. This network includes 289 drug–target interactions connecting berberine and 51 protein targets encoded by significantly mutated genes (SMGs).

various phases of the tumor development, including tumor cell proliferation, survival, invasion, immunosuppression, and inducing and maintaining a pro-carcinogenic inflammatory microenvironment (Fan et al., 2013). A previous study has showed that berberine suppressed tumorigenicity and growth of nasopharyngeal carcinoma (NPC) cells by inhibiting STAT3 activation (Tsang et al., 2013). Recently, a strategy targeting tumor suppressors and apoptosis-related genes provides a rationale for developing more effective approaches and agents for cancer prevention (Sun et al., 2017; López-Cortés et al., 2018; Yamaguchi et al., 2019). Berberine has been observed to activate expression of many tumor apoptosis-related proteins, including caspase-8 (CASP8), tumor necrosis factor-a (TNF-a), and p38 MAPK, and thus induced apoptosis of HeLa cells (Lu et al., 2010). Besides, it has been reported that berberine can decrease expression of mitochondrial-dependent anti-apoptotic factors such as B-cell lymphoma-2 (Bcl-2) and Bcl-2-like protein 1 (BCL2L1) in KB human oral cancer cells (Kim et al., 2015).

Taken together, the observed polypharmacological profiles of berberine motivated us to elucidate its anti-cancer mechanism through systems pharmacology analysis on the interaction between berberine and 51 SMGs.

Elucidating Molecular Mechanisms of Berberine in Cancer Prevention and Treatment

Target–Function Network

As depicted in **Figure 4**, the target–function (T-F) network is composed of 230 T-F pairs connecting 51 SMG targets and 8 cancer-related functional modules based on the DAVID analysis (**Supplementary Table S5**). The eight functional modules include anti-cancer action associated with sustaining proliferative signaling (Huang et al., 2015), resisting cell death (Chidambara Murthy et al., 2012), deregulating cellular energetics (Tan et al., 2015), enabling replicative immortality (Xiong et al., 2015), avoiding immune destruction (Jiang et al., 2017), genome instability and mutation (Li et al., 2014), angiogenesis (Jie et al., 2011), and activating invasion and metastasis (Tang et al., 2009). On average, each SMG target is involved in six cancer-related functional modules. We found that 25 out of 51 SMG targets are associated with more than five functional modules, indicating the higher potential role of these SMG targets related to cancers. Previous studies of berberine in cancer validated the functional analysis of our T-F network. For instance, berberine could induce cell cycle arrest involved in sustaining proliferative signaling in

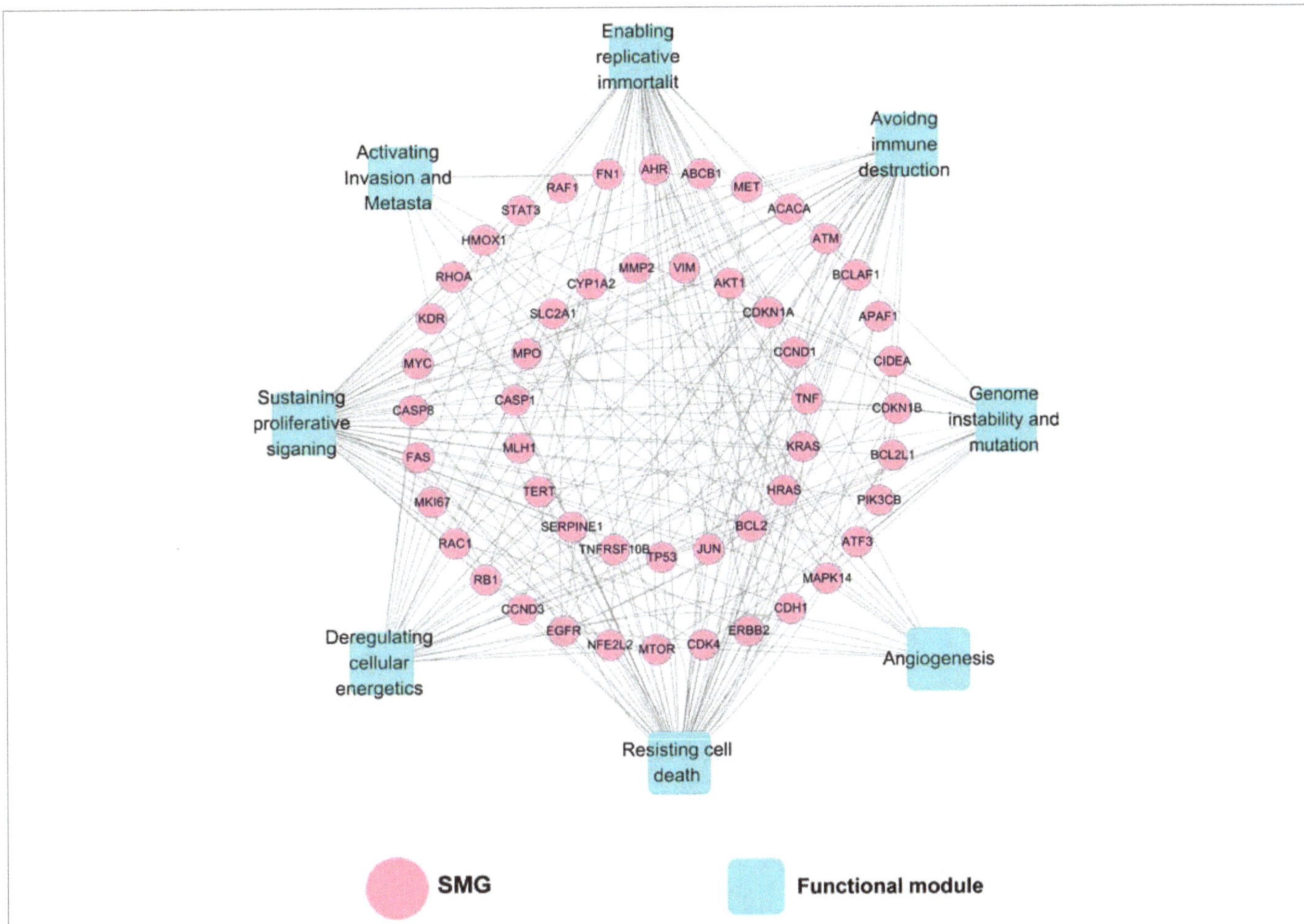

FIGURE 4 | Target–function (T-F) network demonstrating the relationship between cancer-related biological processes and SMGs. A functional module is linked to a target if the target is involved in mechanism of anti-cancer action.

cholangiocarcinoma KKU-213 and KKU-214 cell lines (Puthdee et al., 2017). Berberine was reported to inhibit metastasis and tumor-induced angiogenesis in human cervical cancer cells as well (Chu et al., 2014).

KEGG Enrichment Analysis

In order to further elucidate molecular mechanisms of berberine in cancer prevention and treatment, we performed KEGG pathway enrichment analysis based on the 51 SMGs. After pathways with adjusted P (q) value higher than 0.05 were excluded, 56 enriched pathways related to cancer pathogenesis were obtained (**Supplementary Table S6**).

Among 56 pathways, PI3K-Akt (hsa04151; $q = 2.0 \times 10^{-12}$), p53 (hsa04115; $q = 2.7 \times 10^{-9}$), HIF-1 (hsa04066; $q = 3.9 \times 10^{-9}$), FoxO (hsa04068; $q = 4.9 \times 10^{-9}$), VEGF (hsa04370; $q = 5.7 \times 10^{-7}$), MAPK (hsa04010; $q = 2.5 \times 10^{-6}$), Ras (hsa04014; $q = 6.4 \times 10^{-6}$), Jak-STAT (hsa04630; $q = 9.9 \times 10^{-4}$), mTOR (hsa04150; $q= 1.5 \times 10^{-2}$), AMPK (hsa04152; $q = 1.9 \times 10^{-2}$), and NF-kappa B (hsa04064; $q = 4.0 \times 10^{-2}$) signaling pathways have been confirmed to be associated with berberine in previous literatures (**Table 1**). For example, berberine was reported to inhibit cellular growth and promotes apoptosis by down-regulating PI3K/Akt signaling pathway in breast cancer SKBR-3 cells and hepatoma HepG2 cells (Liu et al., 2011; Kuo et al., 2011). *In vitro* and *in vivo* assays revealed that berberine sensitized drug-resistant breast cancer to doxorubicin (DOX) chemotherapy and directly induced apoptosis through the dose-orchestrated AMPK signaling pathway (Pan et al., 2017). Berberine also induces autophagic cell death through inhibition of mTOR-signaling pathway by suppressing Akt activity and up-regulating P38 MAPK signaling in HepG2 and MHCC97-L cells (Wang et al., 2010). The rest of the 45 enriched pathways prompt the potential anti-cancer acting mechanisms that may be mediated by berberine, which deserve to be validated by experimental assays in the future.

Drug–Target–Diseases Network

We further built a drug–target–diseases (D-T-D) network *via* mapping 51 SMGs targeted by berberine into multiple cancers. As shown in **Figure 5**, the 51 SMGs are related to 24 types of cancer. On average, each cancer links to nine SMGs, while each SMG is connected to 4.6 cancer types. Network analysis showed that the top 6 SMGs connected to the largest number of cancer types are

TABLE 1 | Summary of the 11 enriched pathways validated to be mediated by berberine in previous literatures.

Pathway ID	Pathway name	Genes	*P*-value	PMID
hsa04151	PI3K-Akt signaling pathway	EGFR, HRAS, PIK3CB, MET, TP53, RAF1, BCL2L1, CDK4, KDR, AKT1, CDKN1A, CCND1, KRAS, CDKN1B, CCND3, BCL2, RAC1, MTOR, MYC, FN1	2.03E−12	27081456|25212656
hsa04115	p53 signaling pathway	CDKN1A, CCND1, CCND3, CASP8, SERPINE1, TP53, APAF1, FAS, CDK4, ATM	2.66E−09	20455200
hsa04066	HIF-1 signaling pathway	AKT1, EGFR, HRAS, CCND1, KRAS, PIK3CB, ERBB2, TP53, RAF1, RB1, CDK4	3.89E−09	28775788
hsa04068	FoxO signaling pathway	AKT1, EGFR, HRAS, CCND1, KRAS, PIK3CB, ERBB2, TP53, RAF1, MLH1, CDH1, MYC	4.88E−09	24766860|29360760
hsa04370	VEGF signaling pathway	TNF, MAPK14, BCL2, RAC1, TP53, APAF1, BCL2L1, CASP1	5.72E−07	23869238
hsa04010	MAPK signaling pathway	AKT1, EGFR, HRAS, CCND1, KRAS, PIK3CB, ERBB2, TP53, RAF1, MLH1, CDH1, MYC	2.45E−06	19492307|25212656
hsa04014	Ras signaling pathway	AKT1, EGFR, HRAS, CCND1, KRAS, PIK3CB, ERBB2, TP53, RAF1, RB1, CDK4	6.42E−06	25212656|23159854
hsa04630	Jak-STAT signaling pathway	AKT1, HRAS, KRAS, PIK3CB, JUN, RAC1, RAF1	9.90E−04	26463023
hsa04150	mTOR signaling pathway	TNF, CASP8, APAF1, CASP1	1.50E−02	23159854|20830746
hsa04152	AMPK signaling pathway	EGFR, MAPK14, JUN, RAC1, MET	1.88E−02	28775788
hsa04064	NF-kappa B signaling pathway	TNF, CASP8, APAF1, CASP1	3.97E−02	19107816

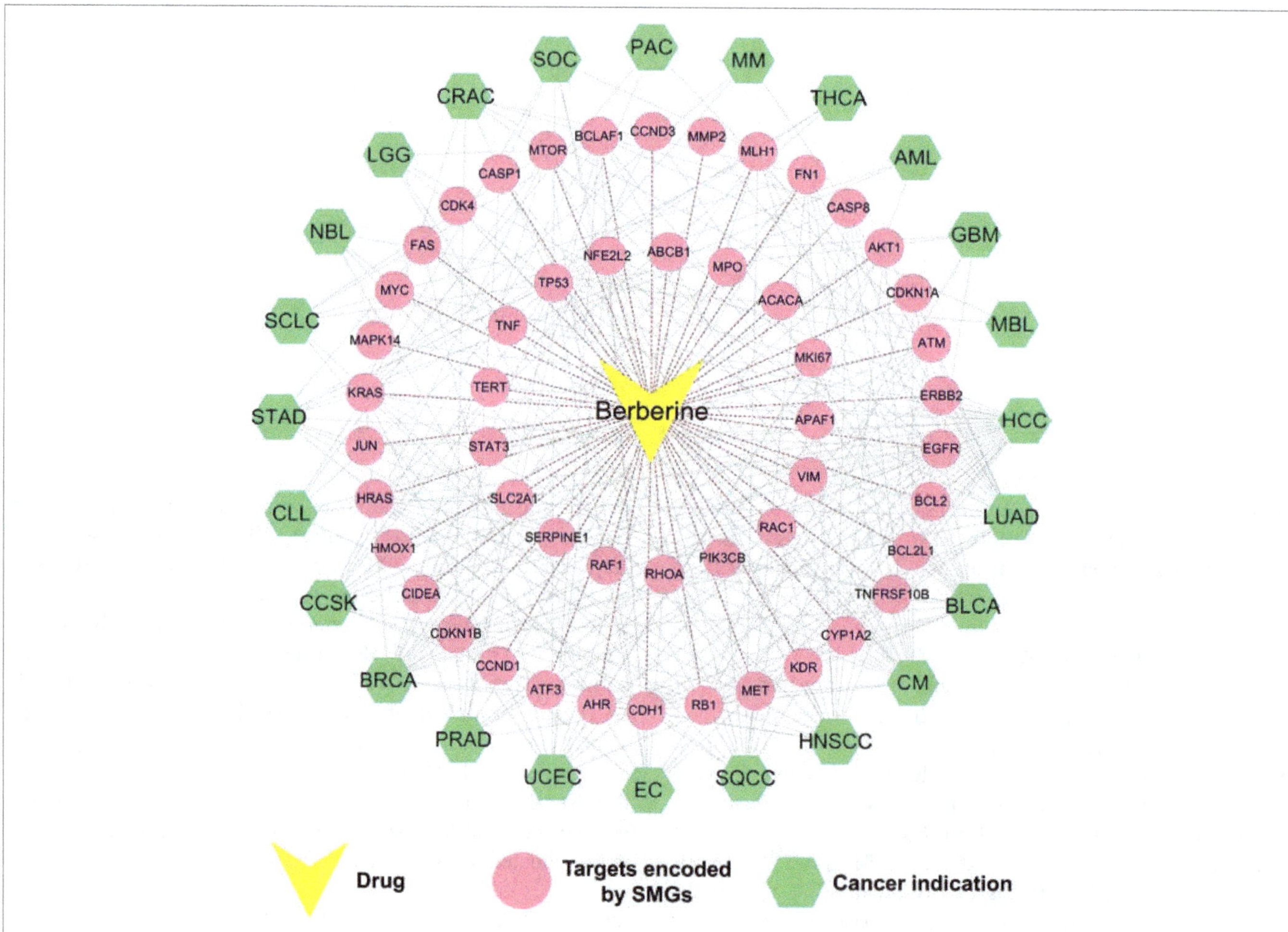

FIGURE 5 | Drug–target–disease (D-T-D) network of berberine. This network shows 51 proteins of berberine encoded by SMGs of 24 types of cancer.

cellular tumor antigen p53 (TP53), gTPase KRas (KRAS), epidermal growth factor receptor (EGFR), retinoblastoma-associated protein (RB1), serine-protein kinase ATM (ATM), and cadherin-1 (CDH1). Among them, EGFR, a key significantly mutated gene of cancer, is involved in the pathological mechanism of 13 cancer types, including LUAD, HNSCC, SQCC, EC, UCEC, PRAD, BRCA, CCSK, CLL,

STAD, LGG, CRAC, and GBM. Previous studies confirmed that berberine can inhibit EGFR signal pathway in several cancer types, including STAD (Wang et al., 2016), PRAD (Huang et al., 2015), and CRAC (Wang et al., 2013). Besides, berberine acts in specific tumor by regulating multiple SMGs. For instance, cellular tumor antigen p53 (TP53) (Wilson et al., 2010), RAC-alpha serine/threonine-protein kinase (AKT1) (López-Cortés et al., 2018), and cyclin-dependent kinase inhibitor 1B (CDKN1B) (Cusan et al., 2018) are highly correlated with breast cancer. Accumulating evidences demonstrated that berberine can inhibit breast cancer by acting on SMGs such as TP53 (Kim et al., 2012; Tan et al., 2015), AKT1 (Kuo et al., 2011), and CDKN1B (Patil et al., 2010).

Briefly, the D-T-D network demonstrated that SMGs targeted by berberine were closely related to multi-cancer types. In the following part, statistical systems pharmacology approach was employed to identify novel cancer indications of berberine and explore the molecular mechanisms.

Systems Pharmacology-Based Prediction of Cancer Indications for Berberine

As shown in **Figure 6**, a statistical systems pharmacology framework is proposed to prioritize novel cancer indications of berberine based on Fisher's exact test analysis. We calculated the therapeutic potential of berberine in 24 cancer indications and obtained 18 cancer indications of which adjusted P (q) values are lower than 0.05 ($q < 0.05$), including HCC ($q < 1.0 \times 10^{-5}$; $-$Log10 (q) = 19.25), LUAD ($q < 1.0 \times 10^{-5}$; $-$Log10 (q) = 9.35), BLCA ($q < 1.0 \times 10^{-5}$; $-$Log10 (q) = 9.31), CM ($q < 1.0 \times 10^{-5}$; $-$Log10 (q) = 9.29), HNSCC ($q < 1.0 \times 10^{-5}$; $-$Log10 (q) = 8.52), SQCC ($q < 1.0 \times 10^{-5}$; $-$Log10 (q) = 6.74), EC ($q < 1.0 \times 10^{-5}$; $-$Log10 (q) = 6.66), UCEC ($q < 1.0 \times 10^{-5}$; $-$Log10 (q) = 6.52), PRAD ($q = 1.15 \times 10^{-5}$; $-$Log10 (q) = 6.32), BRCA ($q = 1.33 \times 10^{-5}$; $-$Log10 (q) = 6.26), CCSK ($q = 2.30 \times 10^{-5}$; $-$Log10 (q) = 6.02), CLL ($q = 0.55 \times 10^{-3}$; $-$Log10 (q) = 4.64), STAD ($q = 1.76 \times 10^{-3}$; $-$Log10 (q) = 4.14), SCLC ($q = 5.33 \times 10^{-3}$; $-$Log10 (q) = 3.65), NBL ($q = 1.29 \times 10^{-2}$; $-$Log10 (q) = 3.27), LGG ($q = 1.67 \times 10^{-2}$; $-$Log10 (q) = 3.16), CRAC ($q = 3.21 \times 10^{-2}$; $-$Log10 (q) = 2.87), and SOC ($q = 3.36 \times 10^{-2}$; $-$Log10 (q) = 2.85) (**Supplementary Table S7**). As listed in **Table 2**, 10 out of the 18 predicted cancer indications of berberine were validated by reported experimental evidences, including HCC, LUAD, BLCA, EC, PRAD, BRCA, STAD, CRAC, and SOC, indicating the high accuracy of our systems pharmacology-based predictive method (success rate = 55.6%).

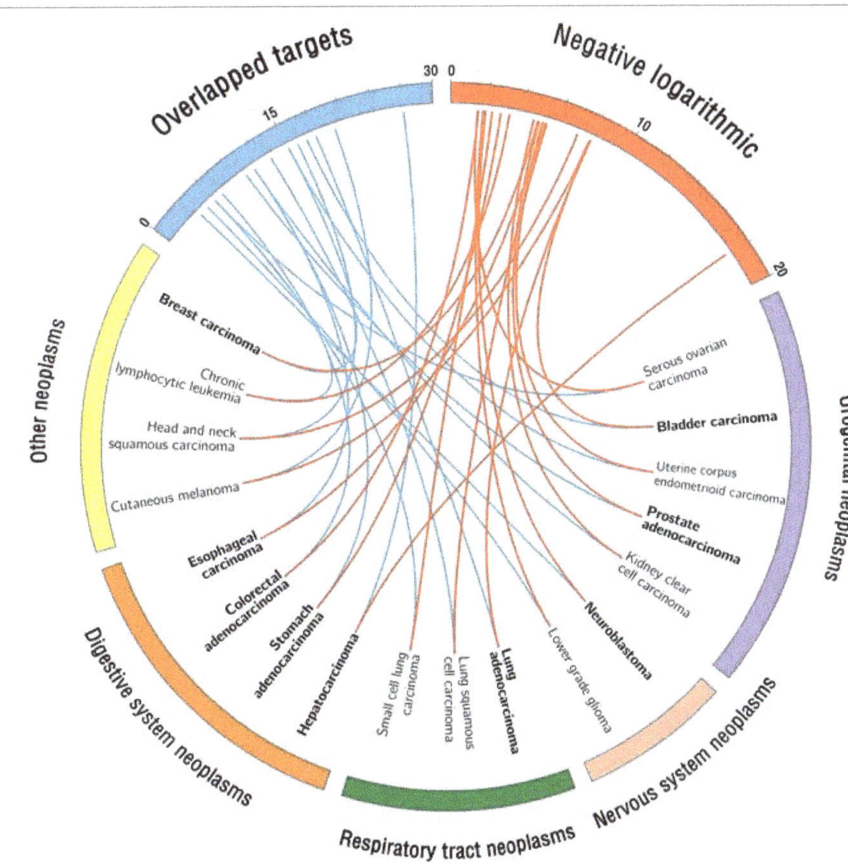

FIGURE 6 | Circos plot visualizes the predicted cancer indications of berberine. The red connected lines represent the calculated $-\text{Log}_{10}(q)$ value of each berberine-cancer type pair based on Fisher's exact test, while the blue ones represent the corresponding number of overlapped targets. The predicted cancer indications with literature validation were highlighted in bold font. We classified the 18 predicted cancer indications into four neoplasm categories according to Medical Subject Headings (MeSH) system (https://www.ncbi.nlm.nih.gov/mesh/68009371).

Among the 18 cancer indications, CM, HNSCC, SQCC, UCEC, CCSK, CLL, SCLC, NBL, and LGG are the unreported cancer indications of berberine, which deserve further preclinical validation. For example, cutaneous melanoma (CM), one of the most aggressive types of cancer, represents a major problem worldwide due to its high incidence and elevated degree of heterogeneity (Jemal et al., 2010; Coricovac et al., 2018). Based on our predictive model, berberine exerted a high potential for anti-CM, with a significant q value [$q < 1.23 \times 10^{-8}$; $-\text{Log10}(q) = 9.29$]. Therefore, the potential of berberine in the prevention and treatment of CM deserves to be further validated.

Case Study: Exploring the MOAs of Berberine on Hepatocarcinoma (HCC), Lung Adenocarcinoma (LUAD), and Bladder Carcinoma (BLCA)

To further validate the accuracy of statistical network models and predicted anti-cancer targets of berberine, we selected three typical cancer types [HCC ($q = 5.63 \times 10^{-20}$), LUAD ($q = 4.52 \times 10^{-10}$), and BLCA ($q = 4.92 \times 10^{-10}$)] as case studies to illustrate their anti-cancer MOAs (**Figure 7**).

Hepatocellular Carcinoma

HCC, the third leading cause of cancer death worldwide, has become one of the most common and prevalent human malignancies in the world (Okubo et al., 2017). *In vitro* assays revealed that berberine can inhibit autophagy in hepatoma cell lines (e.g., HepG2 cells and MHCC97-L cells) by regulating multiple proteins [e.g., mitogen-activated protein kinase 14 (MAPK14), TP53, and phosphatidylinositol 4,5-bisphosphate 3-kinase catalytic subunit beta isoform (PIK3CB)] and pathways (e.g., P38 MAPK signaling), stimulating further development of derivatives for drug-base cancer prevention and treatment (Wang et al., 2010; Liu et al., 2011; Wang et al., 2014). In this study, Fisher's test showed that berberine played a significant role in treatment of liver cancer ($q = 5.63 \times 10^{-20}$). In addition, network analysis revealed that berberine bound with 27 HCC-related SMG targets, suggesting its underlying anti-cancer mechanisms of berberine (**Figure 7**). *In vivo* or *in vitro* data have demonstrated that these SMGs are closely relevant to the treatment of cancer by berberine. For example, berberine can inhibit cell proliferation of HepG2, Hep3B, and SNU-182 through up-regulating protein expression of tumor suppressor genes, such as activating transcription factor 3 (ATF3) (Chuang et al., 2017). Furthermore, study revealed that berberine inhibited expression of BCL2, thus reducing autophagic cell death and mitochondrial apoptosis in liver cancer cells, such as HepG2 and MHCC97-L cells (Hur et al., 2010).

Lung Adenocarcinoma

LUAD is one of the leading causes of cancer-related death both men and women in the United States. Approximately two million people are diagnosed with lung cancer each year (Torre et al., 2016). Berberine was predicted to have anti-LUAD potential ($q = 4.52 \times 10^{-10}$). Some previous *in vivo* and *in vitro* studies confirmed our prediction (Mitani et al., 2001; Zheng et al., 2014). Furthermore, berberine is currently being assessed as an anti-LUAD drug in clinical trials (NCT03486496). As shown in **Figure 7**, berberine interacts with 13 LUAD-related SMGs (e.g., matrix metalloproteinase-2), indicating the underlying MOAs of anti-LUAD of berberine. Matrix metalloproteinases (MMPs), one target displayed in our network, is the major protease of LUAD and is associated with tumor invasion and metastasis (Herbst et al., 2000). Study on human lung cancer cell line A549 confirmed that berberine inhibited invasion and growth of tumor cells through decreasing productions of matrix metalloproteinase-2 (MMP2) (Peng et al., 2006).

Bladder Carcinoma

BLCA is the most common cancer of the urinary system in the United States (Kaufman et al., 2009). In our network model, berberine is predicted to have a significant relationship with

TABLE 2 | Relevant literature evidences of the 18 predicted cancer indications of berberine.

Cancer type	*P*-value (Fisher test)	Adj-*P*	Negative logarithmic	PMID
HCC	5.63E−20	1.35E−18	17.87	26081696|25496992|24942805
LUAD	4.52E−10	1.08E−08	7.96	24766860|26672764|26503561
BLCA	4.92E−10	1.18E−08	7.93	21545798|23065570|10418949
CM	5.12E−10	1.23E−08	7.91	N/A
HNSCC	3.03E−09	7.27E−08	7.14	26503508
SQCC	1.82E−07	4.37E−06	5.36	N/A
EC	2.18E−07	5.23E−06	5.28	28465635|26667771|21858113
UCEC	3.03E−07	7.27E−06	5.14	N/A
PRAD	4.77E−07	1.15E−05	4.94	16505103|26698234|25572870
BRCA	5.53E−07	1.33E−05	4.88	29143794|29414799|28926092
CCSK	9.58E−07	2.30E−05	4.64	N/A
CLL	2.28E−05	5.47E−04	3.26	N/A
STAD	7.32E−05	1.76E−03	2.76	27142767|25837881|18468407
SCLC	2.22E−04	5.33E−03	2.27	N/A
NBL	5.36E−04	1.29E−02	1.89	27235712|19189664|19096576
LGG	6.95E−04	1.67E−02	1.78	N/A
CRAC	1.34E−03	3.21E−02	1.49	23604974|26463023|25954974
SOV	1.40E−03	3.36E−02	1.47	N/A

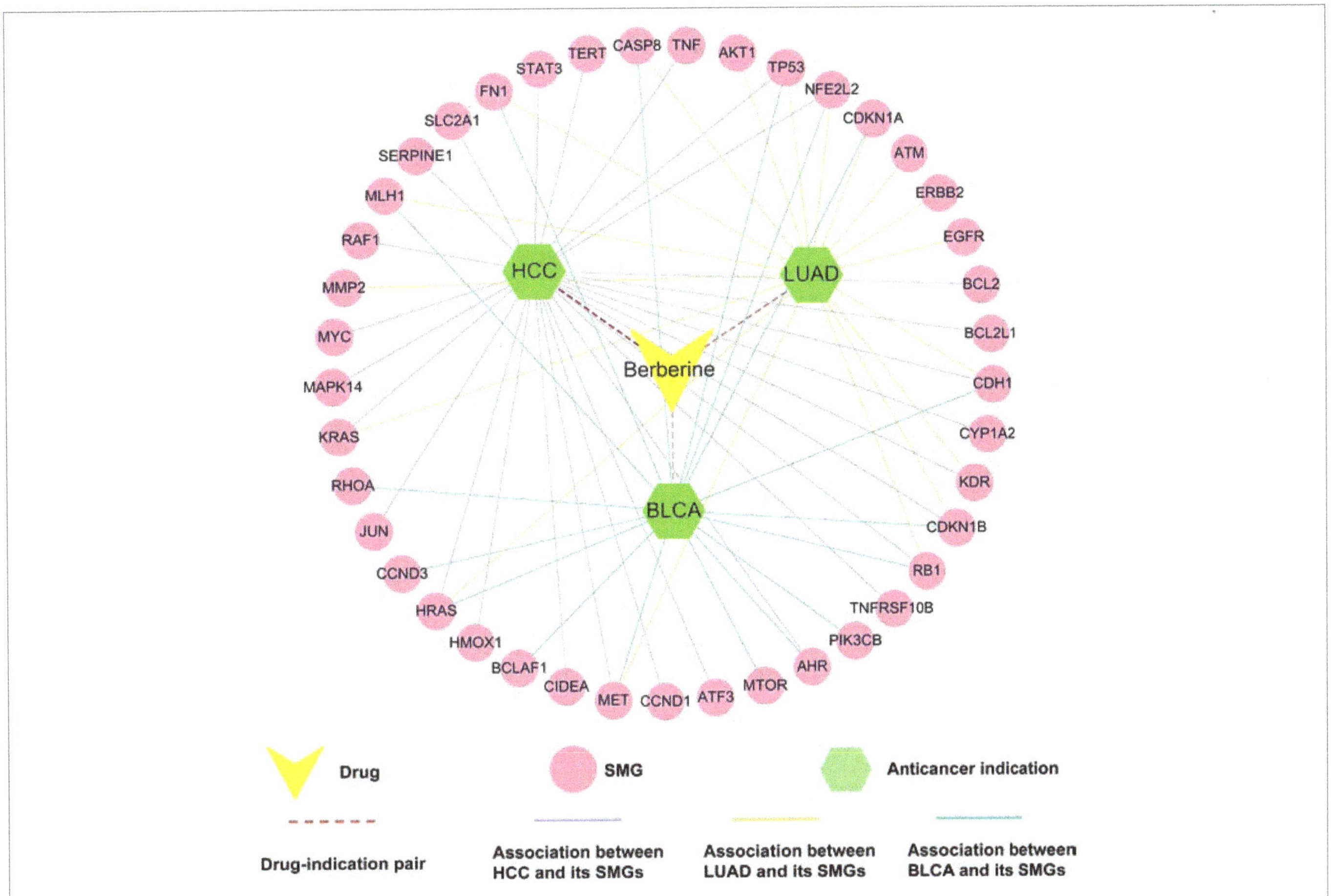

FIGURE 7 | Drug–target–disease (D-T-D) network of berberine on hepatocarcinoma (HCC), lung adenocarcinoma (LUAD), and bladder carcinoma (BLCA). The thickness of the red dotted line represents the predicted association between berberine and three types of tumors.

BLCA ($q = 4.92 \times 10^{-10}$). Meanwhile, our network indicated that berberine interacts with 17 BLCA-related SMGs (e.g., HRAS). According to previous study, the oncogenic ras genes GTPase HRas (HRAS) mutations, endogenously expressed in T24 bladder cancer cell line, were associated with grades and stages of BLCA detected in more than 35% of patients (Buyru et al., 2003). Berberine inhibited cell proliferation and induced cell cycle arrest and apoptosis in BLCA by inhibiting oncogenic H-Ras pathway in BIU-87 and T24 cell lines (Yan et al., 2011).

Taken together, these three case studies against different cancer types (HCC, LUAD, and BLCA) indicate that systems pharmacology approach applied in this study is an effective method for exploring molecular mechanisms of anti-cancer effect of berberine. Meanwhile, the newly predicted tumor types might be promising to further investigate MOAs of berberine.

CONCLUSION

Berberine had been observed to exert multiple biological and pharmacological activities with potential benefits to a variety of complex diseases, including cancer. In this study, we proposed an integrated systems pharmacology infrastructure to identify cancer indications of berberine and explore the underlying molecular mechanisms. This work explores the following new anti-cancer characteristics of berberine: i) Through literature mining, we summarize eight mechanisms of anti-cancer effect of berberine; ii) global drug–target network of berberine is constructed by integrating large-scale experimentally reported targets and computationally predicted targets. Mechanisms of action (MOAs) of various anti-cancer effects of berberine are discussed through current drug–target network; iii) a statistical model is developed to prioritize novel cancer indications of berberine through integrating target profiles of berberine and significantly mutated genes in cancer.

Yet several limitations of our approach should be acknowledged. First, although we have integrated a wide range of DTIs from published literatures and publicly available databases, the incompleteness of current drug-target networks may still exist. Recent studies proved that integration of large-scale gene expression profiles of natural products may help to improve the performance of drug–target network model (Yamanishi et al., 2010; Cheng et al., 2012). Second, as it is extremely difficult to obtain information on the active sites of berberine and mutated domain of proteins from public sources, the current study could not explain the MOAs from a microcosmic point of view. Third, experimental assays should be performed to further validate the predicted targets and MOAs of anti-cancer effects of berberine in the future.

In summary, the systems pharmacology framework in this study has provided potential strategies to discover the polypharmacology effects of berberine for the prevention and treatment towards multiple cancers.

AUTHOR CONTRIBUTIONS

JF and YZ provided the concept and designed the study. PG and CC conducted the experiments and wrote the manuscript. XW, JZ, XF, QWu, YH, WZ, WH, and FZ participated in the experiments. JF and QWa contributed to revision and proofreading of the manuscript. All authors read and approved the final manuscript.

FUNDING

This work was supported by the National Natural Science Foundation of China (Grants 81603318), the youth scientific research training project of GZUCM (2019QNPY05), Research Fund for Characteristic Innovation Projects of Guangdong Province (2016KTSCX013), and Open Tending Project for the Construction of High-Level University (A1-AFD018171Z11027; A1-AFD018171Z11029).

REFERENCES

1. Ayati, S. H., Fazeli, B., Momtazi-Borojeni, A. A., Afg, C., Pirro, M., and Sahebkar, A. (2017). Regulatory effects of berberine on microRNome in cancer and other conditions. *Crit. Rev. Oncol. Hematol.* 116, 147–158. doi: 10.1016/j.critrevonc.2017.05.008
2. Bento, A. P., Gaulton, A., Hersey, A., Bellis, L. J., Chambers, J., Davies, M., et al. (2014). The ChEMBL bioactivity database: an update. *Nucleic Acids Res.* 42, 1083–1090. doi: 10.1093/nar/gkt1031
3. Buyru, N., Tigli, H., Ozcan, F., and Dalay, N. (2003). Ras oncogene mutations in urine sediments of patients with bladder cancer. *J. Biochem. Mol. Biol.* 36, 399– 402. doi: 10.5483/BMBRep.2003.36.4.399
4. Benjamini, Y., and Yekutieli, D. (2001). The control of the false discovery rate in multiple testing under dependency. *Ann. Stat.* 29, 1165–1188. doi: 10.1214/aos/1013699998
5. Chen, Z. Z. (2016). Berberine induced apoptosis of human osteosarcoma cells by inhibiting phosphoinositide 3 kinase/protein kinase B (PI3K/Akt) signal pathway activation. *Iran. J. Public Health* 45, 578–585.
6. Cheng, F., Liu, C., Jiang, J., Lu, W., Li, W., Liu, G., et al. (2012). Prediction of drug-target interactions and drug repositioning *via* network- based inference. *PLoS Comput. Biol.* 8, e1002503. doi: 10.1371/journal. pcbi.1002503
7. Cheng, F., Zhao, J., Fooksa, M., and Zhao, Z. (2016). A network-based drug repositioning infrastructure for precision cancer medicine through targeting significantly mutated genes in the human cancer genomes. *J. Am. Med. Inform. Assoc.* 23, 681–691. doi: 10.1093/jamia/ocw007
8. Chidambara Murthy, K. N., Jayaprakasha, G. K., and Patil, B. S. (2012). The natural alkaloid berberine targets multiple pathways to induce cell death in cultured human colon cancer cells. *Eur. J. Pharmacol.* 688, 14–21. doi: 10.1016/j. ejphar.2012.05.004
9. Chu, S. C., Yu, C. C., Hsu, L. S., Chen, K. S., Su, M. Y., and Chen, P. N. (2014). Berberine reverses epithelial-to-mesenchymal transition and inhibits metastasis and tumor-induced angiogenesis in human cervical cancer cells. *Mol. Pharmacol.* 86, 609–623. doi: 10.1124/mol.114.094037
10. Chuang, T. Y., Wu, H. L., Min, J., Diamond, M., Azziz, R., and Chen, Y. H. (2017). Berberine regulates the protein expression of multiple tumorigenesis-related genes in hepatocellular carcinoma cell lines. *Cancer Cell Int.* 17, 59. doi: 10.1186/s12935-017-0429-3
11. Coricovac, D., Dehelean, C., Moaca, E. A., Pinzaru, I., Bratu, T., Navolan, D., et al. (2018). Cutaneous melanoma—a long road from experimental models to clinical outcome: a review. *Int. J. Mol. Sci.* 19, E1566. doi: 10.3390/ijms19061566
12. Cusan, M., Mungo, G., De Marco Zompit, M., Segatto, I., Belletti, B., and Baldassarre, G. (2018). Landscape of CDKN1B mutations in luminal breast cancer and other hormone-driven human tumors. *Front. Endocrinol.* 9, 393. doi: 10.3389/fendo.2018.00393
13. Dennis, G., Sherman, B. T., Hosack, D. A., Yang, J., Gao, W., Lane, H. C., et al. (2003). DAVID: Database for Annotation, visualization, and Integrated Discovery. *Genome Biol.* 4, R60. doi: 10.1186/gb-2003-4-9-r60
14. Fan, Q. W., Cheng, C. K., Gustafson, W. C., Charron, E., Zipper, P., Wong, R. A., et al. (2013). EGFR phosphorylates tumor-derived EGFRvIII driving STAT3/5 and progression in glioblastoma. *Cancer Cell* 24, 438–449. doi: 10.1016/j.ccr.2013.09.004
15. Fang, J., Cai, C., Chai, Y., Zhou, J., Huang, Y., Gao, L., et al. (2019). Quantitative and systems pharmacology 4. Network-based analysis of drug pleiotropy on coronary artery disease. *Eur. J. Med. Chem.* 161, 192–204. doi: 10.1016/j.ejmech.2018.10.020
16. Fang, J., Cai, C., Wang, Q., Lin, P., Zhao, Z., and Cheng, F. (2017a). Systems pharmacology-based discovery of natural products for precision oncology through targeting cancer mutated genes. *CPT Pharmacometrics Syst. Pharmacol.* 6, 177–187. doi: 10.1002/psp4.12172
17. Fang, J., Gao, L., Ma, H., Wu, Q., Wu, T., Wu, J., et al. (2017b). Quantitative and systems pharmacology 3. Network-based identification of new targets for natural products enables potential uses in aging-associated disorders. *Front. Pharmacol.* 8, 747. doi: 10.3389/fphar.2017.00747
18. Fang, J., Liu, C., Wang, Q., Lin, P., and Cheng, F. (2018). In silico polypharmacology of natural products. *Brief. Bioinform.* 19, 1153–1171. doi: 10.1093/bib/bbx045
19. Fang, J., Wu, Z., Cai, C., Wang, Q., Tang, Y., and Cheng, F. (2017c). Quantitative and systems pharmacology. 1. In silico prediction of drug-target interaction of natural products to enable of new targeted cancer therapy. *J. Chem. Inf. Model.* 57, 2657–2671. doi: 10.1021/acs.jcim.7b00216
20. Gilson, M. K., Liu, T., Baitaluk, M., Nicola, G., Hwang, L., and Chong, J. (2016). BindingDB in 2015: a public database for medicinal chemistry, computational chemistry and systems pharmacology. *Nucleic Acids Res.* 44, D1045–D1053. doi: 10.1093/nar/gkv1072
21. Hamsa, T. P., and Kuttan, G. (2012). Antiangiogenic activity of berberine is mediated through the downregulation of hypoxia-inducible factor-1, VEGF, and proinflammatory mediators. *Drug Chem. Toxicol.* 35, 57–70. doi: 10.3109/01480545.2011.589437
22. Herbst, R. S., Yano, S., Kuniyasu, H., Khuri, F. R., Bucana, C. D., Guo, F., et al. (2000). Differential expression of E-cadherin and type IV collagenase genes predicts outcome in patients with stage I non-small cell lung carcinoma. *Clin. Cancer Res.* 6, 790–797. doi: 10.1159/000007270
23. Huang, Y., Fang, J., Lu, W., Wang, Z., Wang, Q., Hou, Y., et al. (2019). A systems pharmacology approach uncovers wogonoside as an angiogenesis inhibitor of triple-negative breast cancer by targeting hedgehog signaling. *Cell Chem. Biol.* 26, 1–16. doi: 10.1016/j.chembiol.2019.05.004
24. Huang, Z. H., Zheng, H. F., Wang, W. L., Wang, Y., Zhong, L. F., Wu, J. L., et al. (2015). Berberine targets epidermal growth factor receptor signaling to suppress prostate cancer proliferation *in vitro*. *Mol. Med. Rep.* 11, 2125–2128. doi: 10.3892/mmr.2014.2929
25. Hur, J. M., Hyun, M. S., Lim, S. Y., Lee, W. Y., and Kim, D. (2010). The

combination of berberine and irradiation enhances anti-cancer effects *via* activation of p38 MAPK pathway and ROS generation in human hepatoma cells. *J. Cell. Biochem.* 107, 955–964. doi: 10.1002/jcb.22198

26. Jemal, A., Siegel, R., Xu, J., and Ward, E. (2010). Cancer statistics, 2010. *CA Cancer J. Clin.* 60, 277–300. doi: 10.3322/caac.20073
27. Jiang, X., Lu, W., Shen, X., Wang, Q., Lv, J., Liu, M., et al. (2018). Repurposing sertraline sensitizes non-small cell lung cancer cells to erlotinib by inducing autophagy. *JCI Insight* 3, 98921. doi: 10.1172/jci.insight.98921
28. Jiang, Y., Huang, K., Lin, X., Chen, Q., Lin, S., Feng, X., et al. (2017). Berberine attenuates NLRP3 inflammasome activation in macrophages to reduce the secretion of interleukin-1β. *Ann. Clin. Lab. Sci.* 47, 720–728.
29. Jie, S., Li, H., Tian, Y., Guo, D., Zhu, J., Gao, S., et al. (2011). Berberine inhibits angiogenic potential of Hep G2 cell line through VEGF down-regulation *in vitro. J. Gastroenterol Hepatol.* 26, 179–185. doi: 10.1111/j.1440-1746.2010.06389.x
30. Kaufman, D. S., Shipley, W. U., and Feldman, A. S. (2009). Bladder cancer. *Lancet* 374, 239–249. doi: 10.1016/S0140-6736(09)60491-8
31. Khalid, E. B., Ayman, E. K., Rahman, H., Abdelkarim, G., and Najda, A. (2016). Natural products against cancer angiogenesis. *Tumour Biol.* 37, 1–24. doi: 10.1007/s13277-016-5364-8
32. Kim, J. B., Lee, K. M., Ko, E., Han, W., Lee, J. E., Shin, I., et al. (2008). Berberine inhibits growth of the breast cancer cell lines MCF-7 and MDA-MB-231. *Planta Med.* 74, 39–42. doi: 10.1055/s-2007-993779
33. Kim, J. S., Oh, D., Yim, M. J., Park, J. J., Kang, K. R., Cho, I. A., et al. (2015). Berberine induces FasL-related apoptosis through p38 activation in KB human oral cancer cells. *Oncol. Rep.* 33, 1775–1782. doi: 10.3892/or.2015.3768
34. Kim, S., Han, J., Kim, N. Y., Lee, S. K., Cho, D. H., Choi, M. Y., et al. (2012). Effect of berberine on p53 expression by TPA in breast cancer cells. *Oncol. Rep.* 27, 210–215. doi: 10.3892/or.2011.1480
35. Kotoku, N., Arai, M., and Kobayashi, M. (2016). Search for anti-angiogenic substances from natural sources. *Chem. Pharm. Bull.* 64, 128–134. doi: 10.1248/cpb.c15-00744
36. Kuhn, M., Szklarczyk, D., Pletscher-Frankild, S., Blicher, T. H., von Mering, C., Jensen, L. J., et al. (2014). STITCH 4: integration of protein-chemical interactions with user data. *Nucleic Acids Res.* 42, D401–D407. doi: 10.1093/nar/gkt1207
37. Kuo, H. P., Chuang, T. C., Yeh, M. H., Hsu, S. C., Way, T. D., Chen, P. Y., et al. (2011). Growth suppression of HER2-overexpressing breast cancer cells by berberine *via* modulation of the HER2/PI3K/Akt signaling pathway. *J. Agric. Food Chem.* 59, 8216–8224. doi: 10.1021/jf2012584
38. Li, J., Li, O., Kan, M., Zhang, M., Shao, D., Pan, Y., et al. (2015). Berberine induces apoptosis by suppressing the arachidonic acid metabolic pathway in hepatocellular carcinoma. *Mol. Med. Rep.* 12, 4572–4577. doi: 10.3892/mmr.2015.3926
39. Li, Z., Geng, Y. N., Jiang, J. D., and Kong, W. J. (2014). Antioxidant and anti-inflammatory activities of berberine in the treatment of diabetes mellitus. *Evid. Based Complement. Alternat. Med.* 2014, 289264. doi: 10.1155/2014/289264
40. Liu, B., Wang, G., Yang, J., Pan, X., Yang, Z., and Zang, L. (2011). Berberine inhibits human hepatoma cell invasion without cytotoxicity in healthy hepatocytes. *PLoS One* 6, e21416. doi: 10.1371/journal.pone.0021416
41. López-Cortés, A., Leone, P. E., Freire-Paspuel, B., Arcos-Villacís, N., Guevara-Ramírez, P., Rosales, F., et al. (2018). Mutational analysis of oncogenic AKT1 gene associated with breast cancer risk in the high altitude ecuadorian mestizo population. *Biomed. Res. Int.* 2018, 1–10. doi: 10.1155/2018/7463832
42. Lu, B., Hu, M., Liu, K., and Peng, J. (2010). Cytotoxicity of berberine on human cervical carcinoma HeLa cells through mitochondria, death receptor and MAPK pathways, and in-silico drug-target prediction. *Toxicol. In Vitro* 24, 1482–1490. doi: 10.1016/j.tiv.2010.07.017
43. Mitani, N., Murakami, K., Yamaura, T., Ikeda, T., and Saiki, I. (2001). Inhibitory effect of berberine on the mediastinal lymph node metastasis produced by orthotopic implantation of Lewis lung carcinoma. *Cancer Lett.* 165, 35–42. doi: 10.1016/S0304-3835(00)00710-2
44. Okubo, S., Uto, T., Goto, A., Tanaka, H., Nishioku, T., Yamada, K., et al. (2017). Berberine induces apoptotic cell death *via* activation of caspase-3 and -8 in HL-60 human leukemia cells: nuclear localization and structure–activity relationships. *Am. J. Chin. Med.* 45, 1497–1511. doi: 10.1142/S0192415X17500811
45. Ola, M. S., Nawaz, M., and Ahsan, H. (2011). Role of Bcl-2 family proteins and caspases in the regulation of apoptosis. *Mol. Cell Biochem.* 351, 41–58. doi: 10.1007/s11010-010-0709-x
46. Pan, Y., Zhang, F., Zhao, Y., Shao, D., Zheng, X., Chen, Y., et al. (2017). Berberine enhances chemosensitivity and induces apoptosis through dose-orchestrated AMPK signaling in breast cancer. *J. Cancer* 8, 1679–1689. doi: 10.7150/ jca.19106
47. Patil, J. B., Kim, J., and Jayaprakashaa, G. K. (2010). Berberine induces apoptosis in breast cancer cells (MCF-7) through mitochondrial-dependent pathway. *Eur. J. Pharmacol.* 645, 70–78. doi: 10.1016/j.ejphar.2010.07.037
48. Peng, P. L., Hsieh, Y. S., Wang, C. J., Hsu, J. L., and Chou, F. P. (2006). Inhibitory effect of berberine on the invasion of human lung cancer cells *via* decreased productions of urokinase-plasminogen activator and matrix metalloproteinase-2. *Toxicol. Appl. Pharmacol.* 214, 8–15. doi: 10.1016/j.taap.2005.11.010
49. Puthdee, N., Seubwai, W., Vaeteewoottacharn, K., Boonmars, T., Cha'On, U., Phoomak, C., et al. (2017). Berberine induces cell cycle arrest in cholangiocarcinoma cell lines *via* inhibition of NF-κB and STAT3 pathways. *Biol. Pharm. Bull.* 40, 751–757. doi: 10.1248/bpb.b16-00428
50. Qing, Y., Hu, H., Liu, Y., Feng, T., Meng, W., Jiang, L., et al. (2014). Berberine induces apoptosis in human multiple myeloma cell line U266 through hypomethylation of p53 promoter. *Cell Biol. Int.* 38, 563–570. doi: 10.1002/cbin.10206
51. Shannon, P., Markiel, A., Ozier, O., Baliga, N. S., Wang, J. T., Ramage, D., et al. (2003). Cytoscape: a software environment for integrated models of biomolecular interaction networks. *Genome Res.* 13, 2498–2504. doi: 10.1101/gr.1239303
52. Song, Y. C., Lee, Y., Kim, H. M., Hyun, M. Y., Lim, Y. Y., Song, K. Y., et al. (2015). Berberine regulates melanin synthesis by activating PI3K/AKT, ERK and GSK3β in B16F10 melanoma cells. *Int. J. Mol. Med.* 35, 1011–1016. doi: 10.3892/ijmm.2015.2113
53. Sun, X., Wang, S. C., Wei, Y., Luo, X., Jia, Y., Li, L., et al. (2017). Arid1a has context- dependent oncogenic and tumor suppressor functions in liver cancer. *Cancer Cell* 33, 151–152. doi: 10.1016/j.ccell.2017.12.011
54. Tan, W., Li, N., Tan, R., Zhong, Z., Suo, Z., Yang, X., et al. (2015). Berberine interfered with breast cancer cells metabolism, balancing energy homeostasis. *Anticancer Agents Med. Chem.* 15, 66–78. doi: 10.2174/187152061466614091 0120518
55. Tang, F., Wang, D., Duan, C., Huang, D., Wu, Y., Chen, Y., et al. (2009). Berberine inhibits metastasis of nasopharyngeal carcinoma 5-8F cells by targeting Rho kinase-mediated Ezrin phosphorylation at threonine 567. *J. Biol. Chem.* 284, 27456–27466. doi: 10.1074/jbc.M109.033795
56. Tsang, C. M., Cheung, Y. C., Lui, V. W., Yip, Y. L., Zhang, G., Lin, V. W., et al. (2013). Berberine suppresses tumorigenicity and growth of nasopharyngeal carcinoma cells by inhibiting STAT3 activation induced by tumor associated fibroblasts. *BMC Cancer* 13, 619. doi: 10.1186/1471-2407-13-619
57. Torre, L. A., Siegel, R. L., and Jemal, A. (2016). Lung cancer statistics. *Adv. Exp. Med. Biol.* 893, 1–19. doi: 10.1007/978-3-319-24223-1
58. Wang, J., Yang, S., Cai, X., Dong, J., Chen, Z., Wang, R., et al. (2016). Berberine inhibits EGFR signaling and enhances the antitumor effects of EGFR inhibitors in gastric cancer. *Oncotarget* 7, 76076–76086. doi: 10.18632/oncotarget.12589
59. Wang, L., Cao, H., Lu, N., Liu, L., Wang, B., Hu, T., et al. (2013). Berberine inhibits proliferation and down-regulates epidermal growth factor receptor through activation of Cbl in colon tumor cells. *PLoS One* 8, e56666. doi: 10.1371/journal.pone.0056666
60. Wang, N., Feng, Y., Zhu, M., Tsang, C. M., Man, K., Tong, Y., et al. (2010). Berberine induces autophagic cell death and mitochondrial apoptosis in liver cancer cells: the cellular mechanism. *J. Cell. Biochem.* 111, 1426–1436. doi: 10.1002/jcb.22869
61. Wang, N., Zhu, M., Wang, X., Tan, H. Y., Tsao, S. W., and Feng, Y. (2014). Berberine-induced tumor suppressor p53 up-regulation gets involved in the regulatory network of MIR-23a in hepatocellular carcinoma. *Biochim. Biophys. Acta.* 1839, 849–857. doi: 10.1016/j.bbagrm.2014.05.027
62. Wilson, J. R. F., Bateman, A. C., Hanson, H., An, Q., Evans, G., Rahman, N., et al. (2010). A novel HER2-positive breast cancer phenotype arising from germline TP53 mutations. *J. Med. Genet.* 47, 771–774. doi: 10.1136/jmg.2010.078113
63. Wu, Z., Cheng, F., Li, J., Li, W., Liu, G., and Tang, Y. (2017). SDTNBI: an integrated network and chemoinformatics tool for systematic prediction of drug–target interactions and drug repositioning. *Brief. Bioinform.* 18, 333–347. doi: 10.1093/bib/bbw012

64. Wu, Z., Lu, W., Wu, D., Luo, A., Bian, H., Li, J., et al. (2016). In silico prediction of chemical mechanism-of-action *via* an improved network- based inference method. *Br. J. Pharmacol.* 173, 3372–3385. doi: 10.1111/bph.13629
65. Xiong, Y. X., Su, H. F., Lv, P., Ma, Y., Wang, S. K., Miao, H., et al. (2015). A newly identified berberine derivative induces cancer cell senescence by stabilizing endogenous G-quadruplexes and sparking a DNA damage response at the telomere region. *Oncotarget* 6, 35625–35635. doi: 10.18632/ oncotarget
66. Yamaguchi, R., Lartigue, L., and Perkins, G. (2019). Targeting Mcl-1 and other Bcl-2 family member proteins in cancer therapy. *Pharmacol. Ther.* 195, 13–20. doi: 10.1016/j.pharmthera.2018.10.009.
67. Yamanishi, Y., Kotera, M., Kanehisa, M., and Goto, S. (2010). Drug–target interaction prediction from chemical, genomic and pharmacological data in an integrated framework. *Bioinformatics* 26, i246–i254. doi: 10.1093/ bioinformatics/btq176
68. Yan, K., Zhang, C., Feng, J., Hou, L., Yan, L., Zhou, Z., et al. (2011). Induction of G1 cell cycle arrest and apoptosis by berberine in bladder cancer cells. *Eur. J. Pharmacol.* 661, 1–7. doi: 10.1016/j.ejphar.2011.04.021
69. Yap, C. W. (2011). PaDEL-descriptor: an open source software to calculate molecular descriptors and fi gerprints. *J. Comput. Chem.* 32, 1466–1474. doi: 10.1002/jcc.21707
70. Ye, H., Ye, L., Kang, H., Zhang, D., Tao, L., Tang, K., et al. (2011). HIT: linking herbal active ingredients to targets. *Nucleic Acids Res.* 39, D1055–D1059. doi: 10.1093/nar/gkq1165
71. Yu, H., Lee, H., Herrmann, A., Buettner, R., and Jove, R. (2014). Revisiting STAT3 signalling in cancer: new and unexpected biological functions. *Nat. Rev. Cancer.* 14, 736–746. doi: 10.1038/nrc3818
72. Zhao, Y., Jing, Z., Lv, J., Zhang, Z., Lin, J., Cao, X., et al. (2017). Berberine activates caspase-9/cytochrome *c*-mediated apoptosis to suppress triple-negative breast cancer cells *in vitro* and in *vivo*. *Biomed. Pharmacother.* 95, 18–24. doi: 10.1016/j. biopha.2017.08.045
73. Zhe, W., and Huang, G. S. (2002). Database resources of the National Center for Biotechnology Information and its application. *Chin. Bull. Life Sci.* 14, 59–62. doi: 10.1007/BF02943277
74. Zheng, F., Tang, Q., Wu, J. J., Zhao, S. Y., Liang, Z. Y., Li, L., et al. (2014). p38α MAPK-mediated induction and interaction of FOXO3a and p53 contribute to the inhibited-growth and induced-apoptosis of human lung adenocarcinoma cells by berberine. *J. Exp. Clin. Cancer Res.* 33, 36. doi: 10.1186/1756-9966-33-36 Zhu, R. X., Seto, W. K., Lai, C. L., and Yuen, M. F. (2016). Epidemiology of hepatocellular carcinoma in the Asia-Pacific region. *Gut. Liver.* 10, 332–339. doi: 10.5009/gnl15257

17

Integrated Bioinformatics Analysis the Function of RNA Binding Proteins (RBPs) and their Prognostic Value in Breast Cancer

Ke Wang[1†], Ling Li[2†], Liang Fu[2], Yongqiang Yuan[2], Hongying Dai[2], Tianjin Zhu[2], Yuxi Zhou[3] and Fang Yuan[3]*

[1] Clinical Laboratory, Yongchuan People's Hospital of Chongqing, Chongqing, China, [2] Clinical Laboratory, Yongchuan Hospital of Chongqing Medical University, Chongqing, China, [3] Yidu Cloud (Beijing) Technology Co., Ltd., Beijing, China

***Correspondence:**
Ke Wang
wk125@126.com

† These authors have contributed equally to this work

Background and Purpose: Breast cancer is one of the leading causes of death among women. RNA binding proteins (RBPs) play a vital role in the progression of many cancers. Functional investigation of RBPs may contribute to elucidating the mechanisms underlying tumor initiation, progression, and invasion, therefore providing novel insights into future diagnosis, treatment, and prognosis.

Methods: We downloaded RNA sequencing data from the cancer genome atlas (TCGA) by UCSC Xena and identified relevant RBPs through an integrated bioinformatics analysis. We then analyzed biological processes of differentially expressed genes (DEGs) by DAVID, and established their interaction networks and performed pathway analysis through the STRING database to uncover potential biological effects of these RBPs. We also explored the relationship between these RBPs and the prognosis of breast cancer patients.

Results: In the present study, we obtained 1092 breast tumor samples and 113 normal controls. After data analysis, we identified 90 upregulated and 115 downregulated RBPs in breast cancer. GO and KEGG pathway analysis indicated that these significantly changed genes were mainly involved in RNA processing, splicing, localization and RNA silencing, DNA transposition regulation and methylation, alkylation, mitochondrial gene expression, and transcription regulation. In addition, some RBPs were related to histone H3K27 methylation, estrogen response, inflammatory mediators, and translation regulation. Our study also identified five RBPs associated with breast cancer prognosis. Survival analysis found that overexpression of DCAF13, EZR, and MRPL13 showed worse survival, but overexpression of APOBEC3C and EIF4E3 showed better survival.

Conclusion: In conclusion, we identified key RBPs of breast cancer through comprehensive bioinformatics analysis. These RBPs were involved in a variety of biological and molecular pathways in breast cancer. Furthermore, we identified five RBPs as a potential prognostic biomarker of breast cancer. Our study provided novel insights to understand breast cancer at a molecular level.

Keywords: breast cancer, RNA binding protein, integrated bioinformatics analysis, survival, prognosis

INTRODUCTION

Breast cancer is the most commonly diagnosed cancer and a main cause of cancer death among women. In 2018, there was an estimated 2.1 million newly diagnosed female breast cancer cases worldwide, accounting for about 25% of cancer cases among women (Bray et al., 2018). In recent years, with great progress in medical technology, the diagnosis incidence of breast cancer has increased year by year, and the age of onset or diagnosis has consequently become younger. Breast cancer is aggressive and has a high recurrence rate. Currently, the diagnosis of breast cancer mainly relies on pathological assessments, imaging tests, and tumor markers (McDonald et al., 2016), which creates difficulty for meeting clinical requirements. In order to reduce the recurrence rate and mortality of breast cancer patients, and to improve their quality of life, it is vital to increase ability in surveillance, early detection and diagnosis. Over the years there has been an increase of molecular research on early diagnosis, drug resistance and prognosis, and it is therefore valuable to find new molecular markers on the occurrence, progression, and prognosis, to further expand this research.

RNA-binding proteins (RBPs) are abundant and ubiquitously expressed in cells. They play a central and conserved role in gene regulation (Gerstberger et al., 2014b), and act as important participants and coordinators to maintain genome integrity (Nishida et al., 2017). RBPs have extensive capabilities including regulating stability, maturation, posttranscriptional regulation of mRNA stability, splicing, editing and translation, mRNA localization and polyadenylation, which ultimately impacts the expression of every gene in the cell (Campos-Melo et al., 2014; Gerstberger et al., 2014a). Although it is known that post-transcription contributes to tumor initiation and progression, the role of RBPs in cancer remain relatively unexplored (Wurth and Gebauer, 2015).

There is a large number of Human RBPs, but very few have been studied in depth, such as AGO2, Nova, PTB, HuR, AUF1, TTP, CUGBP2 which are known for their role in many regulation processes, including interacting with non-coding RNAs (Iadevaia and Gerber, 2015), controlling intracellular localization of non-coding RNAs (Glisovic et al., 2008), methylation (Harvey et al., 2017), forming the RNA induce silencing complex (Connerty et al., 2015), and alternative splicing (Paronetto et al., 2010). RBPs participate in comprehensive biological processes, such as reproductive development, tumorigenesis and apoptosis, and is therefore closely related to many human diseases. A systematic functional study of RBPs will be helpful to understand the function and mechanism of non-coding RNA, but will also have a significant applied value in studying the pathogenesis of diseases and in the screening of innovative drug targets.

Currently, genes and signaling pathways that participate in breast cancer tumorigenesis and progression remain to be further investigated. Exploring new genes and pathways associated with breast cancer may help to identify potential molecular mechanisms, diagnostic markers and therapeutic targets (Wang et al., 2018). High-throughput genomic analysis techniques can be applied to screening for differentially expressed genes (DEGs) and to understand the relevant pathways and protein interaction networks (Vogelstein et al., 2013). In this study, we downloaded breast cancer data from the cancer genome atlas (TCGA), and selected differential expressed RBPs to perform gene ontology (GO), KEGG pathways and an interaction network and survival analysis. The study identified a number of RBPs involved in breast cancer. Some of which might be used as potential prognostic biomarkers in the future.

RESULTS

Identification of Differently Expressed RBPs (DEGs)

The database analysis contained 1092 breast tumor samples and 113 no-tumor control samples. We conducted a deep analysis of 1912 RBPs and a total of 205 RBPs were identified, including 90 upregulated and 115 downregulated RBPs (**Supplementary Table S1**). We also constructed an expression heat map for all DEGs (**Figure 1**).

Functional and Pathway Enrichment Analysis of DEGs

To determine the function and mechanisms of these RBPs, all DEGs were divided into two groups (upregulated group and down-regulated group), and submitted to the David database for

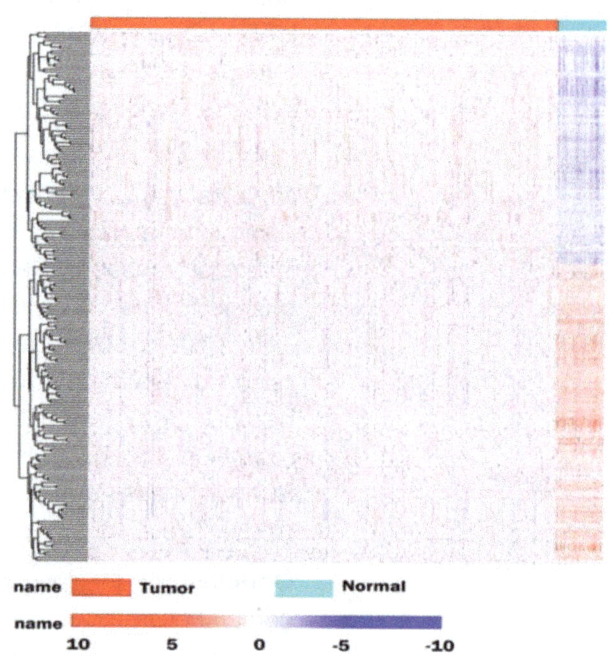

FIGURE 1 | Differentially expressed RBPs in BRCA cancer. Unsupervised clustering analysis was performed using the pheatmap function, using complete and Euclidean as metrics in R, based on log2-transformed FPKM values. The columns are samples and the rows are RBPs. The blue represents down-regulation, while red represents up-regulation.

GO analysis. We then conducted a KEGG pathway analysis for all DEGs. We found that upregulated DEGs were significantly enriched in RNA processing, RNA binding, mRNA binding, and located in the non-membrane-bounded organelle, intracellular non-membrane-bounded organelle, ribonucleoprotein complex, intracellular organelle lumen, organelle lumen, membrane-enclosed lumen, nuclear lumen, and the nucleolus (**Table 1**). The GO result of down-regulated DEGs were significantly enriched in the RNA processing, posttranscriptional regulation of gene expression, mRNA metabolic process, mRNA processing, regulation of translation and the RNA binding, and these genes mainly consisted of the chromatoid body, P granule, germ plasm, pole plasm, intracellular non-membrane-bounded organelle and the non-membrane-bounded organelle (**Table 1**).

TABLE 1 | GO enrichment analysis results of differentially up-regulated genes and down-regulated genes (DEGs).

	Term	*P* value	FDR
Up-regulated genes (DEGs)	RNA processing	3.23E-06	0.00478286
	Non-membrane-bounded organelle	4.53E-13	5.56E-10
	Intracellular non-membrane-bounded organelle	4.53E-13	5.56E-10
	Ribonucleoprotein complex	5.00E-11	6.15E-08
	Intracellular organelle lumen	1.81E-09	2.22E-06
	Organelle lumen	3.09E-09	3.80E-06
	Membrane-enclosed lumen	4.90E-09	6.02E-06
	Nuclear lumen	1.32E-06	0.00162684
	Nucleolus	1.59E-06	0.00194848
	RNA binding	5.78E-16	6.77E-13
	mRNA binding	2.37E-05	0.02904478
Down-regulated genes (DEGs)	RNA processing	1.41E-10	2.21E-07
	Posttranscriptional regulation of gene expression	2.29E-09	3.58E-06
	mRNA metabolic process	1.81E-08	2.82E-05
	mRNA processing	2.40E-07	3.74E-04
	Regulation of translation	1.05E-06	0.00164623
	Chromatoid body	2.05E-06	0.00250038
	P granule	3.57E-06	0.00436073
	Germ plasm	3.57E-06	0.00436073
	Pole plasm	3.57E-06	0.00436073
	Intracellular non-membrane-bounded organelle	1.94E-05	0.02370618
	Non-membrane-bounded organelle	1.94E-05	0.02370618
	RNA binding	1.46E-23	1.83E-20

TABLE 2 | The KEGG pathway analysis of all DEGs.

Term	*P* value
Dorso-ventral axis formation	4.18E-03
Fatty acid elongation in mitochondria	3.11E-02
Pathogenic *Escherichia coli* infection	2.06E-02

According to the KEGG pathway enrichment analysis, all DEGs mainly participated in Dorso-ventral axis formation, fatty acid elongation in mitochondria and pathogenic *Escherichia coli* infection (**Table 2**).

Protein-Protein Interaction Network Building and Interrelation Analysis Between Pathways

To better understand the role of these differentially expressed RBPS in breast cancer development, we constructed co-expression networks. All DEGs were submitted to STRING 10.5, we obtained 294 PPI nodes, 174 edges, and a *p*-value of PPI concentration <1.00–16, while also including the result of the GO and KEGG pathway. In the biological process, there was mainly enrichment in the regulation of transcription, translation level and epigenetics, and it also played an important role in histone modification, mitochondrial gene expression, cell metabolism, production of inflammatory mediators and estrogen response. The cellular components are significantly located in the ribosome, mitochondria, chromosomes, and the telomeres, etc. Molecular functions showed that they can bind to a variety of RNA and specific regions, and were closely related to regulated enzymes activity, including various metabolic and gene expressions, modification and regulation of enzymes, and also bound to steroid hormones and estrogen receptors. For KEGG pathway analysis, it was mainly enriched in Glycolysis/Gluconeogenesis, mRNA surveillance pathway, RNA degradation and pathogenic *E. coli* infection. Then, we constructed the PPI network of these DEGs using Cytoscape (**Figure 2A**). Two topological features, degree and betweenness, were calculated to identify candidate hub nodes. The higher the two quantitative values of a gene, the greater the importance within the network (Liu et al., 2018b). The co-expression network revealed that ELAVL2, VIM, MRPS12, HSPE1, EZH2, HIST1H4B, and MRPL13 played a vital role in the progression of breast cancer, and we further selected important modules of target genes through MCODE (**Figures 2B,C**). Finally, we used the ClueGO to externalize all biological processes (**Figures 3A,B**) and the interaction modes of molecular functions (**Figures 4A,B**).

Survival Analysis

The correlation between RBP expression and overall survival was assessed using both the Cox regression analysis and the Kaplan-Meier estimation method. Then, survival correlation $P < 0.05$ and key RBPs were selected to analyze their correlation with survival prognosis. After that we used both the Kaplan-Meier estimates and the log-rank test to assess the significant differences of the two-group survival curves. As shown in the **Figure 5**, the expression of selected target genes in tumor and normal tissues was significantly different. In addition, patients with highly expressed RBPs of EZR, DCAF13, and MRPL13 showed lower survival, but patients with highly expressed RBPs of APOBEC3C, EIF4E3 showed better survival (**Figure 5**). Therefore these genes could be potential biomarkers for breast cancer prognosis.

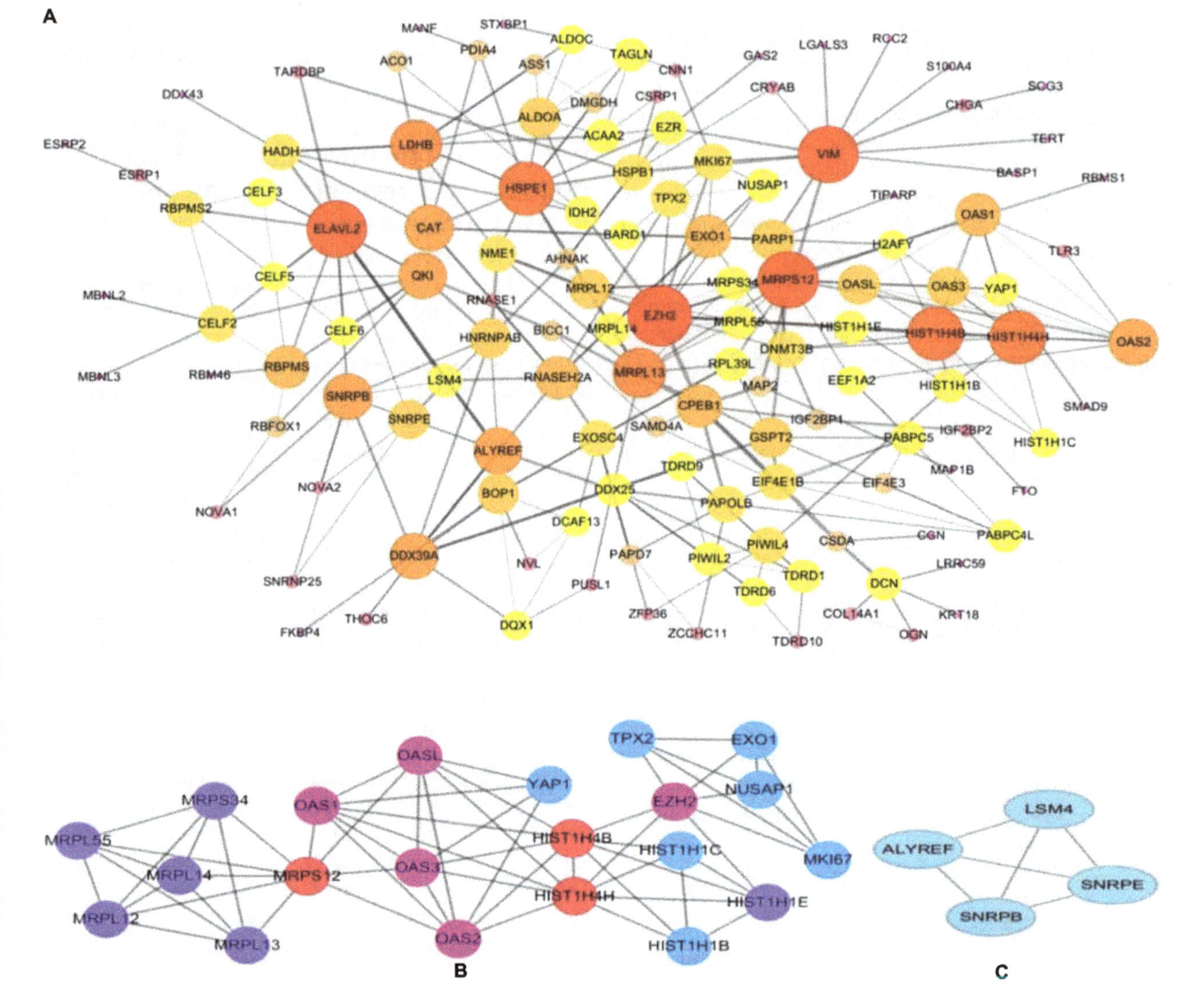

FIGURE 2 | Construction of protein-protein interaction (PPI) network. **(A)** Modules inferred from protein-protein interaction network. Elected important modules of target gene **(B,C)** MCODE score >4, nodes >4.

MATERIALS AND METHODS

Data Sources Analysis

The corresponding clinical data was downloaded from the following website http://gdac.broadinstitute.org/. Combined with the RNA-seq expression data set, 1075 patients had clinical information available including age, gender and disease stage. The details have been listed in **Supplementary Table S1**. We downloaded the RBPs expression data (TOIL RSEM expected count and FPKM) processed by the Toil pipeline (Vivian et al., 2017) based on RNA sequencing (RNA-Seq) for TCGA Pan-Cancer cohort from the website https://xena.ucsc.edu/. The data included the 60498 genes annotated by GENCODE version 23. We then used custom Perl script to extract the data from BRCA cancer, for subsequent analysis. We applied the Voom function (Law et al., 2014) in the Limma package, to estimate DEGs between tumor and normal tissues for BRCA cancer. Those with a fold change ≥ 1 and FDR < 0.05 were considered to have statistical significance. We further identified significantly dysregulated RBPs based on our RBP catalog. Unsupervised clustering of differentially expressed RBPs was performed based on log2-transformed FPKM values using the "pheatmap" package in R.

GO Functional and Pathway Enrichment Analysis

In order to comprehensively analyze the biological functions of these RBPS, we used the GO and kyoto encyclopedia of genes and genomes (KEGG) analysis by The database for annotation, visualization and integrated discovery (DAVID) version 6.7. The GO Term analysis included the

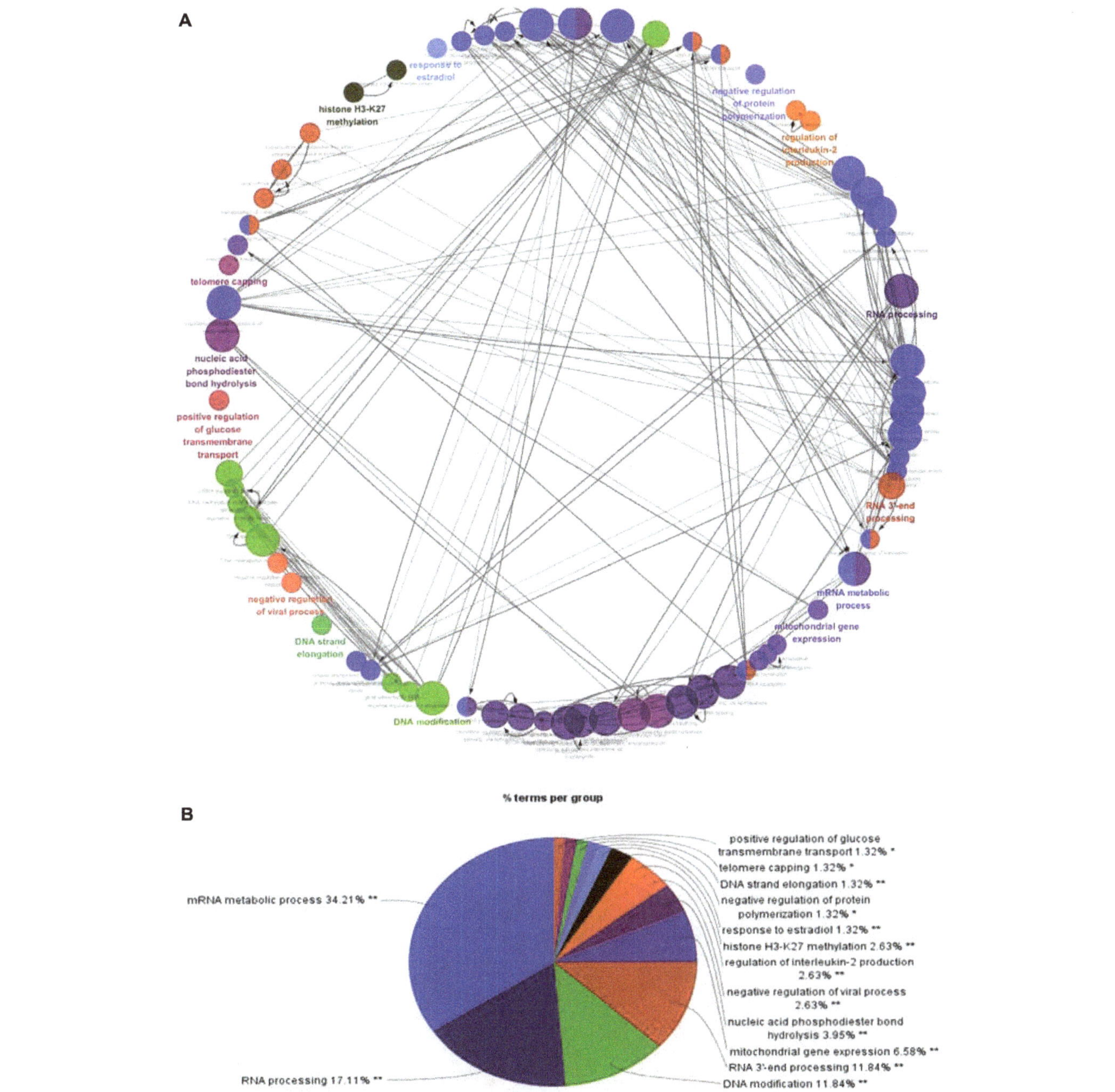

FIGURE 3 | Interrelation analysis between pathways (biological process). **(A)** Interrelation between biological process pathways. **(B)** The proportion of each pathway.

biological process, cellular component and the molecular function. Both $P < 0.05$ and FDR < 0.05 were considered statistically significant.

Protein Interaction Network (PPI) and Pathways Interaction Analysis Building

SRTING version 10.5 was used to evaluate the protein interaction information of all DEGs, and their biological functions were also obtained. Then, the interaction network of these proteins was visualized by Cytoscape3.6.0, and important modules both MCODE score and node number > 4 were selected by the MCODE plug in to Cytoscape version 3.6.0. Furthermore, the pathway enrichment of $P < 0.05$ was analyzed by the ClueGO plug to Cytoscape version 3.6.0.

Statistical Analysis

The correlation of RBP expression and overall survival was assessed using both the Cox regression analysis and the Kaplan-Meier estimation method, based on the "survival"

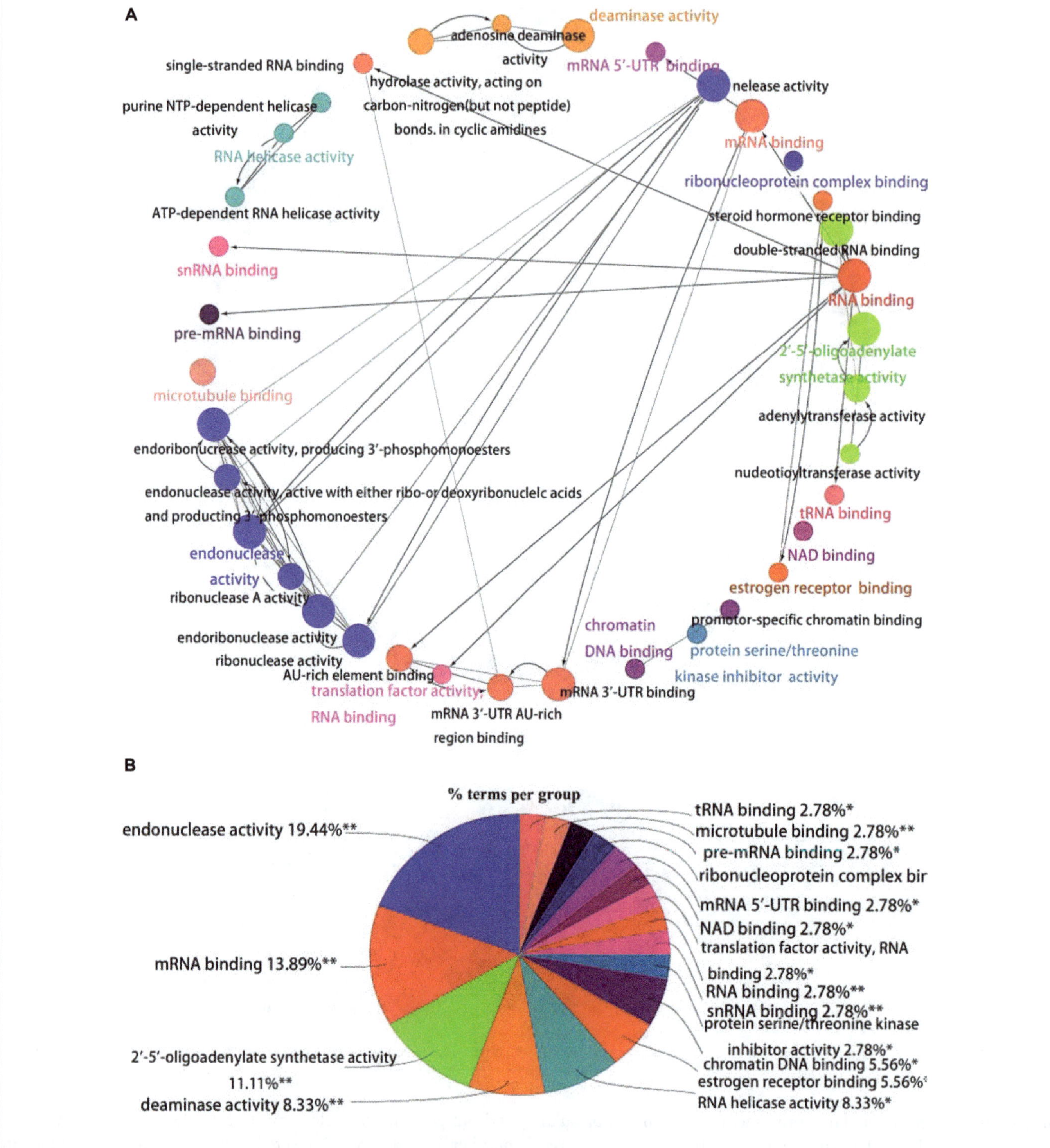

FIGURE 4 | Interrelation analysis between pathways molecular functions. **(A)** Interrelation between molecular functions pathways. **(B)** The proportion of each pathway.

package in R. For the Cox regression analysis, the RBP was evaluated as a continuous variable with age and gender as additional covariables. For the Kaplan-Meier estimates, we defined the high-expression group and low-expression group using the median RBP expression value as a cut-off point. A significant difference of two-group survival curves was assessed by a log-rank test. $P < 0.05$ was considered as statistically significant.

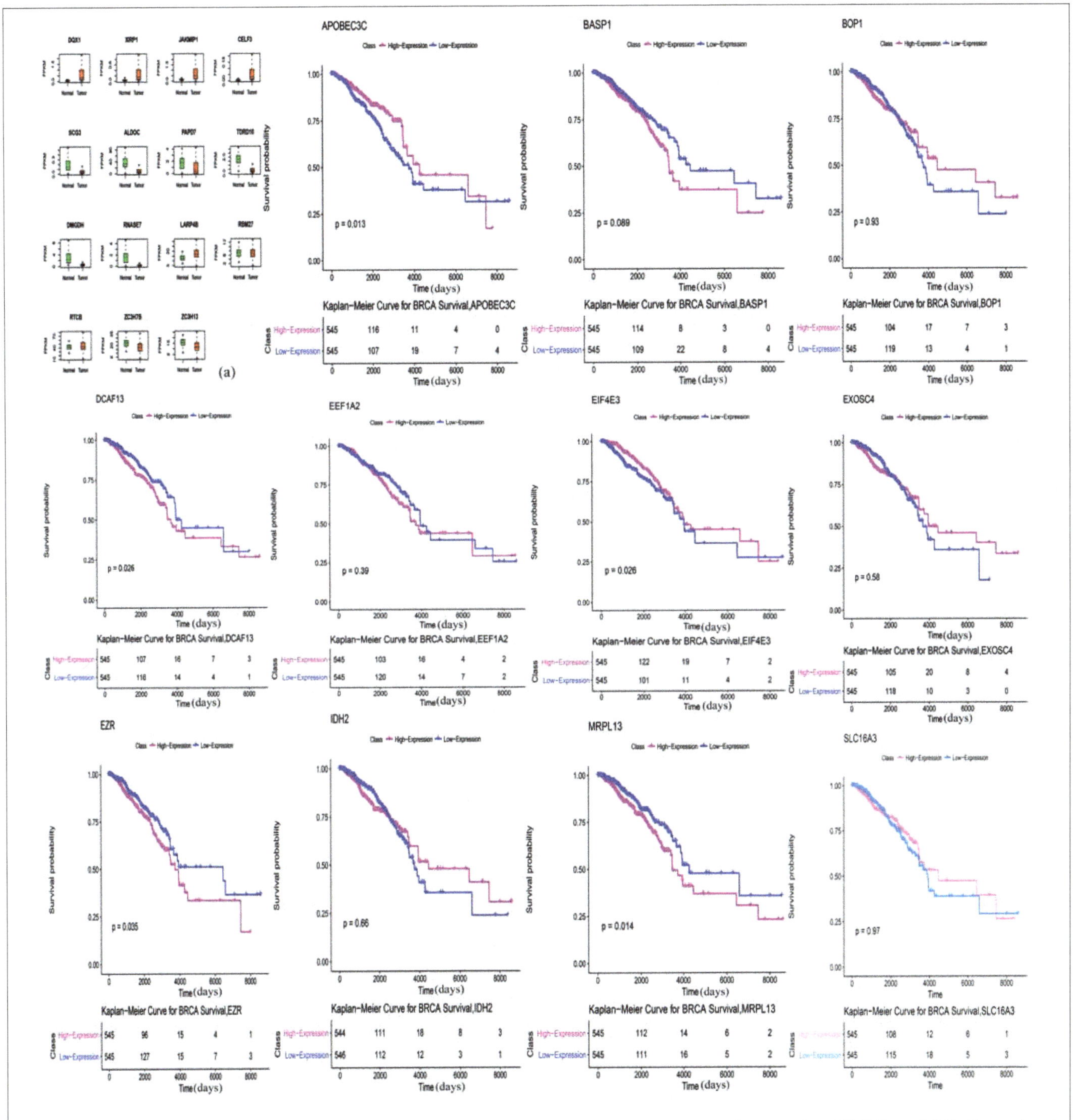

FIGURE 5 | Survival Kaplan-Meier Estimate (EZR $p = 0.035$, DCAF13 $p = 0.026$, MRPL13 $p = 0.014$, APOBEC3C $p = 0.013$, and EIF4E3 $p = 0.026$). Expression of selected target genes in tumor and normal tissues was significantly different.

DISCUSSION

Currently, cancer causes more death than coronary heart diseases or stroke does (Lin et al., 2017a). In recent years, although molecular targeted therapy has improved treatment effect, breast cancer is still the primary cause of death among women. During clinical practice, biomarkers that indicate the grade malignancy, metastasis and the prognosis of breast cancer are needed. Microarray and high-throughput sequencing technologies provide effective tools for deciphering key genetic or epigenetic changes in the occurrence of cancer, as well as promising biomarkers for cancer diagnosis, treatment, and prognosis (Kulasingam and Diamandis, 2008; Cancer Genome Atlas Research and Network, 2014). Our study integrated TCGA RNA sequencing data, and identified DEGs between tumor and normal tissue. We analyzed relevant biological pathways, constructed protein interaction networks and performed survival analyses to explore biological functions and clinical application of these RBPs.

The biological functions of these DEGs were obtained using the GO and KEGG pathway analysis. Firstly, the enrichment of cell components is mainly located in the ribosome, exonuclease, endonuclease, spliceosome and the ribonuclease, which are important sites protecting the transmission of biological information. The ribosome is a key organelle that performs protein synthesis. The mutation of the ribosomal protein regulates the translation and activity of p53, finally resulting in diseases, and cancers (Goudarzi and Lindstrom, 2016). A number of RBPs exist in exonuclease, endonuclease and sites with DNA damage, which may participate in DNA damage repair (Goudarzi and Lindstrom, 2016). In addition, RBPs are widely present in spliceosome. Expression of eukaryotic genes is often accompanied by the RNA splicing process, especially in the alternative splicing of RNA, which could produce tissue and development specific mRNA. For example, Sam68 can result in drug resistance and poor prognosis by regulating the expression ratio of cyclinD1, an alternative splicing in breast cancer (Paronetto et al., 2010). Some RBPs also expressed in the telomere and telomerase and regulate their activity. Telomere play an important role in regulating cell growth and division. Some studies have found that telomerase activity was suppressed in normal tissues but was reactivated in tumors. Telomerase is overexpressed in 80–95% of cancers and is likely to participate in cell malignant transformation (Ruden and Puri, 2013). During the analysis of cellular components, we also found the occurrence of RBPs in the exosome, which could cause tumor invasion and metastasis, immune escape and therapeutic resistance. For example, SYNCRIP, as a component of the miRNA sorting mechanism, in hepatocyte exosomes, can directly bind to specific miRNA rich in exosomes, and regulates miRNA localization (Santangelo et al., 2016).

Secondly, in terms of molecular function, RPBs can bind to various RNAs such as pre-mRNA, Sn RNA, tRNA, mRNA and regulates the activity of various enzymes, such as hydrolytic enzyme, purine metabolic enzyme, and enzymes involved in DNA synthesis, repair, and RNA metabolism. Furthermore, some RBPs also bind to estrogen and steroid hormone receptors. For example, MSI2 is highly expressed in ER(+) breast cancer, and its expression is significantly correlated with ESR1 expression, which affects the growth of breast cancer cells, by changing the function of ESR1 (Kang et al., 2017).

Next, for the biological process, the function enrichment of differential RBPs mainly occurred in RNA processing, splicing, localization, transport, hydrolysis, and RNA silencing. It participates in transposition regulation, methylation, and alkylation of DNA. Some RBPs were also related to histone H3K27 methylation, inflammatory mediators, and translation regulation. Our findings are consistent with the consensus that multiple genes, multiple molecules, and multiple pathways are involved in breast cancer. Although the relationship with breast cancer remains unclear, some RBPs have been reported in other cancers. HuR can promote the growth of colorectal cancer cell by regulating mRNA expression (Lopez de Silanes et al., 2003). CRD-BP can regulate many mRNAs with coding for cancer-related genes, including Gli1, PTEN, PTEN, ptlcp1, MAPK4, MDR1, IGF2, H19, c-myc, etc. (Fakhraldeen et al., 2015). HNRNPA2B1 controls the replacement splicing for the pre-mRNA of cancer-related genes, and which is up-regulated in diverse cancers (Stockley et al., 2014). HuR can bind with DNMT3b and maintain its stability, thus affecting abnormal DNA methylation (Lopez de Silanes et al., 2009). Numerous studies reported that a change of mitochondrial function plays a key role in all kinds of cancers (Tao et al., 2015; Lin et al., 2017b; Zhang J.Y. et al., 2017; Zhang J. et al., 2017), and RBPs involved in the expression and transcription regulation of mitochondrial genes, such as LRPPRC, GRSF1, SLIRP, and other RBPs can interact with mt-RNA to affect the expression and metabolism of mitochondrial transcripts (Dong et al., 2017). The incidence of breast cancer and female estrogen levels are closely related. Some RBPs can respond with estrogen, for example, through Nova1, 17-b estradiol can regulate the replacement splicing of estrogen receptor b in the brain of aging female mice (Shults et al., 2018). Then, the results of the KEGG pathway analysis indicated that these RBPs may affect the occurrence and development of breast cancer through glycolysis, glycosylation, mRNA monitoring pathways, and RNA degradation regulation. RPBs have various basic biological functions, especially the function of RNA which has been studied widely. Other RBPs functions should therefore be studies further.

By constructing a protein network for DEGs, we found that breast cancer is associated with immune response, splicing, transcript regulation, and intercellular signaling transduction. HSPE1 is a member of the heat shock protein family (Hsp10) E, which usually acts as a chaperone to assist protein folding in the mitochondria, which is highly expressed in various cancers, such as lung cancer, pancreatic cancer and bladder cancer. Some studies reported that it may protect cancer cells from apoptosis, and facilitate the immune escape of cancer, by down-regulating the immune response (Rappa et al., 2016; Liu et al., 2018a). ELAVL2 is a neurospecific RNA binding protein, which is involved in splicing and transcript trafficking to regulate protein localization (Berto et al., 2016). Elevated methylation of ELAVL2 was shown in high Gleason scores of prostate tumors (Wu et al., 2016). VIM is expressed in a variety of cell types and is responsible for maintaining cell shape, cytoplasmic integrity, and stabilizing cytoskeletal. It is also involved in immune responses, attachment, migration, and cell signaling in tissues. Previous studies have shown that vimentin regulated Ras, Slug and TGF glows in cancer cells, which is necessary for EMT induction. It is also highly expressed in various tumors such as lung cancer, breast cancer and gastric cancer, and is closely related to invasion, metastasis and the poor prognosis of tumors (Satelli and Li, 2011; Virtakoivu et al., 2015). High expressions of EZH2 is associated with malignancy and hyper-invasiveness in a variety of cancers. EZH2 can activate NF-κB targets and NOTCH1 in breast cancer cells, which has also been implicated in the transcriptional activation of gene expression in breast cancer. Research has shown that it induces the expression of genes that are regulated by the estrogen receptor (ER) and Wnt signaling transcription factors, by physically bridging between the ER and components of Wnt signaling (Kim and Roberts, 2016).

These RBPS may lead to breast cancer by regulating mitochondrial translation, splicing of pre-mRNA, activation of RNase L, and histone modifications through two modules selected from the PPI network. It has been reported that the upregulation of mitochondrial translation may meet the energy needs of cancer cells in human tumors, but the mechanism of its tumorigenesis remains unclear. There are many studies targeting the inhibition of mitochondrial translation in various cell types, to obliterate cancer stem cells. Currently, suppressing mitochondrial translation is considered a valuable therapeutic target (Kim et al., 2017). RNase L was activated through the synthesis of 2′, 5′ -oligoadenylic acid by OAS (OAS1, OAS2, and OAS3). It was found that the activated OAS-RNase L system can degrade virus and cell RNA, promote cell apoptosis, and inhibit protein synthesis (Bhosle et al., 2016). In addition, single nucleotide polymorphisms of OAS are associated with cancer, such as OAS1 SNP rs2660 AA (Mandal et al., 2011). However, no studies reported the exact role of OAS in breast cancer. As we know, epigenetic change is involved in the initiation and progression of cancer, which includes histone modifications and DNA methylation. Studies have shown that the regulation of histone is gene specific, but their function is diversified. Histone cluster 1 can interact with some regulatory factors, such as inhibiting p53-dependent chromatin transcription, and maintaining or establishing specific DNA methylation patterns (Perez-Magan et al., 2010). It has been demonstrated that the function of protecting DNA with histone may be an independent prognostic factor for better survival of cervical cancer patients (Li et al., 2017). Furthermore, splicing affects the expression of most genes, and eventually influences the levels of proteins. In the module, SNRPE, SNRPB, and ALYREF participate in the splicing of pre-mRNA. Knockdown SNRPE significantly reduces the expressed level of mTOR mRNA and protein, and is accompanied by the imbalance of the mTOR pathway, which activates abnormal mTOR signaling and which can result in the growth and metastasis of tumor cells (Quidville et al., 2013).

Finally, we performed a survival analysis and found five genes that are associated with survival in breast cancer patients. The overexpression of DCAF13, EZR, and MRPL13 in patients were associated with lower survival, which reveals that these genes might be associated with tumor invasion, progression and poor prognosis. Whereas, overexpression of APOBEC3C and EIF4E3 in patients were associated with better survival, suggesting their potential role as tumor suppressor genes. DCAF13 is amplified in all kinds of cancers. Studies have shown that overexpression of DCAF13 in hepatocellular carcinoma is significantly correlated with low survival and it may be involved in the regulation of cell cycle (Cao et al., 2017). It also reported that the E3 ligase formed by DCAF13, CUL4B and DDB1, could induce ubiquitination of tumor suppressor PTEN *in vivo* and *in vitro* (Chen et al., 2018). Mutated or inactivated PTEN was helpful to infiltrate and spread cancer cells. As a member of the ERM protein family, Ezrin has been linked to molecules that control the phosphatidylinositol-3-kinase, AKT, Erk1/2 MAPK and Rho pathways, which are functionally involved in regulating cell survival, proliferation and migration, and it is an indicator of poor prognosis of multiple cancers (Hunter, 2004). It has been shown that overexpressed EZR in a nude mice phantom of pancreatic cancer, can increase the number of metastasis and is closely related to the progression of malignant cancer (Meng et al., 2010). MRPL13 is a mitochondrial ribosomal protein. Loss of MRPL13 can lead to the loss of mitochondrial DNA, and eventually lead to the loss of the ability of mitochondrial coding proteins (Gruschke et al., 2010). In a study, reduced MRPL13 expression in hepatocellular carcinoma was a key factor in the regulation of mitochondrial ribosome and subsequent OXPHOS deficiency, which regulates the aggressive activity of liver cancer cells (Lee et al., 2017). APOBEC can mediate c-to-t mutagenesis in various cancers, while the APOBEC3 gene family is overexpressed in breast cancer and other cancer cells and tissues. Some studies suggest that it is regulated by estrogen in breast cancer (Long et al., 2013). At present, there are few studies about APOBEC3C in breast cancer, and some studies have found that it should play a positive role in the invasiveness and prognosis of hepatocellular carcinoma (Zhang et al., 2015). EIF4E3 belongs to the EIF4E family of translational initiation factors that interact with the 5-prime cap structure of mRNA. A study demonstrated that EIF4E3 relies on cap-binding activity to act as a tumor suppressor and compete with the growth-promoting functions of EIF4E. In fact, reduced EIF4E3 levels in high-expressed EIF4E cancers suggests that EIF4E3 underlies a clinically relevant inhibitory mechanism that is lost in some malignancies (Osborne et al., 2013). Other studies also found that EIF4E3 can impede oncogenic transformation (Volpon et al., 2013).

Over all, we identified key genes and related pathways through bioinformatics analysis of differential expressions of RBPs in breast cancer. These RBPs may be involved in the occurrence, development, invasion and metastasis of breast cancer. The survival analysis suggested that DCAF13, EZR, MRPL13, APOBEC3C, and EIF4E3 might have a prognostic value for breast cancer. Future *in vitro* and *in vivo* studies are needed to verify the functions of these genes.

AUTHOR CONTRIBUTIONS

LL and KW conceived and designed the experiments. LF, YY, TZ, and HD analyzed the data. LL, YZ, and FY wrote the manuscript. All authors reviewed and approved the final manuscript.

FUNDING

This study was supported by the Natural Science Foundation Project of Yongchuan People's Hospital of Chongqing (Grant No. YCPH2019001). Chongqing Health and the Health Committee and Chongqing Science and Technology Commission (Grant No. 2018MSXM020) and the Natural Science Foundation Project of Yongchuan (Grant No. Ycstc.2017nc5020).

REFERENCES

1. Berto, S., Usui, N., Konopka, G., and Fogel, B. L. (2016). ELAVL2-regulated transcriptional and splicing networks in human neurons link neurodevelopment and autism. *Hum. Mol. Genet.* 25, 2451–2464. doi: 10.1093/hmg/ddw110
2. Bhosle, S. M., Hunt, A., and Chaudhary, J. (2016). A modified coupled spectrophotometric method to detect 2-5 oligoadenylate synthetase activity in prostate cell lines. *Biol. Proced. Online* 18:9. doi: 10.1186/s12575-016-0038-x
3. Bray, F., Ferlay, J., Soerjomataram, I., Siegel, R. L., Torre, L. A., and Jemal, A. (2018). Global cancer statistics 2018: GLOBOCAN estimates of incidence and mortality worldwide for 36 cancers in 185 countries. *CA Cancer. J. Clin.* 68, 394–424. doi: 10.3322/caac.21492
4. Campos-Melo, D., Droppelmann, C. A., Volkening, K., and Strong, M. J. (2014). RNA-binding proteins as molecular links between cancer and neurodegeneration. *Biogerontology* 15, 587–610. doi: 10.1007/s10522-014-9531-2
5. Cancer Genome Atlas Research and Network (2014). Comprehensive molecular characterization of gastric adenocarcinoma. *Nature* 513, 202–209. doi: 10.1038/nature13480
6. Cao, J., Hou, P., Chen, J., Wang, P., Wang, W., Liu, W., et al. (2017). The overexpression and prognostic role of DCAF13 in hepatocellular carcinoma. *Tumour Biol.* 39:1010428317705753. doi: 10.1177/1010428317705753
7. Chen, Z., Zhang, W., Jiang, K., Chen, B., Wang, K., Lao, L., et al. (2018). MicroRNA-300 regulates the ubiquitination of PTEN through the CRL4B(DCAF13) E3 ligase in osteosarcoma cells. *Mol. Ther. Nucleic Acids* 10, 254–268. doi: 10.1016/j.omtn.2017.12.010
8. Connerty, P., Ahadi, A., and Hutvagner, G. (2015). RNA Binding Proteins in the miRNA Pathway. *Int. J. Mol. Sci.* 17:31. doi: 10.3390/ijms17010031
9. Dong, Y., Yoshitomi, T., Hu, J. F., and Cui, J. (2017). Long noncoding RNAs coordinate functions between mitochondria and the nucleus. *Epigen. Chromatin* 10:41. doi: 10.1186/s13072-017-0149-x
10. Fakhraldeen, S. A., Clark, R. J., Roopra, A., Chin, E. N., Huang, W., Castorino, J., et al. (2015). Two isoforms of the RNA binding protein, coding region determinant-binding protein (CRD-BP/IGF2BP1), are expressed in breast epithelium and support clonogenic growth of breast tumor cells. *J. Biol. Chem.* 290, 13386–13400. doi: 10.1074/jbc.M115.655175
11. Gerstberger, S., Hafner, M., Ascano, M., and Tuschl, T. (2014a). Evolutionary conservation and expression of human RNA-binding proteins and their role in human genetic disease. *Adv. Exp. Med. Biol.* 825, 1–55. doi: 10.1007/978-1-4939-1221-6-1
12. Gerstberger, S., Hafner, M., and Tuschl, T. (2014b). A census of human RNA-binding proteins. *Nat. Rev. Genet.* 15, 829–845. doi: 10.1038/nrg3813
13. Glisovic, T., Bachorik, J. L., Yong, J., and Dreyfuss, G. (2008). RNA-binding proteins and post-transcriptional gene regulation. *FEBS Lett.* 582, 1977–1986. doi: 10.1016/j.febslet.2008.03.004
14. Goudarzi, K. M., and Lindstrom, M. S. (2016). Role of ribosomal protein mutations in tumor development. *Int. J. Oncol.* 48, 1313–1324. doi: 10.3892/ijo.2016. 3387
15. Gruschke, S., Grone, K., Heublein, M., Holz, S., Israel, L., Imhof, A., et al. (2010). Proteins at the polypeptide tunnel exit of the yeast mitochondrial ribosome. *J. Biol. Chem.* 285, 19022–19028. doi: 10.1074/jbc.M110. 113837
16. Harvey, R., Dezi, V., Pizzinga, M., and Willis, A. E. (2017). Post-transcriptional control of gene expression following stress: the role of RNA-binding proteins. *Biochem. Soc. Trans.* 45, 1007–1014. doi: 10.1042/BST20160364
17. Hunter, K. W. (2004). Ezrin, a key component in tumor metastasis. *Trends Mol. Med.* 10, 201–204. doi: 10.1016/j.molmed.2004.03.001
18. Iadevaia, V., and Gerber, A. P. (2015). Combinatorial control of mRNA fates by RNA-binding proteins and non-coding RNAs. *Biomolecules* 5, 2207–2222. doi: 10.3390/biom5042207
19. Kang, M. H., Jeong, K. J., Kim, W. Y., Lee, H. J., Gong, G., Suh, N., et al. (2017). Musashi RNA-binding protein 2 regulates estrogen receptor 1 function in breast cancer. *Oncogene* 36, 1745–1752. doi: 10.1038/onc.2016.327
20. Kim, H.-J., Maiti, P., and Barrientos, A. (2017). Mitochondrial ribosomes in cancer. *Semin. Cancer Biol.* 47, 67–81. doi: 10.1016/j.semcancer.2017.04.004
21. Kim, K. H., and Roberts, C. W. (2016). Targeting EZH2 in cancer. *Nat. Med.* 22, 128–134. doi: 10.1038/nm.4036
22. Kulasingam, V., and Diamandis, E. P. (2008). Strategies for discovering novel cancer biomarkers through utilization of emerging technologies. *Nat. Clin. Pract. Oncol.* 5, 588–599. doi: 10.1038/ncponc1187
23. Law, C. W., Chen, Y., Shi, W., and Smyth, G. K. (2014). Voom: precision weights unlock linear model analysis tools for RNA-seq read counts. *Genome Biol.* 15:R29. doi: 10.1186/gb-2014-15-2-r29
24. Lee, Y. K., Lim, J. J., Jeoun, U. W., Min, S., Lee, E. B., Kwon, S. M., et al. (2017). Lactate-mediated mitoribosomal defects impair mitochondrial oxidative phosphorylation and promote hepatoma cell invasiveness. *J. Biol. Chem.* 292, 20208–20217. doi: 10.1074/jbc.M117.809012
25. Li, X., Tian, R., Gao, H., Yang, Y., Williams, B. R. G., Gantier, M. P., et al. (2017). Identification of a histone family gene signature for predicting the prognosis of cervical cancer patients. *Sci. Rep.* 7:16495. doi: 10.1038/s41598-017-16472-5
26. Lin, M., Bi, H., Yan, Y., Huang, W., Zhang, G., Zhang, G., et al. (2017a). Parthenolide suppresses non-small cell lung cancer GLC-82 cells growth via B-Raf/MAPK/Erk pathway. *Oncotarget* 8, 23436–23447. doi: 10.18632/oncotarget.15584
27. Lin, M., Tang, S., Zhang, C., Chen, H., Huang, W., Liu, Y., et al. (2017b). Euphorbia factor L2 induces apoptosis in A549 cells through the mitochondrial pathway. *Acta Pharm. Sin. B* 7, 59–64. doi: 10.1016/j.apsb.2016.06.008
28. Liu, X., Weng, Y., Liu, P., Sui, Z., Zhou, L., Huang, Y., et al. (2018a). Identification of PGAM1 as a putative therapeutic target for pancreatic ductal adenocarcinoma metastasis using quantitative proteomics. *Onco Targets Ther.* 11, 3345–3357. doi: 10.2147/OTT.S162470
29. Liu, X., Wu, J., Zhang, D., Bing, Z., Tian, J., Ni, M., et al. (2018b). Identification of potential key genes associated with the pathogenesis and prognosis of gastric cancer based on integrated bioinformatics analysis. *Front. Genet.* 9:265. doi: 10.3389/fgene.2018.00265
30. Long, J., Delahanty, R. J., Li, G., Gao, Y. T., Lu, W., Cai, Q., et al. (2013). A common deletion in the APOBEC3 genes and breast cancer risk. *J. Natl. Cancer Inst.* 105, 573–579. doi: 10.1093/jnci/djt018
31. Lopez de Silanes, I., Fan, J., Yang, X., Zonderman, A. B., Potapova, O., Pizer, E.

S., et al. (2003). Role of the RNA-binding protein HuR in colon carcinogenesis. *Oncogene* 22, 7146–7154. doi: 10.1038/sj.onc.1206862

32. Lopez de Silanes, I., Gorospe, M., Taniguchi, H., Abdelmohsen, K., Srikantan, S., Alaminos, M., et al. (2009). The RNA-binding protein HuR regulates DNA methylation through stabilization of DNMT3b mRNA. *Nucleic Acids Res.* 37, 2658–2671. doi: 10.1093/nar/gkp123
33. Mandal, S., Abebe, F., and Chaudhary, J. (2011). 2^1 -5^1 oligoadenylate synthetase 1 polymorphism is associated with prostate cancer. *Cancer* 117, 5509–5518. doi: 10.1002/cncr.26219
34. McDonald, E. S., Clark, A. S., Tchou, J., Zhang, P., and Freedman, G. M. (2016). Clinical diagnosis and management of breast cancer. *J. Nucl. Med.* 57(Suppl. 1), 9S–16S. doi: 10.2967/jnumed.115.157834
35. Meng, Y., Lu, Z., Yu, S., Zhang, Q., Ma, Y., and Chen, J. (2010). Ezrin promotes invasion and metastasis of pancreatic cancer cells. *J. Transl. Med.* 8:61. doi: 10.1186/1479-5876-8-61
36. Nishida, K., Kuwano, Y., Nishikawa, T., Masuda, K., and Rokutan, K. (2017). RNA binding proteins and genome integrity. *Int. J. Mol. Sci.* 18:1341. doi: 10.3390/ijms18071341
37. Osborne, M. J., Volpon, L., Kornblatt, J. A., Culjkovic-Kraljacic, B., Baguet, A., and Borden, K. L. (2013). eIF4E3 acts as a tumor suppressor by utilizing an atypical mode of methyl-7-guanosine cap recognition. *Proc. Natl. Acad. Sci. U.S.A.* 110, 3877–3882. doi: 10.1073/pnas.1216862110
38. Paronetto, M. P., Cappellari, M., Busa, R., Pedrotti, S., Vitali, R., Comstock, C., et al. (2010). Alternative splicing of the cyclin D1 proto-oncogene is regulated by the RNA-binding protein Sam68. *Cancer Res.* 70, 229–239. doi: 10.1158/0008-5472. CAN-09-2788
39. Perez-Magan, E., Rodriguez de Lope, A., Ribalta, T., Ruano, Y., Campos-Martin, Y., Perez-Bautista, G., et al. (2010). Differential expression profiling analyses identifies downregulation of 1p, 6q, and 14q genes and overexpression of 6p histone cluster 1 genes as markers of recurrence in meningiomas. *Neuro Oncol.* 12, 1278–1290. doi: 10.1093/neuonc/noq081
40. Quidville, V., Alsafadi, S., Goubar, A., Commo, F., Scott, V., Pioche-Durieu, C., et al. (2013). Targeting the deregulated spliceosome core machinery in cancer cells triggers mTOR blockade and autophagy. *Cancer Res.* 73, 2247–2258. doi: 10.1158/0008-5472.Can-12-2501
41. Rappa, F., Pitruzzella, A., Marino Gammazza, A., Barone, R., Mocciaro, E., Tomasello, G., et al. (2016). Quantitative patterns of Hsps in tubular adenoma compared with normal and tumor tissues reveal the value of Hsp10 and Hsp60 in early diagnosis of large bowel cancer. *Cell Stress Chaperones* 21, 927–933. doi: 10.1007/s12192-016-0721-5
42. Ruden, M., and Puri, N. (2013). Novel anticancer therapeutics targeting telomerase. *Cancer Treat. Rev.* 39, 444–456. doi: 10.1016/j.ctrv.2012.06.007
43. Santangelo, L., Giurato, G., Cicchini, C., Montaldo, C., Mancone, C., Tarallo, R., et al. (2016). The RNA-binding protein SYNCRIP is a component of the hepatocyte exosomal machinery controlling microRNA sorting. *Cell Rep.* 17, 799–808. doi: 10.1016/j.celrep.2016.09.031
44. Satelli, A., and Li, S. (2011). Vimentin in cancer and its potential as a molecular target for cancer therapy. *Cell. Mol. Life Sci.* 68, 3033–3046. doi: 10.1007/s00018-011-0735-1
45. Shults, C. L., Dingwall, C. B., Kim, C. K., Pinceti, E., Rao, Y. S., and Pak, T. R. (2018). 17beta-estradiol regulates the RNA-binding protein Nova1, which then regulates the alternative splicing of estrogen receptor beta in the aging female rat brain. *Neurobiol. Aging* 61, 13–22. doi: 10.1016/j.neurobiolaging.2017.09.005
46. Stockley, J., Villasevil, M. E., Nixon, C., Ahmad, I., Leung, H. Y., and Rajan, P. (2014). The RNA-binding protein hnRNPA2 regulates beta-catenin protein expression and is overexpressed in prostate cancer. *RNA Biol.* 11, 755–765. doi: 10.4161/rna.28800
47. Tao, Y. W., Lin, Y. C., She, Z. G., Lin, M. T., Chen, P. X., and Zhang, J. Y. (2015). Anticancer activity and mechanism investigation of beauvericin isolated
48. from secondary metabolites of the mangrove endophytic fungi. *Anticancer Agents Med. Chem.* 15, 258–266. doi: 10.2174/1871520614666140825112255
49. Virtakoivu, R., Mai, A., Mattila, E., De Franceschi, N., Imanishi, S. Y., Corthals, G., et al. (2015). Vimentin-ERK signaling uncouples slug gene regulatory function. *Cancer Res.* 75, 2349–2362. doi: 10.1158/0008-5472.CAN-14-2842
50. Vivian, J., Rao, A. A., Nothaft, F. A., Ketchum, C., Armstrong, J., Novak, A., et al. (2017). Toil enables reproducible, open source, big biomedical data analyses. *Nat. Biotechnol.* 35, 314–316. doi: 10.1038/nbt.3772
51. Vogelstein, B., Papadopoulos, N., Velculescu, V. E., Zhou, S., Diaz, L. A. Jr., and Kinzler, K. W. (2013). Cancer genome landscapes. *Science* 339, 1546–1558. doi: 10.1126/science.1235122
52. Volpon, L., Osborne, M. J., Culjkovic-Kraljacic, B., and Borden, K. L. (2013). eIF4E3, a new actor in mRNA metabolism and tumor suppression. *Cell Cycle* 12, 1159–1160. doi: 10.4161/cc.24566
53. Wang, Y., Zhang, Y., Huang, Q., and Li, C. (2018). Integrated bioinformatics analysis reveals key candidate genes and pathways in breast cancer. *Mol. Med. Rep.* 17, 8091–8100. doi: 10.3892/mmr.2018.8895
54. Wu, Y., Davison, J., Qu, X., Morrissey, C., Storer, B., Brown, L., et al. (2016). Methylation profiling identified novel differentially methylated markers including OPCML and FLRT2 in prostate cancer. *Epigenetics* 11, 247–258. doi: 10.1080/15592294.2016.1148867
55. Wurth, L., and Gebauer, F. (2015). RNA-binding proteins, multifaceted translational regulators in cancer. *Biochim. Biophys. Acta* 1849, 881–886. doi: 10.1016/j.bbagrm.2014.10.001
56. Zhang, J. Y., Huang, W. J., Sun, H. M., Liu, Y., Zhao, X. Q., Tang, S. L., et al. (2017). Structure identification and in vitro anticancer activity of lathyrol-3-phenylacetate-5,15-diacetate. *Molecules* 22:1412. doi: 10.3390/molecules22091412
57. Zhang, J., Lai, Z., Huang, W., Ling, H., Lin, M., Tang, S., et al. (2017). Apicidin inhibited proliferation and invasion and induced apoptosis via mitochondrial pathway in non-small cell lung cancer GLC-82 cells. *Anticancer Agents Med. Chem.* 17, 1374–1382. doi: 10.2174/1871520617666170419120044
58. Zhang, Y., Delahanty, R., Guo, X., Zheng, W., and Long, J. (2015). Integrative genomic analysis reveals functional diversification of APOBEC gene family in breast cancer. *Hum. Genomics* 9:34. doi: 10.1186/s40246-015-0056-9

18

PD-1/PD-L1 Inhibitors in Cervical Cancer

Yuncong Liu[1,2†], Li Wu[2†], Ruizhan Tong[1], Feiyue Yang[2], Limei Yin[1,3], Mengqian Li[1,3], Liting You[1,3], Jianxin Xue[1,3] and You Lu[1,3*]*

[1] West China School of Medicine, Sichuan University, Chengdu, China, [2] Department of Gynaecological Oncology, Guizhou Provincial People's Hospital, Guiyang, China, [3] Department of Thoracic Oncology, Cancer Center, West China Hospital, Sichuan University, Chengdu, China

***Correspondence:**
Jianxin Xue
radjianxin@163.com
You Lu
radyoulu@hotmail.com

† These authors have contributed equally to this work

Cervical cancer is one of the most common gynecological tumors, and the majority of early-stage cervical cancer patients achieve good recovery through surgical treatment and concurrent chemoradiotherapy (CCRT). However, for patients with recurrent, persistent, metastatic cervical cancer, effective treatment is rare, except for bevacizumab combined with chemotherapy. Programmed cell death-1/programmed cell death-ligand 1 (PD-1/PD-L1) inhibitors might be a novel choice to improve the clinical outcomes of these patients. Thus far, some pivotal trials, including Keynote 028, Keynote 158 and Checkmate 358, have indicated established clinical benefit of PD-1/PD-L1 inhibitors in cervical cancer. In light of these data, the FDA has approved pembrolizumab for patients with recurrent or metastatic cervical cancer with disease progression during or after chemotherapy. There are also some ongoing studies that may provide more evidence for the PD-1/PD-L1 pathway as a therapeutic target in cervical cancer. In this review, we have summarized the status and application of PD-1/PD-L1 inhibitors in clinical trials for the treatment of cervical cancer and suggested some future directions in this field.

Keywords: cervical cancer, programmed cell death-1/programmed cell death-ligand 1 (PD-1/PD-L1), immune checkpoint inhibitors, immunotherapy, human papillomavirus (HPV)

INTRODUCTION

Cervical cancer is one of the most common gynecological tumors. More than 569,847 women are diagnosed with cervical cancer annually worldwide, resulting in over 311,365 deaths (Bray et al., 2018). Although the incidence of cervical cancer has been greatly reduced by the use of HPV vaccines and cervical cancer screening (Goodman, 2015), cervical cancer is second in terms of morbidity among gynecological tumors in developing countries (Sahasrabuddhe et al., 2012). Over 70% of cervical cancer cases diagnosed in developing countries are locally invasive or metastatic, contributing to the high mortality rate of cervical cancer. The 5-year OS rate of local cervical cancer can achieve approximately 75–85% through effective treatments such as surgery CCRT, etc. (Chen et al., 2015). Nevertheless, the 5-year OS of recurrent, persistent, metastatic cervical cancer is only approximately 15%. The poor prognosis is mainly due to limited therapeutic options (Guitarte et al., 2014). The majority of these patients can only be treated with palliative

Abbreviations: AE, adverse event; APCs, antigen-presenting cells; CCRT, concurrent chemoradiotherapy; CRs, complete responses; CRT, chemoradiotherapy; CTLA-4, cytotoxic T-lymphocyte-associated protein-4; hfRT, hyperfraction radiotherapy; HNSCC, head and neck squamous cell carcinoma; HPV, human papillomavirus; mAb, monoclonal antibody; NSCLC, non-small cell lung cancer; ORR, objective response rate; OS, overall survival rate; PD-1/PD-L1, programmed cell death-1/programmed cell death-ligand 1; PFS, progression-free survival; PRs, partial responses; SCCs, squamous cell cancers; TILs, tumor infiltrating lymphocytes; uPRs, unconfirmed partial responses.

chemotherapy (Boussios et al., 2016), in which platinum-based chemotherapies were the prior choice (Monk et al., 2009). In 2014, the GOG 240 trial indicated that when bevacizumab was added to the chemotherapy, the ORR was improved from 36 to 48% (Tewari et al., 2014), and the OS could be prolonged from 13 to 17 months for recurrent, persistent, metastatic cervical cancer, thus laying the foundation for the first-line choice of combining bevacizumab with chemotherapy for this population (Tewari et al., 2017). However, for those who progress during the first-line treatment, the lack of effective second-line treatment remains to be the main reason for the high mortality rate (Minion and Tewari, 2018). Currently, immune checkpoint inhibitors (Schumacher and Schreiber, 2015), especially PD-1/PD-L1 inhibitors (Constantinidou et al., 2018), have achieved favorable efficacy in treating multiple solid tumors (Gettinger et al., 2018), including cervical cancer (Borcoman and Le Tourneau, 2017). Accumulating evidence has demonstrated that PD-1/PD-L1 inhibitors may be a promising approach for cervical cancer treatment.

IMMUNE CHECKPOINT INHIBITORS

Numerous immunomodulatory therapies are being investigated in clinical trials with diverse potential targets, including PD-1/PD-L1, CTLA-4, Tim-3, ICOS, 4-1BB, and OX-40. Among these novel targets, ICOS (Amatore et al., 2018), 4-1BB (Compte et al., 2018), and OX-40 (Polesso et al., 2018) are costimulatory receptors, while PD-1/PD-L1 (Raedler, 2015), CTLA-4 (Lheureux et al., 2018), and Tim-3 (Gorris et al., 2018) are negative immune regulators of T cells. Currently, only CTLA-4 inhibitors (Hodi et al., 2010) and PD-1/PD-L1 inhibitors (Bagcchi, 2014) have been approved by the FDA. CTLA-4 integrates with the costimulatory molecules CD80 (B7-1) and CD86 (B7-2) that express on the surfaces of APCs (Fife and Bluestone, 2008), while PD-L1 is expressed on a wide variety of cell types, including tumor-associated fibroblasts, tumor cells, APCs, etc. (Boussiotis, 2016). As a result, CTLA-4 inhibits T cell activation within secondary lymphoid organs (Kurup et al., 2017), but PD-1/PD-L1 chiefly regulates T cell function within peripheral tissues and the tumor microenvironment (Pardoll, 2012). Therefore, PD-1/PD-L1 signaling is more specific to tumor than CTLA-4 signaling, and inhibitors of PD-1/PD-L1 may cause less damage to healthy tissue (Boussiotis, 2016; Minion and Tewari, 2018) (**Figure 1**).

Based on the above mechanism, ipilimumab (monoclonal anti-CTLA-4), the first immune checkpoint inhibitor, approved for melanoma, had little clinical benefit until the emergence of pembrolizumab, and the combination of the two drugs further improved treatment efficacy in malignant melanoma (Wang et al., 2017). To date, another mAb for CTLA-4, tremelimumab, has not been approved for the treatment in any type of cancer. However, mAbs targeting PD-1 [pembrolizumab (Paz-Ares et al., 2018), nivolumab (Long et al., 2018), and cemiplimab (Sidaway, 2018)] and PD-L1 [atezolizumab (Hsu et al., 2018), durvalumab (Siu et al., 2018), and avelumab (Le Tourneau et al., 2018)] have presented clinical advantages in malignant melanoma, advanced NSCLC, urothelial cancer (Zhang and Li, 2018) and other tumors (Lim et al., 2018) (**Table 1**). In addition, extensive research has been carried out on gynecological tumors, such as ovarian cancer (Liu and Zamarin, 2018) and breast cancer (Julia et al., 2018), and clinical researches on cervical cancer are ongoing. At present, some initial results have been achieved.

THEORETICAL BASIS FOR PD-1/PD-L1 INHIBITORS IN CERVICAL CANCER

The PD-1/PD-L1 axis is one of the most well-known immune-checkpoint pathways with a mechanism of immune evasion for cancer cells and thus inhibiting the immune response in various kinds of solid tumors, including cervical cancer Cancer Genome Atlas Research Network et al. (2017). In brief, PD-L1 expresses on the surface of cervical tumor cells, APCs and TILs, while the PD-1-positive cells were mostly identified as T cells in the stroma of cervical tumors. For the expression of PD-1 in the tumor stroma of cervical cancer, Meng et al. (2018) reported that 60.82% (59/97) of the patients exhibited PD-1 expression, while another study showed PD-1 expression in 46.97% (31/66) of the patients (Feng et al., 2018).

To date, numerous studies have investigated the expression of PD-L1 in cervical cancer (Yang et al., 2013; Chen et al., 2016). The expression of PD-L1 has been reported in 34.4–96% of cervical carcinoma tissues, while expression of PD-L1 in histologically normal cervical tissues was rarely found (Enwere et al., 2017). Opal Reddy et al. (2017) showed that PD-L1 expression was positive in 32 of 93 (34.4%) cervical carcinoma samples, subcategorically in 28 of 74 (37.8%) SCCs, 2 of 7 (28.6%) adenosquamous carcinomas, and 2 of 12 (16.7%) endocervical adenocarcinomas. In another study, PD-L1 expression was found in 96% of the samples (Enwere et al., 2017). Specifically, for cervical SCC, PD-L1 expression was found in 80% (56/70) cases (Mezache et al., 2015). In the TCGA database for cervical SCCs, the amplification or gain of PD-L1 was found in 28 of 129 (22%) cases (Dijkstra et al., 2016). In addition, PD-L1 can also be expressed on TILs, which plays a role in antitumor response inhibition. A study found that for cervical SCCs samples, the expression rates of PD-L1 on cancer cells and TILs were 59.1 and 47.0%, respectively (Feng et al., 2018). Collectively, these data suggest that both PD-L1 and PD-1 are widely expressed in cervical cancer tumor cells and stroma, providing potential therapeutic targets for PD-1/PD-L1 inhibitors.

Notoriously, persistent HPV infection is involved in the pathogenesis of cervical cancer and is related to its prognosis. Several teams have interrogated whether HPV infection could affect PD-L1 expression in cervical cancer and found that HPV positivity was positively correlated with increased PD-L1 expression (Mezache et al., 2015; Liu et al., 2017).

Considerable effort has been made to dissect the underlying mechanism of the association between HPV status and PD-L1 expression in HPV-related solid tumors, mainly HNSCC and cervical cancer. In HPV-HNSCCs, membranous expression of PD-L1 and significant increased levels of mRNA of IFN-γ were found in the tonsillar crypts, As tonsillar crypts witnesses the initial HPV infection, and IFN-γ induces PD-L1 expression, this

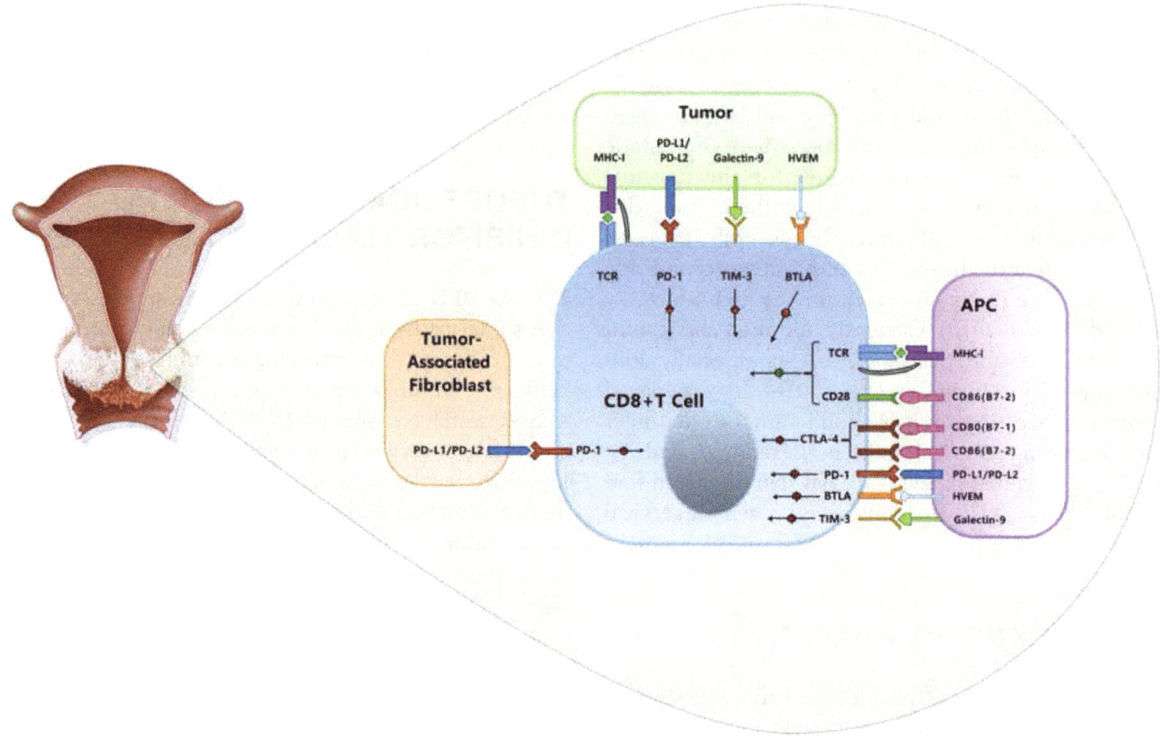

FIGURE 1 | The CTLA-4 and PD-1/PD-L1 pathways in cervical cancer.

evidence might support the role of the PD-1/PD-L1 interaction in creating an "immune-privileged" site for initial viral infection and subsequent adaptive immune resistance (Franzen et al., 2018). In another study, DNA methylation of PD-L1 was inversely correlated with PD-L1 mRNA expression ($p \leq 0.002$) and was further significantly associated with HPV infection in the TCGA cohort, indicating that DNA methylation of PD-L1 is associated with transcriptional silencing and HPV infection in HNSCCs (Balermpas et al., 2017). In cervical cancer, Qin et al. (2017) indicated that HPV-induced somatic mutations and a multitude of neoantigens, which played a crucial role in the inhibitory tumor microenvironment and could lead to notable alterations among checkpoint-related genes such as CTLA-4, PD-1, and PD-L1. Specifically, PD-L1 showed a positive correlation with ENO1, PRDM1, OVOL1, and MNT, all of which are related master regulators of HPV16 E6 and E7 (Qin et al., 2017). Of

TABLE 1 | The characteristics of the clinical application of monoclonal antibodies (mAbs) of immune checkpoint inhibitors in cervical cancer.

Target	Drug (trade name)	Antibody type	Formerly name	Manufacturer	Time to market (FDA)	Indications
CTLA-4	Ipilumumab (Yervoy)	IgG1	–	BMS	March, 2011	Melanoma, colorectal cancer, renal cell carcinoma
	Tremelimumab	IgG2	Ticilimumb, CP-675,206	Pfizer	–	Undergoing human trials has not attained approval for any
PD-1	Pembrolizumab (Keytruda)	IgG4	MK-3475 Lambrolizumab	MSD	September, 2014	Advanced melanoma, non-small cell lung cancer, Hodgkin's lymphoma, and head and neck SCC[1]
	Nivolumab (Opdivo)	IgG4	BMS-9365580 NO-4538	BMS	December, 2014	Metastatic melanoma, squamous non-small cell lung cancer, renal cell carcinoma
	Cemiplimab (REGN2810)	IgG4	–	Sanofi	September, 2018 (EMA[2])	squamous cell skin cancer (EMPOWER-CSCC 1)
PD-L1	Durvalumab (Imfiniz)	IgGIK	–	AstraZeneca	May, 2017	Bladder cancer, NSCLC[3]
	Atezolizumab (Tecentriq)	IgGI	–	Roche	April, 2016	Lung cancer, bladder cancer, advanced triple negative breast cancer

[1]SCC, squamous cell cancers; [2]EMA, European Medicines Agency; [3]NSCLC, non-small cell lung cancer.

TABLE 2 | Clinical research outcomes on PD-1/PD-L1 inhibitors in cervical cancer.

Study	Author	Study population (n)	Phase	Treatment arm(s)	Principal results	Toxicity	Significance
REGN2810	Papadopoulos et al., 2016	Advanced solid tumors	I	Cemiplimab	62.8% patients had disease control	No dose-limiting toxicities	Higher response rate when combined with radiation suggesting abscopal responses
Keynote 028	Frenel et al., 2017	Recurrent cervical cancer with PD-L1 positive tumors (24)	Ib	Pembrolizumab 10 mg/kg q2w	ORR[1] 17% (95% CI: 5–37%)	Grade=3 AE[2] including rash and proteinuria	Well-tolerated and active in cervical cancer
Keynote 158	Schellens et al., 2017	Recurrent cervical cancer with progression or intolerance to standard therapy (82)	II	Pembrolizumab 200 mg/kg q2w	Preliminary results: ORR[1] 17% (95% CI: 8–31%); patients with >27 weeks of follow up, ORR 27% (95% CI: 8–55%)	Grades 3–4 AE[2] included AST/ALT[3] elevation and pyrexia	Demonstrates activity in cervical cancer and increasing response with a longer duration of follow-up
Checkmate 358	Hollebecque et al., 2017	Recurrent or metastatic HPV[4]-related cancers (19)	I–II	Nivolumab 240 mg q2w	Preliminary results: ORR[1] 26% (95% CI: 9.1–51.2%) in cervical cancer patients	Grade 3–4 AE[2] included hyponatremia, syncope, diarrhea and hepatocellular injury	Durable responses demonstrated in cervical cancer patients, with at least 6 months duration

[1]*ORR, objective response rate;* [2]*AE, adverse event;* [3]*AST/ALT, aspartate transaminase/alanine transaminase;* [4]*HPV, human papillomavirus.*

note, a single-arm, phase II study investigated durvalumab in patients with recurrent/metastatic HNSCCs (n = 112) and found that HPV-positive patients had a higher response rate and better survival than that of the HPV-negative patients (Zandberg et al., 2018). Nevertheless, for cervical cancer, the association of HPV status and the efficacy of PD-1/PD-L1 inhibitors is not yet certain due to the paucity of available data.

Several studies have probed the role of PD-L1 expression in the prognosis and therapeutic efficacy of cervical cancer. These results separately proved that an increase in PD-L1 expression was positively associated with tumor metastasis (Yang et al., 2017), tumor progression (Hsu et al., 2018) and poor prognosis in cervical cancer (Heeren et al., 2016). In this regard, the negative relationship between HPV infection and the clinical outcomes of cervical cancer may be partially attributed to the PD-L1 expression induced by HPV infection (Yang et al., 2017). For patients with locally advanced cervical adenocarcinoma and adenosquamous carcinoma treated with CRT, the underexpression of PD-L1 was a prognostic factor for tumor relapse (p = 0.041), indicating that PD-L1 expression might be a novel biomarker for CRT outcome (Lai et al., 2017).

CLINICAL RESEARCH OUTCOMES OF PD-1/PD-L1 INHIBITORS IN CERVICAL CANCER

Since 2015, multiple clinical trials have been conducted to explore the application of PD-1/PD-L1 antibodies in cervical cancer. To date, four studies have yielded preliminary results (**Table 2**). Keynote 028 (a phase Ib study) and Keynote 158 (a phase II study) evaluated pembrolizumab at the dose of 10 mg/kg and 200 mg/kg, respectively, in recurrent, metastatic cervical cancer. In Keynote 028 (Frenel et al., 2017), 24 patients were enrolled, and the overall response rate (RECIST v1.1) was 17% (95% CI: 5 to 37%). In terms of toxicity, 5 patients experienced grade 3 AEs (NCI-CTCAE 3.0), while no grade 4 AEs was observed. In Keynote 158 (Schellens et al., 2017), 98 patients with recurrent or metastatic cervical cancer were enrolled. With a median follow-up time of 11.7 months, the ORR in 77 patients was 14.3% (95% CI: 7.4 to 24.1%), including 2.6% of the patients with CRs and 11.7% of patients with PRs, whereas no response was observed in patients without PD-L1 expression in tumor cells. The most frequent serious adverse reactions included anemia (7%), fistula (4.1%), hemorrhage (4.1%), and infection (4.1%). Based on Keynote 158, the FDA approved pembrolizumab on June 12, 2018, for advanced cervical cancer with disease progression during or after chemotherapy[1]. Checkmate 358 (Hollebecque et al., 2017) (phases I–II studies) adopted nivolumab (200 mg/kg q2w) for the treatment of recurrent, metastatic cervical cancer and resulted in an ORR of 26.3%. The disease control rate was 70.8%. The related grades 3–4 toxic effects included hyponatremia, syncope, diarrhea, and hepatocellular injury. From these three studies, pembrolizumab and nivolumab showed promising antitumor effects and were well-tolerated in patients with recurrent or metastatic cervical cancer. However, due to a limited follow-up time, PFS and OS were not reported. Additionally, the REGN2810 study (Papadopoulos et al., 2016), a phase I multicenter study, assessed REGN2810 (a PD-1 mAb) as a monotherapy and in combination with hfRT, in combination with cyclophosphamide (CTX) or with CTX + hfRT in patients with advanced solid tumors, including cervical cancer. This study adopted a dose escalation design, and as of February 2016, no dose-limiting

[1]https://www.fda.gov/Drugs/InformationOnDrugs/ApprovedDrugs/ucm610572.htm

TABLE 3 | Ongoing clinical research on PD-1/PD-L1 in cervical cancer.

Clinical trial code	Study	Study population (n)	Phase	Treatment arm(s)	Primary outcome measures	Secondary outcome measures
NCT02257528	Nivolumab in Treating Patients with Persistent, Recurrent, or Metastatic Cervical Cancer (NRG-GYO-02)	Recurrent or metastatic cervical cancer (25)	II	Nivolumab	ORR[1] [5 y]; AE[2] [100 d]	PFS[3] [5 y], OS[4] [5 y]
NCT03298893	Nivolumab in Association with Radiotherapy and Cisplatin in Locally Advanced Cervical Cancers Followed by Adjuvant Nivolumab for up to 6 Months (NiCOL)	Locally advanced cervical cancer (21)	III	Nivolumab	DLT[5] [11 w]	ORR[1] [2 m], PFS[3] [2 y], DFS[6] [2 y], SAE[7] [100 d], AE[2] [100 d], etc.
NCT03257267	Study of REGN2810 in Adults with Cervical Cancer (GOG 3016/ENGOT-cx9) (EMPOWER-Cervical)	Recurrent or metastatic platinum-refractory cervical cancer (436)	III	Cemiplimab (REGN2810)	OS[4] [32 m]	PFS[3] [32 m], ORR[1] [32 m], DOR[8] [32 m], Quality of life (QOL) [100 w]
NCT03104699	Phase 1/2 Study of AGEN2034 in Advanced Tumors and Cervical Cancer	Advanced cervical cancer (75)	I–II	AGEN2034	DLTs[5] [3 w], MTD[9] [1 y], BOR[10] [1 y]	Cmax[11] [1 y], AUC[12] [1 y], PFS[3] [1 y], DOR[8] [1 y], OS[4] [1 y]
NCT03518606	Metronomic Oral Vinorelbine Plus Anti-PD-L1/Anti-CTLA4 ImmunothErapy in Patients with Advanced Solid Tumors (MOVIE)	Advanced solid tumors (150) including cervical cancer	I–II	Durvalumab +Tremelimumab +metronomic Vinorelbine	Phase I: MTD[9] and RP2D[13] [9 m] Phase II: CBR[14] [24 m]	None
NCT03556839	Platinum Chemotherapy Plus Paclitaxel with Bevacizumab and Atezolizumab in Metastatic Carcinoma of the Cervix	Carcinoma of the cervix, stage IVB (404)	III	Atezolizumab	OS[4] [48 m]	PFS[3] [48 m], ORR[1] [48 m], DOR[8] [48 m], AE[2] [48 m], etc.
NCT01975831	A Phase 1 Study to Evaluate MEDI4736 in Combination with Tremelimumab	Solid tumors (106) including cervical cancer	I	MEDI4736 (Durvalumab)+Tremelimumab	AE[2] [1 y]	AUC[12], Cmax[11] [15 m], PFS[3] [15 m], OS[4] [15 m], etc.
NCT02914470	Pilot Study of Durvalumab and Vigil in Advanced Women's Cancers (PROLOG)	Solid tumors (12) including cervical cancer	I	Durvalumab and Vigil	Toxicity [30 d]	ORR[1] [120 m]
NCT02725489	Pilot Study of Durvalumab and Vigil in Advanced Women's Cancers	Solid tumors (15) including cervical cancer	II	Vigil+durvalumab	AEs[2] [90 d]	ORR[1] [12 m], Disease status [12 m], IFNγ-ELISPOT conversion rate [12 w]
NCT02921269	Atezolizumab and Bevacizumab in Treating Patients with Recurrent, Persistent, or Metastatic Cervical Cancer	Recurrent, persistent, or metastatic cervical cancer (22)	II	Atezolizumab +Bevac izumab	ORR[1] [2 y]	PFS[3] [2 y], OS[4] [2 y] AE[2] [30 d], PD-L1, etc.
NCT03635567	Efficacy and Safety Study of First-line Treatment with Pembrolizumab (MK-3475) Plus Chemotherapy Versus Placebo Plus Chemotherapy in Women with Persistent, Recurrent, or Metastati Cervical Cancer (MK-3475-826/KEYNOTE-826)	Cervical cancer (600) c	I–II	Pembrolizumab	PFS[3] [2y] OS[4] [2 y]	ORR[1] [2 y], DOR[8] [2 y], etc.
NCT03144466	A Study of Pembrolizumab And Platinum with Radiotherapy in Cervix Cancer (PAPAYA)	Cervical cancer (26)	I	Pembrolizum	MTD[9] [2 y] ab Efficacy [2 y]	OS[4] [2 y], PFS[3] [2 y], etc.
NCT03255252	Assessment Study to Evaluate Specific Immune Response in Locally Advanced Cervix Cancer After Radio-chemotherapy (IMMUVIX)	Cervical cancer (100)	II	Cisplatin	Expression of CD8+CD39+PD1+	Effect on 1-year DFS[6] of other putative biomarkers (CD73, CD39, PD1 and Tim3)
NCT03559803	A Prospective Study of Monitoring Immune Response in Locally Advanced Cervix Cancer(GHR002)	Cervical cancer(50)	Not appli cable	Cisplatin	PD-L1 [3w, 2 m]	PD1+CD4+T [3w, 2 m], PD1+CD8+T [3w, 2 m], TCR[3w, 2 m]

[1]ORR, objective response rate; [2]AE, adverse event; [3]PFS, progression-free survival; [4]OS, overall survival rate; [5]DLT, dose limiting toxicity; [6]DFS, disease-free survival; [7]SAE, serious adverse event; [8]DOR, duration of response; [9]MTD, maximum tolerated dose; [10]BOR, best overall response; [11]Cmax, maximum plasma concentration; [12]AUC, area under curve; [13]RP2D, phase II recommended dose; [14]CBR, clinical benefit response.

toxicity (DLT) was observed. The most common treatment-related AEs were fatigue (n = 14, 24.1%), arthralgia (n = 7, 12.1%), and nausea (n = 6, 10.3%). Additionally, 4 patients experienced grade $\geq$ 3 AEs. For 9/22 (40.9%) patients who received REGN2810 + hfRT and 2/21 (9.5%) patients who received REGN2810 monotherapy, they were determined to have partial/uPRs, suggesting that the treatment response was augmented by the addition of hfRT.

ONGOING CLINICAL RESEARCH ON PD-1/PD-L1 IN CERVICAL CANCER

As of September 2018, 11 clinical trials have been conducted, mainly in patients with persistent, recurrent, or metastatic cervical cancer, with only three studies on patients with locally advanced cervical cancer. Twenty to thirty cases were intended to be included in the majority of these studies, while there were only three studies (Keynote 826, GOG 3016/ENGOT-cx9, and NCT03556839) in which more than 200 cases were intended to be included. Except for the two studies (IMMUVIX, GHR002) aimed at exploring the immune status of PD-1/PD-L1 in patients with locally advanced cervical cancer, the remaining 12 studies all looked into the applicability of PD-1/PD-L1 inhibitors in cervical cancer. Of these 12 studies, there are 2 studies on nivolumab, 2 on pembrolizumab, 4 on durvalumab, 2 on atezolizumab, 1 on cemiplimab (REGN2810) and 1 on AGEN2034. For PD-1 inhibitors, the difference between the 2 studies on nivolumab is the study population. NRG-GYO-02 was conducted in patients with persistent, recurrent, or metastatic cervical cancer, while the NiCOL study enrolled more patients with locally advanced cervical cancer. The main difference between the two studies on pembrolizumab is that KEYNOTE-826 adopted pembrolizumab in combination with chemotherapy versus placebo, while PAPAYA mainly adopted pembrolizumab in combination with platinum and radiotherapy. The GOG 3016/ENGOT-cx9 (EMPOWER-Cervical) study is an important phase III clinical study to advance the clinical application of cemiplimab (REGN2810) in advanced cervical cancer. NCT03104699 is a phase I/II clinical study on AGEN2034, another PD-1 inhibitor, in advanced solid tumors that includes 75 cases of cervical cancer. In terms of treatment combinations, tremelimumab (a fully human mAb against CTLA-4), Vigil vaccine for cervical cancer, bevacizumab, and chemotherapy were paired with PD-1/PD-L1 inhibitors throughout these studies (**Table 3**).

CONCLUSION

Although there are a few studies suggesting the potential feasibility of PD-1/PD-L1 inhibitors for the treatment of cervical cancer, a consideration should be made for the clinical application of PD-1/PD-L1 inhibitors. The inadequate number of cases included and the insufficient follow-up time are the main defects of all the studies, leading to the unavailability of data regarding OS, PFS, AEs, drug resistance and the treatment mechanism as well. These data are very pivotal not only for obtaining a more convincing result, but also for guiding physicians to select the appropriate patients for PD-1/PD-L1 inhibitors.

Currently, most of these studies, including ongoing studies, are mostly limited to recurrent, persistent, metastatic cervical cancer, which accounts for only a minor portion of patients with cervical cancer. There are several future directions that can be given more attention. First, the latest evidence suggests a clinical benefit of PD-1/PD-L1 inhibitors as neoadjuvant therapy in lung cancer (Lommatzsch et al., 2018). For patients with early-stage cervical cancer, studies in a small sample size can be conducted to investigate PD-1/PD-L1 inhibitors with attempted surgical treatment or to prevent post-operative recurrence. Second, for patients with locally advanced cervical cancer who are not sensitive to CCRT or who relapse in the short term after initial treatment, PD-1/PD-L1 inhibitors may be a useful treatment, and we are looking forward to the research targeting this population. Third, for locally advanced cervical cancer patients, whether PD-1/PD-L1 inhibitors can achieve better therapeutic efficacy in tumors with higher PD-L1 expression before CCRT begins will provide a better understanding of the effects of these inhibitors. Finally, since PD-L1 expression is correlated with HPV status, more studies are warranted to provide further insights into the association of HPV status and the efficacy of PD-1/PD-L1 inhibitors in patients with cervical cancer. Combining the level of HPV DNA with the expression of PD-L1 may also provide a novel predictive biomarker of the efficacy of PD-1/PD-L1 inhibitors and the prognosis of patients with cervical cancer.

AUTHOR CONTRIBUTIONS

JX and YoL conceived the review. YuL and LYi searched the literature. YuL, LYi, LW, FY, ML, LY, and RT critically appraised the literature and wrote and all authors approved the final version of the manuscript.

FUNDING

This work was supported by National Natural Science Foundation of China (grants 81672982 and 81602670) and Sichuan Provincial Research Foundation for Basic Research (No. 18YYJC1284).

REFERENCES

1. Amatore, F., Gorvel, L., and Olive, D. (2018). Inducible co-stimulator (ICOS) as a potential therapeutic target for anti-cancer therapy. *Expert. Opin. Ther. Targets* 22, 343–351. doi: 10.1080/14728222.2018.1444753
2. Bagcchi, S. (2014). Pembrolizumab for treatment of refractory melanoma. *Lancet Oncol.* 15:e419. doi: 10.1016/S1470-2045(14)70348-1
3. Balermpas, P., Martin, D., Wieland, U., Rave-Frank, M., Strebhardt, K., Rodel, C., et al. (2017). Human papilloma virus load and PD-1/

PD-L1, CD8(+) and FOXP3 in anal cancer patients treated with chemoradiotherapy: rationale for immunotherapy. *Oncoimmunology* 6:e1288331. doi: 10.1080/2162402X.2017. 1288331

4. Borcoman, E., and Le Tourneau, C. (2017). Pembrolizumab in cervical cancer: latest evidence and clinical usefulness. *Ther. Adv. Med. Oncol.* 9, 431–439. doi: 10.1177/1758834017708742
5. Boussios, S., Seraj, E., Zarkavelis, G., Petrakis, D., Kollas, A., Kafantari, A., et al. (2016). Management of patients with recurrent/advanced cervical cancer beyond first line platinum regimens: where do we stand? A literature review. *Crit. Rev. Oncol. Hematol.* 108, 164–174. doi: 10.1016/j.critrevonc.2016.11.006
6. Boussiotis, V. A. (2016). Molecular and biochemical aspects of the PD-1 checkpoint pathway. *N. Engl. J. Med.* 375, 1767–1778. doi: 10.1056/NEJMra1514296
7. Bray, F., Ferlay, J., Soerjomataram, I., Siegel, R. L., Torre, L. A., and Jemal, A. (2018). Global cancer statistics 2018: globocan estimates of incidence and mortality worldwide for 36 cancers in 185 countries. *CA Cancer J. Clin.* 68, 394–424. doi: 10.3322/caac.21492
8. Cancer Genome Atlas Research Network, Albert Einstein College of Medicine, Analytical Biological Services, Barretos Cancer Hospital, Baylor College of Medicine, Beckman Research Institute of City of Hope, et al. (2017). Integrated genomic and molecular characterization of cervical cancer. *Nature* 543, 378–384. doi: 10.1038/nature21386
9. Chen, J., Gu, W., Yang, L., Chen, C., Shao, R., Xu, K., et al. (2015). Nanotechnology in the management of cervical cancer. *Rev. Med. Virol.* 25(Suppl. 1), 72–83. doi: 10.1002/rmv.1825
10. Chen, Z., Pang, N., Du, R., Zhu, Y., Fan, L., Cai, D., et al. (2016). Elevated expression of programmed death-1 and programmed death ligand-1 negatively regulates immune response against cervical cancer cells. *Med. Inflamm.* 2016:6891482. doi: 10.1155/2016/6891482
11. Compte, M., Harwood, S. L., Munoz, I. G., Navarro, R., Zonca, M., Perez-Chacon, G., et al. (2018). A tumor-targeted trimeric 4-1BB-agonistic antibody induces potent anti-tumor immunity without systemic toxicity. *Nat. Commun.* 9:4809. doi: 10.1038/s41467-018-07195-w
12. Constantinidou, A., Alifieris, C., and Trafalis, D. T. (2018). Targeting programmed cell death -1 (PD-1) and ligand (PD-L1): a new era in cancer active immunotherapy. *Pharmacol. Ther.* 18, 30173–30176. doi: 10.1016/j.pharmthera.2018.09.008
13. Dijkstra, K. K., Voabil, P., Schumacher, T. N., and Voest, E. E. (2016). Genomics- and transcriptomics-based patient selection for cancer treatment with immune checkpoint inhibitors: a review. *JAMA Oncol.* 2, 1490–1495. doi: 10.1001/jamaoncol.2016.2214
14. Enwere, E. K., Kornaga, E. N., Dean, M., Koulis, T. A., Phan, T., Kalantarian, M., et al. (2017). Expression of PD-L1 and presence of CD8-positive T cells in pre treatment specimens of locally advanced cervical cancer. *Mod. Pathol.* 30, 577–586. doi: 10.1038/modpathol.2016.221
15. Feng, Y. C., Ji, W. L., Yue, N., Huang, Y. C., and Ma, X. M. (2018). The relationship between the PD-1/PD-L1 pathway and DNA mismatch repair in cervical cancer and its clinical significance. *Cancer Manag. Res.* 10, 105–113. doi: 10.2147/CMAR.S152232
16. Fife, B. T., and Bluestone, J. A. (2008). Control of peripheral T-cell tolerance and autoimmunity via the CTLA-4 and PD-1 pathways. *Immunol. Rev.* 224, 166–182. doi: 10.1111/j.1600-065X.2008.00662.x
17. Franzen, A., Vogt, T. J., Muller, T., Dietrich, J., Schrock, A., Golletz, C., et al. (2018). PD-L1 (CD274) and PD-L2 (PDCD1LG2) promoter methylation is associated with HPV infection and transcriptional repression in head and neck squamous cell carcinomas. *Oncotarget* 9, 641–650. doi: 10.18632/oncotarget. 23080
18. Frenel, J. S., Le Tourneau, C., O'neil, B., Ott, P. A., Piha-Paul, S. A., Gomez-Roca, C., et al. (2017). Safety and efficacy of pembrolizumab in advanced, programmed death ligand 1-positive cervical cancer: results from the phase Ib KEYNOTE-028 trial. *J. Clin. Oncol.* 35, 4035–4041. doi: 10.1200/JCO.2017.74. 5471
19. Gettinger, S., Horn, L., Jackman, D., Spigel, D., Antonia, S., Hellmann, M., et al. (2018). Five-year follow-up of nivolumab in previously treated advanced non- small-cell lung cancer: results from the CA209-003 study. *J. Clin. Oncol.* 36, 1675–1684. doi: 10.1200/JCO.2017.77.0412
20. Goodman, A. (2015). HPV testing as a screen for cervical cancer. *BMJ* 350:h2372. doi: 10.1136/bmj.h2372
21. Gorris, M. A. J., Halilovic, A., and Rabold, K. (2018). Eight-color multiplex immunohistochemistry for simultaneous detection of multiple immune checkpoint molecules within the tumor microenvironment. *J. Immunol.* 200, 347–354. doi: 10.4049/jimmunol.1701262
22. Guitarte, C., Alagkiozidis, I., Mize, B., Stevens, E., Salame, G., and Lee, Y. C. (2014). Glassy cell carcinoma of the cervix: a systematic review and meta-analysis. *Gynecol. Oncol.* 133, 186–191. doi: 10.1016/j.ygyno.2014.01.048
23. Heeren, A. M., Punt, S., Bleeker, M. C., Gaarenstroom, K. N., Van Der Velden, J., Kenter, G. G., et al. (2016). Prognostic effect of different PD-L1 expression patterns in squamous cell carcinoma and adenocarcinoma of the cervix. *Mod. Pathol.* 29, 753–763. doi: 10.1038/modpathol.2016.64
24. Hodi, F. S., O'day, S. J., Mcdermott, D. F., Weber, R. W., Sosman, J. A., Haanen, J. B., et al. (2010). Improved survival with ipilimumab in patients with metastatic melanoma. *N. Engl. J. Med.* 363, 711–723. doi: 10.1056/NEJMoa1003466
25. Hollebecque, A., Meyer, T., Moore, K. N., Machiels, J.-P. H., De Greve, J., López- Picazo, J. M., et al. (2017). An open-label, multicohort, phase I/II study of nivolumab in patients with virus-associated tumors (CheckMate 358): efficacy and safety in recurrent or metastatic (R/M) cervical, vaginal, and vulvar cancers. *J. Clin. Oncol.* 35:5504. doi: 10.1200/JCO.2017.35.15_suppl.5504
26. Hsu, P. C., Li, S. H., and Yang, C. T. (2018). Recurrent pneumonitis induced by atezolizumab (anti-programmed death ligand 1) in NSCLC patients who previously experienced anti-programmed death 1 immunotherapy-related pneumonitis. *J. Thorac. Oncol.* 13, e227–e230. doi: 10.1016/j.jtho.2018.06.022
27. Julia, E. P., Amante, A., Pampena, M. B., Mordoh, J., and Levy, E. M. (2018). Avelumab, an IgG1 anti-PD-L1 immune checkpoint inhibitor, triggers NK cell-mediated cytotoxicity and cytokine production against triple negative breast cancer cells. *Front. Immunol.* 9:2140. doi: 10.3389/fimmu.2018.02140
28. Kurup, S. P., Obeng-Adjei, N., Anthony, S. M., Traore, B., Doumbo, O. K., Butler, N. S., et al. (2017). Regulatory T cells impede acute and long-term immunity to blood-stage malaria through CTLA-4. *Nat. Med.* 23, 1220–1225. doi: 10.1038/nm.4395
29. Lai, Y. L., Chen, L. C., Huang, C. Y., Chiang, S. F., Liang, J. A., Chao, K. S. C., et al. (2017). PD-L1 as the prognostic immune biomarker for predicting the relapse of locally advanced cervical adenocarcinoma and adenosquamous carcinoma treated with definitive chemoradiation therapy. *Int. J. Radiat. Oncol. Biol. Phys.* 99, E299–E300. doi: 10.1016/j.ijrobp.2017.06.1318
30. Le Tourneau, C., Hoimes, C., Zarwan, C., Wong, D. J., Bauer, S., Claus, R., et al. (2018). Avelumab in patients with previously treated metastatic adrenocortical carcinoma: phase 1b results from the JAVELIN solid tumor trial. *J. Immunother. Cancer* 6:111. doi: 10.1186/s40425-018-0424-9
31. Lheureux, S., Butler, M. O., Clarke, B., Cristea, M. C., Martin, L. P., Tonkin, K., et al. (2018). Association of ipilimumab with safety and antitumor activity in women with metastatic or recurrent human papillomavirus-related cervical carcinoma. *JAMA Oncol.* 4:e173776. doi: 10.1001/jamaoncol.2017.3776
32. Lim, M., Xia, Y., Bettegowda, C., and Weller, M. (2018). Current state of immunotherapy for glioblastoma. *Nat. Rev. Clin. Oncol.* 15, 422–442. doi: 10. 1038/s41571-018-0003-5
33. Liu, C., Lu, J., Tian, H., Du, W., Zhao, L., Feng, J., et al. (2017). Increased expression of PDL1 by the human papillomavirus 16 E7 oncoprotein inhibits anticancer immunity. *Mol. Med. Rep.* 15, 1063–1070. doi: 10.3892/mmr.2017.6102
34. Liu, Y. L., and Zamarin, D. (2018). Combination immune checkpoint blockade strategies to maximize immune response in gynecological cancers. *Curr. Oncol. Rep.* 20:94. doi: 10.1007/s11912-018-0740-8
35. Lommatzsch, M., Bratke, K., and Stoll, P. (2018). Neoadjuvant PD-1 blockade in resectable lung cancer. *N. Engl. J. Med.* 379:e14. doi: 10.1056/NEJMc1808251
36. Long, G. V., Tykodi, S. S., Schneider, J. G., Garbe, C., Gravis, G., Rashford, M., et al. (2018). Assessment of nivolumab exposure and clinical safety of 480 mg every 4 weeks flat-dosing schedule in patients with cancer. *Ann. Oncol.* 29, 2208–2213. doi: 10.1093/annonc/mdy408
37. Meng, Y., Liang, H., Hu, J., Liu, S., Hao, X., Wong, M. S. K., et al. (2018). PD-L1 Expression correlates with tumor infiltrating lymphocytes and response to neoadjuvant chemotherapy in cervical cancer. *J. Cancer* 9, 2938–2945. doi: 10.7150/jca.22532
38. Mezache, L., Paniccia, B., Nyinawabera, A., and Nuovo, G. J. (2015). Enhanced expression of PD L1 in cervical intraepithelial neoplasia and cervical cancers. *Mod. Pathol.* 28, 1594–1602. doi: 10.1038/modpathol.2015.108
39. Minion, L. E., and Tewari, K. S. (2018). Cervical cancer - state of the science: from angiogenesis blockade to checkpoint inhibition. *Gynecol. Oncol.* 148, 609–621. doi: 10.1016/j.ygyno.2018.01.009

40. Monk, B. J., Sill, M. W., Mcmeekin, D. S., Cohn, D. E., Ramondetta, L. M., Boardman, C. H., et al. (2009). Phase III trial of four cisplatin-containing doublet combinations in stage IVB, recurrent, or persistent cervical carcinoma: a gynecologic oncology group study. *J. Clin. Oncol.* 27, 4649–4655. doi: 10.1200/JCO.2009.21.8909
41. Papadopoulos, K. P., Crittenden, M. R., Johnson, M. L., Lockhart, A. C., Moore, K. N., and Falchook, G. S. (2016). A first-in-human study of REGN2810, a monoclonal, fully human antibody to programmed death-1 (PD-1), in combination with immunomodulators including hypofractionaed radiotherapy (hfRT). *J. Clin. Oncol.* 34:3024. doi: 10.1200/JCO.2016.34.15_suppl.3024
42. Pardoll, D. M. (2012). The blockade of immune checkpoints in cancer immunotherapy. *Nat. Rev. Cancer* 12, 252–264. doi: 10.1038/nrc3239
43. Paz-Ares, L., Luft, A., Vicente, D., Tafreshi, A., Gumus, M., Mazieres, J., et al. (2018). Pembrolizumab plus chemotherapy for squamous non-small- cell lung cancer. *N. Engl. J. Med.* 379, 2040–2051. doi: 10.1056/NEJMoa181 0865
44. Polesso, F., Weinberg, A., and Moran, A. E. (2018). Late stage tumor regression after PD-L1 blockade with a concurrent OX40 agonist. *Cancer Immunol. Res.* doi: 10.1158/2326-6066.CIR-18-0222 [Epub ahead of print].
45. Qin, Y., Ekmekcioglu, S., Forget, M. A., Szekvolgyi, L., Hwu, P., Grimm, E. A., et al. (2017). Cervical cancer neoantigen landscape and immune activity is associated with human papillomavirus master regulators. *Front. Immunol.* 8:689. doi: 10. 3389/fimmu.2017.00689
46. Raedler, L. A. (2015). Opdivo (Nivolumab): second PD-1 inhibitor receives FDA approval for unresectable or metastatic melanoma. *Am. Health Drug Benefits* 8, 180–183.
47. Reddy, O. L., Shintaku, P. I., and Moatamed, N. A. (2017). Programmed death-ligand 1 (PD-L1) is expressed in a significant number of the uterine cervical carcinomas. *Diagn. Pathol.* 12:45. doi: 10.1186/s13000-017-0631-6
48. Sahasrabuddhe, V. V., Parham, G. P., Mwanahamuntu, M. H., and Vermund, S. H. (2012). Cervical cancer prevention in low- and middle-income countries: feasible, affordable, essential. *Cancer Prevent. Res.* 5, 11–17. doi: 10.1158/1940-6207.CAPR-11-0540
49. Schellens, J. H. M., Marabelle, A., Zeigenfuss, S., Ding, J., Pruitt, S. K., and Chung, H. C. (2017). Pembrolizumab for previously treated advanced cervical squamous cell cancer:preliminary results from the phase 2 KEYNOTE-158 study. *J. Clin. Oncol.* 35:5514. doi: 10.1200/JCO.2017.35.15_suppl.5514
50. Schumacher, T. N., and Schreiber, R. D. (2015). Neoantigens in cancer immunotherapy. *Science* 348, 69–74. doi: 10.1126/science.aaa4971
51. Sidaway, P. (2018). Cemiplimab effective in cutaneous SCC. *Nat. Rev. Clin. Oncol.* 15:472. doi: 10.1038/s41571-018-0056-5
52. Siu, L. L., Even, C., Mesia, R., Remenar, E., Daste, A., Delord, J. P., et al. (2018). Safety and efficacy of durvalumab with or without tremelimumab in patients with PD-L1-low/negative recurrent or metastatic HNSCC: the phase 2 CONDOR randomized clinical trial. *JAMA Oncol.* doi: 10.1001/jamaoncol. 2018.4628[Epub ahead of print].
53. Tewari, K. S., Sill, M. W., Long, H. J. III, Penson, R. T., Huang, H., Ramondetta, L. M., et al. (2014). Improved survival with bevacizumab in advanced cervical cancer. *N. Engl. J. Med.* 370, 734–743. doi: 10.1056/NEJMoa1309748
54. Tewari, K. S., Sill, M. W., Penson, R. T., Huang, H., Ramondetta, L. M., Landrum, L. M., et al. (2017). Bevacizumab for advanced cervical cancer: final overall survival and adverse event analysis of a randomised, controlled, open-label, phase 3 trial (gynecologic oncology group 240). *Lancet* 390, 1654–1663. doi: 10.1016/S0140-6736(17)31607-0
55. Wang, J., Chmielowski, B., Pellissier, J., Xu, R., Stevinson, K., and Liu, F. X. (2017). Cost-Effectiveness of pembrolizumab versus ipilimumab in ipilimumab-naive patients with advanced melanoma in the United States. *J. Manag. Care Spec. Pharm.* 23, 184–194. doi: 10.18553/jmcp.2017.23.2.184
56. Yang, W., Lu, Y. P., Yang, Y. Z., Kang, J. R., Jin, Y. D., and Wang, H. W. (2017). Expressions of programmed death (PD)-1 and PD-1 ligand (PD-L1) in cervical intraepithelial neoplasia and cervical squamous cell carcinomas are of prognostic value and associated with human papillomavirus status. *J. Obstet. Gynaecol. Res.* 43, 1602–1612. doi: 10.1111/jog.13411
57. Yang, W., Song, Y., Lu, Y. L., Sun, J. Z., and Wang, H. W. (2013). Increased expression of programmed death (PD)-1 and its ligand PD-L1 correlates with impaired cell-mediated immunity in high-risk human papillomavirus-related cervical intraepithelial neoplasia. *Immunology* 139, 513–522. doi: 10.1111/imm. 12101
58. Zandberg, D. P., Algazi, A. P., Jimeno, A., Good, J. S., Fayette, J., Bouganim, N., et al. (2018). Durvalumab for recurrent or metastatic head and neck squamous cell carcinoma: results from a single-arm, phase II study in patients with $> / =$ 25% tumour cell PD-L1 expression who have progressed on platinum- based chemotherapy. *Eur. J. Cancer* 107, 142–152. doi: 10.1016/j.ejca.2018. 11.015
59. Zhang, S., and Li, W. (2018). The effort in exploration of a definitive predictive factor from PD-1/PD-L1 blockade in advanced or metastatic urothelial cancer. *J. Clin. Oncol.* 36, 3056–3057. doi: 10.1200/JCO.2018.79.1400

19

Inhibitors of Human ABCG2: From Technical Background to Recent Updates with Clinical Implications

Yu Toyoda, Tappei Takada and Hiroshi Suzuki*

Department of Pharmacy, The University of Tokyo Hospital, Faculty of Medicine, The University of Tokyo, Tokyo, Japan

Correspondence:
Tappei Takada
tappei-tky@umin.ac.jp

The ATP-binding cassette transporter G2 (ABCG2; also known as breast cancer resistance protein, BCRP) has been suggested to be involved in clinical multidrug resistance (MDR) in cancer like other ABC transporters such as ABCB1 (*P*-glycoprotein). As an efflux pump exhibiting a broad substrate specificity localized on cellular plasma membrane, ABCG2 excretes a variety of endogenous and exogenous substrates including chemotherapeutic agents, such as mitoxantrone and several tyrosine kinase inhibitors. Moreover, in the normal tissues, ABCG2 is expressed on the apical membranes and plays a pivotal role in tissue protection against various xenobiotics. For this reason, ABCG2 is recognized to be an important determinant of the pharmacokinetic characteristics of its substrate drugs. Although the clinical relevance of reversing the ABCG2-mediated MDR has been inconclusive, an appropriate modulation of ABCG2 function during chemotherapy should logically enhance the efficacy of anti-cancer agents by overcoming the MDR phenotype and/or improving their pharmacokinetics. To confirm this possibility, considerable efforts have been devoted to developing ABCG2 inhibitors, although there is no clinically available substance for this purpose. As a clue for addressing this issue, this mini-review provides integrated information covering the technical backgrounds necessary to evaluate the ABCG2 inhibitory effects on the target compounds and a current update on the ABCG2 inhibitors. This essentially includes our recent findings, as we serendipitously identified febuxostat, a well-used agent for hyperuricemia as a strong ABCG2 inhibitor, that possesses some promising potentials. We hope that an overview described here will add value to further studies involving in the multidrug transporters.

Keywords: BCRP, cancer chemotherapy, drug repurposing, febuxostat, Ko143, multidrug resistance, tumor lysis syndrome, vesicle transport

INTRODUCTION

Two decades ago, the ABC transporter G2 (ABCG2) was discovered in drug-resistant cancer cells and human placenta (Allikmets et al., 1998; Doyle et al., 1998; Miyake et al., 1999). Thereafter, many studies were conducted to determine the role of ABCG2 in developing MDR in cancer. Moreover, in the first decade, *in vivo* studies using *Abcg2* knockout mice (Jonker et al., 2002)

Abbreviations: ABC, ATP-binding cassette; BBB, blood–brain barrier; CML, chronic myeloid leukemia; EC_{50}, half-maximal effective concentration; FTC, fumitremorgin C; IC_{50}, half-maximal inhibitory concentration; MDR, multidrug resistance; TKI, tyrosine kinase inhibitor, TLS, tumor lysis syndrome.

coupled with biochemical characterizations revealed the importance of ABCG2 in the biological defense mechanisms against xenobiotics (Vlaming et al., 2009). Indeed, ABCG2—a 655-amino acid protein working as a homodimer on cellular plasma membranes (Robey et al., 2009)—is expressed not only in cancer cells but also in several normal tissues, such as brush border membranes of epithelium in the intestine and of proximal tubules in the kidney, bile canalicular membranes of the hepatocytes in the liver, luminal membranes of the mammary gland epithelium, and blood-facing membranes of the endothelial cells forming the BBB. In these tissues ABCG2 plays a pivotal role in the extrusion of various endogenous and exogenous substrates including drugs (Mizuno et al., 2004, 2007; Adachi et al., 2005; Hirano et al., 2005; Jonker et al., 2005; Ando et al., 2007). Hence, this transporter is recognized as an important determinant of the pharmacokinetic characteristics profiles of various drugs (Giacomini et al., 2010).

In the next decade, after identifying ABCG2 as a physiologically important urate transporter, a positive relationship between ABCG2 dysfunction and increased risk of human diseases, such as gout and hyperuricemia was revealed (Matsuo et al., 2009; Woodward et al., 2009; Ichida et al., 2012; Higashino et al., 2017). In addition to the sulfate conjugates of endogenous steroids (Suzuki et al., 2003) and porphyrins (Zhou et al., 2005; Robey et al., 2009), phytoestrogen sulfate conjugates (van de Wetering and Sapthu, 2012) and a uremic toxin indoxyl sulfate (Takada et al., 2018) were added in the growing list of ABCG2 substrates. Contrary to these advances in understanding the pathophysiological importance of ABCG2, the clinical relevance of reversing ABCG2-mediated MDR has been inconclusive (Robey et al., 2018).

ABCG2 overexpression can render the cancer cells resistant to the ABCG2 substrate chemotherapy agents, such as mitoxantrone, doxorubicin, SN-38, and several TKIs. To the best of our knowledge, no published clinical trial has ever succeeded in reversing the ABCG2-mediated MDR. This is because, despite a lot of efforts in ABCG2 inhibitor development, chemical knock-out/down of ABCG2 in clinical situations has not been achieved yet due to the lack of an appropriate candidate molecule. We herein describe some well-used experimental systems to evaluate the ABCG2 inhibitory activity, followed by a recent update on the ABCG2 inhibitors that includes a potent substance, febuxostat.

TECHNICAL BACKGROUND FOR FUNCTIONAL VALIDATION

Various experimental models are available to examine the functions of the ABC transporters. Mainly focusing on ABCG2, with a current update this section introduces some *in vitro* and *in vivo* models that have been used in ABC transporter field. Broadly, the *in vitro* models are classified into two types, namely membrane-based systems and cell-based systems (**Figure 1**).

Plasma Membrane Vesicle-Based Methods

Preparation of Plasma Membrane Vesicles

In mammals, most of the ABC transporters are membrane proteins and work as an efflux pump involved in the transport of its substrates from the cytosol, either to the extracellular space or into organelles by an ATP-dependent manner. Therefore, isolation of the target ABC protein-enriched cell membrane is the first step for biochemical analyses. For ABCG2, sucrose density gradient ultracentrifugation for the isolation of plasma membrane fraction is generally employed to prepare plasma membrane vesicles from ABCG2-expressing cells (related notes are inscribed in the legend of **Figure 1**). For this purpose, not only mammalian cells but also insect cells [e.g., baculovirus-infected Sf9 cells (Saito et al., 2006)] could be used as host cells. Nonetheless, for easy and convenient preparation of ABCG2-expressing cells, we here recommend plasmid-based overexpression in non-polarized cells exhibiting high transfection efficiency, such as HEK293 cells (Miyata et al., 2016).

Vesicle Transport Assay

Vesicle transport assay is a well-established *in vitro* method employed to quantitatively evaluate ABC transporter function. The presence of ATP-dependent active transport across the cell membrane was directly proved using this method (Ishikawa, 1989). In this assay, ATP-regeneration components—enough amount of creatine phosphate and creatine kinase—are employed to maintain ATP levels in the reaction mixtures during prolonged incubation, and AMP is used as an alternative of ATP for the ATP-deficient controls. After incubation for the transport reaction, the plasma membrane vesicles are washed by filtration and then the intravesicularly accumulated substances are detected. To make this process more convenient and sensitive, radiolabeled or fluorescent substrates are usually used; alternatively, mass spectrometry is used (Toyoda et al., 2016; Takada et al., 2018). With ABCG2, [^{14}C]-urate (Miyata et al., 2016; Stiburkova et al., 2016; Higashino et al., 2017) and [^{3}H]-estrone sulfate (Suzuki et al., 2003) are well-used radiolabeled substrates that exhibit comparatively lower background signal for the quantitative detection due to their relatively hydrophilic properties. Additionally, non-radiolabeled experiments are conducted by the combined use of hematoporphyrin (a fluorescent ABCG2 substrate) and gel filtration techniques (Tamura et al., 2006).

ATPase Assay

Since ABC protein is driven by the free energy of ATP hydrolysis, ATPase activity is recognized as an indicator of the substrate transport. In this assay, the release of inorganic phosphate from ATP coupled with the transport of substrates is estimated using a colorimetric method, such as malachite green procedure (Baykov et al., 1988). This catalytic assay is relatively convenient for estimating the activity of some ABC proteins that prefer lipophilic compounds as their substrates because the non-specifically adsorbed substrates on the vesicles interfere with the measurement of direct transport. Considering that ABCB1 activity has been well

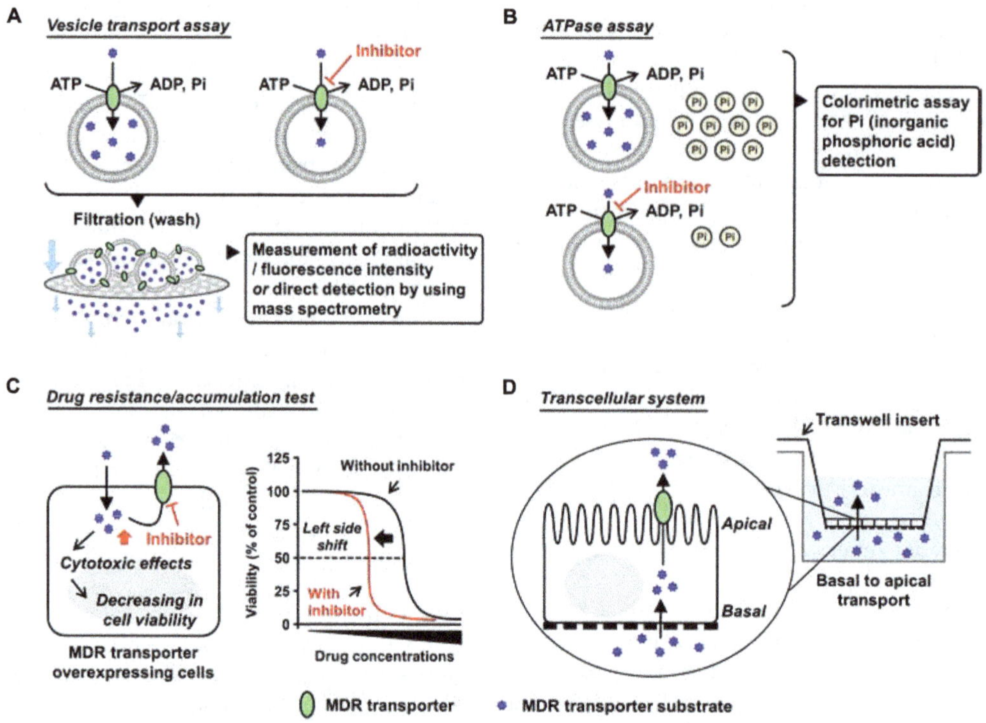

FIGURE 1 | Schematic illustrations of each *in vitro* assay. Generally used *in vitro* models which are classified into membrane-based systems and cell-based systems (Hegedus et al., 2009) are shown. In the former systems, investigators can use culture cell-derived plasma membrane vesicles or reconstituted proteoliposomes as described in the main text. In the latter systems, aside from a couple of exceptions using *Xenopus laevis* oocytes (Nakanishi et al., 2003; Woodward et al., 2009), mammalian cells expressing target ABC protein are generally used. **(A,B)** Plasma membrane vesicle- or proteoliposome-based methods: vesicle transport assay **(A)** and ATPase assay **(B)**. Both plasma membrane vesicles and reconstituted proteoliposomes are applicable to the vesicle transport assay and the ATPase assay. Of note, the final step of the vesicle preparation—gentle homogenization of isolated membrane fraction—is empirically important for the formation of inside-out plasma membrane vesicles, whose outer faces are the cytoplasmic aspects of the parent membranes. Although the resulting plasma membrane vesicles are the mixture of inside-out and right-side-out components, without any separation of the right-side-out vesicles they are generally stored at –80°C and subjected to further assays. This is because that in these *in vitro* assays, only ABC proteins embedded in the inside-out vesicles have their ABCs outside of the vesicles and can use ATP in the reaction mixture for their transport function. In other words, the ABC proteins in the right-side-out vesicles cannot work due to an inaccessibility of the ABCs with ATP. Additionally, ABCG2-enriched plasma membrane vesicles are used for a biochemical analysis to study interactions of candidate chemicals with ABCG2 at the substrate-binding sites, known as the photoaffinity labeling of ABCG2 with $[^{125}I]$-iodoarylazido-prazosin (Shukla et al., 2006). **(C,D)** Cell-based methods: drug resistance/accumulation test **(C)** and transcellular system **(D)**. MDR, multidrug resistance.

studied based on the ATPase assay, this method will be appropriate when investigators would need to compare the inhibitory effects of target compounds on ABCB1 and ABCG2 (Zhang et al., 2016; Guo et al., 2018). Nonetheless, since the ATPase assay does not evaluate the direct transport, regarding ABCG2, we recommend the vesicle transport assay for more precise evaluation.

Proteoliposome-Based Methods

An artificial lipid membrane system characterized by the reconstitution of purified ABC protein into proteoliposomes (Ambudkar et al., 1998; Jackson et al., 2018) is also a powerful technique. The ABC protein-contained proteoliposomes can be used as an alternative to the plasma membrane vesicles, and their detailed preparation methods are described previously (Geertsma et al., 2008). Additionally, this approach serves as the first choice in the functional studies involving the ABC proteins localized on the organelle membrane (Okamoto et al., 2018).

Cell-Based Methods

Drug Resistance/Accumulation Test

The cells overexpressing MDR machinery show lower sensitivity against its substrate drugs exhibiting cytotoxic or anti-proliferative effects compared to their parent cells, indicating that the ABC protein-expressing cells have higher half maximal effective concentration (EC_{50}) values for cytotoxic transporter substrates. In such situations, co-treatment of the transporter inhibitors with the substrate decreases the EC_{50} values, which is depicted as a left-side shift of cell viability curve in the cytotoxic assay. Additionally, if fluorescence transporter substrates are available, flow cytometry analyses addressing their intracellular accumulation will be useful for inhibitor screening (Murakami et al., 2017; Wu et al., 2017).

Transcellular System

To investigate the transcellular transport of substances, monolayer culture of polarized cells expressing target transporter(s) in Transwell® inserts system has been used (Hegedus et al.,

2009). For instance, using double-transfected Madin-Darby canine kidney II cells overexpressing both organic anion-transporting polypeptide 1B1 (OATP1B1, a basal uptake transporter) and ABCG2 (an apical efflux transporter), an earlier study has observed an enhanced vectorial transport of [^{3}H]estrone sulfate—an ABCG2 substrate that cannot passively penetrate the plasma membrane—from the basal to the apical side (Matsushima et al., 2005). A similar strategy employing ABCG2-expressing polarized cells was used for *in vitro* studies investigating the active secretion of drugs and toxins into milk via ABCG2 (Wassermann et al., 2013; Ito et al., 2015). Of note, in this transcellular system, endogenous transporters and metabolic reactions in the cells may affect apparent transport activities of target transporters.

In vivo Evaluation Methods

Xenograft Models

Athymic nude mice models with MDR-xenografts have been used to test whether co-administration of a potential MDR inhibitor with an anti-cancer agent can reverse the MDR phenotype (Tiwari et al., 2013; Zhang et al., 2017, 2018). In such models, the obtained results could be affected by the difference in the origin of the transplanted cancer cells. This concern might be important while xenograft models are studied.

Focusing on Pharmacokinetic Characteristics

To examine the *in vivo* effects of different chemicals on the target ABC transporter, its pharmacokinetic role has been focused (Robey et al., 2018). With ABCG2, the pharmacokinetic parameters related to the intestinal absorption or the brain distribution of ABCG2 substrate drugs will be good indicators for ABCG2 activity *in vivo*. For example, pre-dosing of enough quantity of ABCG2 inhibitors increased the bioavailability of sulphasalazine—an ABCG2 substrate—in wild-type mice. This was, however, not observed in *Abcg2*-knockout mice, suggesting the *in vivo* inhibition of Abcg2 (Kusuhara et al., 2012; Miyata et al., 2016). Interestingly, the utility of a combination of brain-specific firefly luciferase transgenic mice and D-luciferin, a chemiluminescent luciferase substrate transported by ABCG2 (Zhang et al., 2007) to investigate the *in vivo* inhibitory effects of test compounds on ABCG2 in the BBB was reported (Bakhsheshian et al., 2016). Further methodological progress will aid evaluation of *in vivo* ABCG2 function.

Structure-Based *in silico* Approaches

A main approach to abolish MDR is to discover specific inhibitors of the drug-efflux pump. For this purpose, quantitative structure-activity relationship (QSAR) analysis among the series of compounds can serve for the design of lead inhibitors (Nicolle et al., 2009; Ishikawa et al., 2012; Marighetti et al., 2013; Shukla et al., 2014). With ABCG2, since three-dimensional structures of this protein determined by cryo-electron microscopy (EM) were very recently presented (Taylor et al., 2017; Jackson et al., 2018), a deeper understanding of the chemicals–ABCG2 interactions will be achieved as described below.

HISTORY AND RECENT UPDATE OF THE ABCG2 INHIBITORS

As a MDR machinery in cancer cells and an important drug gatekeeper in tissues like the intestine and the brain, ABCG2 is involved in the efficacy of cancer chemotherapy in patients treated with ABCG2 substrate anti-cancer drugs. To achieve appropriate modulation of ABCG2 by small molecules, the inhibitory potency of various compounds against ABCG2 activity has been extensively evaluated. In this section, we highlight the history and recent update of ABCG2 inhibitors.

Overview of the History of ABCG2 Inhibitors

The first ABCG2 inhibitor reported was FTC, a mycotoxin produced by *Aspergillus fumigatus* (Rabindran et al., 1998, 2000). The *in vivo* use of FTC was unfortunately precluded due to its neurotoxicity. Among the FTC derivatives, Ko143 was identified as a highly potent ABCG2 inhibitor *in vivo* as it was less neurotoxic than the native FTC and was not overtly toxic to mice (Allen et al., 2002). Cell-based assays showed that the EC_{90} concentrations of Ko143 were 23 nM (Abcg2-mediated mitoxantrone resistance), 5.5 μM (ABCB1-mediated paclitaxel resistance) and >8 μM (ABCC1-mediated etoposide resistance), respectively; these results indicated that Ko143 inhibits ABCG2 stronger than ABCB1 and ABCC1, but is not selective to ABCG2 (Allen et al., 2002). Furthermore, from a series of ABCB1 inhibitors, some ABCG2 inhibitors, such as elacridar (GF120918) (Allen et al., 1999; Kruijtzer et al., 2002) and tariquidar (XR9576) (Robey et al., 2004) are frequently used in basic research as well as Ko143.

To date, the molecular bases relating to the chemical inhibition of ABCG2 are not fully understood. The cryo-EM structures of ABCG2 (Taylor et al., 2017) and ABCG2 bound to Ko143 derivatives or tariquidar (Jackson et al., 2018) will be an important to address this issue. Besides, another group of researchers has revealed the structural characteristics of ABCG2 protein critical for its function based on a molecular modeling approach combined with biochemical characterizations of ABCG2 mutants (Khunweeraphong et al., 2017). Previous studies employing the QSAR approaches predicted some structural requirements of compounds for interacting with ABCG2 as an inhibitor (Ishikawa et al., 2012; Mao and Unadkat, 2015); not being true for all ABCG2 inhibitors, the representative features are lipophilicity, planner structure, and amine bonded to one carbon of a heterocyclic ring. Furthermore, a virtual screening strategy employing a ligand-based *in silico* classification model to predict the inhibitory potential of drugs toward ABCG2 presented some favorable outcomes (Montanari et al., 2017). Integration of these findings will contribute to providing a basis for the design of new ABCG2 inhibitors.

Hitherto, many studies focusing on the chemicals–ABCG2 interactions identified a large number of ABCG2 inhibitors with diverse chemical structures (Mao and Unadkat, 2015; Wiese, 2015; Pena-Solorzano et al., 2017; Silbermann et al., 2019). An expanding list of the ABCG2 inhibitors, which include ABCG2

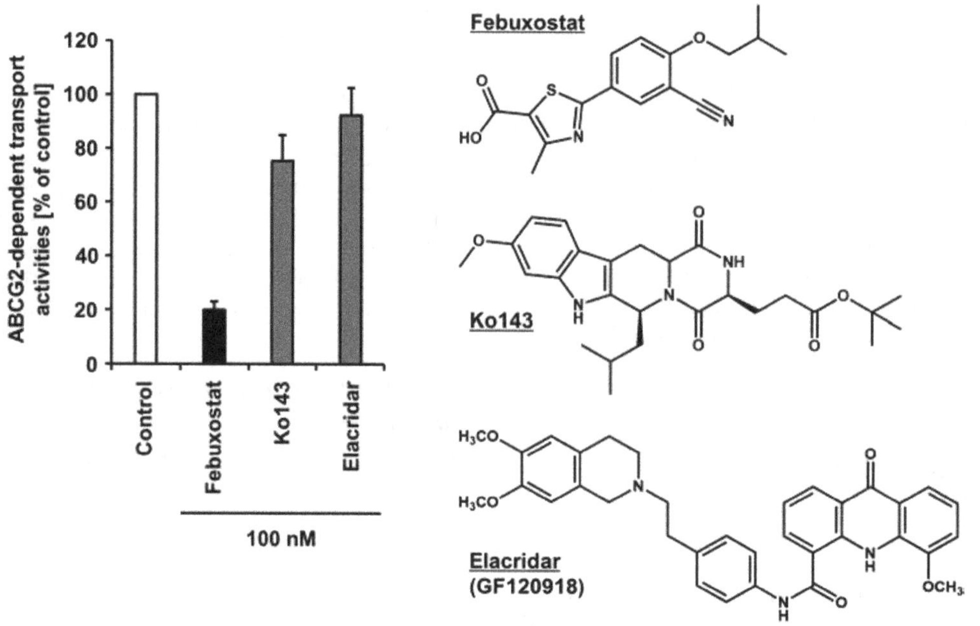

FIGURE 2 | Inhibitory effect of febuxostat against ABCG2 is stronger than that of Ko143 and elacridar, two well-used ABCG2 inhibitors. Febuxostat is known as an oral hypouricemic agent inhibiting xanthine oxidoreductase, a key enzyme for uric acid production. **(Left)** Effect of each compound on the transport activity of ABCG2 are shown. Data from our previous study under CC BY license (Miyata et al., 2016) are shown graphically, in which in the absence (vehicle control) or presence of 100 nM of each compound, the ATP-dependent urate transport activities of ABCG2 were measured using the vesicle transport assay. Data are expressed as the mean ± SD, $n = 3$. Of note, the half-maximal inhibitory concentration (IC_{50}) of febuxostat against the urate transport activity of ABCG2 was 27 nM in the previous study. **(Right)** Chemical structures of each compound are depicted.

substrates (competitive inhibitors), contains such drugs on the market as TKIs and anti-HIV drugs [some of them are often ABCG2 substrates (Polgar et al., 2008; Mao and Unadkat, 2015)] and such dietary phytochemicals as flavonoids and rotenoids. Nevertheless, to the best of our knowledge, the clinical use of such chemicals for ABCG2 inhibition has not yet been achieved probably due to concerns on safety and/or *in vivo* efficacy of them, which may have been common reasons responsible for the failure of the clinical development of ABCG2 inhibitors. Recent studies importantly showed that two potential anti-cancer compounds under clinical development could competitively inhibit both ABCG2 and ABCB1 (Ji et al., 2018a,b).

Febuxostat, a Highly Potent ABCG2 Inhibitor Applicable in Clinical Situations

Regarding the difficulty in the clinical applications of existing ABCG2 inhibitors, our recent study may open up further avenues, in which febuxostat—an approved agent for hyperuricemia globally used in clinical situations—was serendipitously identified as a strong ABCG2 inhibitor both *in vitro* and *in vivo* (Miyata et al., 2016). Using the vesicle transport assay, we revealed that febuxostat inhibits ABCG2 more strongly than Ko143 and elacridar (**Figure 2**). This indicates that febuxostat has a superior safety profile and better inhibitory ability against ABCG2 compared to these two compounds. Moreover, the study demonstrated that the IC_{50} of febuxostat against urate transport activity of ABCG2 (0.027 μM) was lower than its maximum plasma unbound concentrations reported in humans (0.09 μM), suggesting that febuxostat might inhibit human ABCG2 at a clinically used dose. Thus, febuxostat can be a promising candidate as a potential ABCG2 inhibitor in humans. The structural characteristics and molecular mechanisms of febuxostat as an ABCG2 inhibitor remain to be elucidated, as well as the effects of febuxostat on the function of other ABC transporters, including ABCB1.

Febuxostat will be used in cancer chemotherapy more frequently because recently this drug has been approved in Europe and Japan for the prophylaxis of TLS. TLS is a potentially life-threatening condition caused by an abrupt release of intracellular metabolites after tumor cell lysis in cancer patients on chemotherapy (Alakel et al., 2017). It is the most common treatment-related emergency in patients with hematologic malignancies and characterized by metabolic abnormalities including hyperuricemia that triggers several mechanisms resulting in acute kidney injury. Appropriate control of serum uric acid is therefore important in the prevention of TLS. Recent studies demonstrated that febuxostat—an oral hypouricemic agent—can successfully prevent TLS in cancer patients (Spina et al., 2015; Tamura et al., 2016). In such situations, since the patients will be treated with febuxostat before and during chemotherapy, there would be drug-drug interactions between febuxostat and ABCG2 substrate anti-cancer agents.

Importantly, ABCG2 is reportedly expressed on the malignant hematopoietic and the lymphoid cells frequently; its expression in several types of human leukemia has been investigated

(Jordanides et al., 2006; Eechoute et al., 2011; Stacy et al., 2013). Considering that initiating cells in CML arises from a multipotent hematopoietic stem cell (HSC), together with high expression of ABCG2 in human HSCs (Zhou et al., 2001; Scharenberg et al., 2002), overexpression of ABCG2 has been considered to confer drug resistance ability to the CML stem cell population (Brendel et al., 2007). However, the clinical relevance of ABCG2 inhibition in CML patients from the view point of reversing MDR remains to be clarified. Since several TKIs used for CML are ABCG2 substrates (Hira and Terada, 2018), the combination use of febuxostat may be a future research topic.

Additionally, ABCG2 expressed in tumor cells is reportedly involved in the efflux of photosensitizers in 5-aminolevulinic acid-based photodynamic therapy (Ishikawa et al., 2015). Hence, febuxostat might enhance the efficacy of this minimally invasive modality for treating solid cancers by accumulating photosensitizers in the target cells. The details are discussed in our previous report (Miyata et al., 2016).

CONCLUSION AND PERSPECTIVE

Here, we summarized some key experimental systems that will continuously contribute to generating novel ABCG2 inhibitors and described an overview of the current update of ABCG2 inhibitors. Among them, febuxostat will be one of the most promising candidates for clinical use. Considering that dysfunctional *ABCG2* genotypes, which are summarized in a recent review (Heyes et al., 2018), alter the pharmacokinetic characteristics of ABCG2 substrate drugs such as several TKIs (Hira and Terada, 2018) and rosuvastatin (Keskitalo et al., 2009), ABCG2 inhibitors will also exert similar effects in humans. As a beneficial application of this clinical possibility, we have proposed a novel concept named febuxostat-boosted therapy (Miyata et al., 2016), in which febuxostat is expected to enhance the bioavailability of ABCG2 substrate drugs. For a similar purpose, ritonavir and cobicistat are used as pharmacokinetic boosters inhibiting cytochrome P450 3A4, a major pathway of drug metabolism, to increase the plasma concentrations of certain drugs (Shah et al., 2013). No pharmacokinetic enhancer targeting transporter proteins has been, however, successfully evaluated in clinical trials. In this context, the potential benefits of the febuxostat-boosted therapy should be validated in the near future. Furthermore, this concept could also be applied to enhance the BBB penetration of ABCG2 substrate drugs for brain cancer chemotherapy. Despite the potential risks of adverse events in the combination therapy, further clinical studies to elucidate whether febuxostat is beneficial in enhancing the efficacy of pharmacotherapy via ABCG2 inhibition are warranted.

AUTHOR CONTRIBUTIONS

YT researched the data for the manuscript, provided substantial contributions to discussion of its content, and wrote the manuscript. TT contributed to the discussion and the writing of the manuscript. HS critiqued the manuscript and provided intellectual inputs. All the authors reviewed and edited the manuscript before submission and have made final approval of the manuscript.

FUNDING

This work and relating our findings were supported by the JSPS KAKENHI Grant Numbers 15H05610 to YT, 16H1808 and 18KK0247 to TT, 22136015 to HS; TT has received research grants from Gout Research Foundation, The Uehara Memorial Foundation, Mochida Memorial Foundation for Medical and Pharmaceutical Research, The Takeda Medical Foundation, and MSD Life Science Foundation, Public Interest Incorporated Foundation.

ACKNOWLEDGMENTS

The authors would like to acknowledge Drs. Hiroshi Miyata, Hirotaka Matsuo, and Kimiyoshi Ichida for their contribution to our studies highlighted in this mini-review article as well as Drs. Toshihisa Ishikawa and Yuichi Sugiyama for their previous mentorships and encouragements.

REFERENCES

1. Adachi, Y., Suzuki, H., Schinkel, A. H., and Sugiyama, Y. (2005). Role of breast cancer resistance protein (Bcrp1/Abcg2) in the extrusion of glucuronide and sulfate conjugates from enterocytes to intestinal lumen. *Mol. Pharmacol.* 67, 923–928. doi: 10.1124/mol.104.007393
2. Alakel, N., Middeke, J. M., Schetelig, J., and Bornhauser, M. (2017). Prevention and treatment of tumor lysis syndrome, and the efficacy and role of rasburicase. *Onco Targets Ther.* 10, 597–605. doi: 10.2147/OTT.S103864
3. Allen, J. D., Brinkhuis, R. F., Wijnholds, J., and Schinkel, A. H. (1999). The mouse Bcrp1/Mxr/Abcp gene: amplification and overexpression in cell lines selected for resistance to topotecan, mitoxantrone, or doxorubicin. *Cancer Res.* 59, 4237–4241.
4. Allen, J. D., Van Loevezijn, A., Lakhai, J. M., Van Der Valk, M., Van Tellingen, O., Reid, G., et al. (2002). Potent and specific inhibition of the breast cancer resistance protein multidrug transporter in vitro and in mouse intestine by a novel analogue of fumitremorgin C. *Mol. Cancer Ther.* 1, 417–425.
5. Allikmets, R., Schriml, L. M., Hutchinson, A., Romano-Spica, V., and Dean, M. (1998). A human placenta-specific ATP-binding cassette gene (ABCP) on chromosome 4q22 that is involved in multidrug resistance. *Cancer Res.* 58, 5337–5339.
6. Ambudkar, S. V., Lelong, I. H., Zhang, J., and Cardarelli, C. (1998). Purification and reconstitution of human P-glycoprotein. *Methods Enzymol.* 292, 492–504. doi: 10.1016/S0076-6879(98)92038-9
7. Ando, T., Kusuhara, H., Merino, G., Alvarez, A. I., Schinkel, A. H., and Sugiyama, Y. (2007). Involvement of breast cancer resistance protein (ABCG2) in the biliary excretion mechanism of fluoroquinolones. *Drug Metab. Dispos.* 35, 1873–1879. doi: 10.1124/dmd.107.014969
8. Bakhsheshian, J., Wei, B. R., Hall, M. D., Simpson, R. M., and Gottesman, M. M. (2016). In vivo bioluminescent imaging of ATP-binding cassette transporter-mediated efflux at the blood-brain barrier. *Methods Mol. Biol.* 1461, 227–239. doi: 10.1007/978-1-4939-3813-1_19
9. Baykov, A. A., Evtushenko, O. A., and Avaeva, S. M. (1988). A malachite

green procedure for orthophosphate determination and its use in alkalinephosphatase-based enzyme immunoassay. *Anal. Biochem.* 171, 266–270. doi: 10.1016/0003-2697(88)90484-8

10. Brendel, C., Scharenberg, C., Dohse, M., Robey, R. W., Bates, S. E., Shukla, S., et al. (2007). Imatinib mesylate and nilotinib (AMN107) exhibit high-affinity interaction with ABCG2 on primitive hematopoietic stem cells. *Leukemia* 21, 1267–1275. doi: 10.1038/sj.leu.2404638
11. Doyle, L. A., Yang, W., Abruzzo, L. V., Krogmann, T., Gao, Y., Rishi, A. K., et al. (1998). A multidrug resistance transporter from human MCF-7 breast cancer cells. *Proc. Natl. Acad. Sci. U.S.A.* 95, 15665–15670. doi: 10.1073/pnas.95.26.15665
12. Eechoute, K., Sparreboom, A., Burger, H., Franke, R. M., Schiavon, G., Verweij, J., et al. (2011). Drug transporters and imatinib treatment: implications for clinical practice. *Clin. Cancer Res.* 17, 406–415. doi: 10.1158/1078-0432.CCR-10-2250
13. Geertsma, E. R., Nik Mahmood, N. A., Schuurman-Wolters, G. K., and Poolman, B. (2008). Membrane reconstitution of ABC transporters and assays of translocator function. *Nat. Protoc.* 3, 256–266. doi: 10.1038/nprot.2007.519
14. Giacomini, K. M., Huang, S. M., Tweedie, D. J., Benet, L. Z., Brouwer, K. L., Chu, X., et al. (2010). Membrane transporters in drug development. *Nat. Rev. Drug Discov.* 9, 215–236. doi: 10.1038/nrd3028
15. Guo, C., Liu, F., Qi, J., Ma, J., Lin, S., Zhang, C., et al. (2018). A novel synthetic dihydroindeno[1,2-b] indole derivative (LS-2-3j) reverses ABCB1- and ABCG2-mediated multidrug resistance in cancer cells. *Molecules* 23:E3264. doi: 10.3390/molecules23123264
16. Hegedus, C., Szakacs, G., Homolya, L., Orban, T. I., Telbisz, A., Jani, M., et al. (2009). Ins and outs of the ABCG2 multidrug transporter: an update on in vitro functional assays. *Adv. Drug Deliv. Rev.* 61, 47–56. doi: 10.1016/j.addr.2008.09.007
17. Heyes, N., Kapoor, P., and Kerr, I. D. (2018). Polymorphisms of the multidrug Pump ABCG2: a systematic review of their effect on protein expression, function, and drug pharmacokinetics. *Drug Metab. Dispos.* 46, 1886–1899. doi: 10.1124/dmd.118.083030
18. Higashino, T., Takada, T., Nakaoka, H., Toyoda, Y., Stiburkova, B., Miyata, H., et al. (2017). Multiple common and rare variants of ABCG2 cause gout. *RMD Open* 3:e000464. doi: 10.1136/rmdopen-2017-000464
19. Hira, D., and Terada, T. (2018). BCRP/ABCG2 and high-alert medications: biochemical, pharmacokinetic, pharmacogenetic, and clinical implications. *Biochem. Pharmacol.* 147, 201–210. doi: 10.1016/j.bcp.2017.10.004
20. Hirano, M., Maeda, K., Matsushima, S., Nozaki, Y., Kusuhara, H., and Sugiyama, Y. (2005). Involvement of BCRP (ABCG2) in the biliary excretion of pitavastatin. *Mol. Pharmacol.* 68, 800–807. doi: 10.1124/mol.105.014019
21. Ichida, K., Matsuo, H., Takada, T., Nakayama, A., Murakami, K., Shimizu, T., et al. (2012). Decreased extra-renal urate excretion is a common cause of hyperuricemia. *Nat. Commun.* 3:764. doi: 10.1038/ncomms1756
22. Ishikawa, T. (1989). ATP/Mg2+-dependent cardiac transport system for glutathione S-conjugates. A study using rat heart sarcolemma vesicles. *J. Biol. Chem.* 264, 17343–17348.
23. Ishikawa, T., Kajimoto, Y., Inoue, Y., Ikegami, Y., and Kuroiwa, T. (2015). Critical role of ABCG2 in ALA-photodynamic diagnosis and therapy of human brain tumor. *Adv. Cancer Res.* 125, 197–216. doi: 10.1016/bs.acr.2014.11.008
24. Ishikawa, T., Saito, H., Hirano, H., Inoue, Y., and Ikegami, Y. (2012). Human ABC transporter ABCG2 in cancer chemotherapy: drug molecular design to circumvent multidrug resistance. *Methods Mol. Biol.* 910, 267–278. doi: 10.1007/978-1-61779-965-5_11
25. Ito, N., Ito, K., Ikebuchi, Y., Toyoda, Y., Takada, T., Hisaka, A., et al. (2015). Prediction of drug transfer into milk considering breast cancer resistance protein (BCRP)-mediated transport. *Pharm. Res.* 32, 2527–2537. doi: 10.1007/s11095-015-1641-2
26. Jackson, S. M., Manolaridis, I., Kowal, J., Zechner, M., Taylor, N. M. I., Bause, M., et al. (2018). Structural basis of small-molecule inhibition of human multidrug transporter ABCG2. *Nat. Struct. Mol. Biol.* 25, 333–340. doi: 10.1038/s41594-018-0049-1
27. Ji, N., Yang, Y., Cai, C. Y., Lei, Z. N., Wang, J. Q., Gupta, P., et al. (2018a). VS-4718 antagonizes multidrug resistance in ABCB1- and ABCG2-overexpressing cancer cells by inhibiting the efflux function of ABC transporters. *Front. Pharmacol.* 9:1236. doi: 10.3389/fphar.2018.01236
28. Ji, N., Yang, Y., Lei, Z. N., Cai, C. Y., Wang, J. Q., Gupta, P., et al. (2018b). Ulixertinib (BVD-523) antagonizes ABCB1- and ABCG2-mediated chemotherapeutic drug resistance. *Biochem. Pharmacol.* 158, 274–285. doi: 10.1016/j.bcp.2018.10.028
29. Jonker, J. W., Buitelaar, M., Wagenaar, E., Van Der Valk, M. A., Scheffer, G. L., Scheper, R. J., et al. (2002). The breast cancer resistance protein protects against a major chlorophyll-derived dietary phototoxin and protoporphyria. *Proc. Natl. Acad. Sci. U.S.A.* 99, 15649–15654. doi: 10.1073/pnas.202607599
30. Jonker, J. W., Merino, G., Musters, S., Van Herwaarden, A. E., Bolscher, E., Wagenaar, E., et al. (2005). The breast cancer resistance protein BCRP (ABCG2) concentrates drugs and carcinogenic xenotoxins into milk. *Nat. Med.* 11, 127–129. doi: 10.1038/nm1186
31. Jordanides, N. E., Jorgensen, H. G., Holyoake, T. L., and Mountford, J. C. (2006). Functional ABCG2 is overexpressed on primary CML CD34+ cells and is inhibited by imatinib mesylate. *Blood* 108, 1370–1373. doi: 10.1182/blood-2006-02-003145
32. Keskitalo, J. E., Zolk, O., Fromm, M. F., Kurkinen, K. J., Neuvonen, P. J., and Niemi, M. (2009). ABCG2 polymorphism markedly affects the pharmacokinetics of atorvastatin and rosuvastatin. *Clin. Pharmacol. Ther.* 86, 197–203. doi: 10.1038/clpt.2009.79
33. Khunweeraphong, N., Stockner, T., and Kuchler, K. (2017). The structure of the human ABC transporter ABCG2 reveals a novel mechanism for drug extrusion. *Sci. Rep.* 7:13767. doi: 10.1038/s41598-017-11794-w
34. Kruijtzer, C. M., Beijnen, J. H., Rosing, H., ten Bokkel Huinink, W. W., Schot, M., Jewell, R. C., et al. (2002). Increased oral bioavailability of topotecan in combination with the breast cancer resistance protein and P-glycoprotein inhibitor GF120918. *J. Clin. Oncol.* 20, 2943–2950. doi: 10.1200/JCO.2002.12.116
35. Kusuhara, H., Furuie, H., Inano, A., Sunagawa, A., Yamada, S., Wu, C., et al. (2012). Pharmacokinetic interaction study of sulphasalazine in healthy subjects and the impact of curcumin as an in vivo inhibitor of BCRP. *Br. J. Pharmacol.* 166, 1793–1803. doi: 10.1111/j.1476-5381.2012.01887.x
36. Mao, Q., and Unadkat, J. D. (2015). Role of the breast cancer resistance protein (BCRP/ABCG2) in drug transport–an update. *AAPS J.* 17, 65–82. doi: 10.1208/s12248-014-9668-6
37. Marighetti, F., Steggemann, K., Hanl, M., and Wiese, M. (2013). Synthesis and quantitative structure-activity relationships of selective BCRP inhibitors. *ChemMedChem* 8, 125–135. doi: 10.1002/cmdc.201200377
38. Matsuo, H., Takada, T., Ichida, K., Nakamura, T., Nakayama, A., Ikebuchi, Y., et al. (2009). Common defects of ABCG2, a high-capacity urate exporter, cause gout: a function-based genetic analysis in a Japanese population. *Sci. Transl. Med.* 1:5ra11. doi: 10.1126/scitranslmed.3000237
39. Matsushima, S., Maeda, K., Kondo, C., Hirano, M., Sasaki, M., Suzuki, H., et al. (2005). Identification of the hepatic efflux transporters of organic anions using double-transfected Madin-Darby canine kidney II cells expressing human organic anion-transporting polypeptide 1B1 (OATP1B1)/multidrug resistance- associated protein 2, OATP1B1/multidrug resistance 1, and OATP1B1/breast cancer resistance protein. *J. Pharmacol. Exp. Ther.* 314, 1059–1067. doi: 10. 1124/jpet.105.085589
40. Miyake, K., Mickley, L., Litman, T., Zhan, Z., Robey, R., Cristensen, B., et al. (1999). Molecular cloning of cDNAs which are highly overexpressed in mitoxantrone- resistant cells: demonstration of homology to ABC transport genes. *Cancer Res.* 59, 8–13.
41. Miyata, H., Takada, T., Toyoda, Y., Matsuo, H., Ichida, K., and Suzuki, H. (2016). Identification of febuxostat as a new strong ABCG2 inhibitor: potential applications and risks in clinical situations. *Front. Pharmacol.* 7:518. doi: 10.3389/fphar.2016.00518
42. Mizuno, N., Suzuki, M., Kusuhara, H., Suzuki, H., Takeuchi, K., Niwa, T., et al. (2004). Impaired renal excretion of 6-hydroxy-5,7-dimethyl-2-methylamino-4-(3-pyridylmethyl) benzothiazole (E3040) sulfate in breast cancer resistance protein (BCRP1/ABCG2) knockout mice. *Drug Metab. Dispos.* 32, 898–901.
43. Mizuno, N., Takahashi, T., Kusuhara, H., Schuetz, J. D., Niwa, T., and Sugiyama, Y. (2007). Evaluation of the role of breast cancer resistance protein (BCRP/ABCG2) and multidrug resistance-associated protein 4 (MRP4/ABCC4) in the urinary excretion of sulfate and glucuronide metabolites of edaravone (MCI-186; 3-methyl-1-phenyl-2-pyrazolin-5-one). *Drug Metab. Dispos.* 35, 2045–2052. doi: 10.1124/dmd.107.016352
44. Montanari, F., Cseke, A., Wlcek, K., and Ecker, G. F. (2017). Virtual screening of DrugBank reveals two drugs as new BCRP inhibitors. *SLAS Discov.* 22, 86–93. doi: 10.1177/1087057116657513
45. Murakami, M., Ohnuma, S., Fukuda, M., Chufan, E. E., Kudoh, K., Kanehara,

K., et al. (2017). Synthetic analogs of curcumin modulate the function of multidrug resistance-linked ATP-binding cassette transporter ABCG2. *Drug Metab. Dispos.* 45, 1166–1177. doi: 10.1124/dmd.117.076000

46. Nakanishi, T., Doyle, L. A., Hassel, B., Wei, Y., Bauer, K. S., Wu, S., et al. (2003). Functional characterization of human breast cancer resistance protein (BCRP, ABCG2) expressed in the oocytes of *Xenopus laevis*. *Mol. Pharmacol.* 64, 1452–1462. doi: 10.1124/mol.64.6.1452
47. Nicolle, E., Boumendjel, A., Macalou, S., Genoux, E., Ahmed-Belkacem, A., Carrupt, P. A., et al. (2009). QSAR analysis and molecular modeling of ABCG2-specific inhibitors. *Adv. Drug Deliv. Rev.* 61, 34–46. doi: 10.1016/j.addr.2008.10.004
48. Okamoto, T., Kawaguchi, K., Watanabe, S., Agustina, R., Ikejima, T., Ikeda, K., et al. (2018). Characterization of human ATP-binding cassette protein subfamily D reconstituted into proteoliposomes. *Biochem. Biophys. Res. Commun.* 496, 1122–1127. doi: 10.1016/j.bbrc.2018.01.153
49. Pena-Solorzano, D., Stark, S. A., Konig, B., Sierra, C. A., and Ochoa-Puentes, C. (2017). ABCG2/BCRP: specific and nonspecific modulators. *Med. Res. Rev.* 37, 987–1050. doi: 10.1002/med.21428
50. Polgar, O., Robey, R. W., and Bates, S. E. (2008). ABCG2: structure, function and role in drug response. *Expert Opin. Drug Metab. Toxicol.* 4, 1–15. doi: 10.1517/17425255.4.1.1
51. Rabindran, S. K., He, H., Singh, M., Brown, E., Collins, K. I., Annable, T., et al. (1998). Reversal of a novel multidrug resistance mechanism in human colon carcinoma cells by fumitremorgin C. *Cancer Res.* 58, 5850–5858.
52. Rabindran, S. K., Ross, D. D., Doyle, L. A., Yang, W., and Greenberger, L. M. (2000). Fumitremorgin C reverses multidrug resistance in cells transfected with the breast cancer resistance protein. *Cancer Res.* 60, 47–50.
53. Robey, R. W., Pluchino, K. M., Hall, M. D., Fojo, A. T., Bates, S. E., and Gottesman,
54. M. M. (2018). Revisiting the role of ABC transporters in multidrug-resistant cancer. *Nat. Rev. Cancer* 18, 452–464. doi: 10.1038/s41568-018-0005-8
55. Robey, R. W., Steadman, K., Polgar, O., Morisaki, K., Blayney, M., Mistry, P., et al. (2004). Pheophorbide a is a specific probe for ABCG2 function and inhibition. *Cancer Res.* 64, 1242–1246. doi: 10.1158/0008-5472.CAN-03-3298
56. Robey, R. W., To, K. K., Polgar, O., Dohse, M., Fetsch, P., Dean, M., et al. (2009). ABCG2: a perspective. *Adv. Drug Deliv. Rev.* 61, 3–13. doi: 10.1016/j.addr.2008.11.003
57. Saito, H., Hirano, H., Nakagawa, H., Fukami, T., Oosumi, K., Murakami, K., et al. (2006). A new strategy of high-speed screening and quantitative structure-activity relationship analysis to evaluate human ATP-binding cassette transporter ABCG2-drug interactions. *J. Pharmacol. Exp. Ther.* 317, 1114–1124. doi: 10.1124/jpet.105.099036
58. Scharenberg, C. W., Harkey, M. A., and Torok-Storb, B. (2002). The ABCG2 transporter is an efficient Hoechst 33342 efflux pump and is preferentially expressed by immature human hematopoietic progenitors. *Blood* 99, 507–512. doi: 10.1182/blood.V99.2.507
59. Shah, B. M., Schafer, J. J., Priano, J., and Squires, K. E. (2013). Cobicistat: a new boost for the treatment of human immunodeficiency virus infection. *Pharmacotherapy* 33, 1107–1116. doi: 10.1002/phar.1237
60. Shukla, S., Kouanda, A., Silverton, L., Talele, T. T., and Ambudkar, S. V. (2014). Pharmacophore modeling of nilotinib as an inhibitor of ATP-binding cassette drug transporters and BCR-ABL kinase using a three-dimensional quantitative structure-activity relationship approach. *Mol. Pharm.* 11, 2313–2322. doi: 10.1021/mp400762h
61. Shukla, S., Robey, R. W., Bates, S. E., and Ambudkar, S. V. (2006). The calcium channel blockers, 1,4-dihydropyridines, are substrates of the multidrug resistance-linked ABC drug transporter, ABCG2. *Biochemistry* 45, 8940–8951. doi: 10.1021/bi060552f
62. Silbermann, K., Shah, C. P., Sahu, N. U., Juvale, K., Stefan, S. M., Kharkar, P. S., et al. (2019). Novel chalcone and flavone derivatives as selective and dual inhibitors of the transport proteins ABCB1 and ABCG2. *Eur. J. Med. Chem.* 164, 193–213. doi: 10.1016/j.ejmech.2018.12.019
63. Spina, M., Nagy, Z., Ribera, J. M., Federico, M., Aurer, I., Jordan, K., et al. (2015). FLORENCE: a randomized, double-blind, phase III pivotal study of febuxostat versus allopurinol for the prevention of tumor lysis syndrome (TLS) in patients with hematologic malignancies at intermediate to high TLS risk. *Ann. Oncol.* 26, 2155–2161. doi: 10.1093/annonc/mdv317
64. Stacy, A. E., Jansson, P. J., and Richardson, D. R. (2013). Molecular pharmacology of ABCG2 and its role in chemoresistance. *Mol. Pharmacol.* 84, 655–669. doi: 10.1124/mol.113.088609
65. Stiburkova, B., Miyata, H., Zavada, J., Tomcik, M., Pavelka, K., Storkanova, G., et al. (2016). Novel dysfunctional variant in ABCG2 as a cause of severe tophaceous gout: biochemical, molecular genetics and functional analysis. *Rheumatology* 55, 191–194. doi: 10.1093/rheumatology/kev350
66. Suzuki, M., Suzuki, H., Sugimoto, Y., and Sugiyama, Y. (2003). ABCG2 transports sulfated conjugates of steroids and xenobiotics. *J. Biol. Chem.* 278, 22644–22649. doi: 10.1074/jbc.M212399200
67. Takada, T., Yamamoto, T., Matsuo, H., Tan, J. K., Ooyama, K., Sakiyama, M., et al. (2018). Identification of ABCG2 as an exporter of uremic toxin indoxyl sulfate in mice and as a crucial factor influencing CKD progression. *Sci. Rep.* 8:11147. doi: 10.1038/s41598-018-29208-w
68. Tamura, A., Watanabe, M., Saito, H., Nakagawa, H., Kamachi, T., Okura, I., et al. (2006). Functional validation of the genetic polymorphisms of human ATP-binding cassette (ABC) transporter ABCG2: identification of alleles that are defective in porphyrin transport. *Mol. Pharmacol.* 70, 287–296.
69. Tamura, K., Kawai, Y., Kiguchi, T., Okamoto, M., Kaneko, M., Maemondo, M., et al. (2016). Efficacy and safety of febuxostat for prevention of tumor lysis syndrome in patients with malignant tumors receiving chemotherapy: a phase III, randomized, multi-center trial comparing febuxostat and allopurinol. *Int. J. Clin. Oncol.* 21, 996–1003. doi: 10.1007/s10147-016-0971-3
70. Taylor, N. M. I., Manolaridis, I., Jackson, S. M., Kowal, J., Stahlberg, H., and Locher, K. P. (2017). Structure of the human multidrug transporter ABCG2. *Nature* 546, 504–509. doi: 10.1038/nature22345
71. Tiwari, A. K., Sodani, K., Dai, C. L., Abuznait, A. H., Singh, S., Xiao, Z. J., et al. (2013). Nilotinib potentiates anticancer drug sensitivity in murine ABCB1-, ABCG2-, and ABCC10-multidrug resistance xenograft models. *Cancer Lett.* 328, 307–317. doi: 10.1016/j.canlet.2012.10.001
72. Toyoda, Y., Takada, T., and Suzuki, H. (2016). Halogenated hydrocarbon solvent- related cholangiocarcinoma risk: biliary excretion of glutathione conjugates of 1,2-dichloropropane evidenced by untargeted metabolomics analysis. *Sci. Rep.* 6:24586. doi: 10.1038/srep24586
73. van de Wetering, K., and Sapthu, S. (2012). ABCG2 functions as a general phytoestrogen sulfate transporter in vivo. *FASEB J.* 26, 4014–4024. doi: 10.1096/fj.12-210039
74. Vlaming, M. L., Lagas, J. S., and Schinkel, A. H. (2009). Physiological and pharmacological roles of ABCG2 (BCRP): recent findings in Abcg2 knockout mice. *Adv. Drug Deliv. Rev.* 61, 14–25. doi: 10.1016/j.addr.2008.08.007
75. Wassermann, L., Halwachs, S., Baumann, D., Schaefer, I., Seibel, P., and Honscha, W. (2013). Assessment of ABCG2-mediated transport of xenobiotics across the blood-milk barrier of dairy animals using a new MDCKII in vitro model. *Arch. Toxicol.* 87, 1671–1682. doi: 10.1007/s00204-013-1066-9
76. Wiese, M. (2015). BCRP/ABCG2 inhibitors: a patent review (2009-present). *Expert Opin. Ther. Pat.* 25, 1229–1237. doi: 10.1517/13543776.2015.1076796
77. Woodward, O. M., Kottgen, A., Coresh, J., Boerwinkle, E., Guggino, W. B., and Kottgen, M. (2009). Identification of a urate transporter, ABCG2, with a common functional polymorphism causing gout. *Proc. Natl. Acad. Sci. U.S.A.* 106, 10338–10342. doi: 10.1073/pnas.0901249106
78. Wu, C. P., Hsiao, S. H., Murakami, M., Lu, Y. J., Li, Y. Q., Huang, Y. H., et al. (2017). Alpha-mangostin reverses multidrug resistance by attenuating the function of the multidrug resistance-linked ABCG2 transporter. *Mol. Pharm.* 14, 2805–2814. doi: 10.1021/acs.molpharmaceut.7b00334
79. Zhang, G. N., Zhang, Y. K., Wang, Y. J., Gupta, P., Ashby, C. R. Jr., Alqahtani, S., et al. (2018). Epidermal growth factor receptor (EGFR) inhibitor PD153035 reverses ABCG2-mediated multidrug resistance in non-small cell lung cancer: in vitro and in vivo. *Cancer Lett.* 424, 19–29. doi: 10.1016/j.canlet.2018.02.040
80. Zhang, W., Chen, Z., Chen, L., Wang, F., Li, F., Wang, X., et al. (2017). ABCG2-overexpressing H460/MX20 cell xenografts in athymic nude mice maintained original biochemical and cytological characteristics. *Sci. Rep.* 7:40064. doi: 10.1038/srep40064
81. Zhang, Y., Bressler, J. P., Neal, J., Lal, B., Bhang, H. E., Laterra, J., et al. (2007). ABCG2/BCRP expression modulates D-Luciferin based bioluminescence imaging. *Cancer Res.* 67, 9389–9397. doi: 10.1158/0008-5472.CAN-07-0944
82. Zhang, Y. K., Zhang, G. N., Wang, Y. J., Patel, B. A., Talele, T. T., Yang, D. H., et al. (2016). Bafetinib (INNO-406) reverses multidrug resistance by inhibiting the efflux function of ABCB1 and ABCG2 transporters. *Sci. Rep.* 6:25694. doi: 10.1038/srep25694

83. Zhou, S., Schuetz, J. D., Bunting, K. D., Colapietro, A. M., Sampath, J., Morris, J. J., et al. (2001). The ABC transporter Bcrp1/ABCG2 is expressed in a wide variety of stem cells and is a molecular determinant of the side-population phenotype. *Nat. Med.* 7, 1028–1034. doi: 10.1038/nm0901-1028
84. Zhou, S., Zong, Y., Ney, P. A., Nair, G., Stewart, C. F., and Sorrentino, B. P. (2005). Increased expression of the Abcg2 transporter during erythroid maturation plays a role in decreasing cellular protoporphyrin IX levels. *Blood* 105, 2571– 2576. doi: 10.1182/blood-2004-04-1566

20

CACNA2D3 Enhances the Chemosensitivity of Esophageal Squamous Cell Carcinoma to Cisplatin via Inducing Ca^{2+}-Mediated Apoptosis and Suppressing PI3K/Akt Pathways

Changjun Nie[1,2,3,4†], Xiaohui Qin[4†], Xiaoyan Li[1,2,3†], Baoqing Tian[1,2,3], Ying Zhao[1,2,3], Yuan Jin[1,2,3], Yadan Li[1,2,3], Qiang Wang[1,2,3], Dingyuan Zeng[4], An Hong[1,2,3] and Xiaojia Chen[1,2,3*]*

[1] Department of Cell Biology, Institute of Biomedicine, Jinan University, Guangzhou, China, [2] National Engineering Research Center of Genetic Medicine, Guangzhou, China, [3] Guangdong Provincial Key Laboratory of Bioengineering Medicine, Guangzhou, China, [4] Department of Medical Genetics, Liuzhou Maternal and Children Healthcare Hospital, Liuzhou, China

***Correspondence:**
An Hong
tha@jnu.edu.cn
Xiaojia Chen
tchenxj@jnu.edu.cn;
carolcxj@qq.com

† These authors have contributed equally to this work

Resistance to platinum-based combination chemotherapy is the main cause of poor prognosis in patients with advanced esophageal squamous cell carcinoma (ESCC). Previously, we showed that CACNA2D3 (voltage-dependent subunit alpha 2 delta 3 of a calcium channel complex) was significantly downregulated and functioned as a tumor suppressor in ESCC, but its role in the chemosensitivity of ESCC to cisplatin remained unknown. Here, we found that the expression of CACNA2D3 was significantly associated with poor platinum response in ESCC patients from the Gene Expression Omnibus database. Overexpression of CACNA2D3 increased sensitivity to cisplatin in ESCC *in vitro*, whereas knockdown of CACNA2D3 increased cisplatin resistance. CACNA2D3 promoted cisplatin-induced apoptosis by modulating intracellular Ca^{2+} stores. *In vivo* experiments further showed that overexpression of CACNA2D3 enhanced cisplatin anti-tumor effects in a xenograft mouse model. CACNA2D3 overexpression also resulted in the attenuation of PI3K and Akt phosphorylation. Treatment with the PI3K/Akt inhibitor LY294002 restored the chemosensitivity of CACAN2D3-knockdown cells to cisplatin. In conclusion, the results of the current study indicate that CACAN2D3 enhances the chemosensitivity of ESCC to cisplatin via inducing Ca^{2+}-mediated apoptosis and suppressing PI3K/Akt pathways. Therefore, regulating the expression of CACNA2D3 is a potential new strategy to increase the efficacy of cisplatin in ESCC patients.

Keywords: CACNA2D3, chemosensitivity, ESCC, voltage-gated calcium channel, LY294002

INTRODUCTION

Esophageal cancer (EC) is a fatal digestive tract malignancy (1). EC is composed of two major histologic subtypes: adenocarcinoma and squamous cell carcinoma. Esophageal squamous cell carcinoma (ESCC) is more common in Southeast and Central Asia (2, 3). China is a high incidence area for ESCC, especially in Linzhou and Cixian of North China (4). Esophagectomy is the usual method for the treatment of early esophageal cancer. However, most ESCC patients are diagnosed at an advanced stage when surgery is no longer effective. Recently, the use of comprehensive perioperative therapies has dramatically improved the therapeutic efficacy of ESCC, particularly with respect to long-term survival (5–7). A cisplatin-based regimen is widely used as the first-line treatment in advanced ESCC (8–10). However, cisplatin chemotherapy is often limited by natural and acquired resistance. Consequently, it is critical to identify potential resistance mechanisms in order to restore tumor cell sensitivity to cisplatin.

The human *CACNA2D3* gene is located on the short arm of chromosome 3 at position 3p21.1, a common region of allelic deletion, and has been found to possess a potential tumor suppressor function in multiple tumor types, including gastric cancer (11–13), nasopharyngeal cancer (14), breast cancer (15), renal cell cancer neuroblastoma (16), lung cancer (17), and glioma (18). The promoter of CACNA2D3 was shown to be highly methylated in gastric cancer, and this was associated with a low survival rate (12). Similarly, suppression of CACNA2D3 by methylation was found to promote the metastatic phenotype of breast cancer (15). Another study showed that CACNA2D3 could increase intracellular Ca^{2+} levels and promote apoptosis in nasopharyngeal cancer and glioma, causing changes in the network of tumor-suppressive properties and inducing upregulation of Nemo-like kinase (NLK) through the non-canonical Wnt/Ca^{2+} signaling pathway (14, 18). In neuroblastomas with poor prognosis, the expression of CACNA2D3 is often downregulated (19, 20). Our previous study also identified CACNA2D3 as a tumor suppressor gene, and methylation of its promoter and allele deletion could inhibit its expression in ESCC (21). Recently, CACNA2D3 was implicated in the development of chemoresistance. The downregulation of CACNA2D3 was detected in five cytarabine-resistant leukemic cell lines compared with parental cells (22). However, the underlying mechanism by which CACNA2D3 might function in chemosensitivity has not been identified.

In this study, we aimed to investigate the function of CACNA2D3 in cisplatin-based chemotherapy of ESCC and discover its underlying mechanisms. We found that the expression of CACNA2D3 was significantly associated with poor platinum response in ESCC patients. Overexpression of CACNA2D3 significantly sensitized ESCC cell lines to cisplatin, while CACNA2D3 knockdown induced cellular resistance to cisplatin. Further research showed that CACNA2D3 overexpression enhanced cisplatin-induced apoptosis by modulating intracellular Ca^{2+}. Moreover, CACNA2D3 overexpression resulted in the attenuation of PI3K and Akt phosphorylation. LY294002 is a commonly used PI3K/AKT pathway inhibitor, and treatment with LY294002 could restore the chemosensitivity of CACAN2D3-knockdown cells to cisplatin.

MATERIALS AND METHODS

Cell Lines and Reagents

Six ESCC cell lines (KYSE30, KYSE140, KYSE180, KYSE410, KYSE510, and KYSE520) were purchased from DSMZ, the German Resource Centre for Biological Material (23). The short tandem repeat (STR) analysis technique was used to periodically identify all cell lines. Cell lines were cultured in RPMI1640 medium (Hyclone, Logan, UT, USA) supplemented with 10% fetal bovine serum and 1 × penicillin/streptomycin (100 units/mL, 100 μg/mL) (Gibco, NY, USA) at 37°C in a humidified incubator (5% CO_2/95% air). Cisplatin was acquired from Sigma. LY294002 was purchased from Selleck.

Plasmid Constructs and Stable Transfection

CACNA2D3 cDNA was amplified from normal human esophageal epithelial cells. The eukaryotic expression vector pcDNA3.1 (+) (Invitrogen, Carlsbad, CA, USA) was used for cloning the human CACNA2D3 gene. Then pcDNA3.1-CACNA2D3 was transfected into the ESCC cell line KYSE30 using Lipofectamine™ 3000 (Invitrogen, Carlsbad, CA, USA). The empty vector was used as a negative control. KYSE30 cells stably expressing CACNA2D3 were screened with 500 μg/ml G418.

RNA Interference

Small interfering RNA (siRNA) (SR310953) targeting CACNA2D3 and scrambled negative control siRNA (SR30004) were purchased from OriGene. After transfection for 48 h, the relative expression of CACNA2D3 was detected by quantitative real-time PCR (qRT-PCR) and western blotting.

Cell Viability Assay

A Cell Counting Kit-8 (CCK-8) assay (Dojindo, Kumamoto, Japan) was performed to measure cell viability. Cells were seeded at a density of 1×10^4 cells/well in 96-well plates and incubated with serial dilutions of cisplatin for 72 h. The CCK-8 reagent and RPMI-1640 were diluted in a 1:9 ratio and used to replace the original medium. After incubation at 37°C for 2.5 h, absorbance at a wavelength of 450 nm was measured using a microplate reader. Three independent experiments were conducted. Half maximal inhibitory concentration (IC50) was calculated to evaluate cell resistance to cisplatin using GraphPad Prism 5.0.

Colony Formation Assay

Cells were seeded at a density of 1.5×10^3 cells/well in six-well plates and treated with respective concentrations of cisplatin. After incubation for 10–14 days, the cell colonies were fixed with ethanol for 30 min and then stained with 0.1% crystal violet for 15 min. Colonies (≥50 cells) were counted. All assays were independently performed in triplicate.

Intracellular Calcium Assay

The fluorescent probe Fluo-3 AM assay (Beyotime, Haimen, China) was used to measure intracellular Ca^{2+} concentrations. Cells were washed twice with phosphate-buffered saline (PBS) and then loaded with Fluo-3 AM (1 μM) for 30 min in the dark at 37°C. When Fluo-3 AM penetrates the cellular membrane, it is hydrolyzed by cellular esterases to Fluo-3. Fluo-3 emits green fluorescence when combined with Ca^{2+}. The intracellular Ca^{2+} concentration was measured by flow cytometric analysis.

Apoptosis Assays

Apoptosis in ESCC cells treated with or without cisplatin were evaluated using an Annexin V-FITC/propidium iodide (PI) kit (Beyotime, Haimen, China). In brief, cells were digested, washed, and centrifuged twice with cold PBS. After fixing in 75% ethanol for 3 h, cells were stained with Annexin V-FITC and PI at room temperature for 30 min. Then, cells were measured by flow cytometry with FL-1 (530 nm) and FL-2 (585 nm) at an excitation wave length of 480 nm. The data were quantified using the FlowJo software.

Mitochondrial Membrane Potential Array

The mitochondrial membrane potential (ΔΨm) was analyzed using a JC-1 assay kit (Beyotime, Haimen, China). JC-1 is a fluorescent probe for detecting mitochondrial membrane potential; it accumulates in the mitochondrial matrix and forms a red fluorescent polymer under high membrane potential. When the mitochondrial membrane potential is low, JC-1 exists as a monomer and produces green fluorescence. The cells were trypsinized and stained with JC-1 (10 mg/mL) at 37°C for 20 min. After being washed twice in PBS, cells were analyzed by flow cytometry using emission wavelengths of 590 and 525 nm.

Quantitative Real-Time PCR

Total RNA was extracted from ESCC cells using TRIzol reagent (Invitrogen, Carlsbad, CA, USA). First-strand cDNA was synthesized using the Reverse Transcription System (Promega, Wisconsin, USA), and mRNA expression levels were measured by qRT-PCR using a CFX96 Touch™ Real-Time PCR Detection System with SYBR Green Dye mixes (Applied Biosystems, Foster City, CA, USA). The PCR primers used for q-PCR were as follows. CACNA2D3: forward (5′-AGGGATTCACGG TTATGCCTT-3′), reverse (5′-GCCACACCTAAACCCTTT GTC-3′); β-Actin, forward (5′-GCTTGTCCAAGAGTGCAT GGT-3′), reverse (5′-CAGGGCTGGTTCTCGATGG-3′). The amplification parameters were: 5 min denaturation at 94°C, 40 cycles of denaturation 15 s at 94°C, 15 s annealing at 60°C, and 15 s elongation at 72°C, with final extension for 10 min at 72°C. The results were normalized to an internal standard with β-actin, and gene expression was analyzed using the $2^{-\Delta\Delta CT}$ method.

Tumor Xenograft Models

BALB/c nude mice (specific pathogen-free grade, 4–5 weeks old, and 15–20 g in weight) were purchased from Guangdong Medical Laboratory Animal Center (Guangzhou, China). The animals were raised at Jinan University Experimental Animal Management Center. KYSE30-CACNA2D3 cells and KYSE30-vector cells (6×10^6) were subcutaneously inoculated into the right armpit of each nude mouse. Tumor-bearing nude mice were randomly assigned to one of two groups of five mice: the treatment group mice received intraperitoneal injection cisplatin (2 mg/kg, twice per week for 4 weeks), and the control group mice were injected with PBS. Tumor volumes (mm^3) were calculated by the formula $V = 0.5 \times L \times W^2$. The mice were sacrificed and the tumors were isolated, weighed, and imaged. This study was carried out in accordance with the principles of the Basel Declaration and recommendations of the Guide for the Care and Use of Laboratory Animals, US National Institutes of Health (NIH Publication No. 85–23, revised 1996). The protocol was approved by the Laboratory Animal Ethics Committee of Jinan University.

Immunohistochemistry

Immunohistochemical staining was performed with primary antibodies against CACNA2D3 (Novus Biological, Littleton, CO, USA). Sections of xenografts from mice were deparaffinized with xylene and rehydrated in alcohol baths, then incubated in 3% hydrogen peroxide for 20 min to block endogenous peroxidase activity. Antigen retrieval was performed by microwave antigen retrieval in a citric acid buffer (pH 6.0). The slides were subsequently incubated with primary antibodies at 4°C overnight and then incubated with biotinylated secondary antibodies at room temperature for 30 min, followed by incubation with horseradish peroxidase (HRP)-streptavidin for 30 min. Finally, diaminobenzidine (DAB) staining and hematoxylin counterstaining were performed. All samples were observed through a high-power light microscope.

TUNEL Analysis

A colorimetric TUNEL apoptosis assay kit (Beyotime, Haimen, China) was used to identify apoptotic cells in the xenograft. Sections of xenograft from mice were deparaffinized, rehydrated, and incubated with proteinase K for 5 min at 37°C. Endogenous peroxidase was inactivated by treatment with 0.3% hydrogen peroxide for 20 min at room temperature. The sections were washed in PBS and incubated with a labeling buffer containing TdT at 37°C for 1 h, before being incubated with HRP-streptavidin for 30 min. Finally, the sections were incubated with DAB solution for coloration. All samples were observed through a high-power light microscope.

RNA Sequencing (RNA-seq) and Sequencing Analysis

Equal amounts of RNA samples were used to construct strand-specific RNA libraries, following the manufacturer's standard procedures. The libraries were sequenced on a HiSeq X Ten (Illumina, San Diego, CA, USA) platform in PE150 mode. The index of the reference genome was built using Bowtie v2.2.3 (24). Differentially expressed genes (DEGs) were identified using DESeq2 (25). The thresholds for DEGs were set as false discovery rate (FDR) ≤ 0.05 and $|\log_2 \text{fold change}| \geq 1$. Gene ontology (GO; http://www.geneontology.org) classification analysis was performed for DEGs, including molecular function, cellular component, and biological process information (26). The Kyoto Encyclopedia of Genes and Genomes (KEGG; http://www.kegg.jp) was used for systematic analysis of the signaling pathways involving the DEGs (27), and related pathways were evaluated by gene set enrichment analysis (GSEA; http://software.broadinstitute.org/gsea/) (28).

Western Blot Assay

Western blot analysis was performed according to conventional methods. Antibodies against Akt, phosphor-Akt, PI3K, phosphor-PI3K, and GAPDH were from Cell Signaling Technology.

Statistical Analysis

Statistical analysis was performed using GraphPad Prism 5.0 and SPSS 19.0. Data were expressed as mean ± standard deviation (S.D.). Significant differences between two independent groups were identified by student's t-test and expressed as $^{*}p < 0.05$, $^{**}p < 0.01$, or $^{***}p < 0.001$.

RESULTS

Downregulation of CACNA2D3 Is Correlated With Chemoresistance in ESCC

To analyze the relationship between the expression of CACNA2D3 and chemoresistance in ESCC, we screened microarray data predicting the response of esophageal cancer patients to neoadjuvant chemotherapy from the Gene Expression Omnibus (GSE45670) (29). As shown in **Figure 1A**, the expression of CACNA2D3 in the neoadjuvant chemotherapy responder group was significantly higher than that in the non-responder group ($p < 0.05$). We further investigated the association of CACNA2D3 expression with chemotherapeutic response in ESCC cell lines by calculating the IC50 values of cisplatin during treatment. Six ESCC cell lines were treated with different concentrations of cisplatin. The IC50 dose was calculated in each cell, and qRT-PCR was used to determine the expression level of CACNA2D3. The results showed that the IC50 value of cisplatin was negatively correlated with CACNA2D3 expression in ESCC cell lines (**Figures 1B,C**). These observations indicated that CACNA2D3 might regulate chemosensitivity in ESCC.

CACNA2D3 Enhances Cisplatin Sensitivity in ESCC

To investigate the role of CACNA2D3 in regulating cisplatin sensitivity in ESCC cells, a KYSE30 cell line stably expressing CACNA2D3 (30-CAC) was constructed. Control cells were transfected with empty vector (30-Vec). The expression of CACNA2D3 was determined by western blotting and qRT-PCR (**Figure 2A**). CCK8 assays showed that overexpression of CACNA2D3 (30-CAC) could significantly increase the cells' chemosensitivity to cisplatin compared with controls (30-Vec) (**Figure 2B**). The sensitivity of 30-CAC cells to cisplatin was more than twice that of 30-Vec control cells, based on the IC50 value (**Figure 2C**). In colony formation experiments, we also found that overexpression of CACNA2D3 combined with cisplatin could inhibit the formation of clones more significantly (**Figure 2D**). We next examined whether knocking down CACNA2D3 would contribute to cisplatin resistance in ESCC. The results showed that specific siRNA against CACNA2D3 could significantly suppress the expression of CACNA2D3 up to 48 h after transfection in KYSE180 (**Figure 2E**). Knockdown of CACNA2D3 (180-siCAC) significantly induced cisplatin resistance compared with the scrambled siRNA (180-scr) (**Figure 2F**). The IC50 value of 180-siCAC was higher than that of 180-scr cells ($p < 0.001$) (**Figure 2G**). CACNA2D3 knockdown resulted in significantly higher colony formation efficiency in 180-siCAC cells than in control cells in the presence of cisplatin (**Figure 2H**). Taken together, the data showed that CACNA2D3 sensitized ESCC cells to cisplatin.

CACNA2D3 Enhances Cisplatin-Induced Apoptosis Through the Mitochondria-Dependent Pathway

CACNA2D3, as a regulatory subunit, has been reported to elevate the influx of extracellular Ca^{2+} into cells. In our study, Ca^{2+} levels were detected by Fluo-3 AM staining to evaluate their relationship with CACNA2D3 expression levels. CACNA2D3-overexpressing KYSE30 cells (30-CAC) showed significantly increased intracellular Ca^{2+} compared with the control cells (30-Vec), whereas knockdown of CACNA2D3 in KYSE180 cells (180-siCAC) caused a decrease in intracellular Ca^{2+} levels compared with control cells (180-scr) (**Figure 3A**). As Ca^{2+} can induce mitochondrial permeability changes and regulate the initiation phase of apoptosis, we performed an apoptosis assay to evaluate the effect of CACNA2D3 on the apoptosis of ESCC cells. Surprisingly, CACNA2D3 overexpression did not affect ESCC cell apoptosis, but promoted cisplatin-induced apoptosis. The percentage of apoptotic cells in 30-CAC cells increased by 24.8 ± 3.9% with cisplatin treatment, compared with 13.3 ± 1.7% in 30-Vec cells. In KYSE180 cells, cisplatin increased apoptosis by 14.2 ± 2.3% in 180-siCAC cells and by 32.3 ± 3.2% in 180-scr cells (**Figures 3B,C**). In addition, the JC-1 probe was used to assess changes in mitochondrial membrane potential in ESCC cells treated with cisplatin. As shown in **Figures 3D,E**, with cisplatin treatment, the membrane potential of 30-Vec cells decreased by 14.3 ± 2.5%, while that of 30-CAC cells decreased by 25.5 ± 1.6%. In KYSE180 cells, the membrane potential decreased by 24.2 ± 1.8% in 180-scr cells and by 9.6 ± 3.4% in 180-siCAC cells. Western blot analysis demonstrated that the ratios of cleaved Caspase9/Caspase9 and cleaved Caspase3/Caspase3 in CACNA2D3-overexpressing KYSE30 cells were higher than those in the control cells. Conversely, these ratios decreased in 180-siCAC cells treated with cisplatin compared with 180-scr cells (**Figure 3F**). Taken together, these results suggested that CACNA2D3 sensitized ESCC cells to cisplatin through enhancing mitochondria-mediated apoptosis.

CACNA2D3 Increases Cisplatin Sensitivity *in vivo*

In order to better understand the role of CACNA2D3 in cisplatin sensitivity *in vivo*, we established a subcutaneous

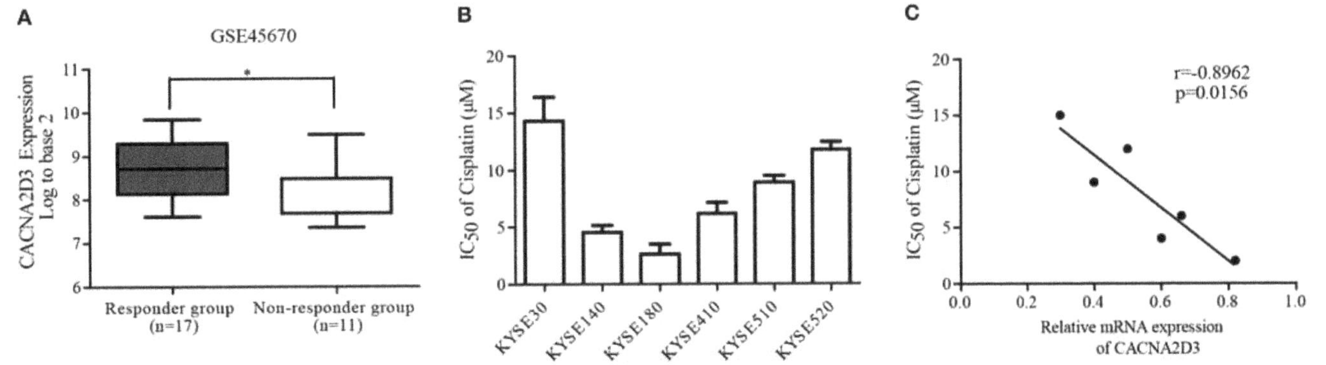

FIGURE 1 | Downregulation of CACNA2D3 is associated with poor chemotherapy response in ESCC. **(A)** Box and whisker plot of CACNA2D3 mRNA levels in neoadjuvant chemotherapy responder and non-responder groups (GSE45670). *$p < 0.05$. **(B)** IC50 values for cisplatin in six ESCC cell lines. Cells were treated with a range of concentrations of cisplatin for 72 h, and IC50 was calculated. Data are represented as the mean ± SD of three independent experiments. **(C)** Correlation of CACNA2D3 mRNA levels and IC50 values for cisplatin in six ESCC cell lines. r, Pearson correlation coefficient.

xenograft model by injecting CACNA2D3-overexpressing cells and control cells into BALB/c-nude mice. When the tumor volumes reached about 100 mm^3, 2 mg/kg cisplatin was injected intraperitoneally twice per week for 4 weeks, while the control group received PBS. As shown in **Figure 4A**, we found that overexpression of CACNA2D3 and cisplatin both inhibited the growth of xenografts. However, CACNA2D3 overexpression in combination with cisplatin could more significantly inhibit the tumorigenic ability of ESCC cells. The mean tumor size (**Figure 4B**) and weight (**Figure 4C**) in the CACNA2D3 overexpression group were significantly lower than those in the vector control group after cisplatin treatment. Moreover, immunohistochemical staining showed that the expression of CACNA2D3 was increased in the CACNA2D3-overexpressing tumors compared with the control tumors (**Figure 4D**). TUNEL analysis also revealed that the apoptosis rate of CACNA2D3 overexpression cells was significantly higher than that of the control cells after cisplatin treatment (**Figure 4E**). These results together indicated that CACNA2D3 increased cisplatin sensitivity *in vivo*.

CACANA2D3 Regulates the Sensitivity of ESCC to Cisplatin Through Inhibiting the PI3K/Akt Pathways

To better understand the molecular mechanism underlying CACNA2D3-enhanced ESCC cisplatin sensitivity, we compared the gene expression profiles of CACNA2D3 stably overexpressed KYSE30 cells with those of control cells using RNA-seq after cisplatin treatment, and identified 2439 DEGs (FDR < 0.05, $|\log_2$ fold change$| \geq 1$) between the two groups. A total of 1,137 genes were upregulated, and 1,302 genes were downregulated (**Figure 5A**). We further explored the biological functions of DEGs by GO, KEGG, and GSEA pathway enrichment analyses. Using the DAVID online GO database for comprehensive analysis, we found that CACNA2D3 was associated with multiple processes, including metabolic processes, biological regulation, regulation of biological processes, and response to stimulus (**Figure 5B**). KEGG database analysis revealed that multiple signaling pathway pathways were highly enriched, including "PI3K-Akt signaling pathway," "Pathways in cancer," "MAPK signaling pathway," and "ABC transporters" (**Figure 5C**). GSEA also showed that the CACNA2D3-regulated genes were enriched in the cell growth pathway and PI3K-Akt-mTOR signaling pathway (**Figure 5D**). Western blotting showed that CACNA2D3 dramatically suppressed the phosphorylation of PI3K and Akt, and the suppression persisted in the presence of cisplatin (**Figure 5E**). These results indicated that CACNA2D3 enhanced cisplatin sensitivity by inhibiting the PI3K/Akt pathway.

LY294002 Restores the Sensitivity of ESCC to Cisplatin in CACNA2D3-Knockdown Cells

For the rescue experiments, we treated CACNA2D3-knockdown cells with Akt inhibitor LY294002. Western blotting showed that LY294002 inhibited Akt activation in 180-siCAC cells and 180-scr cells (**Figure 6A**). The CACNA2D3-knockdown cells showed significantly higher sensitivity to cisplatin after treatment with LY294002 (**Figure 6B**). The effect of LY294002 on the IC50 reduction caused by cisplatin was significantly stronger in 180-siCAC cells than in 180-scr cells (**Figure 6C**). The colony formation assays also demonstrated that the combination of cisplatin and LY294002 suppressed colony formation more significantly in 180-siCAC cells than in control cells (**Figure 6D**). These results suggest that inhibition of the Akt signaling pathway can restore the chemosensitivity of CACNA2D3-knockdown cells to cisplatin.

DISCUSSION

ESCC is a cancer of the digestive system with high incidence in China. Although therapeutic strategies for ESCC have advanced considerably, its mortality rate remains high, and further efforts are needed to improve patient prognosis. Cisplatin is widely used

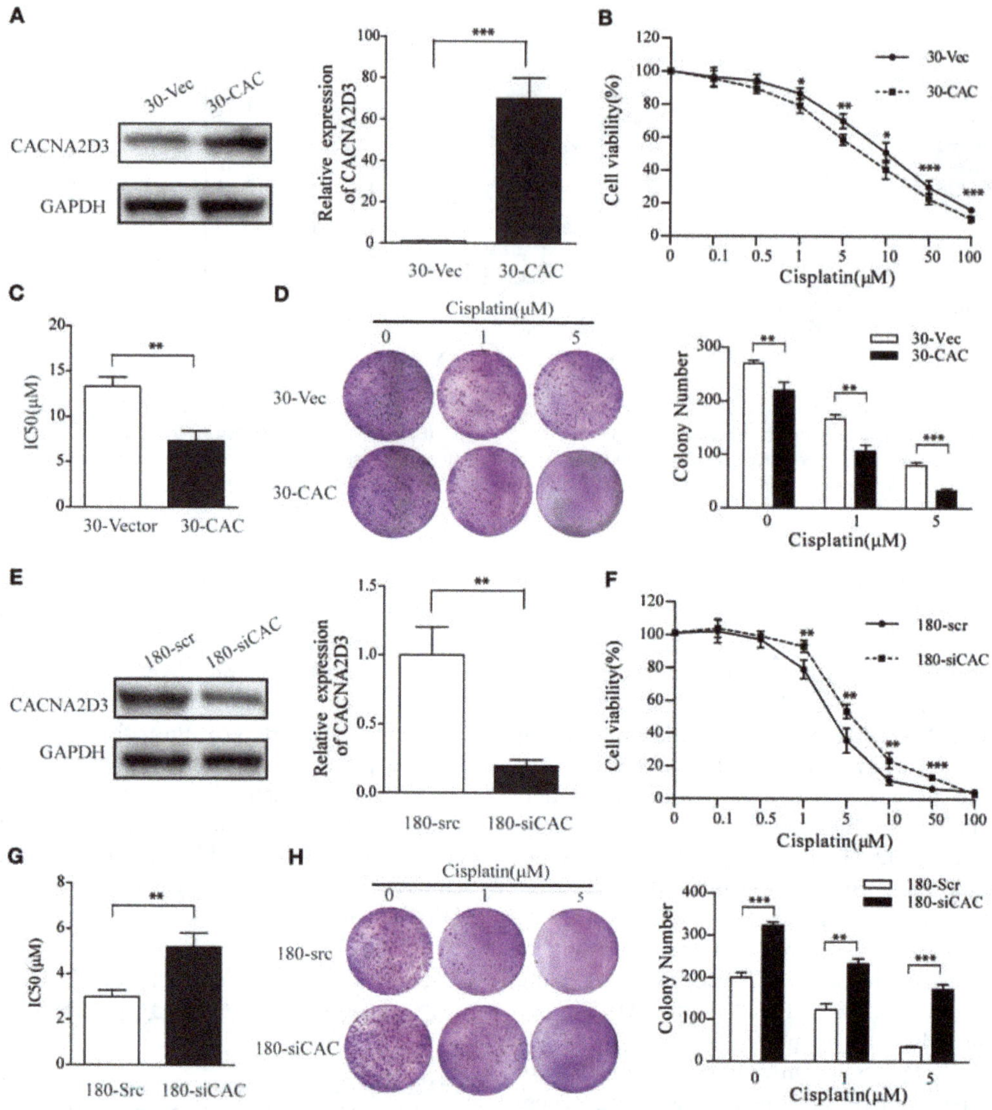

FIGURE 2 | CACNA2D3 promotes chemosensitivity to cisplatin *in vitro*. **(A,E)** Stable expression of CACNA2D3 in KYSE30 cells generated by pCDNA3.1-CACNA2D3 transfection and silencing of CACNA2D3 in KYSE180 cells by siRNA were examined by western blotting and qRT-PCR. GAPDH and β-Actin were employed as a loading control. **(B,F)** CACNA2D3-overexpressing KYSE30 cells and CACNA2D3-knockdown cells were treated with cisplatin at the indicated concentrations for 72 h. The number of viable cells was measured by CCK-8 assay. **(C,G)** IC50 values were calculated using linear or logarithmic regression ($R^2 > 0.9$). Values are presented as the mean ± SD of three wells. **(D,H)** Colony forming assays were used to determine colony forming ability after cisplatin treatment. Data are presented as the mean ± SD of three wells. $^{**}p < 0.01$, $^{***}p < 0.001$.

in the clinical chemotherapy of various types of human tumors, including esophageal, gastric, testicular, bladder, ovarian, and lung cancers (30–32). However, cisplatin resistance is often the biggest obstacle to the success of chemotherapy. Therefore, it is extremely important to be able to predict cisplatin response before chemotherapy, in order to select the most appropriate treatment strategy for patients.

Calcium ions (Ca^{2+}) are vital intracellular second messengers involved in multiple functions of cells, including proliferation, differentiation, fertilization, development, muscle contraction, cell death, learning, and memory (33–35). The voltage-gated calcium channel is a multi-subunit protein complex consisting of a channel-forming α1 subunit and three regulatory subunits, α2δ, β, and γ (36–38). CACNA2D3 encodes one of the α2δ subunits. Our previous study identified CACNA2D3 as a novel tumor suppressor gene for ESCC. Downregulation of CACNA2D3 predicted poor prognosis. Exogenous expression of CACNA2D3 can strongly inhibit cell growth, migration, and invasion, and induce apoptosis (21). In the current study, we first found that the expression of CACNA2D3 was higher in a platinum-based neoadjuvant chemotherapy responder group than in the non-responder group. Based on a serious of assays *in vitro* and *in vivo*, we confirmed the effect of CACNA2D3 on the chemosensitivity of cisplatin in ESCC cells.

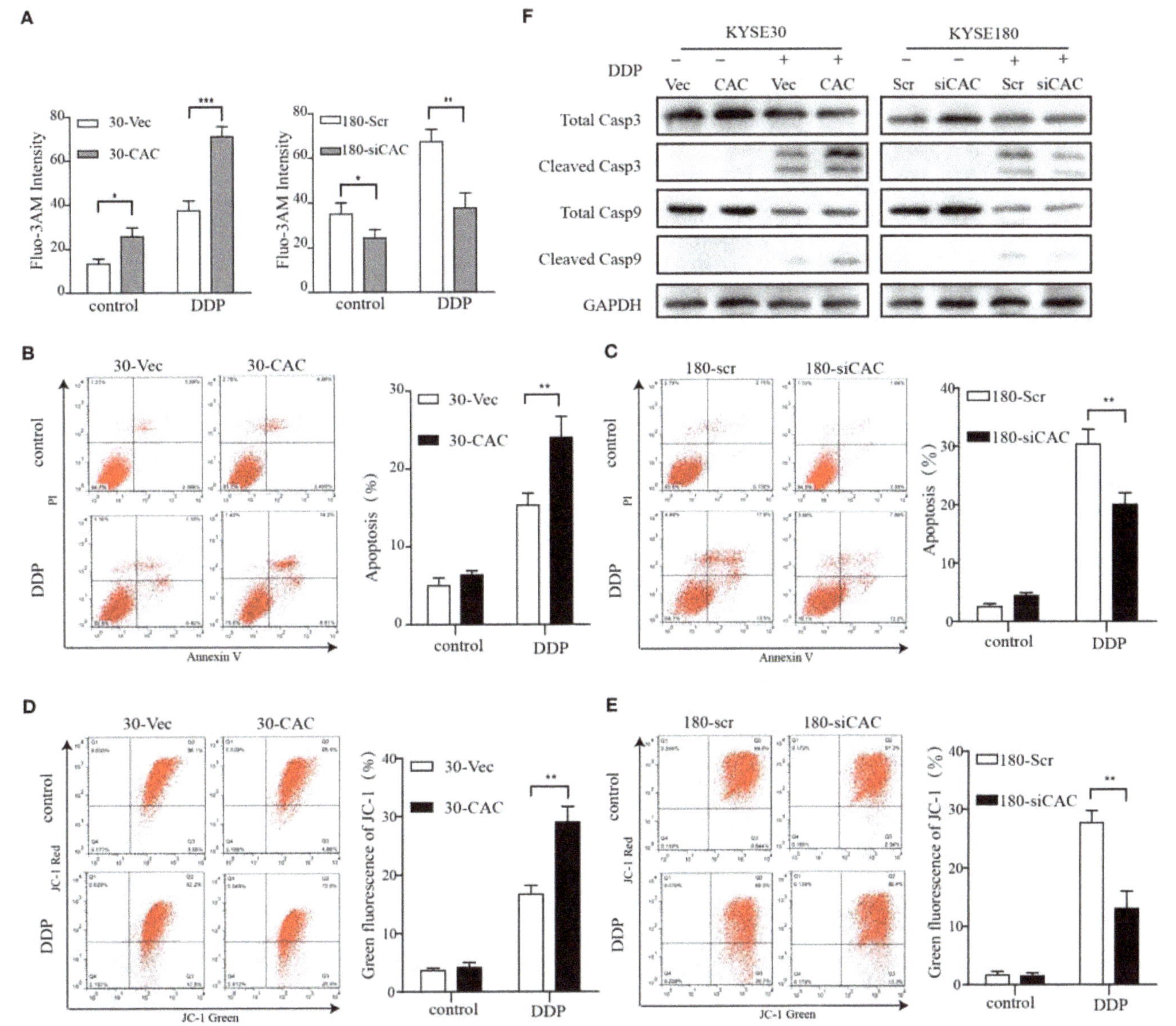

FIGURE 3 | CACNA2D3 enhances cisplatin-induced apoptosis through mitochondria-dependent pathway. **(A)** Intracellular Ca^{2+} levels were detected by fluorescence-activated cell sorting (FACS) with Fluo-3 AM. **(B,C)** Annexin V/PI staining in CACNA2D3 overexpression and knockdown cell lines treated with cisplatin for 48 h; apoptosis was analyzed by FACS. The percentages of apoptotic cells are presented as the mean ± SD of three independent experiments. **(D,E)** The mitochondrial membrane potential was measured using fluorescent dye JC-1 after treatment with cisplatin for 48 h. Percentages of green fluorescence from JC-1 in cells are presented as the mean ± SD of three independent experiments. **(F)** Levels of cleaved caspase-3, total caspase-3, cleaved caspase-9, and total caspase-9 proteins were analyzed by western blotting in CACNA2D3-overexpressing and knockdown cell lines treated with or without cisplatin. $^{*}p < 0.05$; $^{**}p < 0.01$; $^{***}p < 0.001$.

Cisplatin is a conventional chemotherapy drug. It is activated upon entering the cell, when its chloride atoms are replaced by water molecules. The resulting hydrolytic product is an effective electrophilic reagent, which can react with any nucleophile, including DNA, RNA, and proteins. DNA is the primary target of cisplatin. Cisplatin tends to bind to the N7 site of purine bases to form a DNA adduct, causing DNA damage in cancer cells, blocking cell division, and leading to apoptosis (39–41). Several mechanisms of cisplatin resistance have been discovered, including reduced intracellular drug accumulation, increased activity of efflux pumps, changed drug targets, lost mismatch-repair ability, and escape apoptosis (42–44). The voltage-dependent calcium channel α2δ subunits have been found to regulate extracellular Ca^{2+} influx (45). Our study consistently demonstrated that the overexpression of CACNA2D3 increased the uptake of intracellular free Ca^{2+} in ESCC. Apoptosis is closely related to increased intracellular Ca^{2+} concentration. Here, we found that CACNA2D3 overexpression

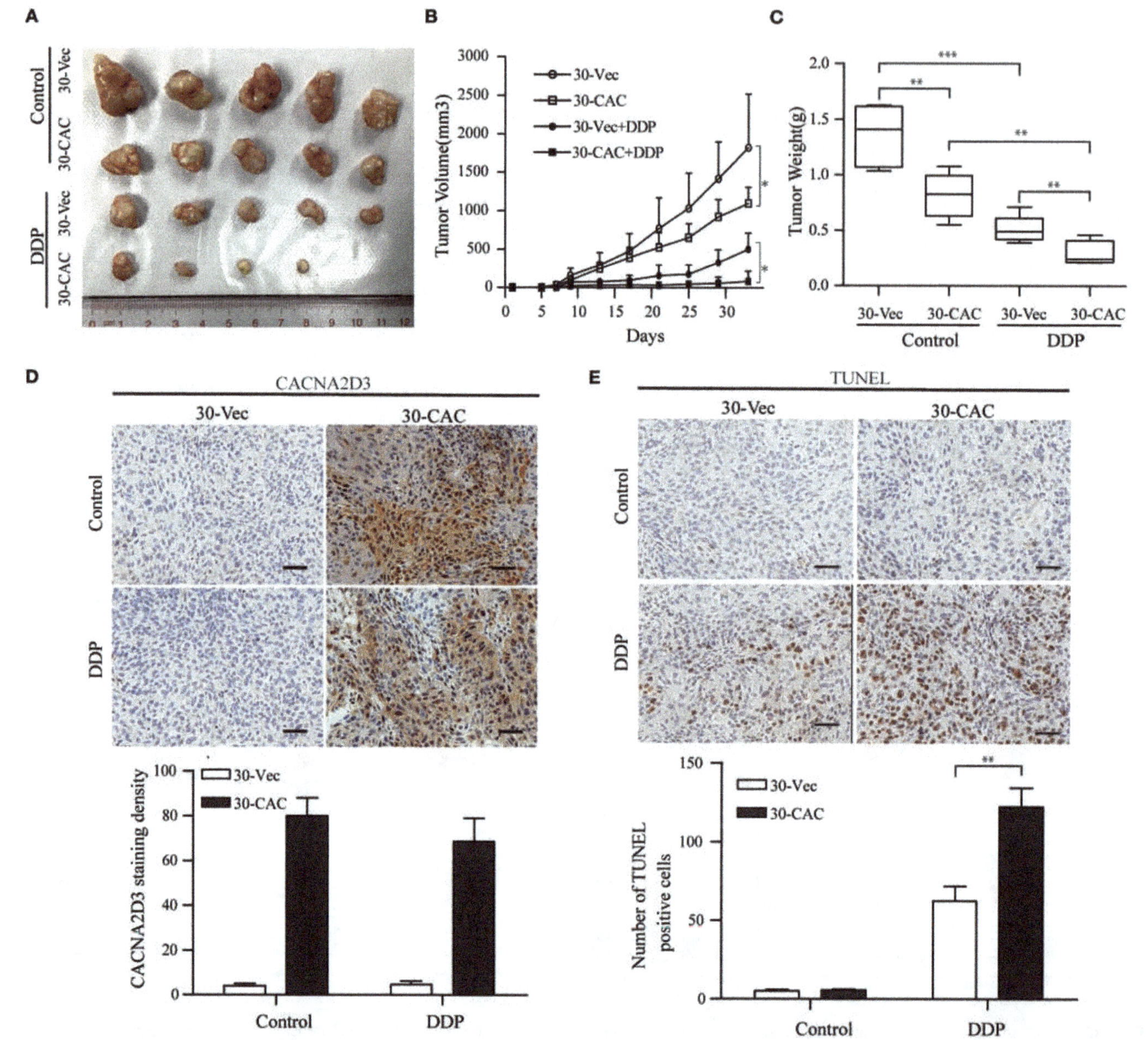

FIGURE 4 | CACNA2D3 increases chemosensitivity of ESCC cells to cisplatin *in vivo*. **(A)** Representative images of xenografted tumors derived from Balb/c-nu mice at day 33. **(B)** The mice in the treatment groups were intraperitoneally injected with 2 mg/kg every 3 days. Tumor volumes were measured at 4 days intervals. Data are presented as mean ± SD. **(C)** Tumor weights were measured after mice were sacrificed. **(D)** Detection of CACNA2D3 from tumor sections by immunohistochemical staining. Quantification was performed by calculating the percentage of the staining intensities using ImageJ. **(E)** TUNEL staining of tumor sections from each group; the number of TUNEL-positive cells was quantified by counting. $^{*}p < 0.05$; $^{**}p < 0.01$; $^{***}p < 0.001$.

did not in itself affect the apoptosis rate of ESCC cells; however, it significantly increased cisplatin-induced apoptosis. Mitochondria often have a decisive role in stimulus-induced apoptosis. Mitochondrial membrane destruction and infiltration are common phenomena related to apoptosis. Excessive Ca^{2+} accumulation inside mitochondria is thought to be a powerful apoptosis stimulator that induces mitochondrial membrane depolarization and activates downstream caspases and finally induces apoptosis (46, 47). We confirmed that ectopic expression of CACNA2D3 led to depolarization of the mitochondrial membrane potential after cisplatin treatment. Moreover, the immunoblotting results showed that CACNA2D3 overexpression activated caspase-3 and caspase-9 in ESCC cells. CACNA2D3 and cisplatin synergistically induce apoptosis by increasing Ca^{2+}-dependent collapse of mitochondrial membrane potential, indicating that CACNA2D3 enhances cisplatin-induced apoptosis by activating the mitochondrial pathway.

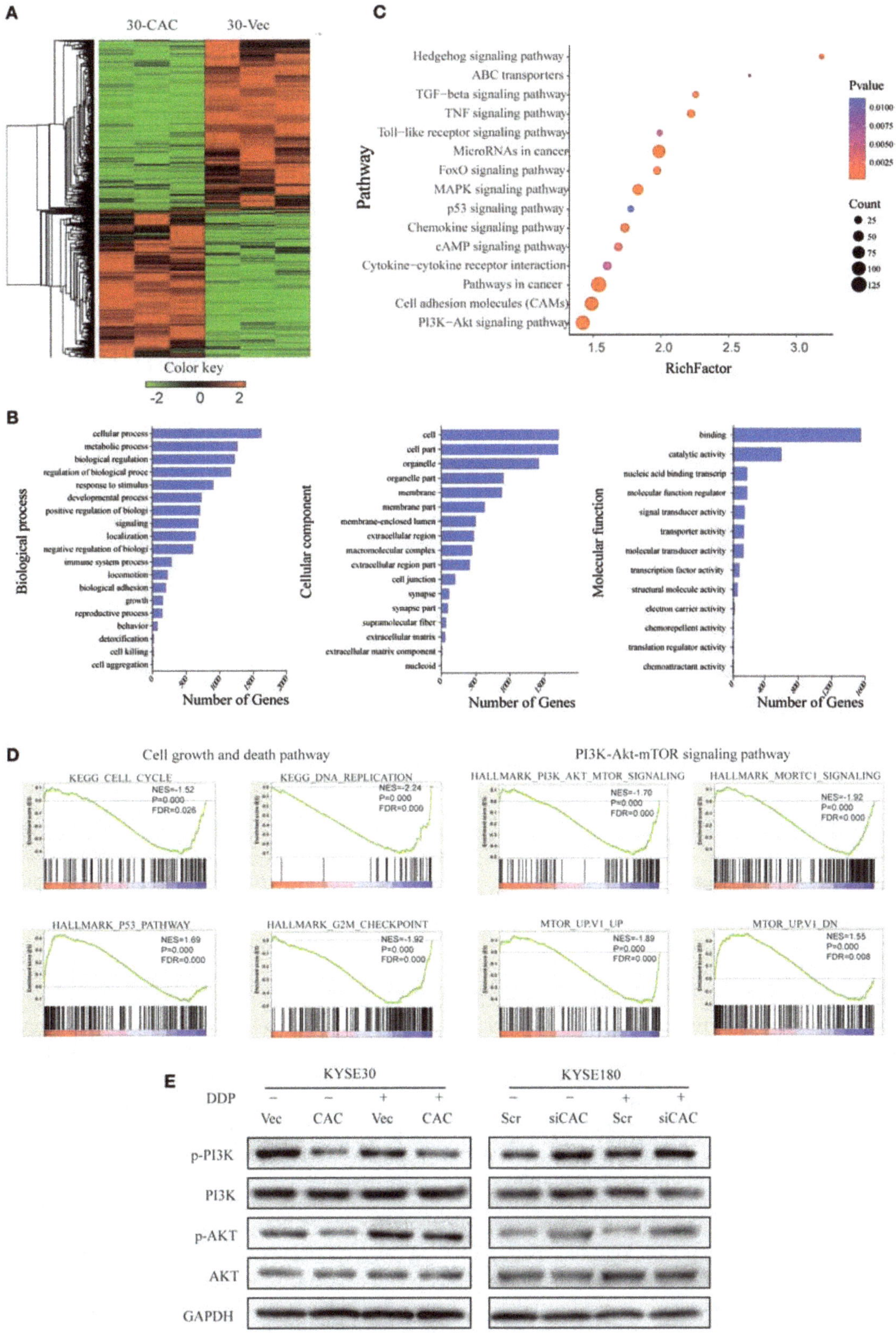

FIGURE 5 | CACANA2D3 regulated the sensitivity of ESCC to cisplatin through inhibiting the PI3K/Akt pathways. **(A)** DEG heatmap and hierarchical clustering results for CACNA2D3-overexpressing KYSE30 ESCC cells. Red and green indicate high and low gene expression, respectively. **(B)** GO enrichment analysis of the DEGs. The genes were divided into three categories: cellular component, biological process, and molecular function genes. **(C)** KEGG pathway enrichment analysis

(Continued)

FIGURE 5 | of differentially expressed pathways upon CACNA2D3 overexpression. The ordinates represent the enriched KEGG pathway. $p < 0.05$ was considered statistically significant. **(D)** GSEA analysis of differentially expressed pathways upon CACNA2D3 overexpression. NES, normalized enrichment score. **(E)** Levels of P-PI3K, PI3K, P-Akt, and Akt proteins were analyzed by western blotting in CACNA2D3-overexpressing and knockdown cell lines treated with or without cisplatin.

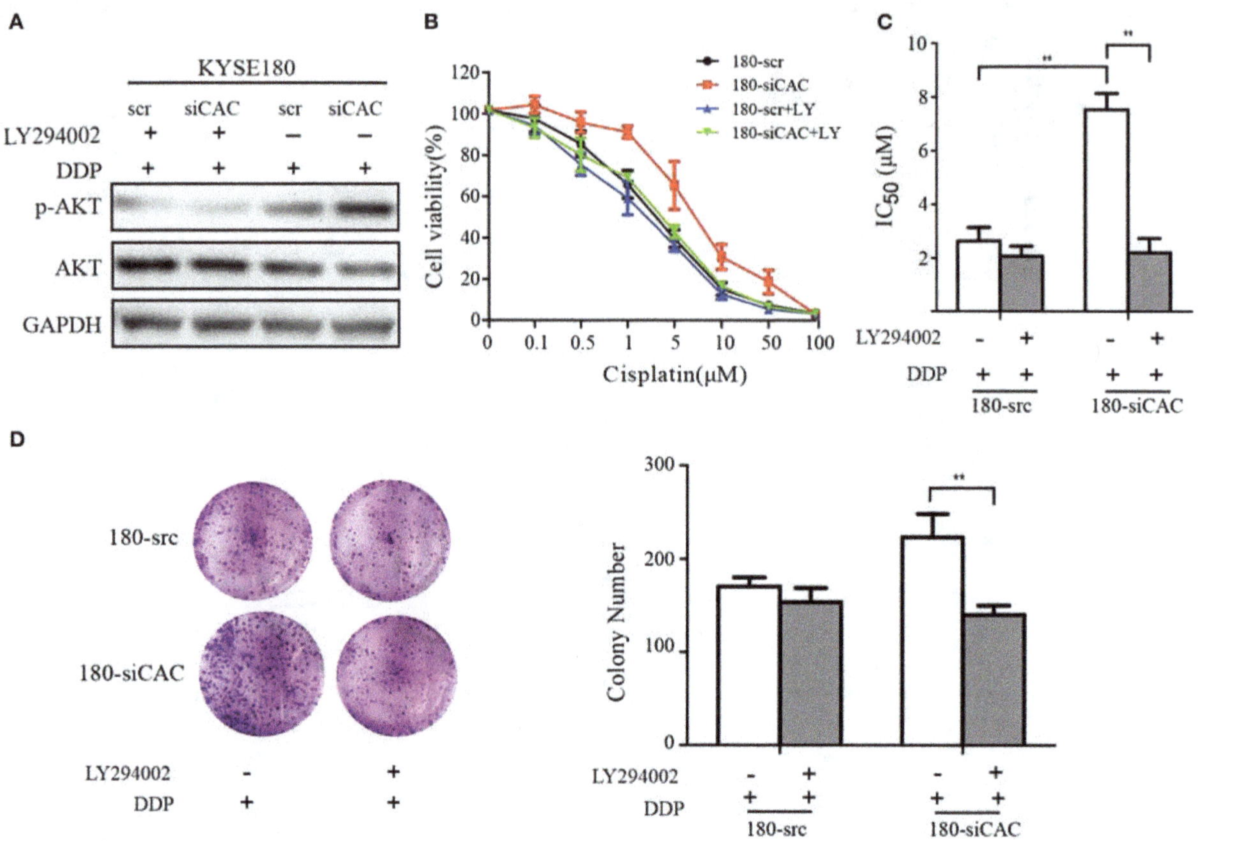

FIGURE 6 | LY294002 restores the sensitivity of ESCC to cisplatin in CACNA2D3-knockdown cells. **(A)** CACNA2D3-knockdown KYSE180 cells and control cells were treated with cisplatin at the indicated concentrations with or without LY294002 for 72 h. Levels of P-Akt and Akt proteins were analyzed by western blotting. **(B)** The number of viable cells was measured by CCK-8 assay. **(C)** IC50 values were calculated using linear or logarithmic regression ($R2 > 0.9$). Data are presented as the mean ± SD from triplicate wells. **(D)** Colony forming assays were used to determine the colony forming ability after cisplatin with or without LY294002 treatment. Data are presented as the mean ± SD from three wells. $^{**}p < 0.01$.

To systematically investigate the underlying molecular mechanism mediating CACNA2D3-induced ESCC cisplatin sensitivity, we compared the expression profiles of KYSE30 cells with and without CACNA2D3 overexpression after cisplatin treatment using RNA-seq. By pathway enrichment analyses, we found that CACNA2D3 could inhibit DNA replication and block ESCC cells in the G2/M phase by inhibiting the expression of p53, as shown in our previous study (21). We also found the PI3K/Akt pathway to be inactivated in CACNA2D3-overexpressing ESCC cells. The PI3K/Akt signaling pathway has important roles in promoting cell growth, proliferation, invasion, angiogenesis, and drug resistance. In-depth studies of the relationship between the PI3K/Akt signaling pathway and drug resistance have led to this pathway being considered as a new target for chemotherapy drug resistance therapy (48, 49). Here, we found that the phosphorylation of PI3K and Akt was blocked in CACNA2D3-overexpressing KYSE30 cells. Consistently, when CACNA2D3 was knocked down in KYSE180 cells, the phosphorylation level of Akt showed a significant increase. Interestingly, our data also showed that blockade of the PI3K/Akt pathway by LY294002 in CACNA2D3-knockdown cells could restore chemosensitivity to cisplatin.

In summary, in this work we first proved that the expression of CACNA2D3 was associated with chemosensitivity in ESCC patients treated with cisplatin-based therapy. Moreover, CACNA2D3 increased chemosensitivity to cisplatin in cell experiments and xenograft tumors, indicating that it could be used as a tumor marker to predict and improve patients' response to cisplatin. We further found that CACNA2D3 regulated cisplatin-induced apoptosis and decreased Akt phosphorylation. Detection of CACNA2D3 expression might be helpful for individualized treatment of ESCC patients.

AUTHOR CONTRIBUTIONS

CN, XC, and AH designed the study. CN, XQ, XL, YZ, YJ, YL, and QW performed the experiments. CN, XQ, XL, DZ, and BT analyzed the data. CN, XL, and XC wrote the paper.

FUNDING

This work was supported by grants from the National Natural Science Foundation of China (grants 81360365, 81472337, 81473131), the National Key Basic Research Program of China (973 Program) (grant 2015CB553706), the Science & Technology Program of Guangdong province (grant 2016A020217012), the Science &Technology Program of Guangzhou (grant 2016201604030039), and the Guangxi Natural Science Foundation of China (grant 2014GXNSFBA118205, 2017GXNSFAA198157). We thank Yuying Zhou and Shujun Guo from the Institute of Biomedicine of Jinan University for technical assistance.

REFERENCES

1. Ferlay J, Soerjomataram I, Dikshit R, Eser S, Mathers C, Rebelo M, et al. Cancer incidence and mortality worldwide: sources, methods and major patterns in GLOBOCAN 2012. *Int J Cancer.* (2015) 136:E359–86. doi: 10.1002/ijc.29210
2. Arnold M, Soerjomataram I, Ferlay J, Forman, D. Global incidence of oesophageal cancer by histological subtype in 2012. *Gut.* (2015) 64:381–7. doi: 10.1136/gutjnl-2014-308124
3. Zhang Y. Epidemiology of esophageal cancer. *World J Gastroenterol.* (2013) 19:5598–606. doi: 10.3748/wjg.v19.i34.5598
4. Lin Y, Totsuka Y, He Y, Kikuchi S, Qiao Y, Ueda J, et al. Epidemiology of esophageal cancer in Japan and China. *J epidemiol.* (2013) 233–42. doi: 10.2188/jea.JE20120162
5. Ando N, Iizuka T, Ide H, Ishida K, Shinoda M, Nishimaki T, et al. Surgery plus chemotherapy compared with surgery alone for localized squamous cell carcinoma of the thoracic esophagus: a Japan clinical oncology group study–JCOG9204. *J Clin Oncol.* (2003) 21:4592–6. doi: 10.1200/JCO.2003.12.095
6. Iinuma H, Fukushima R, Inaba T, Tamura J, Inoue T, Ogawa E, et al. Phase I clinical study of multiple epitope peptide vaccine combined with chemoradiation therapy in esophageal cancer patients. *J Transl Med.* (2014) 12:84. doi: 10.1186/1479-5876-12-84
7. Lyu X, Huang J, Mao Y, Liu Y, Feng Q, Shao K, et al. Adjuvant chemotherapy after esophagectomy: is there a role in the treatment of the lymph node positive thoracic esophageal squamous cell carcinoma? *J Surg Oncol.* (2014) 110:864–8. doi: 10.1002/jso.23716
8. Kato K, Muro K, Minashi K, Ohtsu A, Ishikura S, Boku N, et al. Phase II study of chemoradiotherapy with 5-fluorouracil and cisplatin for Stage II-III esophageal squamous cell carcinoma: JCOG trial (JCOG 9906). *Int J Rad Oncol Biol Phys.* (2011) 81: 684–90. doi: 10.1016/j.ijrobp.2010.06.033
9. Miyazaki T, Sohda M, Tanaka N, Suzuki S, Ieta K, Sakai M, et al. Phase I/II study of docetaxel, cisplatin, and 5-fluorouracil combination chemoradiotherapy in patients with advanced esophageal cancer. *Cancer Chemother Pharmacol.* (2015) 75:449–55. doi: 10.1007/s00280-014-2659-6
10. Hashimoto J, Kato K, Ito Y, Kojima T, Akimoto T, Daiko H, et al. Phase II feasibility study of preoperative concurrent chemoradiotherapy with cisplatin plus 5-fluorouracil and elective lymph node irradiation for clinical stage II/III esophageal squamous cell carcinoma. *Int J Clin Oncol.* (2018) 24:60–7. doi: 10.1007/s10147-018-1336-x
11. Yuasa Y, Nagasaki H, Akiyama Y, Hashimoto Y, Takizawa T, Kojima K, et al. DNA methylation status is inversely correlated with green tea intake and physical activity in gastric cancer patients. *Int J Cancer.* (2009) 124:2677–82. doi: 10.1002/ijc.24231
12. Wanajo A, Sasaki A, Nagasaki H, Shimada S, Otsubo T, Owaki S, et al. Methylation of the calcium channel-related gene, CACNA2D3, is frequent and a poor prognostic factor in gastric cancer. *Gastroenterology.* (2008) 135:580–90. doi: 10.1053/j.gastro.2008.05.041
13. Qu Y, Dang S, Hou P. Gene methylation in gastric cancer. *Clin Chim Acta.* (2013) 424:53–65. doi: 10.1016/j.cca.2013.05.002
14. Wong AM, Kong KL, Chen L, Liu M, Wong AM, Zhu C, et al. Characterization of CACNA2D3 as a putative tumor suppressor gene in the development and progression of nasopharyngeal carcinoma. *Int J Cancer.* (2013) 133:2284–95. doi: 10.1002/ijc.28252
15. Palmieri C, Rudraraju B, Monteverde M, Lattanzio L, Gojis O, Brizio R, et al. Methylation of the calcium channel regulatory subunit alpha2delta-3 (CACNA2D3) predicts site-specific relapse in oestrogen receptor-positive primary breast carcinomas. *Br J Cancer.* (2012) 107:375–81. doi: 10.1038/bjc.2012.231
16. Hanke S, Bugert P, Chudek J, Kovacs G. Cloning a calcium channel alpha2delta-3 subunit gene from a putative tumor suppressor gene region at chromosome 3p21.1 in conventional renal cell carcinoma. *Gene.* (2001) 264: 69–75. doi: 10.1016/S0378-1119(00)00600-4
17. Tai AL, Mak W, Ng PK, Chua DT, Ng MY, Fu L, et al. High-throughput loss-of-heterozygosity study of chromosome 3p in lung cancer using single-nucleotide polymorphism markers. *Cancer Res.* (2006) 66:4133–8. doi: 10.1158/0008-5472.CAN-05-2775
18. Jin Y, Cui D, Ren J, Wang K, Zeng T, Gao L. CACNA2D3 is downregulated in gliomas and functions as a tumor suppressor. *Mol Carcinogene.* (2017) 56: 945–59. doi: 10.1002/mc.22548
19. De Preter K, Vandesompele J, Heimann P, Yigit N, Beckman S, Schramm A, et al. Human fetal neuroblast and neuroblastoma transcriptome analysis confirms neuroblast origin and highlights neuroblastoma candidate genes. *Genome Biol.* (2006) 7:R84. doi: 10.1186/gb-2006-7-9-r84
20. Thorell K, Bergman A, Caren H, Nilsson S, Kogner P, Martinsson T, et al. Verification of genes differentially expressed in neuroblastoma tumours: a study of potential tumour suppressor genes. *BMC Med Genom.* (2009) 2:53. doi: 10.1186/1755-8794-2-53
21. Li Y, Zhu CL, Nie CJ, Li JC, Zeng TT, Zhou J, et al. Investigation of tumor suppressing function of CACNA2D3 in esophageal squamous cell carcinoma. *PLoS ONE.* (2013) 8:e60027. doi: 10.1371/journal.pone.0060027
22. Negoro E, Yamauchi T, Urasaki Y, Nishi R, Hori H, Ueda T. Characterization of cytarabine-resistant leukemic cell lines established from five different blood cell lineages using gene expression and proteomic analyses. *Int J Oncol.* (2011) 38:911–9. doi: 10.3892/ijo.2011.933
23. Shimada Y, Imamura M, Wagata T, Yamaguchi N, Tobe T. Characterization of 21 newly established esophageal cancer cell lines. *Cancer.* (1992) 69:277–84. doi: 10.1002/1097-0142(19920115)69:2<277::AID-CNCR2820690202>3.0.CO;2-C
24. Langmead B, Trapnell C, Pop M, Salzberg SL. Ultrafast and memory-efficient alignment of short DNA sequences to the human genome. *Genome Biol.* (2009) 10:R25. doi: 10.1186/gb-2009-10-3-r25
25. Love MI, Huber W, Anders S. Moderated estimation of fold change and dispersion for RNA-seq data with DESeq2. *Genome Biol.* (2014) 15:550. doi: 10.1186/s13059-014-0550-8
26. Ashburner M, Ball CA, Blake JA, Botstein D, Butler H, Cherry JM, et al. Gene ontology: tool for the unification of biology. The gene ontology consortium. *Nat Genet.* (2000) 25:25–9. doi: 10.1038/75556
27. Huang da W, Sherman BT, Lempicki RA. Systematic and integrative analysis of large gene lists using DAVID bioinformatics resources. *Nat Protocol.* (2009) 4: 44–57. doi: 10.1038/nprot.2008.211
28. Subramanian A, Tamayo P, Mootha VK, Mukherjee S, Ebert BL, Gillette MA, et al. Gene set enrichment analysis: a knowledge-based approach for interpreting genome-wide expression profiles. *Proc Natl Acad Sci USA.* (2005) 102:15545–50. doi: 10.1073/pnas.0506580102
29. Wen J, Yang H, Liu MZ, Luo KJ, Liu H, Hu Y, et al. Gene expression analysis of pretreatment biopsies predicts the pathological response of esophageal

squamous cell carcinomas to neo-chemoradiotherapy. *Ann Oncol.* (2014) 25:1769–74. doi: 10.1093/annonc/mdu201

30. Sersa G, Stabuc B, Cemazar M, Miklavcic D, Rudolf Z. Electrochemotherapy with cisplatin: clinical experience in malignant melanoma patients. *Clin Cancer Res.* (2000) 6:863–7.
31. Kelland L. The resurgence of platinum-based cancer chemotherapy. *Nat Rev Cancer.* (2007) 7:573–84. doi: 10.1038/nrc2167
32. Galluzzi L, Vitale I, Michels J, Brenner C, Szabadkai G, Harel-Bellan A, et al. Systems biology of cisplatin resistance: past, present and future. *Cell Death Dis.* (2014) 5: e1257. doi: 10.1038/cddis.2013.428
33. Berridge MJ, Bootman MD, and Lipp P. Calcium-a life and death signal. *Nature.* (1998) 395: 645–8. doi: 10.1038/27094
34. Webb SE, Miller AL. Calcium signalling during embryonic development. *Nat Rev Mol Cell Biol.* (2003) 4:539–51. doi: 10.1038/nrm1149
35. Monteith GR, McAndrew D, Faddy HM, Roberts-Thomson SJ. Calcium and cancer: targeting Ca^{2+} transport. *Nat Rev Cancer.* (2007) 7:519–30. doi: 10.1038/nrc2171
36. Gong HC, Hang J, Kohler W, Li L, Su TZ. Tissue-specific expression and gabapentin-binding properties of calcium channel alpha2delta subunit subtypes. *J Membr Biol.* (2001) 184:35–43. doi: 10.1007/s00232-001-0072-7
37. Davies A, Hendrich J, Van Minh AT, Wratten J, Douglas L, Dolphin AC. Functional biology of the alpha(2)delta subunits of voltage-gated calcium channels. *Trends Pharmacol Sci.* (2007) 28:220–8. doi: 10.1016/j.tips.2007.03.005
38. Qin N, Yagel S, Momplaisir ML, Codd EE, D'Andrea MR. Molecular cloning and characterization of the human voltage-gated calcium channel alpha(2)delta-4 subunit. *Mol Pharmacol.* (2002) 62: 485–96. doi: 10.1124/mol.62.3.485
39. Siddik ZH. Cisplatin: mode of cytotoxic action and molecular basis of resistance. Oncogene (2003) 22: 7265-79. doi: 10.1038/sj.onc.1206933
40. Wang D, Lippard SJ. Cellular processing of platinum anticancer drugs. *Nat Rev Drug Disc.* (2005) 4:307–20. doi: 10.1038/nrd1691
41. Johnstone TC, Suntharalingam K, Lippard SJ. The next generation of platinum drugs: targeted Pt(II) agents, nanoparticle delivery, and Pt(IV) prodrugs. *Chem Rev.* (2016) 116:3436–86. doi: 10.1021/acs.chemrev.5b00597
42. Hall MD, Okabe M, Shen DW, Liang XJ, Gottesman MM. The role of cellular accumulation in determining sensitivity to platinum-based chemotherapy. *Ann Rev Pharmacol Toxicol.* (2008) 48: 495–535. doi: 10.1146/annurev.pharmtox.48.080907.180426
43. Holohan C, Van Schaeybroeck S, Longley DB, Johnston PG. Cancer drug resistance: an evolving paradigm. *Nat Rev Cancer.* (2013) 13:714–26. doi: 10.1038/nrc3599
44. Ferreira JA, Peixoto A, Neves M, Gaiteiro C, Reis CA, Assaraf YG, et al. Mechanisms of cisplatin resistance and targeting of cancer stem cells: Adding glycosylation to the equation. *Drug Resist Updates.* (2016) 24:34–54. doi: 10.1016/j.drup.2015.11.003
45. Dolphin AC. The alpha2delta subunits of voltage-gated calcium channels. *Biochim Biophys Acta.* (2013) 1828:1541–9. doi: 10.1016/j.bbamem.2012.11.019
46. Wang X. The expanding role of mitochondria in apoptosis. *Genes Dev.* (2001) 15:2922–33.
47. Gogvadze V, Orrenius S, Zhivotovsky B. Multiple pathways of cytochrome c release from mitochondria in apoptosis. *Biochim Biophys Acta.* (2006) 1757: 639–47. doi: 10.1016/j.bbabio.2006.03.016
48. West KA, Castillo SS, Dennis PA Activation of the PI3K/Akt pathway and chemotherapeutic resistance. *Drug Resist Updates.* (2002) 5:234–48. doi: 10.1016/S1368-7646(02) 00120-6
49. Burris HA III. Overcoming acquired resistance to anticancer therapy: focus on the PI3K/AKT/mTOR pathway. *Cancer Chemother Pharmacol.* (2013) 71:829–42. doi: 10.1007/s00280-012-2043-3

21

Inhibition of SMYD2 Sensitized Cisplatin to Resistant Cells in NSCLC Through Activating p53 Pathway

Lei Shang [1,2] *and Minjie Wei* [1*]

[1] *School of Pharmacy, China Medical University, Shenyang, China,* [2] *Shenyang Medical College, Shenyang, China*

Correspondence:
Minjie Wei
mjwei@cmu.edu.cn

The protein lysine methyltransferase SMYD2 has recently emerged as a new enzyme modulate gene transcription or signaling pathways, and involved into tumor progression. However, the role of SMYD2 in drug resistant is still not known. Here, we found that inhibition of SMYD2 by specific inhibitor could enhance the cell sensitivity to cisplatin (CDDP), but not paclitaxel, NVB, and VCR in non-small cell lung cancer (NSCLC). Further study showed that SMYD2 and its substrates were overexpressed in NSCLC resistant cells, and the inhibition of SMYD2 or knockdown by specific siRNA could reverse the cell resistance to cisplatin treatment in NSCLC/CDDP cells. In addition, our data indicated that the inhibition or knockdown SMYD2 inhibit tumor sphere formation and reduce cell migration in NSCLC/CDDP cells, but not in NSCLC parental cells. Mechanistically, inhibition of SMYD2 could enhance p53 pathway activity and induce cell apoptosis through regulating its target genes, including p21, GADD45, and Bax. On the contrary, the sensitivity of cells to cisplatin was decreased after knockdown p53 or in p53 deletion NSCLC cells. The synergistically action was further confirmed by *in vivo* experiments. Taken together, our results demonstrate SMYD2 is involved into cisplatin resistance through regulating p53 pathway, and might become a promising therapeutic target for cisplatin resistance in NSCLC.

Keywords: SMYD2, cisplatin resistance, lung cancer, p53, apoptosis

INTRODUCTION

The incidence and mortality of lung cancer ranks at the NO.1 among all kinds of cancer (1). Non-small cell lung cancer (NSCLC) accounts for about 85% of lung cancer (1, 2). The surgery, radiotherapy, chemotherapy, molecular targeting therapy, and immunotherapy are possible choice for NSCLC treatment (2). However, most of NSCLCs are found at advanced stage, so drug-based therapy, mainly including chemotherapy, is considered as the most important approach to treat NSCLCs (3).

The platinum-based chemotherapy, such as cisplatin plus paclitaxel, cisplatin plus NVB, and cisplatin plus VCR, is the first-line treatment approach in NSCLCs (2, 3). However, drug resistance will be inevitable happened after treatment for 1–2 years, which limit the application of chemotherapeutic agents (4, 5). To solve this problem, we should first understand the resistant mechanisms for chemotherapy in NSCLCs. In fact, many previous studies have shown that the upregulation of efflux protein, the mutation of drug target, the activation of by-pass oncogenic pathway, and the accumulation of phenotype change cells contributed to the resistance of chemotherapeutic agents in NSCLCs (6, 7). However, there is still unknown for a large part of NSCLC resistant patients.

SMYD2 was identified as protein methyltransferase which adds methyl-group to its histone and non-histone substrates and epigenetically regulates their function (8, 9). Recently, SMYD2 was observed to involve into the upset and progression of various tumors including leukemia, breast cancer, teratocarcinoma, gastric cancer, and head and neck cancer (10–14). Mechanistically, SMYD2 was found to prompt cell proliferation, block apoptosis, and enhance cell migration and invasion through regulating its substrates methylation status, such as p53 and histone4 (13–15). However, whether this enzyme is involved into drug resistance is still not known.

Here, NSCLC was used to as an example to investigate the role of SMYD2 in chemotherapeutic resistance. Our data showed that SMYD2 was involved into cisplatin resistance, but not paclitaxel, NVB, and VCR. Further study indicated that SMYD2 expression and its activity were increasing in cisplatin resistant NSCLC cells. Mechanistically, SMYD2 prompt cell migration, increase the tumor sphere and block apoptosis, which is dependent on the methylation of $p53^{K370}$. The inhibition or knockdown of SMYD2 model would result in the increasing of sensitivity to cisplatin *in vitro* and *in vivo*. Our results not only elucidate the role of SMYD2 in cisplatin resistance and provide a potential method to reverse cisplatin resistance in NSCLC.

MATERIALS AND METHODS

Cell Lines, Cell Culture, and Treatment

A549 (p53 wide type, KRAS mutation), NCI-H460 (p53 wide type, KRAS mutation), and NCI-H1299 (p53 deletion, KRAS wide type) human lung adenocarcinoma cell lines were purchased from the American Type Culture Collection (ATCC; Manassas, VA, USA). These cancer cells were routinely cultured in RPMI-1640 medium (Gibco, Grand Island, NY, USA) supplemented with 10% fetal bovine serum (FBS; Gibco) and were maintained at 37°C in a humidified incubator with 5% CO_2. The cells were treated with Cisplatin (J&K Scientific Ltd, Beijing, China) at increasing concentrations (ranging from 0.5 to 4 μM) for 3 months.

Compounds and Reagents

BAY-498(SMYD2 inhibitor), AZ505(SMYD2 inhibitor), Cisplatin(CDDP), Vinorelbine(NVB), Paclitaxel (Taxol), and Vincristine sulfate(VCR) was obtained from MedChem Express (Princeton, NJ, USA). The primary antibodies against SMYD2, p53, Cleaved-PARP, and β-actin were obtained from Cell Signaling Technology (Danvers, MA, USA), and the primary antibodies against $p53^{K370Me}$ was purchased from Immunoway Technology (Plano, TX, USA). The pcDNA3-p53 vector was obtained from Addgene.

Cell Viability Assay

In vitro cell viability was determined using the MTT assay. Cells (1×10^5 cells/ml) were seeded in 96-well culture plates. After incubating overnight, the cells were treated with various concentrations of the appropriate agents for 48 h, after which 10 μl of MTT solution (2.5 mg/ml in PBS) was added to each well, and the plates were incubated for an additional 4 h at 37°C. After the samples were centrifuged (2,500 rpm, 10 min), the medium supplemented with MTT was aspirated, and then 100 μl of DMSO was added to each well. The optical density of each well was measured at 570 nm with a Biotek Synergy™ HT Reader (BioTek Instruments, Winooski, VT, USA).

Western Blot Analysis

Western blotting was performed as previously described (14). Briefly, equal amounts of total protein extracts from cultured cells or tissues were fractionated by 10–15% SDS-PAGE before being electrically transferred onto polyvinylidene difluoride (PVDF) membranes, which were sequentially incubated with mouse or rabbit primary antibodies and horseradish peroxidase (HRP)-conjugated secondary antibodies designed to detect the proteins of interest. The indicated secondary antibodies were subsequently reacted with ECL detection reagents (Pierce, Thermo Fisher Scientific, Waltham, MA, USA) and then incubated in a dark room. The relative expression levels of the indicated proteins were normalized to those of β-actin.

Flow Cytometry Analysis

Analyses for apoptosis were conducted with an Annexin V-FITC Apoptosis Detection Kit (BioVision, Mountain View, CA, USA). Cells (1×10^6) were exposed to various inhibitors for 48 h. They were collected by centrifugation and resuspended in 500 μL of 1 × binding buffer. Annexin V-fluorescein isothiocyanate (FITC; 5 μL) and PI (5 μL) were added to the cells. After incubation at room temperature for 5 min in the dark, cells were analyzed by FACS using a flow cytometer (BD Biosciences, San Jose, CA, USA). Cells that stained Annexin V-FITC (apoptosis) were analyzed.

siRNA-Mediated Gene Knockdown

SMYD2 and *p53* knockdown was performed using specific siRNAs purchased from Santa Cruz Biotechnology (Santa Cruz Biotechnology, Santa Cruz, CA, USA). Scramble non-target siRNAs served as negative controls. siRNA was introduced into the indicated cell lines with Lipofectamine RNAiMAX reagent (Thermo Fisher Scientific), according to the manufacturer's instructions, and knockdown efficiency was assessed by western blotting.

Transwell Migration Assay

NCI-H460/CDDP and its parental cell lines migration capacities were tested by Corning transwell assay, according to the manufacturer's instructions. Briefly, the indicated lung cancer cells were treated DMSO, BAY-598 (200 nM), Scramble siRNA, and SMYD2 siRNA (50 nM) for 48 h and then seeded in the upper chamber of the system at a density of 5×10^4 cells/well in serum-free medium (100 μl). The wells in the lower chamber of the system were filled with complete medium. After incubating for 48 h, the cells remaining in the upper chamber were carefully removed with a cotton swab, and the cells that had migrated through the membrane and adhered to its lower surface were fixed with 100% methanol and stained with 0.2% crystal violet. The membrane was then photographed under a microscope,

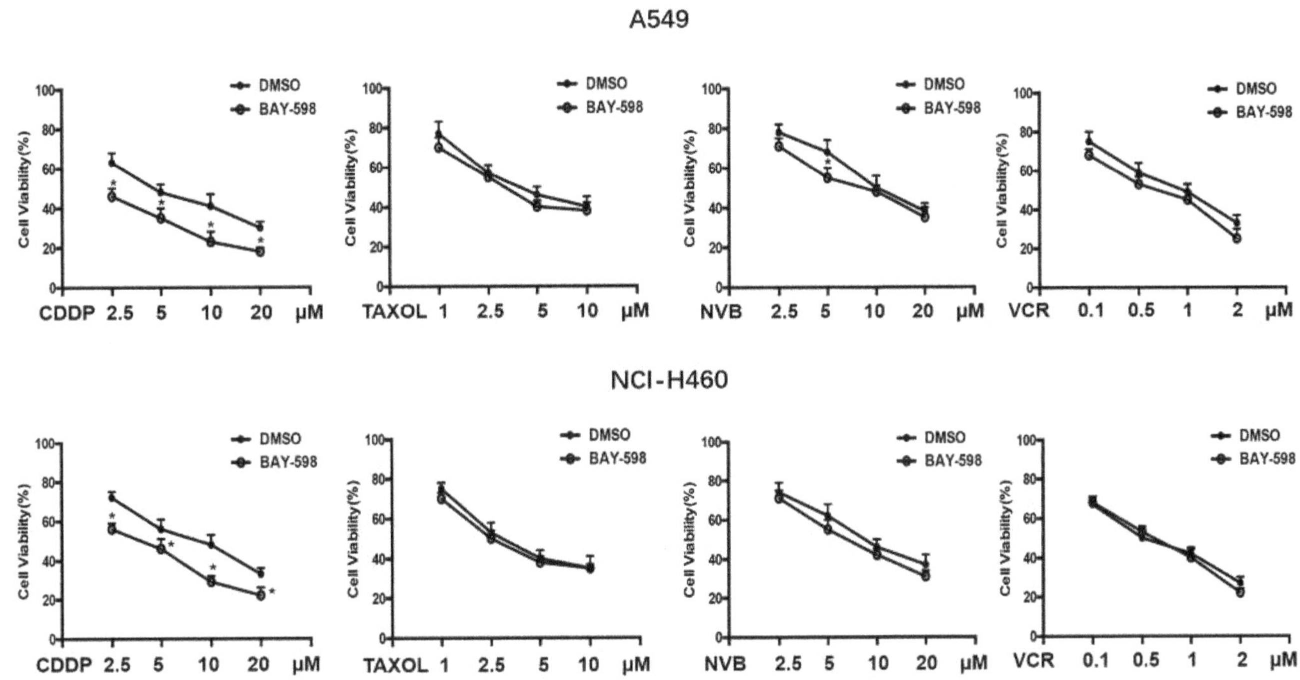

FIGURE 1 | Effects of the combination of chemotherapeutic agents and SMYD2 inhibitor on cell growth in NSCLC cells. The growth of A549 and NCI-H460 cells treated with chemotherapeutic agents, including CDDP, Taxol, NVB, and VCR at different concentrations or combination with SMYD2 inhibitor BAY-598. Cell lines treated with DMSO were used as controls.

and the cells in five predetermined fields were counted at 200× magnification.

Tumor Sphere Formation Assay

NCI-H460/CDDP and its parental cell lines were treated DMSO, BAY-598 (200 nM), Scramble siRNA, and SMYD2 siRNA (50 nM) for 48 h, after which single cells prepared by mechanical and enzymatic dissociation were seeded in 6-well ultra-low attachment plates (Corning, NY, USA) at a density of 1,000 cells/well in serum-free DMEM/F-12 medium supplemented with B27 (1×, Invitrogen, Thermo Fisher Scientific), 20 ng/ml human recombinant bFGF (PeproTech, Rocky Hill, NJ, USA), and 20 ng/ml EGF (PeproTech) for 10–14 days. The cells were then photographed under a microscope.

Luciferase Reporter Gene Assays

NCI-H460/CDDP and its parental cells were plated in 96-well plates. Cells in 96-well plates were transfected with 2 ng pRL-tk (Promega) and 50 ng p53 reporter plasmid (Addgene) for 24 h with the lipofectamine 3000. Cells were treated with DMSO or BAY-598 at indicated concentrations for 24 h. Luciferase activities were evaluated with the Berthold LB960 system (Berthold, DE).

Quantitative PCR Analysis

Total RNA was isolated using an RNeasy Mini Kit (Qiagen, Hilden, Germany), as described in the product insert, and then reverse transcribed with a RevertAid First Strand cDNA Synthesis Kit (Thermo Fisher Scientific). PCR was performed with iQ SYBR Green SuperMix (Bio-Red Laboratories, Hercules, CA, USA) and a CFX96 Real-Time PCR Detection System (Bio-Rad Laboratories). The following primers were used for the experiment: glyceraldehyde-3-phosphate dehydrogenase (*GAPDH*): reverse: 5′-CCCTCAACGACCACTTTGTCA-3′ and forward: 5′-TTCCTCTTGTGCTCTTGCTGG-3′; p21 forward: 5′-TGTACCCTTGTGCCTCGCTC-3′ and reverse: 5′- TGGAGA AGATCAGCCGGCGT-3′; Bax forward: 5′- TTTGCTTCAGGG TTTCATCC-3′ and reverse: 5′- CAGTTGAAGTTGCCGTCA GA-3′; and GADD45 forward: 5′-GGATGCCCTGGAGGAAGT GCT-3′ and reverse: 5′- GGCAGGATCCTTCCATTGAGATGA ATGTG-3′.

Xenografts in Mice

To assess the characteristics of chemotherapy-resistant tumors, we subcutaneously injected viable NCI-H460/CDDP cells (5×10^6/100 μl PBS per mouse), as confirmed by trypan blue staining, into the right flank of 7–8 weeks-old male BALB/C mice. When the average tumor volume reached 100 mm^3, the mice were randomly divided into the following four treatment groups: a control group (saline only, $n = 6$), a AZ505 group (40 mg/kg/qd, i.p.; $n = 6$), an CDDP group (4.0 mg/kg/3 day, i.p.; $n = 6$), and a combination treatment group (AZ505 plus CDDP). After 2 weeks, the mice were sacrificed, and the tumors were excised and stored at −80°C. These experiments were performed in strict accordance with the recommendations in the Guide for the Care and Use of Laboratory Animals of the National Institutes of Health, and the corresponding protocol was approved by the

Animal Experimental Ethics Committee of Shenyang Medical College (Shenyang, Liaoning Province, China).

Statistical Analysis

Differences between the indicated experimental groups were evaluated by one-way ANOVA or Turkey's *post hoc* test with the SPSS 11.5 software package for Windows (SPSS, Chicago, IL, USA). $P < 0.05$ were considered statistically significant ($P < 0.05$, two-tailed test).

RESULTS

The Inhibition of SMYD2 Enhanced the Antigrowth Action of Cisplatin in NSCLC Cells

To explore the possible action of SMYD2 in chemotherapeutic agents in NSCLC, A549 and NCI-H460 cells were treated with various concentrations of the first-line chemotherapeutic agents, including CDDP, Taxol, NVB, and VCR, and combined treatment with SMYD2 inhibitor BAY-598 with non-cytotoxicity concentration (2 μM, cell viability>90%, **Supplementary Figure 1A**). As shown in **Figure 1**, single treatment with CDDP, Taxol, NVB, and VCR could inhibit cell growth at concentration-dependent manner in both cell lines. Addition of SMYD2 inhibitor had no effect on the cell viability when combined with Taxol and VCR, and owned a slightly enhanced inhibition when combined with NVB. Notably, the combination of BAY-598 and CDDP could significantly retard cell growth in both A549 and NCI-H460 cells ($P < 0.05$), suggesting SMYD2 inhibition might be involved into the cell sensitivity to CDDP but not Taxol, VCR, and NVB.

The Expression and Function of SMYD2 in Cisplatin Resistant NSCLC Cells

To clarify the role and function of SMYD2 in CDDP sensitivity of NSCLC cells, we established A549 and NCI-H460 CDDP resistant cell lines. First, we detected the expression level of SMYD2 in parental cell lines and resistant cell lines. Western blot data indicated that SMYD2 was increased in both resistant cell lines as compared to parental cell lines. In consistent with the SMYD2 upregulation in resistant cell lines, the non-histone substrate of SMYD2, $p53^{K370me}$, was also increased in resistant cell lines. The above data demonstrated that the expression and activity of SMYD2 were increased in CDDP resistant cells. Next, to further elucidate the role of SMYD2 in CDDP resistance, we measured the cell viability of NCI-H460/CDDP cells to CDDP after suppression of SMYD2 by specific inhibitor and siRNA. Our data showed, whether inhibition by SMYD2 inhibitor BAY-598 or knockdown by specific siRNA, the cell sensitivity to CDDP would be significantly increased as compared to DMSO or Scramble treated groups ($P < 0.05$). The above data was confirmed by flow cytometry experiments. Treatment with BAY-598 at non-cytotoxic concentration would prompt the apoptosis induced action of CDDP in NCI-H460/CDDP cells. Similarly, knockdown SMYD2 also resulted in the increase of cell apoptosis in CDDP treated NCI-H460/CDDP cells when compared to scramble treated cells. Notably, although the addition of SMYD2 inhibitor or knockdown of SMYD2 could enhance the induction of apoptosis by CDDP in NCI-H460 cells, the level was decreased as compared with resistant cells (**Figure 2C**). The above data indicated that SMYD2 play an important role in CDDP resistance of NSCLC cells.

Inhibition of SMYD2 Reversed Malignant Phenotype of Cisplatin Resistant NSCLC Cells

To further elucidate the role of SMYD2 in CDDP resistance of NSCLC cells, we next assessed the effect of inhibition or knockdown of SMYD2 on cell migration and tumor sphere formation, which are considered as the crucial characteristics of CDDP resistant NSCLC cells (16, 17). Our results showed that cell migration number of NCI-H460/CDDP cells was significant decreased after treated with SMYD2 inhibitor or SMYD2 siRNA as compared to DMSO and Scramble siRNA control, respectively. Furthermore, tumor sphere number of NCI-H460/CDDP cells was also obviously reduced by SMYD2 inhibitor and SMYD2 siRNA. It should be noted that whether addition of BAY-598 or specific siRNA could not significantly affect cell migration number and tumor sphere ability in NCI-H460 cells (**Supplementary Figures 1B–D**). The above results demonstrated that SMYD2 was also involved into the formation of malignant phenotype in CDDP resistant NSCLC cells.

SMYD2 Mediated Cisplatin Resistance Dependent on p53 Regulation in NSCLC Cells

In view of the crucial role of p53 and its epigenetic regulation by SMYD2 (18), we next explore possible role of p53 in SMYD2 mediated CDDP resistance. As shown in **Figure 4A**, knockdown p53 by specific siRNA contributed to the decrease of cell sensitivity to CDDP in NCI-H460/CDDP cells, which owned wide type p53 expression. In addition, the restore of p53 in NCI-H1299 cells (p53 deletion) could lead to the increase of cell sensitivity to CDDP. The above data indicates that the status and expression level of p53 will affect the cell sensitivity of NSCLC cells to CDDP.

In order to explore the effect of SMYD2 on p53 activity, we detected the transcriptional regulation activity of p53 by luciferase assay after treated with BAY-598 in NCI-H460/CDDP and its parental cells. The results showed that BAY-598 could concentration-dependently enhance p53 reporter activity in NCI-H460/CDDP cells (**Figure 4B**). In consistent with reporter assay, BAY-598 treatment also significantly resulted in the upregulation in mRNA level of p53 targeting genes, including p21, GADD45, and Bax (**Figure 4C**), in NCI-H460/CDDP cells. In consistent with resistant cell lines, BAY-598 also could increase p53 reporter activity, p21 and GADD45 expressions in NCI-H460 cells to some extent (**Figure 4B**). On the contrary, BAY-598 treatment could not induce the BAX expression in NCI-H460 cells, suggesting the role of SMYD2 in BAX regulation is different in parental and resistant cells (**Figure 4C**). Furthermore,

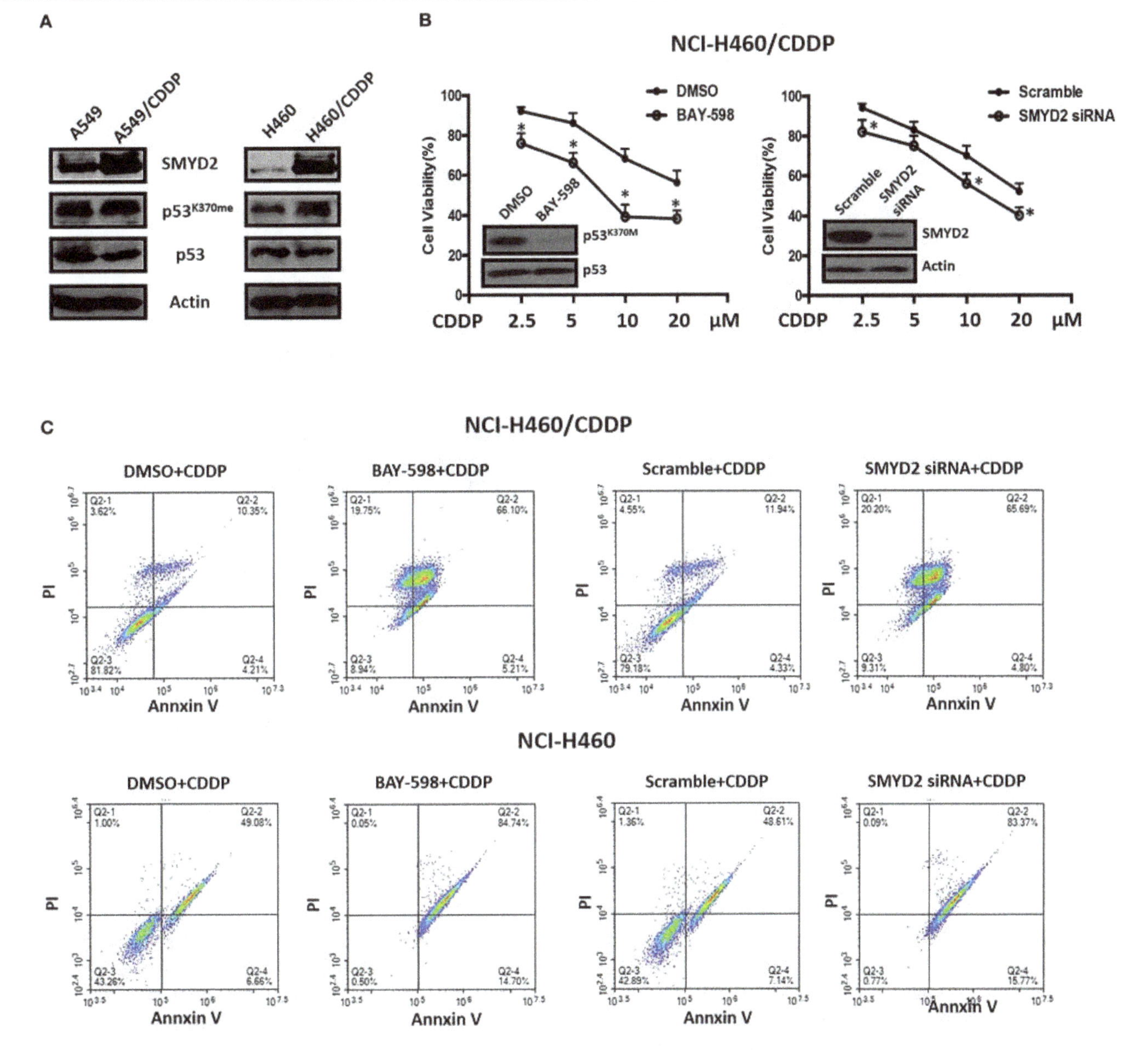

FIGURE 2 | The expression level of SMYD2-related proteins and the effects of genetic or chemical manipulation of SMYD2 on the cell growth of CDDP-resistant and parental NSCLC cells. **(A)** SMYD2, p53, and p53^{K370me} expression levels were measured in CDDP resistant and parental NSCLC cell lines. β-actin was used as a loading control. **(B)** Cell viability was measured in BAY-598-treated or SMYD2-knockdown NCI-H460/CDDP cells treated with CDDP at different concentrations for 36 h. Scramble siRNA or DMSO was used as a control. The efficacy of genetic or chemical manipulation of SMYD2 was confirmed by Western blot in NCI-H460/CDDP cells. **(C)** Cell apoptosis was assessed using Annexin V/PI double staining in BAY-598-treated or SMYD2-knockdown CDDP resistant and parental NCI-H460 cells after treated with CDDP at 10 μM for 48 h. *$P < 0.05$, compared to corresponding control cells.

we also detected the cell apoptosis status of NCI-H460/CDDP and NCI-H460 cells after treated with BAY-598. Our results indicated BAY-598 at 10 μM could induce cell apoptosis in NCI-H460/CDDP cells, but not in NCI-H460 cells (**Figure 4D**), which confirmed the regulation action of Bax, a pro-apoptosis gene, by SMYD2. Taken together, our data suggested that the SMYD2 mediated CDDP resistance through epigenetic regulation of p53.

Inhibition of SMYD2 Sensitized Cisplatin Through Epigenetic Regulation of p53 *in vivo*

To clarify the therapeutic meaning of the above finding, we assessed anti-tumor effect of the combination of SMYD inhibitor and CDDP in NCI-H1299/CDDP xenograft mice. As shown in **Figure 5A**, single treatment with CDDP has no significant effect on tumor growth, indicating the resistant phenotype of

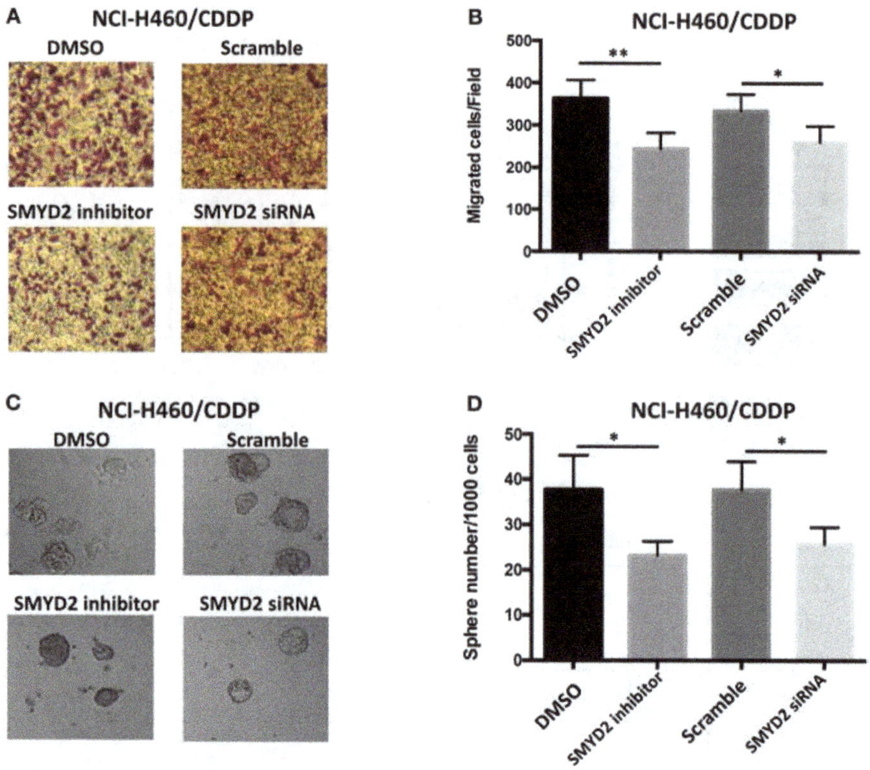

FIGURE 3 | Effects of genetic or chemical manipulation of SMYD2 on the biological characteristics of CDDP-resistant NSCLC cells. **(A,B)** Cell migration was measured in NCI-H460/CDDP cells treated with 2 μM BAY-598 or 50 nM SMYD2 siRNA. Scramble siRNA or DMSO was used as a control. **(C,D)** Tumor sphere was counted in NCI-H460/CDDP cells treated with 2 μM BAY-598 or 50 nM SMYD2 siRNA. Scramble siRNA or DMSO was used as a control. (Scale bars, 100 μm) $^{*}P < 0.05$, $^{**}P < 0.001$, compared to corresponding control cells.

NCI-H1299/CDDP xenograft mice. Similar to CDDP single treatment, single treatment with AZ505, an *in vivo* available SMYD2 inhibitor, only displayed a slightly inhibition on tumor growth. Interestingly, the combination of AZ505 and CDDP could obviously inhibit tumor growth of NCI-H1299/CDDP xenograft mice when compared to vehicle control and single treatment group. In addition, we didn't find the body weight loss in the combination treated group (data not shown), suggesting the combination has no effect on gross toxicity. Next, we further explored the underlying mechanisms using tumor tissue. Western blot data showed that AZ505 single treatment could lead to the decrease of p53^{K370me}, whereas CDDP single treatment could slightly increase the level of p53^{K370me} (**Figure 5B**). The combination treatment contributed to a decrease of p53^{K370me}. In addition, we found the expression of the clv-PARP, an apoptosis biomarker, was increased in the combination group (**Figure 5B**). In summary, our *in vivo* data showed the inhibition of SMYD2 by AZ505 could sensitize cisplatin antitumor action through epigenetic regulation of p53.

DISCUSSION

Cisplatin(CDDP) is the first line drug for NSCLC patients, therefore, understanding and preventing CDDP resistance are considered as the crucial issue with respect to the treatment of NSCLC (5). Here, we found that SMYD2, a protein methyltransferase, was involved into cisplatin resistance. Furthermore, out data showed that SMYD2 expression and its activity were increasing in cisplatin resistant NSCLC cells. Mechanistically, SMYD2 prompt cell migration, increase the tumor sphere, and block apoptosis, which is dependent on the methylation of p53^{K370}. The inhibition or knockdown of SMYD2 model would result in the increasing of sensitivity to cisplatin *in vitro* and *in vivo*. Our findings provide us with a novel perspective epigenetic regulation mechanisms underlying CDDP resistance and define that the combination of SMYD2 inhibitor and CDDP may have promise as treatments for patients with CDDP-resistant NSCLC.

SMYD2 is a protein methyltransferase that catalyzes the methylation of histone substrates, such as H3K4 and H3K36 (18), and non-histone substrates, including p53 (19), Rb (20), HSP90 (21), STAT3, and NF-κB (22). It has been reported that SMYD2 was involved into the upset and progression of various tumors, including leukemia, breast cancer, gastric cancer, and head and neck cancer. Recently, Wang et al. reported SMYD2 inhibition also led to the suppression of cell growth in NSCLC cells (23), suggesting SMYD2 might be involved into lung cancer. Our results demonstrated that SMYD2

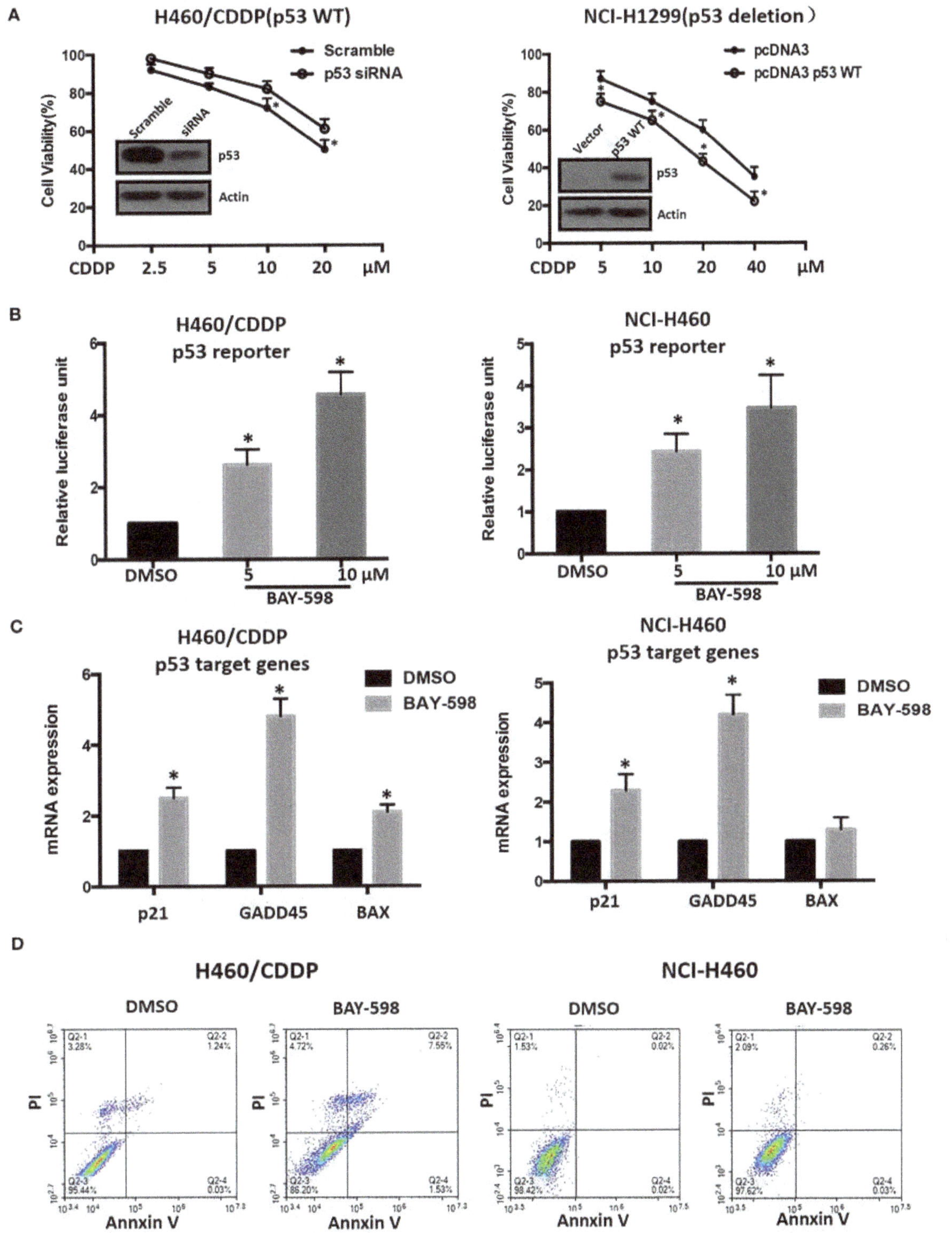

FIGURE 4 | Epigenetic regulation of p53 and its role in CDDP resistance in NSCLC. **(A)** Cell viability in NCI-H460/CDDP (p53 wide type) and NCI-H1299(p53 deletion) cells, with p53 gene manipulation, which were treated with CDDP at different concentrations for 48 h. Scramble siRNA or mock vector was used as a control. The p53 knock-down or restoration efficacy was confirmed by Western Blot. **(B)** The p53 reporter activity was measured in CDDP resistant and parental NCI-H460 cells after treated with BAY-598. The relative luciferase unit was calculated by Luciferase/Renilla and DMSO was considered as 100%. **(C)** The mRNA expression levels of p21, GADD45, and Bax were assessed by real-time RT-PCR in CDDP resistant and parental NCI-H460 cells treated with 10 μM BAY-598. GAPDH was used as a control. **(D)** Cell apoptosis was assessed using Annexin V/PI double staining in CDDP resistant and parental NCI-H460 cells which were treated with BAY-598 at 10 μM concentrations for 48 h. *$P < 0.05$, compared to corresponding control cells.

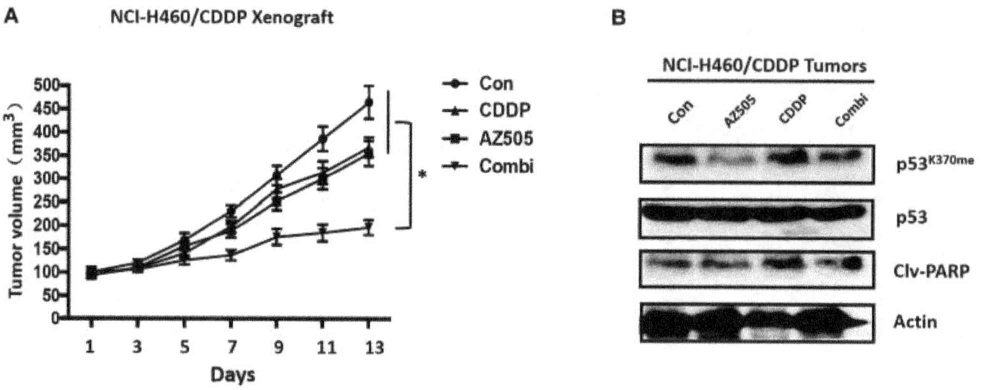

FIGURE 5 | Effects of SMYD2 inhibition and/or CDDP on tumor growth in an CDDP-resistant xenograft model. **(A)** Tumor volume was measured in NCI-H460/CDDP xenografts treated with AZ505, CDDP, or the combination of AZ505 and CDDP. **(B)** The p53 and $p53^{K370me}$, and cleaved PARP(clv-PARP) expression levels were measured in NCI-H460/CDDP xenograft tumor tissues. β-actin was used as a loading control. $^{*}P < 0.05$, combined treatment group compared to single treatment group and vehicle control.

expression and enzymatic activity levels were upregulated in NSCLC CDDP-resistant cells as compared to parental cells. In addition, either suppressing SMYD2 activity or knocking down SMYD2 would contribute to the increases in sensitivity to CDDP, and the reduction in cell migration and self-renewal ability in CDDP-resistant NSCLC cells, indicating that SMYD2 executes a crucial role in CDDP resistance of NSCLC.

SMYD2 methylates H3K4 and H3K36 would contribute the change of chromatin structure, and subsequently lead to the alteration of its target genes (18). In fact, the important function of SMYD2 was reported to related methylate to its non-histone substrates (9, 24). SMYD2 monomethylates Lys-370 of p53, leading to decreased DNA-binding activity and subsequent transcriptional regulation activity of p53. We found that, as long as the SMYD2 upregulation, the $p53^{K370me}$ level was also increased in CDDP resistant NSCLC cells. Importantly, our data showed that cell sensitivity to CDDP was dependent on wild type p53 level. Inhibition of SMYD2 could induce the increasing of p53 transcription activity and its target gene expression. Taken together, these findings indicate that epigenetic regulation by SMYD2 plays an important role in p53 transcriptional activity and is involved in processes associated with CDDP resistance.

K-RAS is one of the most frequently mutated in human NSCLC (25). Mutation of K-RAS usually results in the activation of oncogenic signaling molecules that regulate cell growth, survival and differentiation by coupling receptor activation to downstream effector pathways (25), and leads to the resistance to tyrosine kinase inhibitors such as gefitinib and erlotinib (26). Therefore, chemotherapy is the standard of treatment for K-RAS mutant NSCLC tumors. Here, our data shown that inhibition of SMYD2 by specific inhibitor can sensitize CDDP efficacy in K-RAS mutated A549 and NCI-H460 cell lines, suggesting epigenetic manipulation might be a promising adjuvant approach to treat K-RAS mutant tumors.

In conclusion, the present study elucidated that the activity of SMYD2 in NSCLC may affect the cell sensitivity to chemotherapeutic agents, especially to CDDP. The elevated SMYD2 mediated CDDP resistance and malignant phenotype in NSCLC, indicating that SMYD2 may be a useful biomarker of CDDP resistance in NSCLC. Inhibition of SMYD2 contributes to the methylation-related activation of p53 and thus results in cell apoptosis. Furthermore, combination treatment with CDDP and an SMYD2 inhibitor had a synergistically antitumor effects in a xenograft model *in vivo*. Given that SMYD2 has reversible effects and is a targetable protein methyltransferase, treatments targeting the protein may be useful for reversing CDDP resistance in NSCLC.

ETHICS STATEMENT

This study was carried out in accordance with the recommendations in the Guide for the Care and Use of Laboratory Animals of the National Institutes of Health, and the corresponding protocol was approved by the Animal Experimental Ethics Committee of Shenyang Medical College (Shenyang, Liaoning Province, China).

AUTHOR CONTRIBUTIONS

All authors listed have made a substantial, direct and intellectual contribution to the work, and approved it for publication.

FUNDING

This work was supported by the National Natural Science Foundation of China (No. 81803476).

SUPPLEMENTARY MATERIAL

Supplementary Figure 1 | The effects of genetic or chemical manipulation of SMYD2 on the cell growth, migration, and tumor sphere ability of NCI-H460 cells. **(A)** The growth of A549 and NCI-H460 cells treated with various concentrations SMYD2 inhibitor BAY-598. Cell viability was detected by MTT assay. **(B)** The efficacy of genetic or chemical manipulation of SMYD2 was confirmed by Western blot in NCI-H460 cells. $p53^{K370me}$ and SMYD2 expression levels were measured in NCI-H460 cell lines. The p53 or β-actin was used as a loading control. **(C)** Cell migration was measured in NCI-H460 cells treated with 2 μM BAY-598 or 50 nM SMYD2 siRNA. Scramble siRNA or DMSO was used as a control. **(D)** Tumor sphere was counted in NCI-H460 cells treated with 2 μM BAY-598 or 50 nM SMYD2 siRNA. Scramble siRNA or DMSO was used as a control.

REFERENCES

1. Siegel RL, Miller KD, Jemal A. Cancer statistics, 2016. *CA Cancer J Clin.* (2016) 66:7–30. doi: 10.3322/caac.21332
2. Hirsch FR, Scagliotti GV, Mulshine JL, Kwon R, Curran WJ Jr., Wu YL, et al. Lung cancer: current therapies and new targeted treatments. *Lancet.* (2017) 389:299–311. doi: 10.1016/S0140-6736(16)30958-8
3. Chang A. Chemotherapy, chemoresistance and the changing treatment landscape for NSCLC. *Lung Cancer.* (2011) 71:3–10. doi: 10.1016/j.lungcan.2010.08.022
4. Rivera G, Wakelee HA. Resistance to therapy. *Cancer Treat Res.* (2016) 170:183–202. doi: 10.1007/978-3-319-40389-2_9
5. Kim ES. Chemotherapy resistance in lung cancer. *Adv Exp Med Biol.* (2016) 893:189–209. doi: 10.1007/978-3-319-33826-2
6. Galluzzi L, Vitale I, Michels J, Brenner C, Szabadkai G, Harel-Bellan A, et al. Systems biology of cisplatin resistance: past, present and future. *Cell Death Dis.* (2014) 5:e1257. doi: 10.1038/cddis.2013.428
7. Hardin C, Shum E, Singh AP, Perez-Soler R, Cheng H. Emerging treatment using tubulin inhibitors in advanced non-small cell lung cancer. *Expert Opin Pharmacother.* (2017) 18:701–16. doi: 10.1080/14656566.2017.1316374
8. Brown MA, Sims RJ III, Gottlieb PD, Tucker PW. Identification and characterization of Smyd2: a split SET/MYND domain-containing histone H3 lysine 36-specific methyltransferase that interacts with the Sin3 histone deacetylase complex. *Mol Cancer.* (2006) 5:26. doi: 10.1186/1476-4598-5-26
9. Hamamoto R, Saloura V, Nakamura Y. Critical roles of non-histone protein lysine methylation in human tumorigenesis. *Nat Rev Cancer.* (2015) 15:110–24. doi: 10.1038/nrc3884
10. Sakamoto LH, Andrade RV, Felipe MS, Motoyama AB, Pittella Silva F. SMYD2 is highly expressed in pediatric acute lymphoblastic leukemia and constitutes a bad prognostic factor. *Leuk Res.* (2014) 38:496–502. doi: 10.1016/j.leukres.2014.01.013
11. Li LX, Zhou JX, Calvet JP, Godwin AK, Jensen RA, Li X. Lysine methyltransferase SMYD2 promotes triple negative breast cancer progression. *Cell Death Dis.* (2018) 9:326. doi: 10.1038/s41419-018-0347-x
12. Zhu J, Dou Z, Sammons MA, Levine AJ, Berger SL. Lysine methylation represses p53 activity in teratocarcinoma cancer cells. *Proc Natl Acad Sci USA.* (2016) 113:9822–7. doi: 10.1073/pnas.1610387113
13. Ohtomo-Oda R, Komatsu S, Mori T, Sekine S, Hirajima S, Yoshimoto S, et al. SMYD2 overexpression is associated with tumor cell proliferation and a worse outcome in human papillomavirus-unrelated nonmultiple head and neck carcinomas. *Hum Pathol.* (2016) 49:145–55. doi: 10.1016/j.humpath.2015.08.025
14. Komatsu S, Ichikawa D, Hirajima S, Nagata H, Nishimura Y, Kawaguchi T, et al. Overexpression of SMYD2 contributes to malignant outcome in gastric cancer. *Br J Cancer.* (2015) 112:357–64. doi: 10.1038/bjc.2014.543
15. Sajjad A, Novoyatleva T, Vergarajauregui S, Troidl C, Schermuly RT, Tucker HO, et al. Lysine methyltransferase Smyd2 suppresses p53-dependent cardiomyocyte apoptosis. *Biochim Biophys Acta.* (2014) 1843:2556–62. doi: 10.1016/j.bbamcr.2014.06.019
16. Wang L, Liu X, Ren Y, Zhang J, Chen J, Zhou W, et al. Cisplatin-enriching cancer stem cells confer multidrug resistance in non-small cell lung cancer via enhancing TRIB1/HDAC activity. *Cell Death Dis.* (2017) 8:e2746. doi: 10.1038/cddis.2016.409
17. Xu Y, Jiang Z, Zhang Z, Sun N, Zhang M, Xie J, et al. HtrA1 downregulation induces cisplatin resistance in lung adenocarcinoma by promoting cancer stem cell-like properties. *J Cell Biochem.* (2014) 115:1112–21. doi: 10.1002/jcb.24751
18. Ferguson AD, Larsen NA, Howard T, Pollard H, Green I, Grande C, et al. Structural basis of substrate methylation and inhibition of SMYD2. *Structure.* (2011) 19:1262–73. doi: 10.1016/j.str.2011.06.011
19. Huang J, Perez-Burgos L, Placek BJ, Sengupta R, Richter M, Dorsey JA, et al. Repression of p53 activity by Smyd2-mediated methylation. *Nature.* (2006) 444:629–32. doi: 10.1038/nature05287
20. Saddic LA, West LE, Aslanian A, Yates JR III, Rubin SM, Gozani O, et al. Methylation of the retinoblastoma tumor suppressor by SMYD2. *J Biol Chem.* (2010) 285:37733–40. doi: 10.1074/jbc.M110.137612
21. Hamamoto R, Toyokawa G, Nakakido M, Ueda K, Nakamura Y. SMYD2-dependent HSP90 methylation promotes cancer cell proliferation by regulating the chaperone complex formation. *Cancer Lett.* (2014) 351:126–33. doi: 10.1016/j.canlet.2014.05.014
22. Li LX, Fan LX, Zhou JX, Grantham JJ, Calvet JP, Sage J, et al. Lysine methyltransferase SMYD2 promotes cyst growth in autosomal dominant polycystic kidney disease. *J Clin Invest.* (2017) 127:2751–64. doi: 10.1172/JCI90921
23. Wang R, Deng X, Yoshioka Y, Vougiouklakis T, Park JH, Suzuki T, et al. Effects of SMYD2-mediated EML4-ALK methylation on the signaling pathway and growth in non-small-cell lung cancer cells. *Cancer Sci.* (2017) 108:1203–9. doi: 10.1111/cas.13245
24. Zhang X, Huang Y, Shi X. Emerging roles of lysine methylation on non-histone proteins. *Cell Mol Life Sci.* (2015) 72:4257–72. doi: 10.1007/s00018-015-2001-4
25. Piva S, Ganzinelli M, Garassino MC, Caiola E, Farina G, Broggini M, et al. Across the universe of K-RAS mutations in non-small-cell-lung cancer. *Curr Pharm Des.* (2014) 20:3933–43. doi: 10.2174/13816128113196660761
26. Duffy MJ, O'Donovan N, Crown J. Use of molecular markers for predicting therapy response in cancer patients. *Cancer Treat Rev.* (2011) 37:151–9. doi: 10.1016/j.ctrv.2010.07.004

22

Targeting TF-AKT/ERK-EGFR Pathway Suppresses the Growth of Hepatocellular Carcinoma

Shan-Zhou Huang[1,2†], *Meng-Ning Wei*[3†], *Jia-Rong Huang*[3†], *Zi-Jian Zhang*[4], *Wen-Ji Zhang*[3], *Qi-Wei Jiang*[3], *Yang Yang*[3], *Huan-Yu Wang*[5], *Hui-Lin Jin*[1], *Kun Wang*[3], *Zi-Hao Xing*[3], *Meng-Ling Yuan*[3], *Yao Li*[3], *Xiao-Shun He*[2*], *Zhi Shi*[2*] and *Qi Zhou*[1,6*]

[1] *Department of Hepatic Surgery, The First Affiliated Hospital, Sun Yat-sen University, Guangzhou, China,* [2] *Organ Transplant Center, The First Affiliated Hospital, Sun Yat-sen University, Guangzhou, China,* [3] *Guangdong Provincial Key Laboratory of Bioengineering Medicine, Department of Cell Biology and Institute of Biomedicine, National Engineering Research Center of Genetic Medicine, College of Life Science and Technology, Jinan University, Guangzhou, China,* [4] *Department of Hepatobiliary Surgery, The Seventh Affiliated Hospital of Sun Yat-sen University, Shenzhen, China,* [5] *Department of Thyroid and Breast Surgery, Nanshan District People's Hospital, Shenzhen, China,* [6] *Department of General Surgery, Hui Ya Hospital of The First Affiliated Hospital, Sun Yat-sen University, Huizhou, China*

***Correspondence:**
Zhi Shi
tshizhi@jnu.edu.cn
Xiao-Shun He
gdtrc@163.com
Qi Zhou
zhouqi@mail.sysu.edu.cn

†These authors have contributed equally to this work

Tissue factor (TF) is a transmembrane glycoprotein to initiate blood coagulation and frequently overexpressed in a variety of tumors. Our previous study has showed that the expression of TF is upregulated and correlated with prognosis in hepatocellular carcinoma (HCC). However, the role and molecular mechanism of TF in the growth of HCC are still unclear. *In vitro* and *in vivo* functional experiments were performed to determine the effect of TF on the growth of HCC cells. A panel of biochemical assays was used to elucidate the underlying mechanisms. TF could promote the growth of HCC *in vitro* and *in vivo* by activating both ERK and AKT signaling pathways. TF induced EGFR upregualtion, and inhibition of EGFR suppressed TF-mediated HCC growth. In addition, TF protein expression was correlated with EGFR in HCC tissues. TF promotes HCC growth by upregulation of EGFR, and TF as well as EGFR may be potential therapeutic targets of HCC.

Keywords: hepatocellular carcinoma, tissue factor, epidermal growth factor receptor, AKT/ERK, tumor growth

INTRODUCTION

Hepatocellular carcinoma (HCC) is the fifth most lethal cancers worldwide, while China accounted for more than half of all cases and deaths in 2012 (1). More than 400,000 people die from liver cancer and over 450,000 new cases are diagnosed in China each year (2). Though the treatments for HCC have been greatly advanced in recent years, the outcome of HCC is still unoptimistic. Postoperative recurrence, the main reason for poor survival of HCC patients, mainly owes to the tendency of the invasion and metastasis of HCC cells (3, 4). Therefore, understanding the mechanism of HCC tumorigenesis and progression is critical to improve the clinical outcome of HCC patients.

Tissue factor (TF, also known as platelet tissue factor, factor III, thromboplastin, or CD142, encoded by the F3 gene) is a 47 kD transmembrane glycoprotein that contains 263 amino acid residues totally including a 219 amino acid extracellular region, a 23 amino acid hydrophobic transmembrane region, and a 21 amino acids C-terminal intracellular tail (5). Originally, TF is found on the surface of intravascular cells, such as platelets, leukocytes, and endothelial cells and functions as the principal initiator of the extrinsic coagulation cascade by binding with circulating factor VII or VIIα (FVII/VIIα) (6). Recently, TF is frequently overexpressed in a variety of tumors, including breast cancer, colorectal carcinoma, gastric cancer, non-small cell lung, and pancreatic ductal carcinoma, etc. (7). We and other groups have reported that the expression of TF is upregulated and correlated with prognosis in HCC (8–10). In the current study, we investigate the role and molecular mechanism of TF in the growth of HCC cells.

MATERIALS AND METHODS

Patients and Tissue Specimens

A total 144 HCC tissues were obtained from patients who underwent curative resection between Jan 2008 and Dec 2010 at the First Affiliated Hospital, Sun Yat-sen University. None of the patients received neoadjuvant radiotherapy or chemotherapy before surgery. Signed informed consents were obtained from all patients. The study was approved by the ethics committee of the First Affiliated Hospital, Sun Yat-sen University.

Cell Culture and Reagents

The human HCC cell lines HepG2, BEL-7402, SK-HEP1, SMMC-7721, and normal hepatic cell line LO2 were from China Center for Type Culture Collection and cultured in Dulbecco's modified Eagle's medium (DMEM) supplemented with 10% fetal bovine serum (FBS), penicillin (100 U/ml) and streptomycin (100 ng/ml) in a humidified incubator at 37°C with 5% CO_2 atmosphere. U0126, LY294002, and Gefitinib were from ApexBio. Anti-TF (ab17375) and Anti-Ki-67 (2724-1) were from Abcam. Anti-pAKT (4060), Anti-AKT (4691), Anti-pERK (4370), and Anti-ERK (4695) antibodies were from Cell Signaling Technologies. Anti-EGFR (SC-03) and Anti-c-Myc (SC-40) antibodies were from Santa Cruz Biotechnology. Anti-β-actin

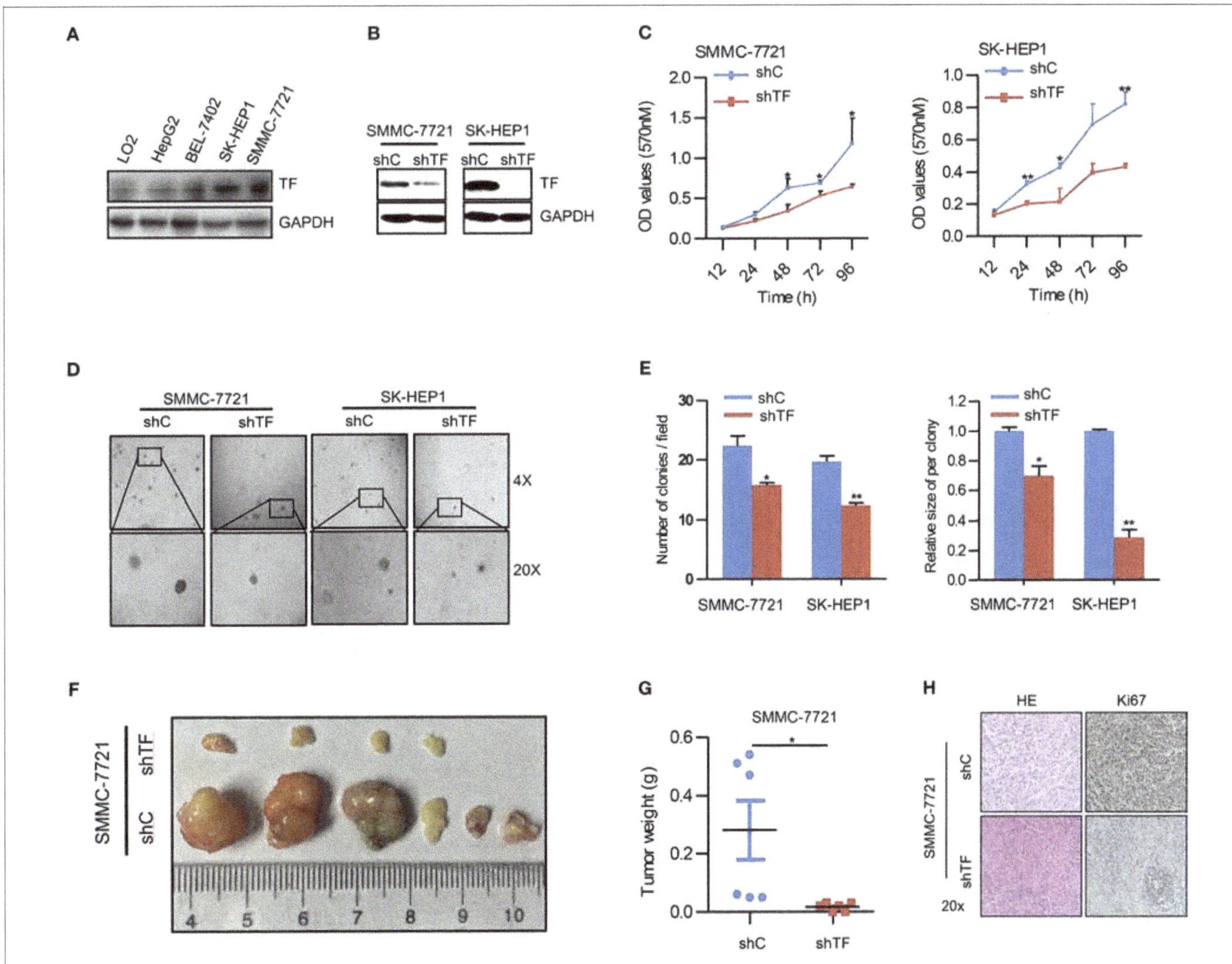

FIGURE 1 | Knockdown of TF inhibits the growth of HCC. **(A,B)** Western blot analysis of the protein expressions in the indicated cells. **(C)** Cell growth of the indicated cells as determined with MTT assay. **(D)** Representative images and **(E)** quantification of the indicated cells sphere as determined with sphere formation assay. **(F)** The indicated subcutaneous tumors and **(G)** tumor weight of nude mice were shown. **(H)** Representative images of H&E and Ki-67 staining in the indicated tumor sections as determined with IHC assay. Error bars, mean ± SD. $^*p < 0.05$ and $^{**}p < 0.01$ [two-tailed Student's *t*-test **(C,E,G)**].

(LK9001T) and Anti-GAPDH (LK9002T) antibodies were from Tianjin Sungene Biotech.

Plasmid Construction and Lentivirus Production

The human TF cDNA was cloned into pLVX-AcGFP1-N1 lentiviral vector, and shRNA targeting human TF mRNA (5′-GCGCUUCAGGCACUACAAA-3′) was cloned into pLKO.1 lentiviral vector. Lentivirus was packaged in HEK293T cells and collected from the medium supernatant. Stable cell lines were established by infecting lentivirus into cells, followed by puromycin selection (11, 12).

siRNA Transfection

The EGFR siRNA (sense sequences: 5′- CUGACUCCGUCCAGUAUUGAU−3′) and negative control siRNA were synthesized by Guangzhou Ribobio. Each siRNA solution was mixed gently with the respective volume of the X-tremeGENE siRNA Transfection Reagent and allowed to form transfection mixture for 20 min. Cells were cultured in 6-well plate with DMEM until 50% of confluence and added with the transfection mixture for 24 h before the next experiment (13, 14).

Western Blot

Cells were harvested and washed twice with cold PBS, then resuspended and lysed in RIPA buffer (1% NP-40, 0.5% sodium deoxycholate, 0.1% SDS, 10 ng/ml PMSF, 0.03% aprotinin, 1 μM sodium orthovanadate) at 4°C for 30 min. Lysates were centrifuged for 10 min at 14,000 × g and supernatants were stored at −80°C as whole cell extracts. Proteins were separated on 12% SDS-PAGE gels and transferred to polyvinylidene difluoride membranes. Membranes were blocked with 5% BSA and incubated with the indicated primary antibodies. Corresponding horseradish peroxidase-conjugated secondary antibodies were used against each primary antibody. Signals were detected using

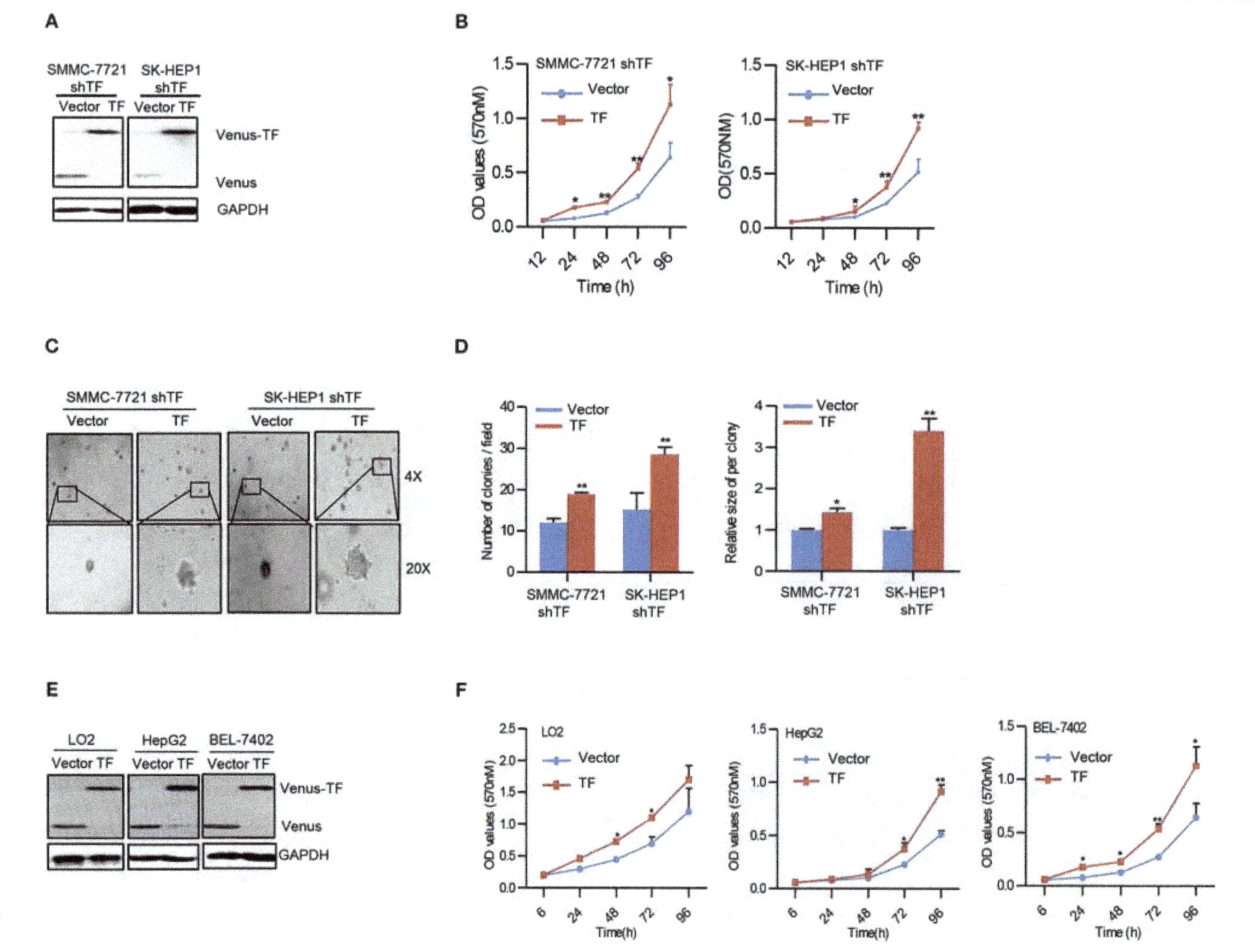

FIGURE 2 | Overexpression of TF promotes the growth of HCC. **(A,E)** Western blot analysis of the protein expressions in the indicated cells. **(B,F)** Cell growth of the indicated cells as determined with MTT assay. **(C)** Representative images and **(D)** quantification of the indicated cells sphere as determined with sphere formation assay. Error bars, mean ± SD. *$p < 0.05$ and **$p < 0.01$ [two-tailed Student's *t*-test **(B,D,F)**].

the ChemiDoc XRS chemiluminescent gel imaging system (Bio-RAD) (15, 16).

MTT Assay

Cells were seeded into a 96-well plate at a density of 0.5–1 × 10^4 cells/well and treated with various concentrations of agents. After 3 days, 3-(4, 5-dimethylthiazolyl-2)-2, 5-diphenyltetrazolium bromide (MTT) was added to each well at a final concentration of 0.5 mg/ml. After incubation for 4 h, the medium and MTT solution were removed from each well, and formazan crystals were dissolved in 100 μl of DMSO. Absorbance was measured at 570 nm by Multiscan Spectrum (Thermofisher) (17, 18).

Sphere Formation Assay

Cells were trypsinized, suspended in medium containing 0.3% agar and 10% FBS and seeded at a density of 5 × 10^2 cells/well in a 12-well plate. The agar–cell mixture was plated onto a bottom layer with 0.5% agar. Then treated cells were incubated in a humidified incubator and fresh medium was added every 3 days. Two weeks later, colonies were analyzed microscopically (19, 20).

Nude Mice Xenograft Tumor Assay

The female Balb/c nude mice with 5 weeks old and 16–18 g weight were obtained from the Shanghai SLAC Laboratory Animal Co and maintained with sterilized food and water. For xenograft tumor assay, 4 × 10^6 cells in 100 μl of DMEM were injected subcutaneously under the shoulder of six mice per group. The mice were anesthetized after experiment, and tumors or lungs were removed, weighed, and sectioned. All experimental procedures were approved by the Institutional Animal Care and Use Committee of Jinan University (21, 22).

Immunohistochemistry Assay

Immunohistochemistry (IHC) assay was performed with a microwave-enhanced avidin-biotin staining method. Formalin-fixed, paraffin embedded human HCC tissue array and subcutaneous tumors in mice were stained with antibodies, respectively, using a microwave-enhanced avidin-biotin staining method. To quantify the protein expression, the following formula was used: IHC score = percentage of positive cells × intensity score. The intensity was scored as follows: 0, negative (no staining); 1, weak (light yellow); 2, moderate (yellow brown); and 3, intense (brown) (23, 24).

Statistical Analysis

Statistical analyses were performed using SPSS 19.0 for Windows (SPSS) and Graph-Pad Prism 6. Data were expressed as the mean ± standard deviation (SD) from at least three independent experiments. Quantitative data between two groups were compared using the Student's *t*-test. Categorical data

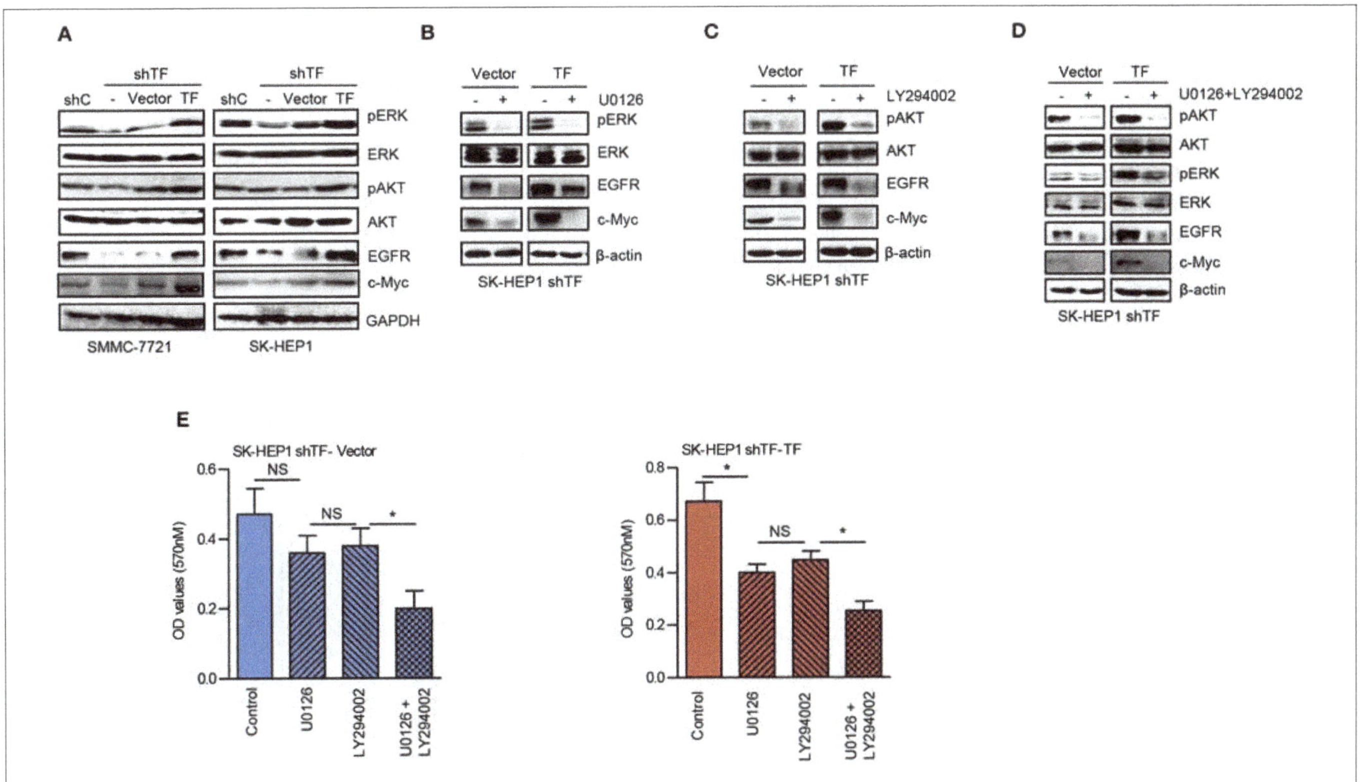

FIGURE 3 | TF promotes the growth of HCC by activating both ERK and AKT signaling pathways. **(A)** Western blot analysis of the protein expressions in the indicated cells. SK-HEP1 shTF-Vector and SK-HEP1 shTF-TF cells were treated with/without U0126 and LY294002 at the concentration of 10 μM for 24 h. **(B–D)** Western blot and **(E)** MTT assay analysis of the protein expressions and cell growth. Error bars, mean ± SD. *$p < 0.05$ (two-tailed Student's *t*-test **E**).

were analyzed by the χ^2 test or Fisher exact test. Correlations between different protein expressions level were determined using Spearman's rank analysis. The $p < 0.05$ was considered as statistical significance. $^{*}p < 0.05$; $^{**}p < 0.01$; NS: no statistical significance.

RESULTS

Knockdown of TF Inhibits the Growth of HCC

To explore the potential biological function of TF in HCC, we first examined the protein expression of TF in human HCC cell lines including HepG2, BEL-7402, SK-HEP1, SMMC-7721, and normal hepatic cell line LO2. Notably, all HCC cell lines displayed higher protein levels of TF than normal hepatic cell line, and SK-HEP1 and SMMC-7721 cells showed the highest protein levels of TF in all cells (**Figure 1A**). To further investigate the role of TF in HCC malignancy, we generated the cells with shRNA-mediated stable knockdown of endogenous TF in both SK-HEP1 and SMMC-7721 cells (**Figure 1B**). Knockdown of TF decreased the cell amounts, sphere numbers and sizes in both SK-HEP1 and SMMC-7721 cells as detected by MTT and sphere formation assays (**Figures 1C–E**). Additionally, the data of subcutaneous tumor models in nude mice showed that TF knockdown inhibited the growth of SMMC-7721 xenografts by decreasing the volumes and weights of tumors as well as the numbers of Ki67^{+} proliferating cells (**Figures 1F–H**).

Overexpression of TF Promotes the Growth of HCC

To confirm the effect of TF on HCC growth, we performed rescue experiments by ectopic expression of TF in both TF-silenced SMMC-7721 and SK-HEP1 cells (**Figure 2A**). Ectopic expression of TF increased the cell amounts, sphere numbers, and sizes in both TF-silenced SMMC-7721 and SK-HEP1 cells (**Figures 2B–D**). Furthermore, overexpression of TF increased the cell amounts in LO2, HepG2, and BEL-7402 cells (**Figures 2E, F**). Taken together, these results suggest that TF can promote the growth of HCC.

TF Promotes the Growth of HCC by Activating Both ERK and AKT Signaling Pathways

To further explore the molecular mechanism of TF-promoted HCC growth, we detected the downstream signaling pathway of TF. As shown in **Figure 3A**, knockdown of TF decreased the protein levels of phosphorylated ERK (pERK), phosphorylated AKT (pAKT), and their downstream transcriptional factor c-Myc in both SMMC-7721 and SK-HEP1 cells. While ectopic expression of TF increased the protein levels of pERK, pAKT and c-Myc in both TF-silenced SMMC-7721 and SK-HEP1 cells. Interesting, the protein level of EGFR was downregulated in TF-silenced HCC cells and upregulated in TF-overexpressed HCC cells (**Figure 3A**). To define the roles of ERK and AKT in TF-mediated HCC growth, we examined the effects of MEK inhibitor U0126 and PI3K inhibitor LY294002 on the growth of both SK-HEP1 shTF-Vector and -TF cells. Treatment with U0126 or/and LY294002 decreased the protein levels of EGFR, c-Myc, pERK or/and pAKT in both SK-HEP1 shTF-Vector and -TF cells (**Figures 3B–D**). However, with U0126 or LY294002 alone inhibited the growth only in SK-HEP1 shTF-TF cells but not in SK-HEP1 shTF-Vector cells. After treating with the combination of U0126 and LY294002 significantly

TABLE 1 | The correlation between TF and EGFR protein expressions in HCC tissues.

		TF expression			P
		High	**Low**	**Total**	**r**
EGFR	High	82	9	91	< 0.001
expression	Low	23	30	53	0.668
		105	39	144	

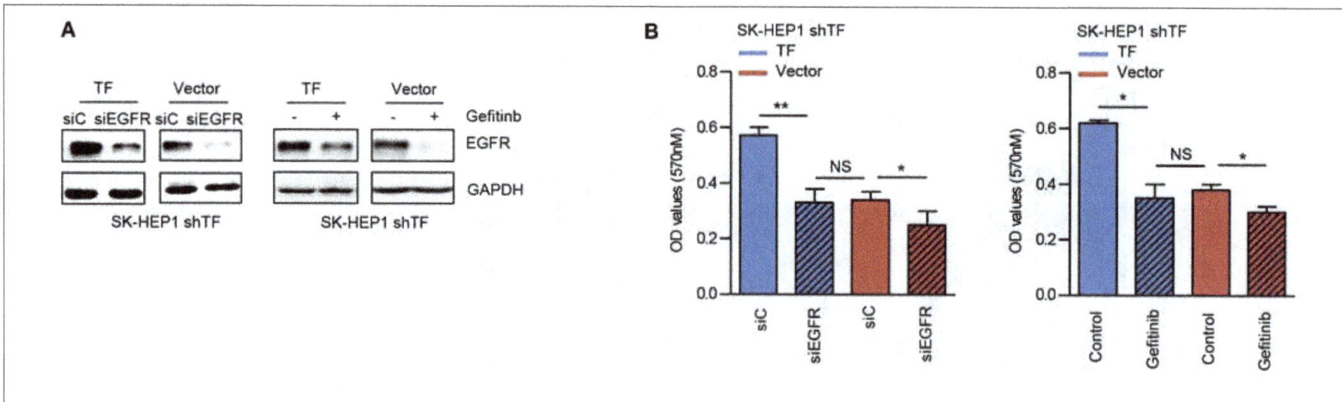

FIGURE 4 | Inhibition of EGFR suppresses TF-mediated HCC growth. SK-HEP1 shTF-Vector and SK-HEP1 shTF-TF cells were transfected with siControl or siEGFR or treated with/without gefinib at the concentration of 10 μM for 24 h. **(A)** Western blot and **(B)** MTT assay analysis of the protein expressions and cell growth. Error bars, mean ± SD. $^{*}p < 0.05$ and $^{**}p < 0.01$ (two-tailed Student's t-test **B**).

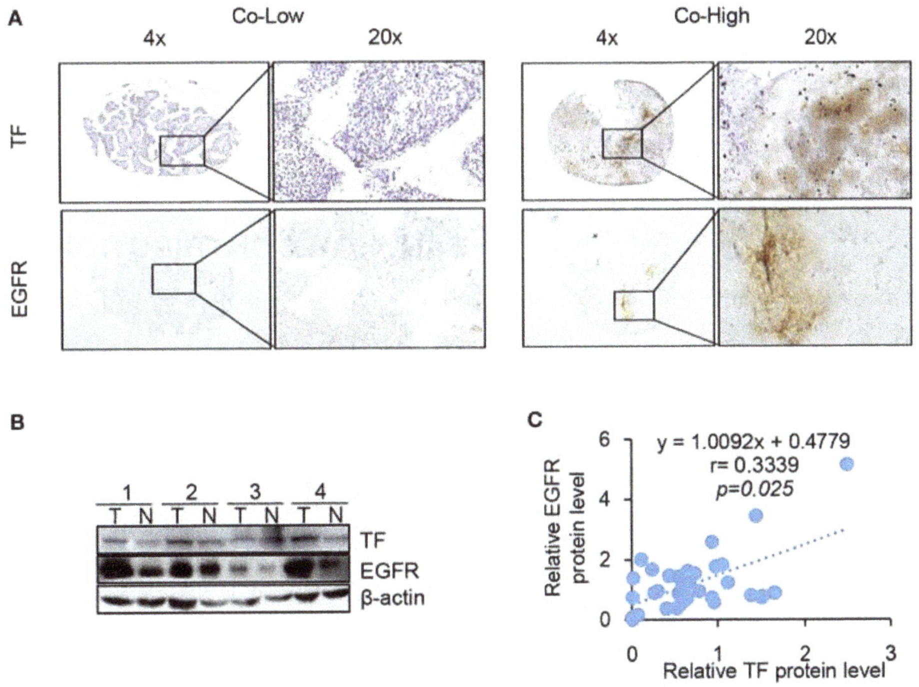

FIGURE 5 | TF protein expression is correlated with EGFR and poor HCC patient prognosis. TF and EGFR protein expressions in 144 HCC tissues were examined with IHC assay. **(A)** Representative images of positive and negative expression of both TF and EGFR were shown at 4 X and 20 X magnification. **(B)** Representative images of western blot analysis of TF and EGFR protein expression in the paired HCC tissues and adjacent normal tissues. **(C)** Spearman's rank correlation test showed the correlation between TF and EGFR protein expressions by Western blot.

inhibited the growth in both SK-HEP1 shTF-Vector and -TF cells (**Figure 3E**). In short, these data suggest that TF promotes the growth of HCC by activating both ERK and AKT signaling pathways.

Inhibition of EGFR Suppresses TF-Mediated HCC Growth

EGFR has been identified as a key player in the development of HCC (25). To verify the role of EGFR in TF-mediated HCC growth, we examined the effects of EGFR siRNA and EGFR inhibitor gefitinib on the growth of both SK-HEP1 shTF-Vector and -TF cells. EGFR siRNA or gefitinib decreased the protein levels of EGFR in both SK-HEP1 shTF-Vector and -TF cells (**Figure 4A**). Furthermore, EGFR siRNA or gefitinib inhibited the growth more significantly in SK-HEP1 shTF-TF cells than in SK-HEP1 shTF-Vector cells, indicating that inhibition of EGFR suppresses TF-mediated HCC growth (**Figure 4B**).

TF Protein Expression Is Correlated With EGFR in HCC Tissues

Our results clearly demonstrate that EGFR is regulated by TF in cell culture. To determine whether this is also the case in tumor tissues, we compared the protein levels of TF and EGFR in human 144 HCC tissues by IHC assay. High TF and EGFR staining were present in 105 (72.9%) and 91 (63.2%) out of 144 HCC tissues, respectively. Results of representative tissues with co-low or co-high staining of TF and EGFR were shown in **Figure 5A**. The expression of TF was highly correlated with the expression of EGFR in HCC tissues (**Table 1** and **Figures 5B, C**).

DISCUSSION

It has been demonstrated that TF-induced tumor progression need the activation of intracellular signaling pathways, where TF cytoplasmic domain couples to proteolytic activation of the protease activated receptor (PAR) 2 and subsequently activates ERK, AKT and other signaling pathways (26). For example, TF was involved in retinoblastoma cell proliferation via activating both ERK and AKT signaling pathways (27). Knockdown of TF suppressed human lung adenocarcinoma growth *in vitro* and *in vivo* through inhibiting both ERK and AKT signaling pathways (28). Similarly, our results showed that TF promoted the growth of HCC *in vitro* and *in vivo* by activating both ERK and AKT signaling pathways. Inhibition of ERK and AKT blocked TF-mediated growth of HCC. Therefore, activation of both ERK and AKT signaling pathways is indispensable for TF-promoted the growth of HCC.

EGFR is a member of ErbB/HER family of transmebrane receptor tyrosine kinases. It is activated by specific ligands resulting in the activation of multiple intracellular signaling pathways including ERK, AKT. Those signaling pathways is related to cell proliferation, migration and invasion (29–31). The gene expression of EGFR is regulated by the transcription factor c-Myc (32). In this study, we found that TF could enhance the expression of c-Myc and EGFR, and inhibition of ERK and AKT could block TF-induced c-Myc and EGFR upregulation. Phosphorylation of serine 62 amino acid residues by ERK prevents c-Myc protein from degradation (33). AKT stabilizes c-Myc protein by phosphorylation and inactivation of GSK-3β which phosphorylated threonine 58 amino acid residues of c-Myc to promote c-Myc degradation (33).

Inhibition of EGFR with either small molecule inhibitors or specific antibodies has achieved promising results in the preclinical HCC models. In human HCC cells, gefitinib, erlotinib or cetuximab could induce growth inhibition, cell cycle arrest and apoptosis (34–36). In the orthotopic HCC models, gefitinib significantly inhibited the growth and metastasis of HCC tumors, and enhanced by the combination with cisplatin (37, 38). However, the outcome of targeting EGFR in HCC was modest in the clinical trials. When used as a single agent in HCC patients, erlotinib only acquired moderate effects (39, 40), and cetuximab showed no antitumor activity (41). Treatment failure with EGFR inhibitors in HCC patients may cause by many reasons, such as the levels and mutations of EGFR, EMT status of tumor cells, etc. (42–44). In the current study, we found that treatment with EGFR siRNA or gefitinib suppressed the growth more significantly in the TF highly expressed HCC cells, suggesting that the levels of TF in tumor cells may influence the effects of EGFR inhibitors. Furthermore, our IHC data showed that both positive ratios of TF and EGFR protein in the HCC tissue were 72.9% (105/144) and 63.2% (91/144), respectively. The expression of TF was highly correlated with the expression of EGFR in HCC tissues. Therefore, it may be valuable to investigate the relation of TF expressions and EGFR inhibitors effects in the future studies.

CONCLUSIONS

Our results provide proof-of-principle insights into a novel mechanism driven by TF on HCC growth and suggest that TF and EGFR may be potential therapeutic targets of HCC.

AUTHOR CONTRIBUTIONS

S-ZH, M-NW, J-RH, Z-JZ, W-JZ, Q-WJ, and YY performed experiments. H-YW, H-LJ, KW, Z-HX, M-LY, and YL collected and analyzed data. X-SH, ZS, and QZ prepared the manuscript.

FUNDING

This work was supported by funds from the National Natural Science Foundation of China Nos. 81661148049 and 81772540 (ZS), the Guangdong Natural Science Funds for Distinguished Young Scholar No. 2014A030306001 (ZS), the Guangdong Special Support Program for Young Talent No. 2015TQ01R350 (ZS), the Science and Technology Program of Guangdong Nos. 201300000187 (QZ) and 2016A050502027 (ZS), the Science and Technology Program of Guangzhou No. 201704030058 (ZS), the Science and Technology Program of Huizhou (170520181743174/2017Y229 and 180529101741637/2018Y305), and the Program Sci-tech Research Development of Guangdong Province 2014A020212717 (QZ).

REFERENCES

1. Torre LA, Bray F, Siegel RL, Ferlay J, Lortet-Tieulent J, Jemal A. Global cancer statistics, 2012. *CA Cancer J Clin.* (2015) 65:87–108. doi: 10.3322/caac.21262
2. Chen W, Zheng R, Baade PD, Zhang S, Zeng H, Bray F, et al. Cancer statistics in China, 2015. *CA Cancer J Clin.* (2016) 66:115–32. doi: 10.3322/caac.21338
3. Sun T, Liu H, Ming L. Multiple roles of autophagy in the sorafenib resistance of hepatocellular carcinoma. *Cell Physiol Biochem.* (2017) 44:716–27. doi: 10.1159/000485285
4. Li C, Chen J, Zhang K, Feng B, Wang R, Chen L. Progress and prospects of long noncoding RNAs (lncRNAs) in hepatocellular carcinoma. *Cell Physiol Biochem.* (2015) 36:423–34. doi: 10.1159/0004 30109
5. Versteeg HH, Spek CA, Peppelenbosch MP, Richel DJ. Tissue factor and cancer metastasis: the role of intracellular and extracellular signaling pathways. *Mol Med.* (2004) 10:6–11. doi: 10.2119/2003-00047.Versteeg
6. Mackman N. Role of tissue factor in hemostasis, thrombosis, and vascular development. *Arterioscler Thromb Vasc Biol.* (2004) 24:1015–22. doi: 10.1161/01.ATV.0000130465.23430.74
7. Ruf W. Tissue factor and cancer. *Thromb Res.* (2012) 130(Suppl. 1):S84–87. doi: 10.1016/j.thromres.2012.08.285
8. Zhou Q, Huang T, Wang YF, Zhou XB, Liang LJ, Peng BG. Role of tissue factor in hepatocellular carcinoma genesis, invasion and metastasis. *Chin Med J.* (2011) 124:3746–51.
9. Kaido T, Oe H, Yoshikawa A, Mori A, Arii S, Imamura M. Tissue factor is a useful prognostic factor of recurrence in hepatocellular carcinoma in 5-year survivors. *Hepatogastroenterology.* (2005) 52:1383–7.
10. Poon RT, Lau CP, Ho JW, Yu WC, Fan ST, Wong J. Tissue factor expression correlates with tumor angiogenesis and invasiveness in human hepatocellular carcinoma. *Clin Cancer Res.* (2003) 9:5339–45.
11. Yang Y, Qiu JG, Li Y, Di JM, Zhang WJ, Jiang QW, et al. Targeting ABCB1-mediated tumor multidrug resistance by CRISPR/Cas9-based genome editing. *Am J Transl Res.* (2016) 8:3986–94.
12. Shi Z, Li Z, Li ZJ, Cheng K, Du Y, Fu H, et al. Cables1 controls p21/Cip1 protein stability by antagonizing proteasome subunit alpha type 3. *Oncogene.* (2015) 34:2538–45. doi: 10.1038/onc.2014.171
13. Luo Y, Jiang QW, Wu JY, Qiu JG, Zhang WJ, Mei XL, et al. Regulation of migration and invasion by toll-like receptor-9 signaling network in prostate cancer. *Oncotarget.* (2015) 6:22564–74. doi: 10.18632/oncotarget.4197
14. Zhang WJ, Li Y, Wei MN, Chen Y, Qiu JG, Jiang QW, et al. Synergistic antitumor activity of regorafenib and lapatinib in preclinical models of human colorectal cancer. *Cancer Lett.* (2017) 386:100–9. doi: 10.1016/j.canlet.2016.11.011
15. Lv M, Qiu JG, Zhang WJ, Jiang QW, Qin WM, Yang Y, et al. Wallichinine reverses ABCB1-mediated cancer multidrug resistance. *Am J Transl Res.* (2016) 8:2969–80.
16. Chen X, Gong L, Ou R, Zheng Z, Chen J, Xie F, et al. Sequential combination therapy of ovarian cancer with cisplatin and gamma-secretase inhibitor MK-0752. *Gynecol Oncol.* (2016) 140:537–44. doi: 10.1016/j.ygyno.2015.12.011
17. Lin M, Bi H, Yan Y, Huang W, Zhang G, Tang S, et al. Parthenolide suppresses non-small cell lung cancer GLC-82 cells growth via B-Raf/MAPK/Erk pathway. *Oncotarget.* (2017) 8:23436–47. doi: 10.18632/oncotarget.15584
18. Gong LH, Chen XX, Wang H, Jiang QW, Pan SS, Qiu JG, et al. Piperlongumine induces apoptosis and synergizes with cisplatin or paclitaxel

in human ovarian cancer cells. *Oxid Med Cell Longev.* (2014) 2014:906804. doi: 10.1155/2014/906804
19. Li P, Yang Y, Liu H, Yang AK, Di JM, Tan GM, et al. MiR-194 functions as a tumor suppressor in laryngeal squamous cell carcinoma by targeting wee1. *J Hematol Oncol.* (2017) 10:32. doi: 10.1186/s13045-017-0402-6
20. Jiang QW, Cheng KJ, Mei XL, Qiu JG, Zhang WJ, Xue YQ, et al. Synergistic anticancer effects of triptolide and celastrol, two main compounds from thunder god vine. *Oncotarget.* (2015) 6:32790–804. doi: 10.18632/oncotarget.5411
21. Zheng DW, Xue YQ, Li Y, Di JM, Qiu JG, Zhang WJ, et al. Volasertib suppresses the growth of human hepatocellular carcinoma *in vitro* and *in vivo*. *Am J Cancer Res.* (2016) 6:2476–88.
22. Mei XL, Yang Y, Zhang YJ, Li Y, Zhao JM, Qiu JG, et al. Sildenafil inhibits the growth of human colorectal cancer *in vitro* and *in vivo*. *Am J Cancer Res.* (2015) 5:3311–24.
23. Shi Z, Park HR, Du Y, Li Z, Cheng K, Sun SY, et al. Cables1 complex couples survival signaling to the cell death machinery. *Cancer Res.* (2015) 75:147–58. doi: 10.1158/0008-5472.CAN-14-0036
24. Qiu JG, Zhang YJ, Li Y, Zhao JM, Zhang WJ, Jiang QW, et al. Trametinib modulates cancer multidrug resistance by targeting ABCB1 transporter. *Oncotarget.* (2015) 6:15494–509. doi: 10.18632/oncotarget.3820
25. Berasain C, Avila MA. The EGFR signalling system in the liver: from hepatoprotection to hepatocarcinogenesis. *J Gastroenterol.* (2014) 49:9–23. doi: 10.1007/s00535-013-0907-x
26. Han X, Guo B, Li Y, Zhu B. Tissue factor in tumor microenvironment: a systematic review. *J Hematol Oncol.* (2014) 7:54. doi: 10.1186/s13045-014-0054-8
27. Lee BJ, Kim JH, Woo SH, Kim DH, Yu YS. Tissue factor is involved in retinoblastoma cell proliferation via both the akt and extracellular signal-regulated kinase pathways. *Oncol Rep.* (2011) 26:665–70. doi: 10.3892/or.2011.1314
28. Xu C, Gui Q, Chen W, Wu L, Sun W, Zhang N, et al. Small interference RNA targeting tissue factor inhibits human lung adenocarcinoma growth *in vitro* and *in vivo*. *J Exp Clin Cancer Res.* (2011) 30:63. doi: 10.1186/1756-9966-30-63
29. Grant S, Qiao L, Dent P. Roles of ERBB family receptor tyrosine kinases, and downstream signaling pathways, in the control of cell growth and survival. *Front Biosci.* (2002) 7:d376–89. doi: 10.2741/grant
30. Normanno N, De Luca A, Bianco C, Strizzi L, Mancino M, Maiello MR, et al. Epidermal growth factor receptor (EGFR) signaling in cancer. *Gene.* (2006) 366:2–16. doi: 10.1016/j.gene.2005.10.018
31. Ma P, Fu Y, Chen M, Jing Y, Wu J, Li K, et al. Adaptive and acquired resistance to EGFR inhibitors converge on the MAPK pathway. *Theranostics.* (2016) 6:1232–43. doi: 10.7150/thno.14409
32. Perini G, Diolaiti D, Porro A, Della Valle G. *In vivo* transcriptional regulation of n-myc target genes is controlled by E-box methylation. *Proc Natl Acad Sci USA.* (2005) 102:12117–22. doi: 10.1073/pnas.0409097102
33. Sears R, Nuckolls F, Haura E, Taya Y, Tamai K, Nevins JR. Multiple ras-dependent phosphorylation pathways regulate Myc protein stability. *Genes Dev.* (2000) 14:2501–14. doi: 10.1101/gad.836800
34. Okano J, Matsumoto K, Nagahara T, Murawaki Y. Gefitinib and the modulation of the signaling pathways downstream of epidermal growth factor receptor in human liver cancer cells. *J Gastroenterol.* (2006) 41:166–76. doi: 10.1007/s00535-005-1736-3
35. Hopfner M, Sutter AP, Huether A, Schuppan D, Zeitz M, Scherubl H. Targeting the epidermal growth factor receptor by gefitinib for treatment of hepatocellular carcinoma. *J Hepatol.* (2004) 41:1008–16. doi: 10.1016/j.jhep.2004.08.024
36. Huether A, Hopfner M, Sutter AP, Schuppan D, Scherubl H. Erlotinib induces cell cycle arrest and apoptosis in hepatocellular cancer cells and enhances chemosensitivity towards cytostatics. *J Hepatol.* (2005) 43:661–9. doi: 10.1016/j.jhep.2005.02.040
37. Matsuo M, Sakurai H, Saiki I. ZD1839, a selective epidermal growth factor receptor tyrosine kinase inhibitor, shows antimetastatic activity using a hepatocellular carcinoma model. *Mol Cancer Ther.* (2003) 2:557–61.
38. Zhu BD, Yuan SJ, Zhao QC, Li X, Li Y, Lu QY. Antitumor effect of gefitinib, an epidermal growth factor receptor tyrosine kinase inhibitor, combined with cytotoxic agent on murine hepatocellular carcinoma. *World J Gastroenterol.* (2005) 11:1382–6. doi: 10.3748/wjg.v11.i9.1382
39. Philip PA, Mahoney MR, Allmer C, Thomas J, Pitot HC, Kim G, et al. Phase II study of erlotinib (OSI-774) in patients with advanced hepatocellular cancer. *J Clin Oncol.* (2005) 23:6657–63. doi: 10.1200/JCO.2005.14.696
40. Thomas MB, Chadha R, Glover K, Wang X, Morris J, Brown T, et al. Phase 2 study of erlotinib in patients with unresectable hepatocellular carcinoma. *Cancer.* (2007) 110:1059–67. doi: 10.1002/cncr.22886
41. Zhu AX, Stuart K, Blaszkowsky LS, Muzikansky A, Reitberg DP, Clark JW, et al. Phase 2 study of cetuximab in patients with advanced hepatocellular carcinoma. *Cancer.* (2007) 110:581–9. doi: 10.1002/cncr.22829
42. Lanaya H, Natarajan A, Komposch K, Li L, Amberg N, Chen L, et al. EGFR has a tumour-promoting role in liver macrophages during hepatocellular carcinoma formation. *Nat Cell Biol.* (2014) 16:972–7. doi: 10.1038/ncb3031
43. Su MC, Lien HC, Jeng YM. Absence of epidermal growth factor receptor exon 18-21 mutation in hepatocellular carcinoma. *Cancer Lett.* (2005) 224:117–21. doi: 10.1016/j.canlet.2004.10.010
44. Fuchs BC, Fujii T, Dorfman JD, Goodwin JM, Zhu AX, Lanuti M, et al. Epithelial-to-mesenchymal transition and integrin-linked kinase mediate sensitivity to epidermal growth factor receptor inhibition in human hepatoma cells. *Cancer Res.* (2008) 68:2391–9. doi: 10.1158/0008-5472.CAN-07-2460

23

Iron-Chelated Polydopamine Decorated Doxorubicin-Loaded Nanodevices for Reactive Oxygen Species Enhanced Cancer Combination Therapy

Xu-Jing Li[1†], Wen-Tong Li[1,2†], Zi-Hao-Ran Li[1], Li-Ping Zhang[3], Cheng-Cheng Gai[1], Wei-Fen Zhang[2,3] and De-Jun Ding[2,3]*

[1] Department of Pathology, Weifang Medical University, Weifang, China, [2] Collaborative Innovation Center for Target Drug Delivery System, Weifang Medical University, Weifang, China, [3] College of Pharmacy, Weifang Medical University, Weifang, China

***Correspondence:**
De-Jun Ding
dejunding@wfmc.edu.cn

† These authors have contributed equally to this work

Combination therapy which enhances efficacy and reduces toxicity, has been increasingly applied as a promising strategy for cancer therapy. Here, a reactive oxygen species (ROS) that enhanced combination chemotherapy nanodevices was fabricated based on the Fe-chelated polydopamine (PDA) nanoparticles (NPs). The structure was characterized by dynamic light scattering-autosizer, transmission electron microscopy, energy dispersive spectroscopy, and Fourier-transform infrared (FT-IR) spectrophotometer. The *in vitro* drug release profile triggered by low intracellular pH indicated that the system demonstrated controlled therapeutic activity. *In vitro* cell uptake studies showed that doxorubicin (DOX)-loaded Fe-PDA/ folic acid (FA)-polyethylene glycol (DOX@Fe-PDA/FA-PEG) had a strong uptake capacity and can be rapidly internalized by MCF-7 cells. The *in vitro* experiments demonstrated that DOX@Fe-PDA/FA-PEG triggered the intracellular ROS overproduction, thereby enhancing its therapeutic effect on breast cancer. In summary, this experiment demonstrated the novel DOX-loaded composite NPs used as a potential targeted nanocarrier for breast cancer treatment, which could be a promising therapeutic strategy against breast cancer.

Keywords: polydopamine, combination therapy, reactive oxygen species, doxorubicin, breast cancer

INTRODUCTION

As one of the most common malignant tumors among women, breast cancer is the second and common cause of cancer-related death in women (Wood et al., 2017; Bray et al., 2018). Chemotherapy has become one of the most mature and common treatment option for breast cancer (Fisher et al., 1998; Miller et al., 2016; Spiegel and Koontz, 2018). Doxorubicin (DOX) is an anthracycline non-specific broad-spectrum anticancer drug that is widely used to treat breast cancer. Doxorubicin can exert its effects by elevating reactive oxygen species (ROS) thereby activating of caspase and ultimately leading to apoptosis (Russell and Cotter, 2015; Chakravarti et al., 2016). However, serious side effects, such as myelosuppression, cardiotoxicity, and drug resistance, are the major clinical chemotherapeutic drawbacks of DOX.

It has been proposed that combination therapeutics plays a synergistic effect and can enhance efficacy and reduce the toxicity of chemotherapy (Xu et al., 2015; Camacho et al., 2016; Kemp et al., 2016; Seo et al., 2017). Dayton et al. (2011) reported that the use of HO-3867, which is a synthetic curcumin analog, combined with DOX, in low doses to achieve enhanced cell death and reduced myocardial toxicity. And the increased generation of ROS, thereby resulting in oxidative damage to the cellular constituents, is widely exploited for therapeutic benefits on cancer (Matés and Sánchez-Jiménez, 2000; Schumacker Paul, 2015; Zhou et al., 2016). Fe, which plays a role in several types of cell death, has long been associated with toxicity because it induces hydroxyl radical (OH·), which is a ROS formed via Fenton reaction (Dixon and Stockwell, 2013; Shen et al., 2018; Zhang et al., 2018). Using ROS-producing agents could enhance the anticancer activity of DOX in cancer therapy through ROS-mediated apoptosis (Xia et al., 2017; Wu et al., 2017), autophagy (Fong et al., 2012), and ferroptosis (Zheng et al., 2017). Fan et al. (2014) identified the synergistic effect of DOX/ selenocystine sensitized to DOX by through ROS overproduction. Dai et al. (2018) fabricated assembled metal-phenolic network Nps as a novel ROS promoted synergistic nanomedicine platform for cancer therapy. This observation inspires us to import an iron-supply system in combination with DOX to elicit a synergistic effect on the cancer therapy.

Recently, researchers attempted to build some drug carrier systems to load and transport DOX overcoming the low bioavailability, poor absorption, and high toxicity of DOX (Xu et al., 2015; Kemp et al., 2016; Indermun et al., 2018). Particularly, polydopamine (PDA), which is a natural-inspired polymer, is an appealing material as drug carrier due to its good biocompatibility (Lynge et al., 2015; Indermun et al., 2018; Ryu et al., 2018). Considering its abundant aromatic rings, PDA NPs could be an efficient platform for loading DOX through π–π stacking and hydrogen-bonding interactiron. Meanwhile, the existence of phenolic hydroxyl groups on the surface makes it suitable for further modification with PEG, which could endow nanoparticles excellent physiological stability of NPs (Liu et al., 2014). More attractively, the phenolic surface have excellent chelating ability with metal ions such as Mn (Miao et al., 2015; Xi et al., 2017), Cu (Ge et al., 2017), and Fe (Li et al., 2016).

Keep all the issues in mind, we hypothesized that the Fe-chelated PDA nanoparticles with DOX loading could act as an Fe-supply system used for Fe and DOX combined cancer theranostics, as shown in **Figure 1**. The designed DOX@Fe-PDA/folic acid (FA)-PEG could be provided with several advantages, as follows: (Wood et al., 2017) Combination therapy. The chemotherapy drug DOX undergoes redox cycles to generate and increase H_2O_2 in living cells. The released Fe from PDA further reacts with H_2O_2 to generate hydroxyl radical via Fenton reaction and induces cell death. In combination with Fe, DOX was prone to kill cancer cells efficiently (Bray et al., 2018). Biocompatibility and safety. PDA, which is a natural biopolymer, possesses biocompatibility. The coated PEG and chelated Fe of PDA Nps were metabolic. Meanwhile, the pH-triggered release performance of PDA in tumor microenvironment, avoids damage to surrounding tissues. The PEG-coating can help Nps to ameliorate long-term circulation (Fisher et al., 1998). Tumor targeted. Considering folate receptor overexpression on the surface of breast cancer cells, the FA conjugated NPs may improve cell uptake via receptor mediated endocytosis. In summary, the DOX@Fe-PDA/FA-PEG system could be used as potential combination chemotherapy nanodevice for breast cancer treatment.

MATERIALS AND METHODS

NPs Synthesis

The synthesis of NPs was modified based on the previously introduced procedure (Li et al., 2016). In brief, 4.08 mg $FeCl_3$ and 15 mg dopamine plus 10 mL of water were mixed and stirred at room temperature for 1 h. Then 500 mg Tris was added, and the mixture was stirred at room temperature for 1.5 h. The mixture was centrifuged at 12000 rpm for 15 min to obtain Fe-PDA NPs. A total of 3.85 mL Fe-PDA NPs (5.2 mg/mL) were mixed with 20 mg FA-PEG-SH, 4.7 mg Tris, and 100 μL *tris*(2-carboxyethyl)phosphine (8 mg/mL). The mixture was vigorously stirred for 1 h at room temperature. Then, the FA-PEG modified NPs (Fe-PDA/PEG-FA) were purified via centrifugation and washed with deionized water.

Drug Loading

A total of 2 mg adriamycin hydrochloride were added into 300 μL of dimethyl sulfoxide and 8.2 μL of triethylamine was added. The mixture was stirred in dark at room temperature for 12 h to desalinate hydrochloride. Then, the neutral DOX (2 mg) above-mentioned was added dropwise to 1 mL of Fe-PDA/FA-PEG NPs (10 mg/mL). Afterward, Tris (2.42 mg) was added and volume of 3 mL was obtained by adding distilled water. After vigorous stirring for 24 h in the dark, free DOX was removed via centrifugation at 12000 rpm for 10 min, then washed with phosphate buffer solution (PBS) and stored at 4°C in the dark. The DOX loading capacity of NPs was determined by UV-Vis spectrophotometer at the wavelength of 480 nm. The encapsulation efficiency (EE) of DOX was calculated by the following equation: EE = (initial amount of feeding drugs − free drugs)/initial amount of feeding drugs.

NPs Characterization

The size and Zeta potential of the prepared NPs were measured by dynamic light scattering-autosizer (DLS) on Zetasizer Nano ZS90 (Malvern Instruments, Malvern, United Kingdom). The liquid sample was sonicated before measurement. Three independent test results were recorded. The shape and surface morphology of the NPs were imaged by a transmission electron microscope (TEM, JEM-1230; JEOL, Tokyo, Japan). TEM, energy dispersive X-ray spectroscopy (EDS) and corresponding EDS-mapping were adopted for morphology and elemental distribution analyses on the JEM-1230 electron microscope operated at 200 kV. The chemical composition and structural changes of NPs were analyzed by Fourier transform infrared (FT-IR) spectroscopy (VERTEX 70; Bruker, Bremen, Germany). The IR spectra

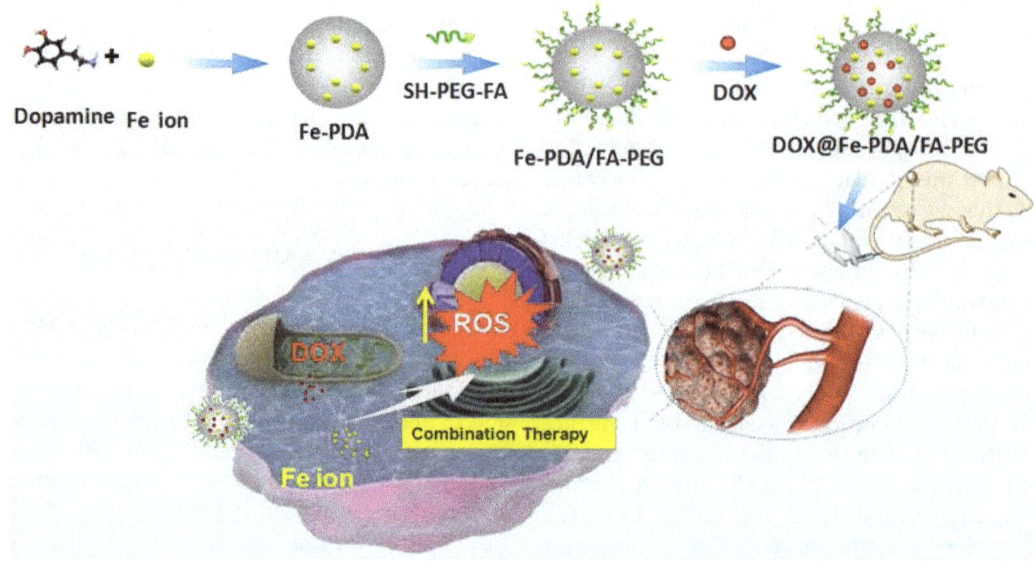

FIGURE 1 | Schematic representation of DOX@Fe-PDA/PEG-FA synthesis, targeted cell uptake and intracellular drug release and combination therapy.

of the samples were obtained in the range of 4000 and 500 cm^{-1}.

In vitro Drug Release Profiles

The *in vitro* DOX release behavior of DOX@Fe-PDA/FA-PEG was tested as reported previously (Liu et al., 2014). Briefly, DOX@Fe-PDA/FA-PEG was dispersed in 2 mL PBS with the pH of either 7.2 or 5.5. The tube was shaken at 37°C with 100 rpm in dark. At appropriate time points, the full release buffer was collected via centrifugation at 12000 rpm for 10 min, and replaced with 2 mL of fresh PBS. The amount of released drug DOX was quantified by a UV spectrophotometer at the wavelength of 480 nm. The correlation between the accumulative DOX released from NPs and time was plotted.

Cell Culture

The *in vitro* cell cytotoxicity cellular uptake and ROS measurement were assessed on human breast cancer cell line MCF-7, which was purchased from American Type Culture Collection. Cells were incubated at 37°C with modified Eagle's medium (MEM) containing 10% fetal bovine serum (FBS), 100 U/mL penicillin, and 100 mg/mL streptomycin in a 5% CO_2 atmosphere.

Cellular Uptake Study

A total of 2 × 10^5 cells/well MCF-7 cells were seeded in 6-well plates for 24 h. Then, the samples (free DOX, DOX@Fe-PDA/FA-PEG) were added to each well (equivalent DOX concentration of 10 μg/mL) and the cells were incubated at 37°C for an appropriate time at an additional of 24 h. Afterward, the cells were washed with PBS and stained by Hoechst 33342 (Sangon Biotech, Shanghai, China). Confocal laser scanning microscopy (CLSM) imaging was performed on LSM 410 fluorescence microscope (Zeiss, Jena, Germany). The fluorescence signal of DOX was excited at 488 nm and measured at 610 nm. The fluorescence signal stained by Hoechst 33342 was excited at 405 nm and detected at 490 nm.

In vitro Cytotoxicity by Using MTT Assay

MCF-7 cells were seeded in 96-well plates at a density of 5000 cells per well and incubated in 100 mL of medium for 24 h to allow attachment. Then, the cells were incubated with free DOX and DOX@Fe-PDA/FA-PEG (DOX concentration of 0.1093, 0.2187, 04375, 0.875, 1.75, and 3.5 μg/mL) for 24 and 48 h, respectively. A total of 20 μL MTT solution (5 mg/mL) were added to each well and incubated for 4 h. The crystals were dissolved by adding DMSO. The optical density value of each well was measured at 490 nm by an iMark plate reader (Bio-Rad, Berkeley, CA, United States). All data were obtained in quadruplicate.

Intracellular ROS Content Measurement

MCF-7 cells were seeded on 6-well plates at a density of 2 × 10^5 cells per well. Then the cells were incubated with free DOX and DOX@Fe-PDA/FA-PEG (equivalent DOX concentration of 10 μg/mL) for 8 h at 37°C. Afterward, diluted 2′,7′-dichlorofluorescein diacetate (DCFH-DA; Solarbio, Beijing, China), which is a cell-permeable fluorescent probe, were added. Then, the cells were placed in a 6-well plate at 37°C and incubated for another 30 min. The cells were washed for three times with serum-free medium to remove DCFH-DA completely and finally observed using fluorescence microscope.

Data Analysis Methodology

All experiments were performed at least three times unless otherwise stated. All experimental data were expressed as mean ± SD and both were treated with SPSS 18.0 (SPSS, Chicago, IL, United States).

RESULTS AND DISCUSSION

DOX@ Fe-PDA/FA-PEG Synthesis and Characterization

The design and synthetic strategy of DOX@Fe-PDA/FA-PEG is shown in **Figure 1**. First, the Fe-PDA was synthesized using an oxidative self-polymerization method according to previously literature (Li et al., 2016). In addition, folic acid conjugated PEG was introduced to modify the PDA in enhancing the targeting effect and improving the stability of the NPs. Finally, DOX was loaded via diffusion in an aqueous media. The mean hydrodynamic sizes of DOX@PDA/FA-PEG, DOX@Fe-PDA/FA-PEG and the unloaded Fe-PDA/FA-PEG were 239.5 ± 28.82, 267.7 ± 34.16, and 283.22 ± 21.6 nm, respectively, with a narrow size distribution as demonstrated in **Figure 2A**. This particle size is theoretically suitable for cellular uptake and tumor cell permeation duo to EPR effect (Maeda, 2015). Zeta potential plays a key role in the stability and penetration through cell membranes for Nps (Bhattacharjee, 2016). Considering the presence of the carboxyl group of FA, the zeta potentials of all NPs are negative (**Supplementary Figure 1**), thereby indicating that these Nps were stable *in vivo* by electrostatic repulsion, which is the basis of drug delivery (Wu et al., 2011). The zeta potential of Fe-PDA/FA-PEG (−30 mV) is slightly lower than that of Fe-PDA/FA-PEG loaded with DOX (−27.2 mV) (**Supplementary Figure 1**), thereby suggesting that the positively charged amino groups on DOX partially neutralized the negative charge.

The morphologies of Fe-PDA/FA-PEG (wihout DOX loaded), DOX@PDA/FA-PEG (without Fe chelated), DOX@Fe-PDA/FA-PEG were observed by TEM. The results revealed that the DOX-loaded PDA/FA-PEG exhibited a spherical and uniform morphology (**Figure 2B**). The particle size observed by TEM was substantially the same as the particle size measured by DLS. Scanning electron microscopy used to perform accurate elemental analysis of Nps. Using dark field image (DFI) characterization, electron energy loss spectroscopy (EELS), energy dispersive spectroscopy (EDS), and corresponding element mapping (EDS mapping) (**Figure 3**) clearly show the morphological structure of the nanoparticles and distribution of four elements (C, N, O, Fe). The results showed that the coexistence of C, N, O, and Fe signals coexisted in the EDS spectra of Fe-PDA and Fe-PDA/FA-PEG. The uniform distribution of C, N, O, and Fe was confirmed by EDS element mapping. This result indicated the success and dispersion loads of Fe, PDA, and PEG in the DOX-loaded Fe-PDA/FA-PEG and unloaded Fe-PDA/FA-PEG. However, in the EDS element mapping of PDA, only C, N, and O signals coexisted and were distributed, thereby indicating the success and dispersion load of PDA and PEG in the DOX-loaded PDA/FA-PEG. Further, the FR-IR was performed to evaluat the surface characterization. As shown in **Supplementary Figure 2**, the, the characteristic peaks of N-H bending vibration appearing at 1512, 1589, and 3250 cm^{-1}. The peaks at 1493 and 1445 cm^{-1} can be ascribed to the existence of FA. Compared with PDA, the peaks of PEG at 1128 cm^{-1} (C-O-C stretching) were observed.

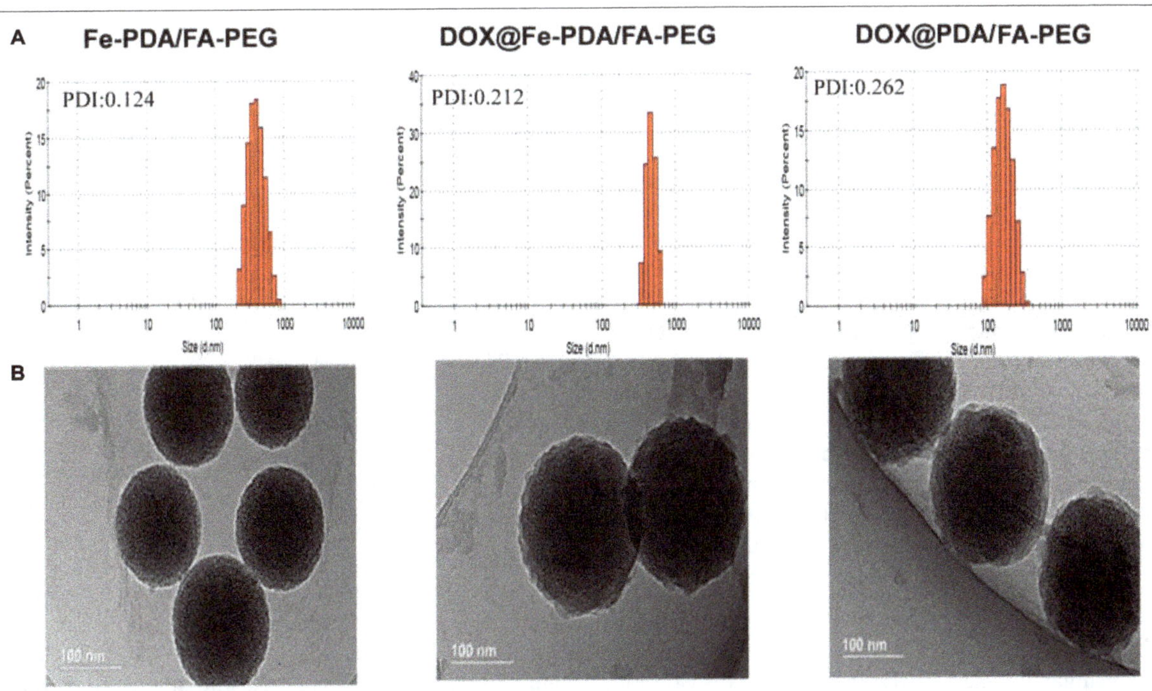

FIGURE 2 | The characterization of different nanopartícl nanoparticles. **(A)** Size distributions of Fe-PDA/FA-PEG, DOX@Fe-PDA/FA-PEG, DOX@PDA/FA-PEG. **(B)** TEM image of PDA/FA-PEG, DOX@Fe-PDA/FA-PEG, DOX@PDA/FA-PEG. Scale bar: 100 nm.

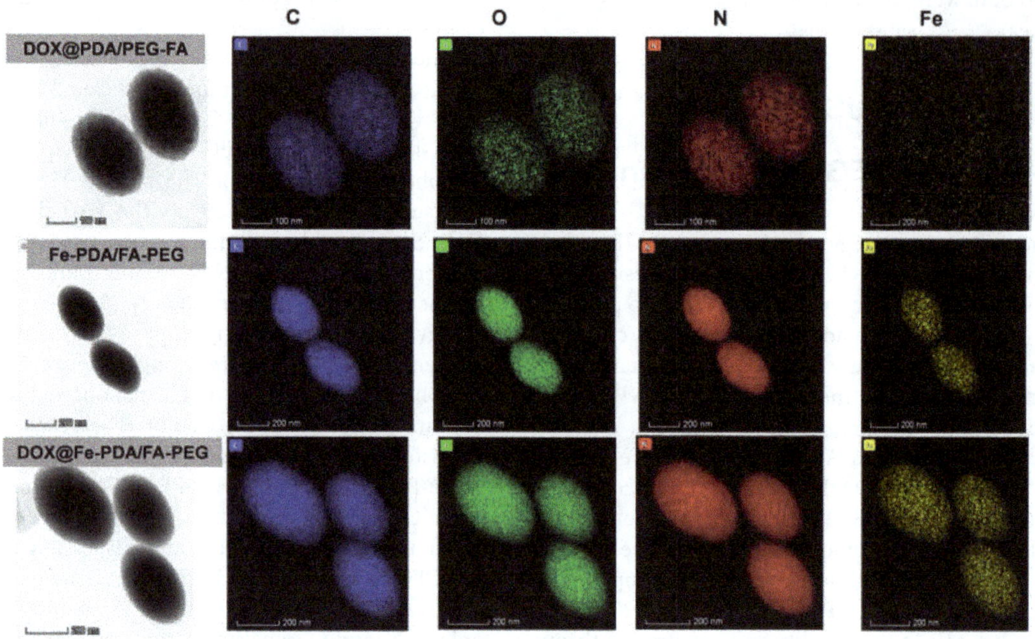

FIGURE 3 | Dark-field image, and corresponding area-elemental mappings of PDA/FA-PEG, DOX@Fe-PDA/FA-PEG, DOX@PDA/FA-PEG. Scale bar: 50 nm.

In vitro pH-Stimuli Release Study

At a drug to Fe-PDA/FA-PEG feeding ratio of 1:5 in weight, the encapsulation efficiency of DOX in the Fe-PDA/FA-PEG was 76.6 ± 5.2% determined by UV-Vis absorption spectrophotometer. As PDA NPs exist abundant aromatic rings and phenolic hydroxyl groups, the DOX was loaded through π−π stacking and hydrogen-bonding interaction. Subsequently, the pH dependent release capability of DOX@Fe-PDA/FA-PEG was investigated at 37°C under the pH levels of 7.2 and 5.5. The accumulative drug release kinetics curves are shown in **Figure 4**. The drug release of both the DOX-loaded Fe-PDA/FA-PEG was significantly pH-dependent. As shown in **Figure 4**, the release of the drug was as low as 25.5% at the of pH 7.2 within 36 h, and even 30.1% within 48 h. However, under acidic conditions, the release amount reached 34.6% within 8 h at the pH of 5.5, and the release rate at 48 h was 47.2%. This indicated that the drug-loaded Nps can cause the drug release under acidic condition, mainly due to the extremely high pH responsiveness of the PDA-modified NPs. This phenomenon allowed the rapid drug release at low pH. Considering the acidic microenvironment of the tumor and intracellular acidic endosomes and lysosomes, drugs are released only after being phagocytized by lysosomes in tumor cells, thereby effectively reducing drug waste and enhancing the antitumor effects by rapidly increasing the lysosome concentration (Duo et al., 2017).

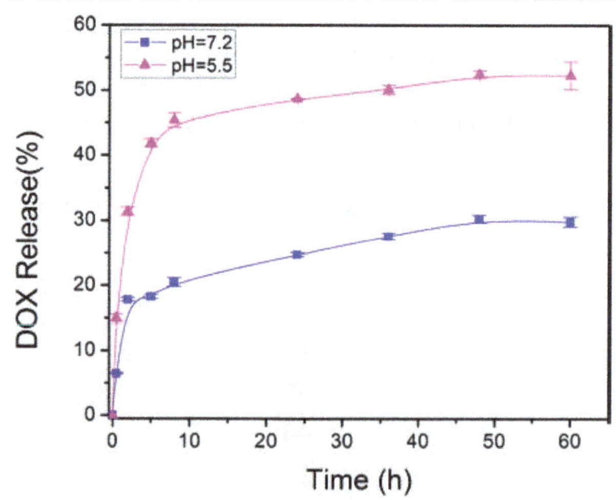

FIGURE 4 | *In vitro* drug release profile of DOX@Fe-PDA/FA-PEG in media with different pH value (pH 7.2 and 5.5).

Cellular Uptake

To study the cellular uptake and the intracellular distribution, we investigated the intracellular delivery of free DOX by using a confocal microscopy. **Figure 5A** shows the fluorescence of DOX distrubuted in the cytoplasm and cell nuclei after incubation with free DOX for 1 h. However the red flourescence with NPS observed in nucleus was not obvious. Based on the different intracellular fates of DOX, it was indicated that the NPs were internalized into cell mainly via endocytic pathway. And then we continued to incubate for another 9 h and observed under a fluorescence microscope as shown in **Figure 5B**. Apparently, the uptake intensities of DOX-loaded NPs was higher than that of free DOX, and it was contributed by the targeting effect of folate receptor. Moreover, the cell uptake intensities of DOX-loaded NPs were positive correlation with incubation time. While the fluorescence intensity of free DOX

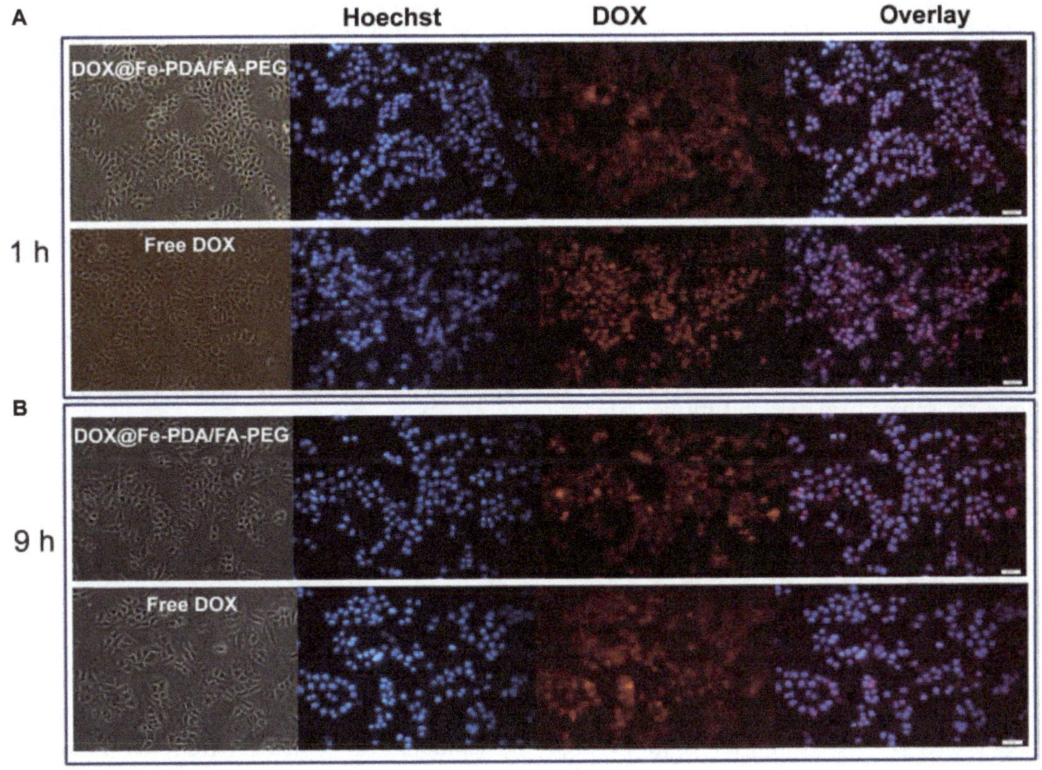

FIGURE 5 | Confocal laser scanning microscopy (CLSM) images of MCF-7 cells after incubation with free DOX, DOX-@ Fe-PDA/FA-PEG for 1 h **(A)**, and 9 h **(B)**. The cells were stained by Hoechst (blue) and drug DOX was red.

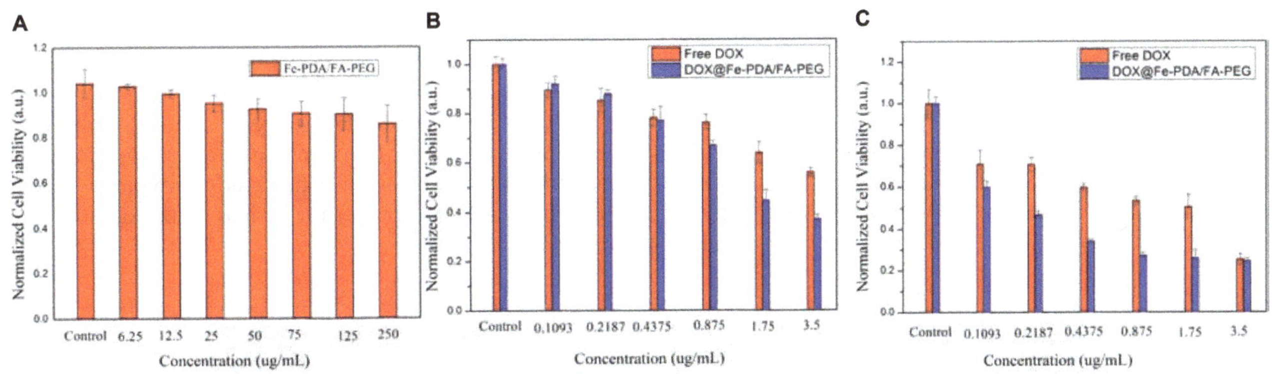

FIGURE 6 | Relative viabilities of MCF-7 cells after incubated with PDA/FA-PEG for 48 h **(A)** and free DOX and DOX@Fe-PDA/FA-PEG at different concentrations 24 h **(B)** and 48 h **(C)**.

in the cells is weaker than that of the doxorubicin-loaded NPs, indicating that the intracellular free DOX decays with time. According to the *in vitro* drug release profiles, this phenomenon proves that the DOX-loaded Nps have a sustained release effect, which may help to enhance the cytotoxicity of DOX.

Cytotoxicity of DOX-Loaded NPs

To assess the cytotoxicity of DOX@Fe-PDA/FA-PEG, we performed the MTT assays. In order to confirm the high biocompatibility and safety of the NPs, we incubated the Fe-PDA/FA-PEG NPs with MCF-7 cells. As shown in **Figure 6A**, the Fe-PDA/FA-PEG NPs without drug-loading exhibited a negligible cytotoxicity the concentration ranging from 0 to 250 μg/mL for 48 h. This result suggested that the prepared material possessed high biocompatibility and low cell cytotoxicity. Then, we compared the results of cytotoxicity of free DOX and DOX-loaded Nps at 24 and 48 h. **Figures 6B,C** shows the cytotoxicity of DOX on MCF-7 was time and dose-dependent. As the DOX concentration and incubation time prolonged, the greater the toxicity of the drug to MCF-7 cell. Apparently, the cytotoxicity of DOX-loaded Fe-PDA/FA-PEG NPs was greater than that free DOX, thereby demonstrating that Fe enhanced the killing effect of DOX on the MCF-7 cells. And it was found that the 48 h of incubation exhibited a considerable killing effect on MCF-7 cells than 24 h. This result further confirmed the sustained release of NPs.

ROS Detection

Reactive oxygen species -induced cell death has been a widely uesed strategy for tumor therapy (Matés and Sánchez-Jiménez, 2000; Dixon and Stockwell, 2013; Schumacker Paul, 2015; Zhou et al., 2016). As we know, DOX could activate nicotinamide adenine dinucleotide phosphate oxidases, and further produce ROS, which contribute to anticancer drug-induced toxicity (Chakravarti et al., 2016; Seo et al., 2017). Recently, synergistic approaches by using ROS-producing agents with DOX have attracted considerable attention (Xia et al., 2017). Intriguingly, the presence of Fe (II and III) contributes to the enhanced chemotherapy efficacy by converting the accumulated H_2O_2 to the hydroxyl radical via Fenton reactions (Dixon and Stockwell, 2013). To explore the underlying mechanism of enhanced antiproliferating effects of DOX@Fe-PDA/FA-PEG further, we quantified the intracellular ROS by using 2′-7′-dichlorofuorescin diacetate. Compared with the control group, green fluorescence was observed after incubation with DOX and DOX@Fe-PDA/FA-PEG (**Figure 7**). In addition, cells treated with DOX-loaded Fe-PDA/FA-PEG had the highest fluorescence intensity, thereby indicating the highest ROS production. The results showed that the cells treated with DOX loaded Fe-PDA/FA-PEG can synergistically produce ROS to kill tumor cells. DOX used to undergo redox cycles to generate high H_2O_2 levels inside the cancer cells. After endocytosis by tumor cells, the DOX@Fe-PDA/FA-PEG was decomposed by the acidic microenvironment. The elevated H_2O_2 of DOX can be further catalyzed by Fe ions via Fenton reaction to generate abundant highly toxic resulting in enhancing anticancer effects of DOX through oxidative damage to DNA, protein, and lipid (Matés and Sánchez-Jiménez, 2000; Schumacker Paul, 2015; Zhou et al., 2016). Previous investigations have developed iron-based nanomaterials, including iron nanometallic glasses and iron oxide, have been employed to upregulation of ROS by using the situ Fenton reaction (Zhang et al., 2016; Liu et al., 2018; Tang et al., 2018). However, current iron-based nanomaterials is far from satisfactory. Some of the nanomaterials such as Fe^0 nanoparticles (Zhang et al., 2016) and iron oxide nanoplatform (Liu et al., 2018), are difficult to fabricate and the synthetic conditions generally are harsh and complicated. In this work, we synthesized the iron-chelated PDA NPs via a one-pot reaction and the FA-PEG as the surface ligand for tumor homing with a low cost and biocompable biocompatibility. And the pH-stimuli release profiles included being highly selective and logical, and amenable to activation by endogenous stimuli. This strategy present an approach for synergistic combination of ROS and chemotherapy to enhance the anticancer efficacy.

CONCLUSION

In this study, we successfully fabricated a novel nanocarrier on the basis of Fe-chelated PDA nanoparticles used for Fe and DOX combined cancer theranostics through ROS over-generation. The obtained DOX@Fe-PDA/FA-PEG Nps had a hydrodynamic size of about 250 nm, and the structure was characterized by DLS, TEM, EDS, and FT-IR. The *in vitro* drug release profile triggered by low intracellular pH indicated that the system demonstrated controlled therapeutic activity. Further, *in vitro* cell uptake studies indicate that DOX-loaded Fe-PDA /FA-PEG can be internalized by MCF-7 cells and exhibited high targeting efficiency due to specific recognition. The *in vitro* experiments demonstrated that DOX@Fe-PDA/FA-PEG trigged the intracellular ROS overproduction, thereby enhancing the therapeutic effect on breast cancer. Taken together, this study provides a strategy to harness Fe-PAD nanocarrier for Fe and DOX combined cancer theranostics.

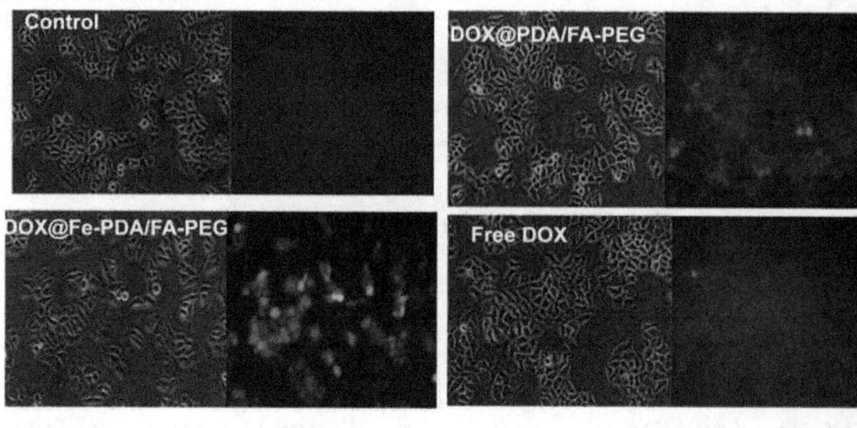

FIGURE 7 | The intracellular ROS stained with DCFH-DA in MCF-7 cells after incubation with free DOX, DOX@Fe-PDA/FA-PEG, DOX@PDA/FA-PEG for 8 h were measured by fluorescence microscopic.

AUTHOR CONTRIBUTIONS

X-JL and W-TL performed the experiments and drafted the manuscript. Z-H-RL and L-PZ prepared and characterized the NPs. C-CG and performed the statistical design of the experiments. W-FZ and D-JD conceived the initial idea. All authors helped to correct and polish the manuscript and read and approved the final manuscript.

FUNDING

The authors are grateful for the generous financial support of the Project of Shandong Province Higher Educational Science and Technology Program (Grant No. J18KA279), National Natural Science Foundation of China (Grant No. 81774125), Project of Collaborative Innovation Center for Target Drug Delivery System of Weifang Medical University (2017), and College Students' Technology Innovation Project of Weifang Medical University (Grant No. KX2017045).

ACKNOWLEDGMENTS

We appreciate the experimental assistance of bachelor students Ling-Yan Liao, Ruo-Bing Liu, Yajing Ji, and Yanan Li.

REFERENCES

1. Bhattacharjee, S. (2016). DLS and zeta potential - what they are and what they are not? *J. Controll. Release* 235, 337–351. doi: 10.1016/j.jconrel.2016.06.017
2. Bray, F., Ferlay, J., Soerjomataram, I., Siegel, R. L., Torre, L. A., and Jemal, A. (2018). Global cancer statistics 2018: GLOBOCAN estimates of incidence and mortality worldwide for 36 cancers in 185 countries. *CA Cancer J. Clin.* 68, 394–424. doi: 10.3322/caac.21492
3. Camacho, K. M., Menegatti, S., Vogus, D. R., Pusuluri, A., Fuchs, Z., Jarvis, M., et al. (2016). DAFODIL: a novel liposome-encapsulated synergistic combination of doxorubicin and 5FU for low dose chemotherapy. *J. Controll. Release* 229, 154–162. doi: 10.1016/j.jconrel.2016.03.027
4. Chakravarti, B., Yang, J., Luo, Z., and Ahlers, K. E. (2016). Contribution of NADPH oxidase (Nox)-derived reactive oxygen species (ROS) to doxorubicin-induced cardiomyopathy mediated by regulator of g protein signaling 6 (RGS6). *FASEB J.* 30:939.3. doi: 10.1096/fasebj.30.1_supplement.939.3
5. Dai, Y., Yang, Z., Cheng, S., Wang, Z., Zhang, R., Zhu, G., et al. (2018). Toxic reactive oxygen species enhanced synergistic combination therapy by self-assembled metal-phenolic network nanoparticles. *Adv. Mat.* 30:1704877. doi: 10.1002/adma.201704877
6. Dayton, A., Selvendiran, K., Meduru, S., Khan, M., Kuppusamy, M. L., Naidu, S., et al. (2011). Amelioration of doxorubicin-induced cardiotoxicity by an anticancer-antioxidant dual-function compound, HO-3867. *J. Pharmacol. Exp. Ther.* 339:350. doi: 10.1124/jpet.111.183681
7. Dixon, S. J., and Stockwell, B. R. (2013). The role of iron and reactive oxygen species in cell death. *Nat. Chem. Biol.* 10:9. doi: 10.1038/nchembio.1416
8. Duo, Y., Li, Y., Chen, C., Liu, B., Wang, X., Zeng, X., et al. (2017). DOX-loaded pH-sensitive mesoporous silica nanoparticles coated with PDA and PEG induce pro-death autophagy in breast cancer. *RSC Adv.* 7, 39641–39650. doi: 10.1039/C7RA05135B
9. Fan, C., Zheng, W., Fu, X., Li, X., Wong, Y.-S., and Chen, T. (2014). Strategy to enhance the therapeutic effect of doxorubicin in human hepatocellular carcinoma by selenocystine, a synergistic agent that regulates the ROS-mediated signaling. *Oncotarget* 5, 2853–2863. doi: 10.18632/oncotarget.1854
10. Fisher, B., Bryant, J., Wolmark, N., Mamounas, E., Brown, A., Fisher, E. R., et al. (1998). Effect of preoperative chemotherapy on the outcome of women with operable breast cancer. *J. Clin. Oncol.* 16, 2672–2685. doi: 10.1200/jco.1998.16.8.2672
11. Fong, M. Y., Jin, S., Rane, M., Singh, R. K., Gupta, R., and Kakar, S. S. (2012). Withaferin a synergizes the therapeutic effect of doxorubicin through ROS-mediated autophagy in ovarian cancer. *PLoS One* 7:e42265. doi: 10.1371/journal.pone.0042265
12. Ge, R., Lin, M., Li, X., Liu, S., Wang, W., Li, S., et al. (2017). Cu2+-loaded polydopamine nanoparticles for magnetic resonance imaging-guided pH- and near-infrared-light-stimulated thermochemotherapy. *ACS Appl. Mat. Interfaces* 9, 19706–19716. doi: 10.1021/acsami.7b05583
13. Indermun, S., Govender, M., Kumar, P., Choonara, Y. E., and Pillay, V. (2018). "2 - Stimuli-responsive polymers as smart drug delivery systems: classifications based on carrier type and triggered-release mechanism," in *Stimuli Responsive Polymeric Nanocarriers for Drug Delivery Applications*, Vol. 1, eds A. S. H. Makhlouf and N. Y. Abu-Thabit (Sawston: Woodhead Publishing), 43–58. doi: 10.1016/B978-0-08-101997-9.00002-3
14. Kemp, J. A., Shim, M. S., Heo, C. Y., and Kwon, Y. J. (2016). "Combo" nanomedicine: co-delivery of multi-modal therapeutics for efficient, targeted, and safe cancer therapy. *Adv. Drug Deliv. Rev.* 98, 3–18. doi: 10.1016/j.addr.2015.10.019
15. Li, Y., Xie, Y., Wang, Z., Zang, N., Carniato, F., Huang, Y., et al. (2016). Structure and function of iron-loaded synthetic melanin. *ACS Nano* 10, 10186–10194. doi: 10.1021/acsnano.6b05502
16. Liu, Y., Ai, K., and Lu, L. (2014). Polydopamine and its derivative materials: synthesis and promising applications in energy, environmental, and biomedical fields. *Chem. Rev.* 114, 5057–5115. doi: 10.1021/cr400407a
17. Liu, Y., Ji, X., Tong, W. W. L., Askhatova, D., Yang, T., Cheng, H., et al. (2018). Engineering multifunctional RNAi nanomedicine to concurrently target cancer hallmarks for combinatorial therapy. *Angew. Chem. Int. Ed.* 57, 1510–1513. doi: 10.1002/anie.201710144
18. Lynge, M. E., Schattling, P., and Städler, B. (2015). Recent developments in poly(dopamine)-based coatings for biomedical applications. *Nanomedicine* 10, 2725–2742. doi: 10.2217/nnm.15.89
19. Maeda, H. (2015). Toward a full understanding of the EPR effect in primary and metastatic tumors as well as issues related to its heterogeneity. *Adv. Drug Deliv. Rev.* 91, 3–6. doi: 10.1016/j.addr.2015.01.002
20. Matés, J. M., and Sánchez-Jiménez, F. M. (2000). Role of reactive oxygen species in apoptosis: implications for cancer therapy. *Int. J. Biochem. Cell Biol.* 32, 157–170. doi: 10.1016/S1357-2725(99)00088-6
21. Miao, Z.-H., Wang, H., Yang, H., Li, Z.-L., Zhen, L., and Xu, C.-Y. (2015). Intrinsically Mn2+-chelated polydopamine nanoparticles for simultaneous magnetic resonance imaging and photothermal ablation of cancer cells. *ACS Appl. Mat. Interfaces* 7, 16946–16952. doi: 10.1021/acsami.5b0 6265
22. Miller, K. D., Siegel, R. L., Lin, C. C., Mariotto, A. B., Kramer, J. L., Rowland, J. H., et al. (2016). Cancer treatment and survivorship statistics, 2016. *CA Cancer J. Clin.* 66, 271–289. doi: 10.3322/caac.21349
23. Russell, E. G., and Cotter, T. G. (2015). "Chapter six - new insight into the role of reactive oxygen species (ROS) in cellular signal-transduction processes," in *International Review of Cell and Molecular Biology*, Vol. 319, ed. K. W. Jeon (Cambridge, MA: Academic Press), 221–254.
24. Ryu, J. H., Messersmith, P. B., and Lee, H. (2018). Polydopamine surface chemistry: a decade of discovery. *ACS Appl. Mat. Interfaces* 10, 7523–7540. doi: 10.1021/acsami.7b19865

25. Schumacker Paul, T. (2015). Reactive oxygen species in cancer: a dance with the devil. *Cancer Cell* 27, 156–157. doi: 10.1016/j.ccell.2015.01.007
26. Seo, S. U., Kim, T. H., Kim, D. E., Min, K.-J., and Kwon, T. K. (2017). NOX4-mediated ROS production induces apoptotic cell death via down-regulation of c-FLIP and Mcl-1 expression in combined treatment with thioridazine and curcumin. *Redox Biol.* 13, 608–622. doi: 10.1016/j.redox.2017.07.017
27. Shen, Z., Song, J., Yung, B. C., Zhou, Z., Wu, A., and Chen, X. (2018). Cancer therapy: emerging strategies of cancer therapy based on ferroptosis. *Adv. Mat.* 30:1870084. doi: 10.1002/adma.201870084
28. Spiegel, D. Y., and Koontz, B. F. (2018). Meeting the needs of long-term survivors: a testament to success in the care of patients with cancer. *Cancer* 124, 2488–2490. doi: 10.1002/cncr.31381
29. Tang, Z., Liu, Y., He, M., and Bu, W. (2018). Chemodynamic therapy: tumour microenvironment-mediated fenton and fenton-like reactions. *Angew. Chem. Int. Ed.* 58, 946–956. doi: 10.1002/anie.201805664
30. Wood, R., Mitra, D., de Courcy, J., and Iyer, S. (2017). Patient-reported quality of life and treatment satisfaction in patients With HR+/HER2-advanced/metastatic breast cancer. *Clin. Ther.* 39, 1719–1728. doi: 10.1016/j.clinthera.2017.07.009
31. Wu, H., Liu, S., Gong, J., Liu, J., Zhang, Q., Leng, X., et al. (2017). VCPA, a novel synthetic derivative of α-tocopheryl succinate, sensitizes human gastric cancer to doxorubicin-induced apoptosis via ROS-dependent mitochondrial dysfunction. *Cancer Lett.* 393, 22–32. doi: 10.1016/j.canlet.2017.02.007
32. Wu, L., Zhang, J., and Watanabe, W. (2011). Physical and chemical stability of drug nanoparticles. *Adv. Drug Deliv. Rev.* 63, 456–469. doi: 10.1016/j.addr.2011. 02.001
33. Xi, J., Da, L., Yang, C., Chen, R., Gao, L., Fan, L., et al. (2017). Mn2+-coordinated PDA@DOX/PLGA nanoparticles as a smart theranostic agent for synergistic chemo-photothermal tumor therapy. *Int. J. Nanomed.* 2017, 3331–3345. doi: 10.2147/IJN.S132270
34. Xia, J., Inagaki, Y., Gao, J., Qi, F., Song, P., Han, G., et al. (2017). Combination of cinobufacini and doxorubicin increases apoptosis of hepatocellular carcinoma cells through the Fas- and mitochondria-mediated pathways. *Am. J. Chin. Med.* 45, 1537–1556. doi: 10.1142/s0192415x17500835
35. Xu, X., Ho, W., Zhang, X., Bertrand, N., and Farokhzad, O. (2015). Cancer nanomedicine: from targeted delivery to combination therapy. *Trends Mol. Med.* 21, 223–232. doi: 10.1016/j.molmed.2015.01.001
36. Zhang, C., Bu, W., Ni, D., Zhang, S., Li, Q., Yao, Z., et al. (2016). Synthesis of iron nanometallic glasses and their application in cancer therapy by a localized fenton reaction. *Angew. Chem. Int. Ed.* 55, 2101–2106. doi: 10.1002/anie.201510031
37. Zhang, W., Gai, C., Ding, D., Wang, F., and Li, W. (2018). Targeted p53 on small- molecules-induced ferroptosis in cancers. *Front. Oncol.* 8:507. doi: 10.3389/fonc.2018.00507
38. Zheng, D.-W., Lei, Q., Zhu, J.-Y., Fan, J.-X., Li, C.-X., Li, C., et al. (2017). Switching apoptosis to ferroptosis: metal–organic network for high-efficiency anticancer therapy. *Nano Lett.* 17, 284–291. doi: 10.1021/acs.nanolett.6b04060
39. Zhou, Z., Song, J., Nie, L., and Chen, X. (2016). Reactive oxygen species generating systems meeting challenges of photodynamic cancer therapy. *Chem. Soc. Rev.* 45, 6597–6626. doi: 10.1039/C6CS00271D

Permissions

All chapters in this book were first published by Frontiers; hereby published with permission under the Creative Commons Attribution License or equivalent. Every chapter published in this book has been scrutinized by our experts. Their significance has been extensively debated. The topics covered herein carry significant findings which will fuel the growth of the discipline. They may even be implemented as practical applications or may be referred to as a beginning point for another development.

The contributors of this book come from diverse backgrounds, making this book a truly international effort. This book will bring forth new frontiers with its revolutionizing research information and detailed analysis of the nascent developments around the world.

We would like to thank all the contributing authors for lending their expertise to make the book truly unique. They have played a crucial role in the development of this book. Without their invaluable contributions this book wouldn't have been possible. They have made vital efforts to compile up to date information on the varied aspects of this subject to make this book a valuable addition to the collection of many professionals and students.

This book was conceptualized with the vision of imparting up-to-date information and advanced data in this field. To ensure the same, a matchless editorial board was set up. Every individual on the board went through rigorous rounds of assessment to prove their worth. After which they invested a large part of their time researching and compiling the most relevant data for our readers.

The editorial board has been involved in producing this book since its inception. They have spent rigorous hours researching and exploring the diverse topics which have resulted in the successful publishing of this book. They have passed on their knowledge of decades through this book. To expedite this challenging task, the publisher supported the team at every step. A small team of assistant editors was also appointed to further simplify the editing procedure and attain best results for the readers.

Apart from the editorial board, the designing team has also invested a significant amount of their time in understanding the subject and creating the most relevant covers. They scrutinized every image to scout for the most suitable representation of the subject and create an appropriate cover for the book.

The publishing team has been an ardent support to the editorial, designing and production team. Their endless efforts to recruit the best for this project, has resulted in the accomplishment of this book. They are a veteran in the field of academics and their pool of knowledge is as vast as their experience in printing. Their expertise and guidance has proved useful at every step. Their uncompromising quality standards have made this book an exceptional effort. Their encouragement from time to time has been an inspiration for everyone.

The publisher and the editorial board hope that this book will prove to be a valuable piece of knowledge for researchers, students, practitioners and scholars across the globe.

List of Contributors

Da Liu, Xue Meng, Donglu Wu, Zhidong Qiu and Haoming Luo
Department of Pharmacy, Changchun University of Chinese Medicine, Changchun, China
Key Laboratory of Effective Components of Traditional Chinese Medicine, Changchun University of Chinese Medicine, Changchun, China

Pier Adelchi Ruffini
Research and Development Department, Dompé farmaceutici S.p.A., Milan, Italy

Tao Li, Xiuxiu Wang, Lijun Jing and Yu Li
Department of Respiratory Diseases, Qilu Hospital of Shandong University, Jinan, China

Bruno Sangiorgi, Felipe Canto de Souza, Ildercílio Mota de Souza Lima, Josiane Lilian dos Santos Schiavinato, Amanda Cristina Corveloni, Wilson Araújo Silva Jr. and Rodrigo Alexandre Panepucci
Center for Cell-Based Therapy (CTC), Regional Blood Center of Ribeirão Preto, Ribeirão Preto, Brazil
Department of Genetics and Internal Medicine, Ribeirão Preto Medical School, University of São Paulo (FMRP-USP), Ribeirão Preto, Brazil

Carolina Hassibe Thomé and Vitor Marcel Faça
Center for Cell-Based Therapy (CTC), Regional Blood Center of Ribeirão Preto, Ribeirão Preto, Brazil
Department of Biochemistry and Immunology, Ribeirão Preto Medical School, University of São Paulo (FMRP-USP), Ribeirão Preto, Brazil

Dimas Tadeu Covas and Marco Antônio Zago
Center for Cell-Based Therapy (CTC), Regional Blood Center of Ribeirão Preto, Ribeirão Preto, Brazil

Kun-kun Xia
Department of Hepatobiliary and Pancreatic Surgery, First Affiliated Hospital of Zhengzhou University, Zhengzhou, China
Department of Colon and Rectal Surgery, First Affiliated Hospital of Zhengzhou University, Zhengzhou, China

Yong Lyu, Wei-tang Yuan and Gui-xian Wang
Department of Colon and Rectal Surgery, First Affiliated Hospital of Zhengzhou University, Zhengzhou, China

Harrison Stratton
Department of Neurobiology, Barrow Neurological Institute, St. Joseph's Hospital and Medical Center, Phoenix, AZ, United States

Shui-jun Zhang
Department of Hepatobiliary and Pancreatic Surgery, First Affiliated Hospital of Zhengzhou University, Zhengzhou, China

Jie Wu
Department of Hepatobiliary and Pancreatic Surgery, First Affiliated Hospital of Zhengzhou University, Zhengzhou, China
Department of Neurobiology, Barrow Neurological Institute, St. Joseph's Hospital and Medical Center, Phoenix, AZ, United States

Chao Hu, Shanli Zhu, Yu Lin, Li Ma, Liufang Zhu, Pengyue Jiang and Zhengli Li
Institute for Infectious Diseases and Vaccine Development, Tongji University School of Medicine, Shanghai, China

Jing Wang
Institute for Infectious Diseases and Vaccine Development, Tongji University School of Medicine, Shanghai, China
Integrative Cancer Centre, the First Affiliated Hospital of Guangzhou University of Chinese Medicine, Guangzhou, China

Weiqing Pan
Institute for Infectious Diseases and Vaccine Development, Tongji University School of Medicine, Shanghai, China
Department of Tropical Diseases, Second Military Medical University, Shanghai, China

Wenjuan Dai
Shenzhen Center for Disease Control and Prevention, Shenzhen, China
Jiangxi Provincial Key Laboratory of Preventive Medicine, School of Public Health, Nanchang University, Nanchang, China

Yingbin Fu, Yanxia Deng, Zhuoying Zeng, Pan Gu, Hailong Liu, Jianjun Liu, Xinyun Xu, Desheng Wu, Xianru Luo, Linqing Yang, Jinzhou Zhang, Kai Lin and Haiyan Huang
Shenzhen Center for Disease Control and Prevention, Shenzhen, China

Gonghua Hu
Jiangxi Provincial Key Laboratory of Preventive Medicine, School of Public Health, Nanchang University, Nanchang, China
Department of Preventive Medicine, Gannan Medical University, Ganzhou, China

Yanping Li, Ronghui Liang, Xiaoya Zhang and Leilei Li
Biomedical Translational Research Institute, Jinan University, Guangzhou, China

Jiyan Wang
State Key Laboratory of Medicinal Chemical Biology, College of Pharmacy and Tianjin Key Laboratory of Molecular Drug Research, Nankai University, Tianjin, China

Changliang Shan
Biomedical Translational Research Institute, Jinan University, Guangzhou, China
State Key Laboratory of Medicinal Chemical Biology, College of Pharmacy and Tianjin Key Laboratory of Molecular Drug Research, Nankai University, Tianjin, China

Shuangping Liu
Department of Pathology, Medical School, Dalian University, Dalian, China

Shuai Zhang
School of Integrative Medicine, Tianjin University of Traditional Chinese Medicine, Tianjin, China
Xu Wu, Jianhua Yin, Mingxing Li, Jing Shen, Yueshui Zhao, Qijie Zhao and Chi Hin Cho
Laboratory of Molecular Pharmacology, Department of Pharmacology, School of Pharmacy, Southwest Medical University, Luzhou, China
South Sichuan Institute of Translational Medicine, Luzhou, China

Jing Li
Department of Oncology and Hematology, Hospital (T.C.M) Affiliated to Southwest Medical University, Luzhou, China

Tao Yi
School of Chinese Medicine, Hong Kong Baptist University, Hong Kong, China

Zhangang Xiao
Laboratory of Molecular Pharmacology, Department of Pharmacology, School of Pharmacy, Southwest Medical University, Luzhou, China

Liping Qu
College of Pharmacy, Chengdu University of Traditional Chinese Medicine, Chengdu, China

Jing Jin, Jingbo Wu and Qinglian Wen
Department of Oncology, The Affiliated Hospital of Southwest Medical University, Southwest Medical University, Luzhou, China

Zhiru Wang
School of Pharmaceutical Sciences, Zhenghzou University, Zhengzhou, China
Collaborative Innovation Centre of New Drug Research and Safety Evaluation, Henan Province, and Key Laboratory of Advanced Drug Preparation Technologies, Zhengzhou University and KeyLaboratory of Henan Province for Drug Quality and Evaluation, Ministry of Education of China, Zhengzhou, China
Pathology, Institute of Clinical Medicine, Faculty of Medicine, University of Oslo, Oslo, Norway

Wenting Kang, Yinghua You, Jingru Pang, Hongmei Ren, Hongmin Liu and Yichao Zheng
School of Pharmaceutical Sciences, Zhenghzou University, Zhengzhou, China
Collaborative Innovation Centre of New Drug Research and Safety Evaluation, Henan Province, and Key Laboratory of Advanced Drug Preparation Technologies, Zhengzhou University and Key Laboratory of Henan Province for Drug Quality and Evaluation, Ministry of Education of China, Zhengzhou, China

Zhenhe Suo
Pathology, Institute of Clinical Medicine, Faculty of Medicine, University of Oslo, Oslo, Norway

Mei Han, Lina Jia, Wencai Lv, Lihui Wang and Wei Cui
Department of Pharmacology, Shenyang Pharmaceutical University, Shenyang, China

Ling-Ling Sun, Chang-Ming Chen, Jue Zhang, Cai-Zhi Yang and Li-Zhu Lin
Integrative Cancer Centre, the First Affiliated Hospital of Guangzhou University of Chinese Medicine, Guangzhou, China

Ning Ji
Tianjin Key Laboratory on Technologies Enabling Development of Clinical Therapeutics and Diagnostics, School of Pharmacy, Tianjin Medical University, Tianjin, China
Department of Pharmaceutical Sciences, College of Pharmacy and Health Sciences, St. John's University, Queens, NY, United States

Yuqi Yang, Chao-Yun Cai, Jing-Quan Wang, Zi-Ning Lei, Zhuo-Xun Wu, Qingbin Cui, Dong-Hua Yang and Zhe-Sheng Chen
Department of Pharmaceutical Sciences, College of Pharmacy and Health Sciences, St. John's University, Queens, NY, United States

Dexin Kong
Tianjin Key Laboratory on Technologies Enabling Development of Clinical Therapeutics and Diagnostics, School of Pharmacy, Tianjin Medical University, Tianjin, China
Research Center, School of Medicine, Tianjin Tianshi College, Tianyuan University, Tianjin, China

Tong Meng
Division of Spine, Department of Orthopedics, Tongji Hospital Affiliated to Tongji University School of Medicine, Shanghai, China
Shanghai Bone Tumor Institution, Shanghai, China
Department of Orthopedics, Shanghai General Hospital, School of Medicine, Shanghai Jiaotong University, Shanghai, China

Jiali Jin
Department of Central Laboratory, Shanghai Tenth People's Hospital of Tongji University, School of Medicine, School of Life Sciences and Technology, Tongji University, Shanghai, China

Cong Jiang
Beth Israel Deaconess Medical Center, BIDMC Cancer Center, Harvard Medical School, Cancer Research Institute, Boston, MA, United States

Runzhi Huang
Division of Spine, Department of Orthopedics, Tongji Hospital Affiliated to Tongji University School of Medicine, Shanghai, China

Huabin Yin and Dianwen Song
Shanghai Bone Tumor Institution, Shanghai, China
Department of Orthopedics, Shanghai General Hospital, School of Medicine, Shanghai Jiaotong University, Shanghai, China

Liming Cheng
Division of Spine, Department of Orthopedics, Tongji Hospital Affiliated to Tongji University School of Medicine, Shanghai, China
Key Laboratory of Spine and Spinal Cord Injury Repair and Regeneration, Ministry of Education, Tongji University, Shanghai, China
Wenzhi Liu, Ruoyu Wang, Yun Bao, Zhiqiang Wang, Dewei Zhao and Fei Wu
The Institute for Translational Medicine, The Affiliated Zhongshan Hospital of Dalian University, Dalian, China

Lili Liu
Department of Oncology, The Second Affiliated Hospital of Dalian Medical University, Dalian, China

Guanyu Gong
The Institute for Translational Medicine, The Affiliated Zhongshan Hospital of Dalian University, Dalian, China
Genomic Future Inc., Lexington, MA, United States

Xinjia Ding
Department of Neurosurgery, The Second Affiliated Hospital of Dalian Medical University, Dalian, China

Bin Yang
Genomic Future Inc., Lexington, MA, United States
Department of Pediatrics, Children's Hospital of Boston, Harvard Medical School, Boston, MA, United States

Bo Zhang
Department of Neurosurgery, The Second Affiliated Hospital of Dalian Medical University, Dalian, China

Yan Ding
The Institute for Translational Medicine, The Affiliated Zhongshan Hospital of Dalian University, Dalian, China
Department of Pediatrics, Children's Hospital of Boston, Harvard Medical School, Boston, MA, United States

Pengfei Guo
Science and Technology Innovation Center, Guangzhou University of Chinese Medicine, Guangzhou, China
Laboratory of Experimental Animal, Guangzhou University of Chinese Medicine, Guangzhou, China

Chuipu Cai
Science and Technology Innovation Center, Guangzhou University of Chinese Medicine, Guangzhou, China
School of Basic Medical Sciences, Guangzhou University of Chinese Medicine, Guangzhou, China

Xiaoqin Wu and Xiude Fan
Lerner Research Institute, Cleveland Clinic, Cleveland, OH, United States

Wei Huang, Jingwei Zhou, Qihui Wu, Yujie Huang and Wei Zhao
Science and Technology Innovation Center, Guangzhou University of Chinese Medicine, Guangzhou, China

Fengxue Zhang
School of Basic Medical Sciences, Guangzhou University of Chinese Medicine, Guangzhou, China

Qi Wang
Science and Technology Innovation Center, Guangzhou University of Chinese Medicine, Guangzhou, China
Institute of Clinical Pharmacology, Guangzhou University of Chinese Medicine, Guangzhou, China

Yongbin Zhang
Laboratory of Experimental Animal, Guangzhou University of Chinese Medicine, Guangzhou, China

Jiansong Fang
Science and Technology Innovation Center, Guangzhou University of Chinese Medicine, Guangzhou, China
Lerner Research Institute, Cleveland Clinic, Cleveland, OH, United States
Institute of Clinical Pharmacology, Guangzhou University of Chinese Medicine, Guangzhou, China

Ke Wang
Clinical Laboratory, Yongchuan People's Hospital of Chongqing, Chongqing, China

Ling Li, Liang Fu, Yongqiang Yuan, Hongying Dai and Tianjin Zhu
Clinical Laboratory, Yongchuan Hospital of Chongqing Medical University, Chongqing, China

Yuxi Zhou and Fang Yuan
Yidu Cloud (Beijing) Technology Co., Ltd., Beijing, China

Yuncong Liu
West China School of Medicine, Sichuan University, Chengdu, China
Department of Gynaecological Oncology, Guizhou Provincial People's Hospital, Guiyang, China

Li Wu and Feiyue Yang
Department of Gynaecological Oncology, Guizhou Provincial People's Hospital, Guiyang, China

Ruizhan Tong
West China School of Medicine, Sichuan University, Chengdu, China

Limei Yin, Mengqian Li, Liting You, Jianxin Xue and You Lu
West China School of Medicine, Sichuan University, Chengdu, China
Department of Thoracic Oncology, Cancer Center, West China Hospital, Sichuan University, Chengdu, China

Yu Toyoda, Tappei Takada and Hiroshi Suzuki
Department of Pharmacy, The University of Tokyo Hospital, Faculty of Medicine, The University of Tokyo, Tokyo, Japan

Changjun Nie
Department of Cell Biology, Institute of Biomedicine, Jinan University, Guangzhou, China
National Engineering Research Center of Genetic Medicine, Guangzhou, China
Guangdong Provincial Key Laboratory of Bioengineering Medicine, Guangzhou, China
Department of Medical Genetics, Liuzhou Maternal and Children Healthcare Hospital, Liuzhou, China

Xiaohui Qin and Dingyuan Zeng
Department of Medical Genetics, Liuzhou Maternal and Children Healthcare Hospital, Liuzhou, China
Xiaoyan Li, Baoqing Tian, Ying Zhao, Yuan Jin, Yadan Li, Qiang Wang, An Hong and Xiaojia Chen
Department of Cell Biology, Institute of Biomedicine, Jinan University, Guangzhou, China
National Engineering Research Center of Genetic Medicine, Guangzhou, China
Guangdong Provincial Key Laboratory of Bioengineering Medicine, Guangzhou, China

Lei Shang
School of Pharmacy, China Medical University, Shenyang, China
Shenyang Medical College, Shenyang, China

Minjie Wei
School of Pharmacy, China Medical University, Shenyang, China

Shan-Zhou Huang
Department of Hepatic Surgery, The First Affiliated Hospital, Sun Yat-sen University, Guangzhou, China
Organ Transplant Center, The First Affiliated Hospital, Sun Yat-sen University, Guangzhou, China

Meng-Ning Wei, Jia-Rong Huang, Wen-Ji Zhang, Qi-Wei Jiang, Yang Yang, Kun Wang, Zi-Hao Xing, Meng-Ling Yuan and Yao Li
Guangdong Provincial Key Laboratory of Bioengineering Medicine, Department of Cell Biology and Institute of Biomedicine, National Engineering Research Center of Genetic Medicine, College of Life Science and Technology, Jinan University, Guangzhou, China

Zi-Jian Zhang
Department of Hepatobiliary Surgery, The Seventh Affiliated Hospital of Sun Yat-sen University, Shenzhen, China

Huan-Yu Wang
Department of Thyroid and Breast Surgery, Nanshan District People's Hospital, Shenzhen, China

Hui-Lin Jin
Department of Hepatic Surgery, The First Affiliated Hospital, Sun Yat-sen University, Guangzhou, China

Xiao-Shun He and Zhi Shi
Organ Transplant Center, The First Affiliated Hospital, Sun Yat-sen University, Guangzhou, China

Qi Zhou
Department of Hepatic Surgery, The First Affiliated Hospital, Sun Yat-sen University, Guangzhou, China
Department of General Surgery, Hui Ya Hospital of The First Affiliated Hospital, Sun Yat-sen University, Huizhou, China

Xu-Jing Li, Zi-Hao-Ran Li and Cheng-Cheng Gai
Department of Pathology, Weifang Medical University, Weifang, China

Wen-Tong Li
Department of Pathology, Weifang Medical University, Weifang, China
Collaborative Innovation Center for Target Drug Delivery System, Weifang Medical University, Weifang, China

Li-Ping Zhang
College of Pharmacy, Weifang Medical University, Weifang, China

Wei-Fen Zhang and De-Jun Ding
Collaborative Innovation Center for Target Drug Delivery System, Weifang Medical University, Weifang, China
College of Pharmacy, Weifang Medical University, Weifang, China

Index

www.ingramcontent.com/pod-product-compliance
Lightning Source LLC
LaVergne TN
LVHW082132200926
848484LV00008B/2042

* 9 7 9 8 8 8 7 4 0 3 5 1 9 *